Calculation of Drug Dosages

Seventh Edition

Sheila J. Ogden, MSN, RN
Orthopaedics Program Director
Clarian Health Partners
Indianapolis, Indiana

Mosby
An Affiliate of Elsevier

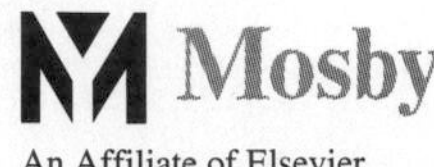

11830 Westline Industrial Drive
St. Louis, Missouri 63146

Calculation of Drug Dosages, Seventh Edition ISBN 0-323-01888-2

NOTICE

Pharmacology is an ever-changing field. Standard safety precautions must be followed, but as new research and clinical experience broaden our knowledge, changes in treatment and drug therapy may become necessary or appropriate. Readers are advised to check the most current product information provided by the manufacturer of each drug to be administered to verify the recommended dose, the method and duration of administration, and contraindications. It is the responsibility of the licensed prescriber, relying on experience and knowledge of the patient, to determine dosages and the best treatment for each individual patient. Neither the publisher nor the editor assumes any liability for any injury and/or damage to persons or property arising from this publication.

Previous editions copyrighted 1999, 1995, 1991, 1987, 1980, and 1977.

Library of Congress Cataloging-in-Publication Data

Ogden, Sheila J., 1949-
Calculation of drug dosages. — 7th ed. / Sheila J. Ogden.
p. ; cm.
Rev. ed. of: Radcliff & Ogden's calculation of drug dosages. 6th ed. 1999.
Includes index.
ISBN 0-323-01888-2
1. Pharmaceutical arithmetic—Programmed instruction. I. Ogden, Sheila J., 1949- Radcliff & Ogden's calculation of drug dosages. II. Title.
[DNLM: 1. Pharmaceutical Preparations—administration & dosage—Problems and Exercises. 2. Mathematics—Problems and Exercises. QV 18.2 O34r 2003]
RS57 .R33 2003
615′.14—dc21 2002042729

Executive Vice President, Nursing and Health Professions, Nursing: Sally Schrefer
Acquisitions Editor: Yvonne Alexopoulos
Associate Developmental Editor: Danielle M. Frazier
Publishing Services Manager: Catherine Jackson
Project Manager: Clay S. Broeker
Designer: Teresa Breckwoldt
Cover Design: Studio Montage

GW/KPT

Printed in the United States of America

Last digit is the print number: 9 8 7 6 5 4 3 2

To
my children, John, Amy, and Justin,
who are all special

and

To
my husband and best friend, David,
for your patience, support, and love

S.J.O

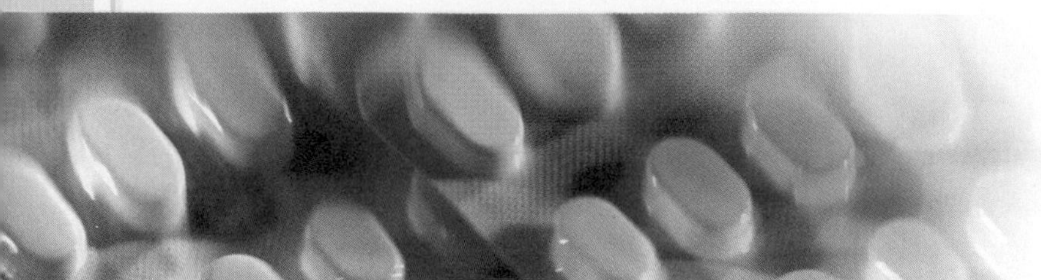

Contributor

Linda K. Fluharty, MSN, RN
Associate Professor
ASN Program
Ivy Tech State College
Indianapolis, Indiana

Reviewers

Janet Tompkins McMahon, RN, MSN
Associate Professor of Nursing
Department of Health Sciences
Pennsylvania College of Technology
Williamsport, Pennsylvania

Robert S. Warner, MS, RN
Assistant Professor
Department of Nursing
Fulton-Montgomery Community College
Johnstown, New York

Mary Welhaven, PhD, RN
Professor
Department of Nursing
Winona State University—Rochester Center
Rochester, Minnesota

Jo A. Voss, RN, PhDc, CNS
Instructor
College of Nursing
South Dakota State University
Rapid City, South Dakota

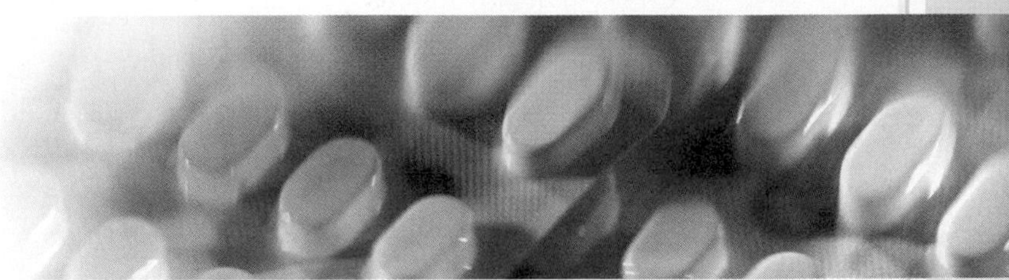

Preface to Instructors

This work text is designed for students in professional and vocational schools of nursing and for nurses returning to practice after being away from the clinical setting. It can be used in the classroom or for individual study. The work text contains an extensive review of basic mathematics to assist students who have not mastered the subject in previous educational experiences. It can also be used by those who have not attended school for a number of years and feel a lack of confidence in the area of mathematics computations.

ORGANIZATION OF MATERIAL

A pretest precedes each chapter in Parts I and II and may be used for evaluating present skills. For those students who are comfortable with basic mathematics, a quick assessment for each area will confirm their competency in the subject matter.

Part II begins with the use of the metric system, which is predominant in the medical field; the apothecary system continues to decline in utilization. However, in remembering that differences in practice exist throughout the United States and the world, it was felt that the content concerning the apothecary system should remain in the text. Still, the number of problems and amount of emphasis have been reduced in this edition. These chapters remain separate because each system must be learned separately before it can be manipulated in conversions.

Part III begins with an emphasis on the interpretation of the physician's orders and how to read drug labels. Chapter 11 presents dimensional analysis as a method to calculate drug dosages. In Chapters 12 through 14, the proportion and alternative formula methods are introduced for the calculation of drug dosage problems. The actual drug labels have been updated and increased in number in all of the chapters dealing with the calculation of drug dosages. Also, content related to dosages measured in units has been expanded. Because of the increased use of IV fluids in health care, Chapter 15, Intravenous Flow Rates, has been expanded. Also, the chapter on pediatric dosages has been expanded and now includes pediatric IV flow rate problems.

Part IV includes content concerning automated medication dispensing systems. The chapter on special considerations for the elderly has been enhanced, as has the chapter on home care considerations. The student needs to remember that the actual calculation of drug dosages does vary based on the setting of the patient. Also, the administration and delivery may be affected by the age and location of the patient in the health care system.

The majority of the calculation problems relating to drug dosages continue to represent actual physicians' orders in various health care settings.

Features in the Seventh Edition

- **Learning objectives** are listed in the beginning of each chapter so the student will know the goals that must be achieved.
- Chapter **work sheets** provide the opportunity to practice solving realistic problems.

- Almost every chapter contains two **posttests** designed to evaluate the student's learning.
- A **comprehensive posttest** at the end of the book will help students assess their total understanding of the process of calculation of drug dosages.
- A **glossary** is included to define important terms.
- **Chapter 16, Critical Care IV Flow Rates,** is a new chapter that has been added to address medication administration for critically ill patients
- Numerous **full-color drug labels** continue to provide a more realistic representation of medication administration

Ancillaries

The ***Instructor's Manual and Test Bank*** is specifically geared toward this edition and includes:
- Teaching outlines
- Teaching tips and strategies
- Transparency masters
- A test bank with over 100 questions

Romans & Daugherty Dosages and Solutions CTB has been **completely updated** and is provided as a gratis item to instructors upon adoption of this text. This is a generic computerized test bank (in CD-ROM format) that contains over 700 questions on general math, converting within systems of measurement, oral dosages, parenteral dosages, flow rates, pediatric dosages, and IV calculations. This provides additional practice problems for instructors to utilize above what is available in the *Instructor's Manual and Test Bank*.

The ***Daugherty & Romans Dosages and Solutions CD-ROM Companion*** is included with each text and provides hundreds of practice problems in the ratio and proportion, formula, dimensional analysis, and fractional equation methods. It also includes information on how to read medication labels, a glossary, quizzes, and a comprehensive exam.

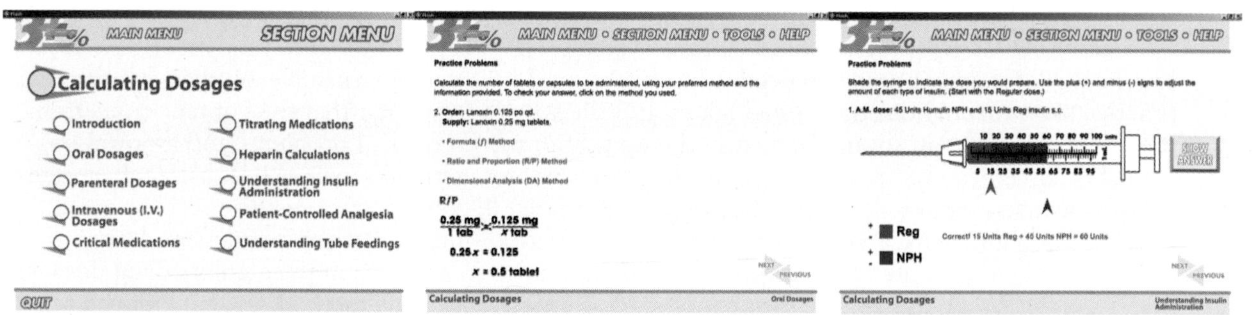

ACKNOWLEDGMENTS

I am grateful to the students and instructors who have chosen to use this book; I continue to learn so much from each of you. You have helped me understand the problems that students have with basic mathematics and with the calculation of drug dosages. I appreciate the physicians, nurses, pharmacists, and representatives of various health care agencies who took the time to discuss topics with me. I hope this book will provide readers with a feeling of confidence when working with a variety of mathematical problems.

I want to give special thanks to the reviewers of this text. Your sincere evaluation and critique played an integral part in the revision of this edition, and your attention to detail was most helpful.

I would also like to acknowledge Danielle Frazier and Yvonne Alexopoulos for their help and support during the writing of this seventh edition. In particular, Danielle supplied answers to many questions, pushed to meet deadlines, and offered her services as needed. She also remained calm and offered guidance during the entire revision process. I also acknowledge the expertise and help of Clay Broeker in the process of reviewing page proofs and readying the book for publication.

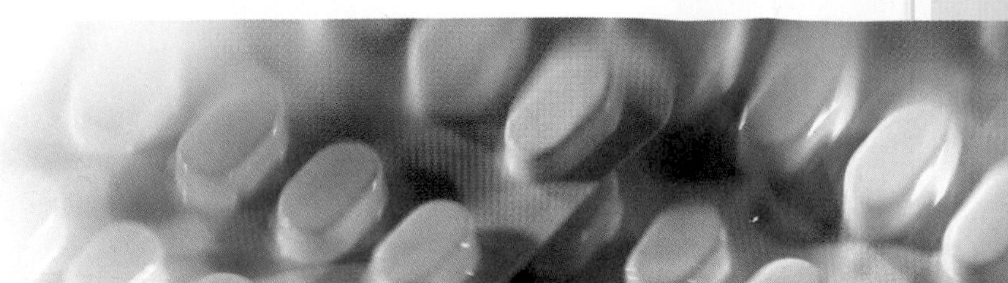

Preface to Students

DESCRIPTION AND FEATURES

Calculation of Drug Dosages is an innovative drug calculation work text designed to provide you with a systematic review of mathematics and a simplified method of calculating drug dosages. It affords you the opportunity to move at a pace that is comfortable and one that ensures success. It includes information on the ratio and proportion, formula, and dimensional analysis methods of drug calculation, as well as numerous practice problems. Take a look at the following features so that you may familiarize yourself with this text and maximize its value.

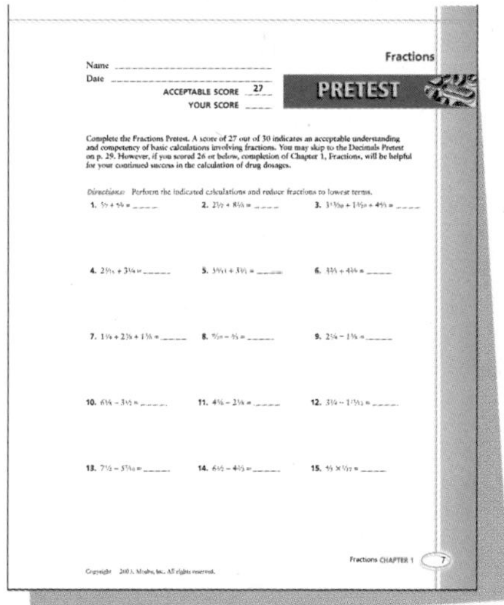

Fractions

Name

Date

ACCEPTABLE SCORE 27

YOUR SCORE

PRETEST

Complete the Fractions Pretest. A score of 27 out of 30 indicates an acceptable understanding and competency of basic calculations involving fractions. You may skip to the Decimals Pretest on p. 29. However, if you scored 26 or below, completion of Chapter 1, Fractions, will be helpful for your continued success in the calculation of drug dosages.

Directions: Perform the indicated calculations and reduce fractions to lowest terms.

Fractions CHAPTER 1 7

Pretests evaluate your present skills in utilizing mathematics, units, and measurements.

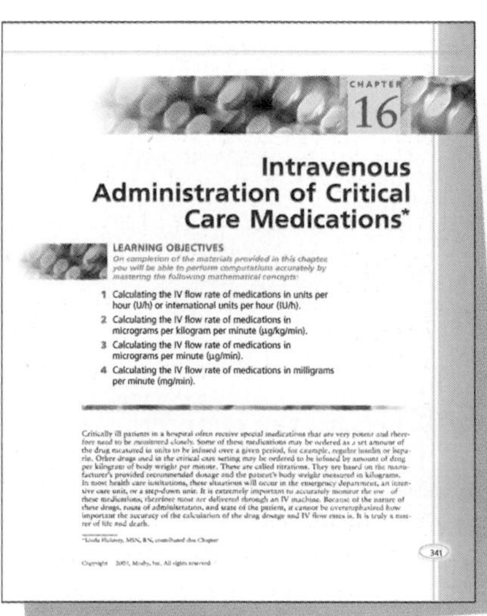

CHAPTER 16

Intravenous Administration of Critical Care Medications*

LEARNING OBJECTIVES

On completion of the materials provided in this chapter you will be able to perform computations accurately by mastering the following mathematical concepts:

1 Calculating the IV flow rate of medications in units per hour (U/h) or international units per hour (IU/h).
2 Calculating the IV flow rate of medications in micrograms per kilogram per minute (µg/kg/min).
3 Calculating the IV flow rate of medications in micrograms per minute (µg/min).
4 Calculating the IV flow rate of medications in milligrams per minute (mg/min).

Critically ill patients in a hospital often receive special medications that are very potent and therefore need to be monitored closely. Some of these medications may be ordered as a set amount of the drug measured in units to be infused over a given period, for example, regular insulin or heparin. Other drugs used in the critical care setting may be ordered to be infused by amount of drug per kilogram of body weight per minute. These are called titrations. They are based on the manufacturer's provided recommended dosage and the patient's body weight measured in kilograms. In most health care institutions, these situations will occur in the emergency department, an intensive care unit, or a step-down unit. It is extremely important to accurately monitor the use of these medications; therefore most are delivered through an IV machine. Because of the nature of these drugs, route of administration, and state of the patient, it cannot be overemphasized how important the accuracy of the calculation of the drug dosage and IV flow rates is. It is truly a matter of life and death.

341

Learning Objectives highlight key content and goals that must be achieved.

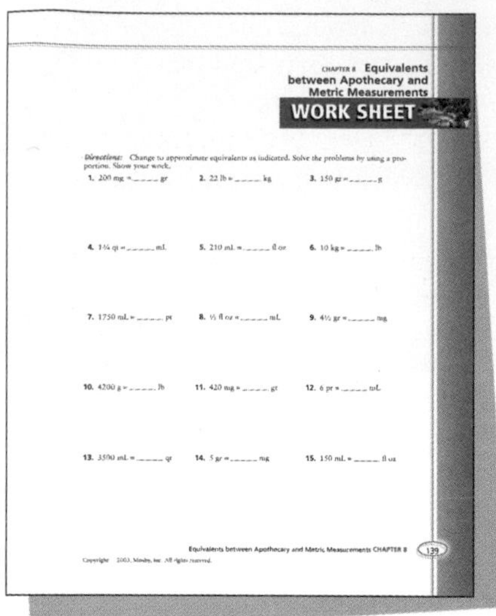

Work Sheets provide you with the opportunity to practice solving realistic problems.

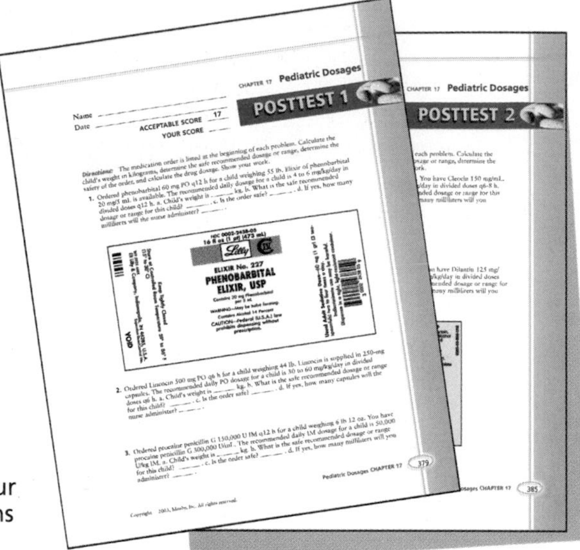

Posttests are designed to assess your learning and identify your strengths and weaknesses.

The ***Daugherty & Romans Dosages and Solutions CD-ROM Companion*** is also included with this text. It provides hundreds of practice problems in the ratio and proportion, formula, dimensional analysis, and fractional equation methods. It also includes information on how to read medication labels, a glossary, quizzes, and a comprehensive exam.

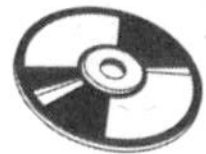

Look for this icon at the end of many of the chapters. It will refer you to the *CD-ROM Companion* for additional practice problems.

USING THIS WORK TEXT

A pretest precedes each chapter in Parts I and II to assess previous learning. If your grade on the pretest is acceptable (an acceptable score is noted at the top of the test), you may continue to the next pretest. If your score on the pretest indicates a need for further study, read the introduction to the chapter, study the method of solving the problems, and complete the work sheet. If you have difficulty with a problem, refer to the examples in the introduction.

On completion of the work sheet, refer to the answer key in the back of the book to verify that your answers are correct. Rework all the incorrect problems to find your errors. It may be necessary to refer again to the examples in each chapter. Then proceed to the first posttest and grade the test. If your grade is acceptable, as indicated at the top of the test, continue to the next chapter. If your grade is less than acceptable, rework all incorrect problems to find your errors. Review as necessary before completing the second posttest. Again verify that your answers are correct. At this point, if you have followed the system of study, your grade on the second posttest should be more than acceptable. Follow the same system of study in each of the chapters.

When all the chapters in the work text are completed with acceptable scores (between 90% and 100%), you should be proficient in solving problems relating to drug dosages; more importantly, you will have completed the first step toward becoming a safe practitioner of medication administration.

On completion of the material provided in this work text, you will have mastered the following mathematical concepts, to be used for the accurate performance of computations:

1. Solving problems using fractions, decimals, percents, ratios, and proportions
2. Solving problems involving the apothecary, metric, and household systems of measurements
3. Solving problems measured in units and milliequivalents
4. Solving problems related to oral and parenteral dosages
5. Solving problems involving intravenous flow rates and critical care intravenous flow rates
6. Solving problems confirming the correct dosage of pediatric medications
7. Solving problems by using the dimensional analysis method

You are now ready to begin Chapter 1!

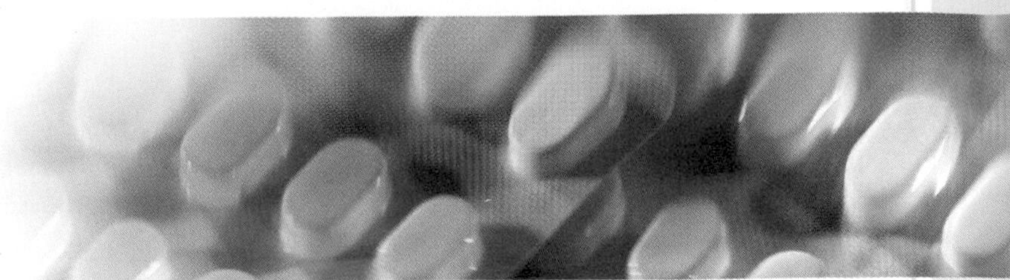

Contents

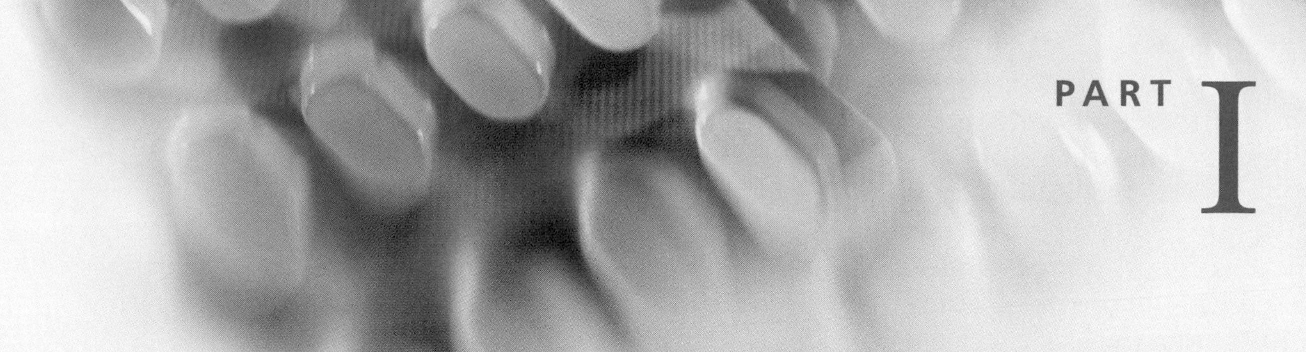

PART I

Review of Mathematics

CHAPTERS

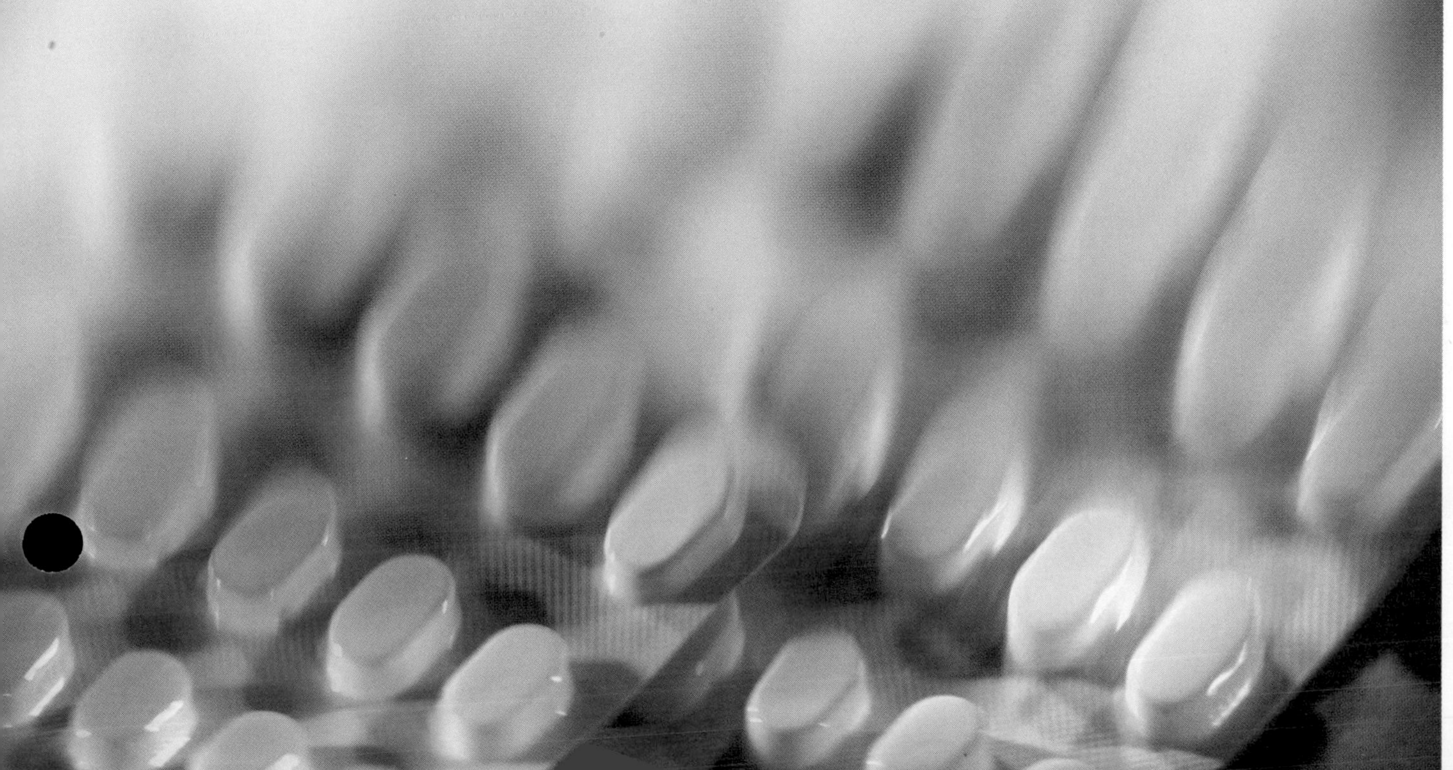

A solid knowledge base of general mathematics is necessary before you will be able to use these concepts in the more complicated calculations of drug dosages. It is this knowledge that allows for the safe administration of medications to your patients and prevents medication errors.

As you prepare to learn how to calculate drug dosages, an assessment of your current basic mathematics understanding and competency is essential. A general mathematics pretest is provided. Allow 1 to 2 hours in a quiet study area to complete the pretest without the use of a calculator. This is your opportunity to assess your true capability of performing basic math problems. Calculators are very useful tools. In some areas of health care, the use of a calculator is actually required to ensure accuracy in the delivery of medications. Follow the direction of your instructor as to the acceptable use of calculators while using this text on your path to safe administration of medications.

The pretest allows you to assess your need for a more extensive review. After completion of the test, check your answers with the key provided. A score of 90%, or 45 out of 50 problems correct, indicates a firm foundation in basic mathematics. You may then skip to Part II, Units and Measurements for the Calculation of Drug Dosages. However, a score of 89 or below indicates a need to review fraction, decimal, percent, ratio, and/or proportion calculations. Chapters 1 through 5 allow you to work on these basic mathematical skills at your leisure.

The pretest and review chapters are provided to ensure your success in the calculation and administration of your future patients' medications. Begin now, and good luck!

Name ______________________

Date ______________________

ACCEPTABLE SCORE 45

YOUR SCORE ______

Review of Mathematics

PRETEST

Directions: Perform the indicated computations. Reduce fractions to lowest terms.

1. $3/8 + 1/3 =$ ______

2. $2\,3/7 + 1\,2/3 =$ ______

3. $1\,3/5 + 7/8 / 1/3 =$ ______

4. $1.03 + 2.2 + 1.134 =$ ______

5. $1.479 + 28.68 + 4.5 =$ ______

6. $14/15 - 1/6 =$ ______

7. $2\,1/3 - 1/2 =$ ______

8. $2.04 - 0.987 =$ ______

9. $8.53 - 7.945 =$ ______

10. $3 \times 4/7 =$ ______

11. $2\frac{1}{2} \times 3\frac{3}{5} =$ _______

12. $0.315 \times 5.8 =$ _______

13. $4.884 \times 6.51 =$ _______

14. $\frac{3}{5} \div \frac{5}{6} =$ _______

15. $\frac{1}{150} \div \frac{1}{20} =$ _______

16. $2\frac{3}{4} \div 6\frac{2}{3} =$ _______

17. $241.73 \div 9.3 =$ _______

18. $128.24 \div 6 =$ _______

19. $22.67 \div 3.5 =$ _______

Directions: Circle the decimal fraction that has the *least* value.

20. 0.3, 0.03, 0.003

21. 0.9, 0.45, 0.66

22. 0.72, 0.721, 0.0072

23. 0.058, 0.1001, 0.07

Directions: Circle the decimal fraction that has the *greatest* value.

24. 0.1, 0.15, 0.155

25. 0.4, 0.8, 0.21

26. 0.249, 0.1587, 0.00633

27. 2.913, 2.99, 2.9

Directions: Change the following fractions to decimals.

28. $5/8$ = _______

29. $17/25$ = _______

Directions: Change the following decimals to fractions reduced to lowest terms.

30. 0.375 = _______

31. 0.05 = _______

32. Express 0.432 as a percent.

33. Express 65% as a proper fraction and reduce to the lowest terms.

34. Express 0.3% as a ratio.

35. What percent of 2.5 is 0.5?

36. What is $1/4$% of 60?

37. What is 65% of 450?

Directions: Change the following fractions and decimals to ratios reduced to lowest terms.

38. $\frac{9}{42}$ = ______ **39.** $1\frac{1}{2}/2\frac{2}{3}$ = ______ **40.** 0.34 = ______

Directions: Find the value of x.

41. $7 : \frac{7}{100} :: x : 4$

42. $x : 40 :: 7 : 56$

43. $2.5 : 6 :: 10 : x$

44. $x : \frac{1}{4}\% :: 9.6 : \frac{1}{300}$

45. $\frac{1}{150} : \frac{1}{100} :: x : 30$

46. $0.10 : 0.20 :: x : 200$

47. $\frac{1}{200} : \frac{1}{40} :: 100 : x$

48. $x : 85 :: 6 : 10$

49. $\frac{1}{20}/\frac{1}{5} : 5 :: x : 50$

50. $100 : 5 :: x : 3.4$

Answers on p. 425.

Fractions

Name ______________________________

Date ______________________________

ACCEPTABLE SCORE 27

YOUR SCORE ______

PRETEST

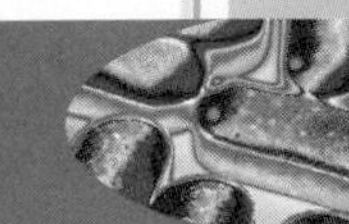

Complete the Fractions Pretest. A score of 27 out of 30 indicates an acceptable understanding and competency of basic calculations involving fractions. You may skip to the Decimals Pretest on p. 29. However, if you scored 26 or below, completion of Chapter 1, Fractions, will be helpful for your continued success in the calculation of drug dosages.

Directions: Perform the indicated calculations and reduce fractions to lowest terms.

1. $\frac{5}{7} + \frac{4}{9} =$ ______

2. $2\frac{1}{2} + 8\frac{1}{6} =$ ______

3. $3\frac{13}{20} + 1\frac{3}{10} + 4\frac{4}{5} =$ ______

4. $2\frac{5}{16} + 3\frac{1}{4} =$ ______

5. $5\frac{6}{11} + 3\frac{1}{2} =$ ______

6. $3\frac{2}{3} + 4\frac{2}{9} =$ ______

7. $1\frac{3}{4} + 2\frac{3}{8} + 1\frac{5}{6} =$ ______

8. $\frac{9}{10} - \frac{3}{5} =$ ______

9. $2\frac{1}{4} - 1\frac{3}{8} =$ ______

10. $6\frac{1}{8} - 3\frac{1}{2} =$ ______

11. $4\frac{5}{6} - 2\frac{1}{8} =$ ______

12. $3\frac{3}{4} - 1\frac{11}{12} =$ ______

13. $7\frac{1}{2} - 5\frac{7}{10} =$ ______

14. $6\frac{1}{2} - 4\frac{2}{3} =$ ______

15. $\frac{4}{5} \times \frac{1}{12} =$ ______

16. $1\frac{1}{3} \times 3\frac{3}{4} =$ ______

17. $3\frac{2}{7} \times 2\frac{2}{9} =$ ______

18. $\frac{5}{8} \times 1\frac{5}{7} =$ ______

19. $\frac{1}{1000} \times \frac{1}{10} =$ ______

20. $2\frac{4}{9} \times 1\frac{3}{4} =$ ______

21. $4\frac{1}{6} \times 2\frac{9}{10} =$ ______

22. $1\frac{1}{8} \times 2\frac{4}{7} =$ ______

23. $\frac{1}{4} \div \frac{4}{5} =$ ______

24. $2\frac{1}{6} \div 1\frac{5}{8} =$ ______

25. $\frac{1}{3} \div \frac{1}{100} =$ ______

26. $1\frac{3}{4} \div 2 =$ ______

27. $\frac{4}{5}/\frac{3}{5} =$ ______

28. $\frac{1}{3}/\frac{3}{5} =$ ______

29. $2\frac{5}{6}/1\frac{2}{3} =$ ______

30. $4\frac{1}{2}/2\frac{1}{4} =$ ______

Answers on p. 425.

CHAPTER

1

Fractions

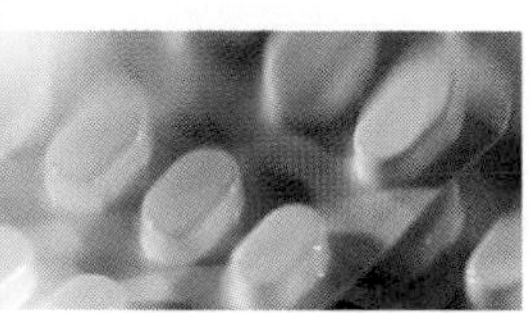

LEARNING OBJECTIVES

On completion of the materials provided in this chapter, you will be able to perform computations accurately by mastering the following mathematical concepts:

1. Changing an improper fraction to a mixed number
2. Changing a mixed number to an improper fraction
3. Changing a fraction to an equivalent fraction with the lowest common denominator
4. Changing a mixed number to an equivalent fraction with the lowest common denominator
5. Adding fractions having the same denominator, having unlike denominators, or involving whole numbers and unlike denominators
6. Subtracting fractions having the same denominator, having unlike denominators, or involving whole numbers and unlike denominators
7. Multiplying fractions and mixed numbers
8. Dividing fractions and mixed numbers
9. Reducing a complex fraction
10. Reducing a complex fraction involving mixed numbers

Study the introductory material for fractions. The processes for the calculation of fraction problems are listed in steps. Memorize the steps for each type of calculation before beginning the work sheet. Complete the work sheet at the end of this chapter, which provides extensive practice in the manipulation of fractions. Check your answers. If you have difficulties, go back and review the steps for that type of calculation. When you feel ready to evaluate your learning, take the first posttest. Check your answers. An acceptable score (number of answers correct) as indicated on the posttest signifies that you are ready for the next chapter. An unacceptable score signifies a need for further study before you take the second posttest.

A **fraction** indicates the number of equal parts of a whole. An example is $\frac{3}{4}$, which means three of four equal parts.

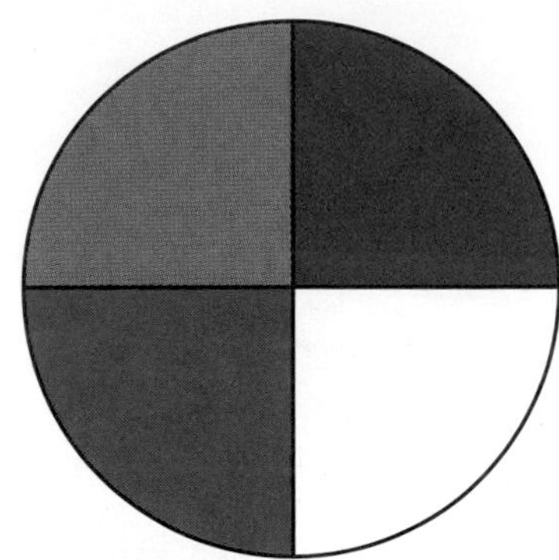

The **denominator** indicates the number of parts into which a whole has been divided. The denominator is the number *below* the fraction line. The **numerator** designates the number of parts that you have of a divided whole. It is the number *above* the fraction line. The line also indicates division to be performed and can be read as "divided by." The example $\frac{3}{4}$, or three fourths, can therefore be read as "three divided by four." In other words the numerator is "divided by" the denominator. The numerator is the **dividend,** and the denominator is the **divisor.**

A fraction can often be expressed in smaller numbers without any change in its real value. This is what is meant by the direction "Reduce to lowest terms." The reduction is accomplished by dividing both numerator and denominator by the same number.

Example 1: $\frac{6}{8}$

$6 \div 2 = 3$

$8 \div 2 = 4$

$$\frac{6}{8} = \frac{3}{4}$$

Example 2: $\frac{3}{9}$

$3 \div 3 = 1$

$9 \div 3 = 3$

$$\frac{3}{9} = \frac{1}{3}$$

Example 3: $\frac{4}{10}$

$4 \div 2 = 2$

$10 \div 2 = 5$

$$\frac{4}{10} = \frac{2}{5}$$

There are several different types of fractions. A **proper fraction** is one in which the numerator is smaller than the denominator. A proper fraction is sometimes called a *common* or *simple fraction.*

Examples: $\frac{2}{3}$, $\frac{1}{8}$, $\frac{5}{12}$

An **improper fraction** is a fraction in which the numerator is larger than or equal to the denominator.

Examples: $\frac{8}{7}$, $\frac{6}{6}$, $\frac{4}{2}$

A **complex fraction** is one that contains a fraction in its numerator, its denominator, or both.

Examples: $2\frac{1}{3}/3$, $2/\frac{1}{2}$, $\frac{3}{4}/\frac{3}{8}$

Sometimes a fraction is seen in conjunction with a whole number. This combination is called a **mixed number.**

Examples: $2\frac{3}{8}$, $4\frac{1}{3}$, $6\frac{1}{2}$

Changing an Improper Fraction to a Mixed Number

1. Divide the numerator by the denominator.
2. Place any remainder over the denominator and write this proper fraction beside the whole number found in step 1.

Example 1: $5/3$

$$3\overline{)5} = 1 \text{ remainder } 2 = 1\frac{2}{3}$$
$$\frac{3}{2}$$

Example 2: $7/2$

$$2\overline{)7} = 3 \text{ remainder } 1 = 3\frac{1}{2}$$
$$\frac{6}{1}$$

When an improper fraction is reduced, it will *always* result in a mixed number or a whole number.

Changing a Mixed Number to an Improper Fraction

1. Multiply the denominator of the fraction by the whole number.
2. Add the product to the numerator of the fraction.
3. Place the sum over the denominator.

Example 1: $3\frac{1}{4}$

$4 \times 3 = 12$

$12 + 1 = 13$

$3\frac{1}{4} = \frac{13}{4}$

Example 2: $1\frac{3}{8}$

$8 \times 1 = 8$

$8 + 3 = 11$

$1\frac{3}{8} = \frac{11}{8}$

Example 3: $2\frac{7}{10}$

$10 \times 2 = 20$

$20 + 7 = 27$

$2\frac{7}{10} = \frac{27}{10}$

If fractions are to be added or subtracted, it is necessary for their *denominators to be the same.*

LOWEST COMMON DENOMINATOR

Computations are facilitated when the lowest common denominator is used. The term **lowest common denominator** is defined as the smallest whole number that can be divided evenly by all denominators within the problem.

When trying to determine the lowest common denominator, first observe whether one of the denominators in the problem is evenly divisible by each of the other denominators. If so, this will be the lowest common denominator for the problem.

Example 1: $2/3$ and $5/12$
You find that 12 is evenly divisible by 3; therefore 12 is the lowest common denominator.

Example 2: $1/2$ and $3/8$
You find that 8 is evenly divisible by 2; therefore 8 is the lowest common denominator.

Example 3: $2/7$ and $5/14$ and $1/28$
You find that 28 is evenly divisible by 7 and 14; therefore 28 is the lowest common denominator.

Changing a Fraction to an Equivalent Fraction with the Lowest Common Denominator

1. Divide the lowest common denominator by the denominator of the fraction to be changed.
2. Multiply the quotient by the numerator of the fraction to be changed.
3. Place the product over the lowest common denominator.

Example 1: $2/3 = ?/12$

$12 \div 3 = 4$

$4 \times 2 = 8$

$\frac{2}{3} = \frac{8}{12}$

Example 2: $1/2 = ?/8$

$8 \div 2 = 4$

$4 \times 1 = 4$

$\frac{1}{2} = \frac{4}{8}$

Example 3: $2/7 = ?/14$

$14 \div 7 = 2$

$2 \times 2 = 4$

$\frac{2}{7} = \frac{4}{14}$

Changing a Mixed Number to an Equivalent Fraction with the Lowest Common Denominator

1. Change the mixed number to an improper fraction.
2. Divide the lowest common denominator by the denominator of the fraction.
3. Multiply the quotient by the numerator of the improper fraction.
4. Place the product over the lowest common denominator.

Example 1: $1\,3/4$ and $5/12$

$1\frac{3}{4} = \frac{?}{12}$

$4 \times 1 = 4$

$4 + 3 = 7$

$\frac{7}{4} = \frac{?}{12}$

$12 \div 4 = 3$

$3 \times 7 = 21$

$1\frac{3}{4} = \frac{21}{12}$

Example 2: $3\,2/3$ and $4/9$

$3\frac{2}{3} = \frac{?}{9}$

$3 \times 3 = 9$

$9 + 2 = 11$

$\frac{11}{3} = \frac{?}{9}$

$9 \div 3 = 3$

$3 \times 11 = 33$

$3\frac{2}{3} = \frac{33}{9}$

If one of the denominators in the problem is not the lowest common denominator for all, you must look further. One suggestion is to multiply two of the denominators together and if possible use that number as the lowest common denominator.

Example: $3\frac{1}{2}$ and $\frac{2}{3}$
Multiply the two denominators: $2 \times 3 = 6$

$3\frac{1}{2} = \frac{?}{6}$	$\frac{2}{3} = \frac{?}{6}$
$2 \times 3 = 6$	$6 \div 3 = 2$
$6 + 1 = 7$	$2 \times 2 = 4$
$\frac{7}{2} = \frac{?}{6}$	$\frac{2}{3} = \frac{4}{6}$
$6 \div 2 = 3$	
$3 \times 7 = 21$	
$3\frac{1}{2} = \frac{21}{6}$	

Another method is to multiply one of the denominators by 2, 3, or 4. Determine whether the resulting number can be used as a common denominator.

Example: $\frac{3}{4}$ and $\frac{1}{8}$ and $\frac{5}{12}$
Multiply the denominator 8 by 3: $8 \times 3 = 24$

$\frac{3}{4} = \frac{?}{24}$	$\frac{1}{8} = \frac{?}{24}$	$\frac{5}{12} = \frac{?}{24}$
$24 \div 4 = 6$	$24 \div 8 = 3$	$24 \div 12 = 2$
$6 \times 3 = 18$	$3 \times 1 = 3$	$2 \times 5 = 10$
$\frac{3}{4} = \frac{18}{24}$	$\frac{1}{8} = \frac{3}{24}$	$\frac{5}{12} = \frac{10}{24}$

ADDITION OF FRACTIONS

Addition of Fractions Having the Same Denominator

1. Add the numerators.
2. Place the sum over the common denominator.
3. Reduce to lowest terms.

Example 1: $\frac{1}{7} + \frac{2}{7} =$ _______

$$\frac{1}{7} + \frac{2}{7} =$$

$$\frac{1+2}{7} =$$

$$\frac{3}{7}$$

Example 2: $\frac{1}{8} + \frac{3}{8} =$ _______

$$\frac{1}{8} + \frac{3}{8} =$$

$$\frac{1+3}{8} =$$

$$\frac{4}{8} = \frac{1}{2}$$

Addition of Fractions with Unlike Denominators

1. Change the fractions to equivalent fractions with the lowest common denominator.
2. Add the numerators.
3. Place the sum over the lowest common denominator.
4. Reduce to lowest terms.

Example 1: $\frac{2}{3} + \frac{1}{5} =$ ______

$$\frac{2}{3} + \frac{1}{5} =$$

To find the lowest common denominator, multiply the two denominators together.

$3 \times 5 = 15$

Change each fraction to an equivalent fraction with 15 as the denominator.

$\frac{2}{3} = \frac{?}{15}$

$15 \div 3 = 5$

$5 \times 2 = 10$

$\frac{2}{3} = \frac{10}{15}$

$\frac{1}{5} = \frac{?}{15}$

$15 \div 5 = 3$

$3 \times 1 = 3$

$\frac{1}{5} = \frac{3}{15}$

$$\frac{10}{15} + \frac{3}{15} =$$

$$\frac{10 + 3}{15} = \frac{13}{15}$$

Example 2: $\frac{1}{6} + \frac{1}{4} + \frac{1}{3} =$ ______

To find a common denominator, try multiplying two of the denominators together and check to see whether that number is divisible by the other denominator.

$4 \times 3 = 12$

Is 12 divisible by the other denominator, 6? The answer is YES.

$\frac{1}{6} = \frac{?}{12}$

$12 \div 6 = 2$

$2 \times 1 = 2$

$\frac{1}{6} = \frac{2}{12}$

$\frac{1}{4} = \frac{?}{12}$

$12 \div 4 = 3$

$3 \times 1 = 3$

$\frac{1}{4} = \frac{3}{12}$

$\frac{1}{3} = \frac{?}{12}$

$12 \div 3 = 4$

$4 \times 1 = 4$

$\frac{1}{3} = \frac{4}{12}$

$$\frac{2}{12} + \frac{3}{12} + \frac{4}{12} =$$

$$\frac{2 + 3 + 4}{12} = \frac{9}{12}$$

$$\frac{9}{12} = \frac{3}{4} \text{ (reduced to lowest terms)}$$

Addition of Fractions Involving Whole Numbers and Unlike Denominators

1. Change the fractions to equivalent fractions with the lowest common denominator.
2. Add the numerators.
3. Place the sum over the lowest common denominator.
4. Reduce to lowest terms.
5. Write the reduced fraction next to the sum of the whole numbers.

Example 1: $1\frac{1}{3} + 2\frac{3}{8} =$ ______

To find the lowest common denominator, multiply the two denominators together.

$3 \times 8 = 24$

Change the fractions $\frac{1}{3}$ and $\frac{3}{8}$ to equivalent fractions with 24 as their denominators.

$\frac{1}{3} = \frac{?}{24}$

$24 \div 3 = 8$

$8 \times 1 = 8$

$\frac{1}{3} = \frac{8}{24}$

$\frac{3}{8} = \frac{?}{24}$

$24 \div 8 = 3$

$3 \times 3 = 9$

$\frac{3}{8} = \frac{9}{24}$

$$1\frac{8}{24} + 2\frac{9}{24} =$$

$$\begin{array}{r} 1\frac{8}{24} \\ +\,2\frac{9}{24} \\ \hline 3\frac{17}{24} \end{array}$$

Example 2: $5\frac{1}{2} + 3\frac{3}{10} =$ ______

Because 10 is evenly divisible by 2, 10 is the lowest common denominator. Therefore $\frac{1}{2}$ needs to be changed to an equivalent fraction with 10 as the denominator.

$\frac{1}{2} = \frac{?}{10}$

$10 \div 2 = 5$

$5 \times 1 = 5$

$\frac{1}{2} = \frac{5}{10}$

$$5\frac{5}{10} + 3\frac{3}{10} =$$

$$\begin{array}{r} 5\frac{5}{10} \\ +\,3\frac{3}{10} \\ \hline 8\frac{8}{10} \end{array} = 8\frac{4}{5} \text{ (reduced to lowest terms)}$$

SUBTRACTION OF FRACTIONS

Subtraction of Fractions Having the Same Denominator

1. Subtract the numerator of the **subtrahend** from the numerator of the **minuend**.
2. Place the difference over the common denominator.
3. Reduce to lowest terms.

Example 1: $6/8 - 4/8 =$ ______

$$\frac{6}{8} - \frac{4}{8} =$$

$$\frac{6-4}{8} =$$

$$\frac{2}{8} = \frac{1}{4} \text{ (reduced to lowest terms)}$$

Example 2: $7/12 - 1/12 =$ ______

$$\frac{7}{12} - \frac{1}{12} =$$

$$\frac{7-1}{12} =$$

$$\frac{6}{12} = \frac{1}{2} \text{ (reduced to lowest terms)}$$

Subtraction of Fractions with Unlike Denominators

1. Change the fractions to equivalent fractions with the lowest common denominator.
2. Subtract the numerator of the subtrahend from that of the minuend.
3. Place the difference over the lowest common denominator.
4. Reduce to lowest terms.

Example 1: $2/3 - 1/6 =$ ______

The lowest common denominator is 6, because 6 is evenly divisible by 3. Therefore the fraction $2/3$ needs to be changed to an equivalent fraction with 6 as the denominator.

Step 1: $\frac{2}{3} = \frac{?}{6}$

$6 \div 3 = 2$

$2 \times 2 = 4$

$\frac{2}{3} = \frac{4}{6}$

Step 2: $\frac{4}{6} - \frac{1}{6} =$

$\frac{4-1}{6} =$

$\frac{3}{6} = \frac{1}{2}$ (reduced to lowest terms)

Example 2: $7/10 - 3/5 =$ ______

The lowest common denominator is 10, because 10 is evenly divisible by 5. Therefore the fraction $3/5$ needs to be changed to an equivalent fraction with 10 as the denominator.

Step 1: $\frac{3}{5} = \frac{?}{10}$

$10 \div 5 = 2$

$2 \times 3 = 6$

$\frac{3}{5} = \frac{6}{10}$

Step 2: $\frac{7}{10} - \frac{6}{10} =$

$\frac{7-6}{10} = \frac{1}{10}$

Subtraction of Fractions Involving Whole Numbers and Unlike Denominators

1. Change the fractions to equivalent fractions with the lowest common denominator.
2. Subtract the numerator of the subtrahend from the minuend, borrowing one from the whole number if necessary.
3. Place the difference over the lowest common denominator.
4. Reduce to lowest terms.
5. Write the reduced fraction next to the difference of the whole numbers.

Example 1: $3\frac{2}{3} - 1\frac{1}{4} =$ ______

The lowest common denominator is 12 (determined by multiplying 3 × 4). Each fraction needs to be changed to an equivalent fraction with 12 as the common denominator.

$\frac{2}{3} = \frac{?}{12}$ $\quad$ $\frac{1}{4} = \frac{?}{12}$

$12 \div 3 = 4$ $\quad$ $12 \div 4 = 3$

$4 \times 2 = 8$ $\quad$ $3 \times 1 = 3$

$\frac{2}{3} = \frac{8}{12}$ $\quad$ $\frac{1}{4} = \frac{3}{12}$

$$3\frac{8}{12} - 1\frac{3}{12} =$$

$$\begin{array}{r} 3\frac{8}{12} \\ -\ 1\frac{3}{12} \\ \hline 2\frac{5}{12} \end{array}$$

Example 2: $8\frac{1}{2} - 3\frac{4}{7} =$ ______

The lowest common denominator is 14 (determined by multiplying 2 × 7). Each fraction needs to be changed to an equivalent fraction with 14 as the common denominator.

$\frac{1}{2} = \frac{?}{14}$ $\quad$ $\frac{4}{7} = \frac{?}{14}$

$14 \div 2 = 7$ $\quad$ $14 \div 7 = 2$

$7 \times 1 = 7$ $\quad$ $2 \times 4 = 8$

$\frac{1}{2} = \frac{7}{14}$ $\quad$ $\frac{4}{7} = \frac{8}{14}$

$$8\frac{7}{14} - 3\frac{8}{14} =$$

To perform the subtraction, it is necessary to borrow one from the whole number. "One" for this problem can be expressed as $\frac{14}{14}$. Therefore $8\frac{7}{14} = 7\frac{21}{14}$. Now the mathematics may be completed.

$$\begin{array}{r} 8\frac{7}{14} \\ -\ 3\frac{8}{14} \\ \hline \end{array} \quad = \quad \begin{array}{r} 7\frac{21}{14} \\ -\ 3\frac{8}{14} \\ \hline 4\frac{13}{14} \end{array}$$

MULTIPLICATION OF FRACTIONS

1. Multiply the numerators.
2. Multiply the denominators.
3. Place the product of the numerators over the product of the denominators.
4. Reduce to lowest terms.

Example 1: $2/3 \times 3/5 =$ ______

$$\frac{2}{3} \times \frac{3}{5} =$$

$$\frac{2 \times 3}{3 \times 5} = \frac{6}{15}$$

$$\frac{6}{15} = \frac{2}{5} \text{ (reduced to lowest terms)}$$

Example 2: $4/9 \times 4/5 =$ ______

$$\frac{4}{9} \times \frac{4}{5} =$$

$$\frac{4 \times 4}{9 \times 5} = \frac{16}{45} \text{ (reduced to lowest terms)}$$

The process of multiplying fractions may be shortened by **canceling**. In other words, numbers common to the numerators and denominators may be divided or canceled out.

Example 1: $2/3 \times 3/5 =$ ______

$$\frac{2}{\overset{}{\underset{1}{\cancel{3}}}} \times \frac{\overset{1}{\cancel{3}}}{5} = \frac{2 \times 1}{1 \times 5} = \frac{2}{5}$$

Example 2: $7/20 \times 2/5 \times 3/14 =$ ______

$$\frac{\overset{1}{\cancel{7}}}{\underset{10}{\cancel{20}}} \times \frac{\overset{1}{\cancel{2}}}{5} \times \frac{3}{\underset{2}{\cancel{14}}} =$$

$$\frac{1 \times 1 \times 3}{10 \times 5 \times 2} = \frac{3}{100}$$

Example 3: $2/6 \times 3/4 =$ ______

$$\frac{\overset{1}{\cancel{2}}}{\underset{2}{\cancel{6}}} \times \frac{\overset{1}{\cancel{3}}}{\underset{2}{\cancel{4}}} = \frac{1 \times 1}{2 \times 2} = \frac{1}{4}$$

Multiplication of Mixed Numbers

1. Change each mixed number to an improper fraction.
2. Multiply the numerators.
3. Multiply the denominators.
4. Place the product of the numerators over the product of the denominators.
5. Reduce to lowest terms.

Example 1: $1\frac{1}{2} \times 2\frac{1}{4} =$ ______

$$\frac{3}{2} \times \frac{9}{4} =$$

$$\frac{3 \times 9}{2 \times 4} = \frac{27}{8} = 3\frac{3}{8} \text{ (reduced to lowest terms)}$$

Example 2: $2 \times 3\frac{5}{6} =$ ______

$$\frac{2}{1} \times \frac{23}{6} =$$

$$\frac{\overset{1}{\cancel{2}}}{1} \times \frac{23}{\underset{3}{\cancel{6}}} =$$

$$\frac{1 \times 23}{1 \times 3} = \frac{23}{3} = 7\frac{2}{3} \text{ (reduced to lowest terms)}$$

DIVISION OF FRACTIONS

1. Invert (or turn upside down) the divisor.
2. Multiply the two fractions.
3. Reduce to lowest terms.

Example 1: $2/3 \div 6/8 =$ ______

$$\frac{2}{3} \div \frac{6}{8} =$$

$$\frac{2}{3} \times \frac{8}{6} =$$

$$\frac{\overset{1}{\cancel{2}}}{3} \times \frac{8}{\underset{3}{\cancel{6}}} = \frac{1 \times 8}{3 \times 3} = \frac{8}{9}$$

Example 2: $3/4 \div 8/9 =$ ______

$$\frac{3}{4} \div \frac{8}{9} =$$

$$\frac{3}{4} \times \frac{9}{8} =$$

$$\frac{3 \times 9}{4 \times 8} = \frac{27}{32}$$

Division of Mixed Numbers

1. Change each mixed number to an improper fraction.
2. Invert (or turn upside down) the divisor.
3. Multiply the two fractions.
4. Reduce to lowest terms.

Example 1: $1\,3/4 \div 2\,1/8 =$ ______

$$\frac{7}{4} \div \frac{17}{8} =$$

$$\frac{7}{\underset{1}{\cancel{4}}} \times \frac{\overset{2}{\cancel{8}}}{17} = \frac{7 \times 2}{1 \times 17} = \frac{14}{17}$$

Example 2: $1/7 \div 7 =$ ______

$$\frac{1}{7} \div \frac{7^*}{1} =$$

$$\frac{1}{7} \times \frac{1}{7} = \frac{1 \times 1}{7 \times 7} = \frac{1}{49}$$

*Remember that the denominator of a whole number is always 1.

$$6 = \frac{6}{1}$$

$$12 = \frac{12}{1}$$

REDUCTION OF A COMPLEX FRACTION

1. Rewrite the complex fraction as a division problem.
2. Invert (or turn upside down) the divisor.
3. Multiply the two fractions.
4. Reduce to lowest terms.

Example 1: $3/8 / 1/4 = \_\_\_\_\_\_$

$$\frac{3}{8} \div \frac{1}{4} =$$

$$\frac{3}{8} \times \frac{4}{1} =$$

$$\frac{3}{\cancel{8}_2} \times \frac{\cancel{4}^1}{1} = \frac{3 \times 1}{2 \times 1} = \frac{3}{2} = 1\frac{1}{2}$$ (reduced to lowest terms)

Example 2: $1/2 / 2/7 = \_\_\_\_\_\_$

$$\frac{1}{2} \div \frac{2}{7} =$$

$$\frac{1}{2} \times \frac{7}{2} =$$

$$\frac{1 \times 7}{2 \times 2} = \frac{7}{4} = 1\frac{3}{4}$$ (reduced to lowest terms)

Reduction of a Complex Fraction with Mixed Numbers

1. Change the mixed numbers to improper fractions.
2. Rewrite the complex fraction as a division problem.
3. Invert (or turn upside down) the divisor.
4. Multiply the two fractions.
5. Reduce to lowest terms.

Example 1: $2\frac{1}{2} / 1\frac{1}{3} = \_\_\_\_\_\_$

$$2\frac{1}{2} \div 1\frac{1}{3} =$$

$$\frac{5}{2} \div \frac{4}{3} =$$

$$\frac{5}{2} \times \frac{3}{4} =$$

$$\frac{5 \times 3}{2 \times 4} = \frac{15}{8} = 1\frac{7}{8}$$ (reduced to lowest terms)

Example 2: $3\frac{3}{4} / 2\frac{1}{6} = \_\_\_\_\_\_$

$$3\frac{3}{4} \div 2\frac{1}{6} =$$

$$\frac{15}{4} \div \frac{13}{6} =$$

$$\frac{15}{4} \times \frac{6}{13} =$$

$$\frac{15 \times \cancel{6}^3}{\cancel{4}_2 \times 13} = \frac{45}{26} = 1\frac{19}{26}$$ (reduced to lowest terms)

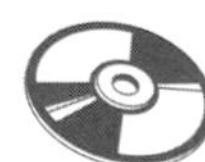

Refer to Mathematics Review: Fractions on the CD for additional help and practice problems.

WORK SHEET

Directions: Change the following improper fractions to mixed numbers.

1. $4/3$ = _______ **2.** $6/2$ = _______ **3.** $16/5$ = _______ **4.** $13/4$ = _______

5. $15/10$ = _______ **6.** $9/8$ = _______ **7.** $10/6$ = _______ **8.** $26/12$ = _______

9. $21/6$ = _______ **10.** $11/8$ = _______ **11.** $7/2$ = _______ **12.** $112/100$ = _______

Directions: Change the following mixed numbers to improper fractions.

1. $1\,1/2$ = _______ **2.** $3\,3/4$ = _______ **3.** $2\,2/3$ = _______ **4.** $2\,5/6$ = _______

5. $1\,3/5$ = _______ **6.** $3\,4/7$ = _______ **7.** $4\,7/8$ = _______ **8.** $3\,7/100$ = _______

9. $2\,7/10$ = _______ **10.** $6\,5/8$ = _______ **11.** $1\,3/25$ = _______ **12.** $4\,1/4$ = _______

Directions: Add and reduce fractions to lowest terms.

1. $\frac{2}{3} + \frac{5}{6} =$ _______ **2.** $\frac{2}{5} + \frac{3}{7} =$ _______ **3.** $3\frac{1}{8} + \frac{2}{3} =$ _______

4. $2\frac{1}{2} + \frac{3}{4} =$ _______ **5.** $2\frac{1}{4} + 3\frac{2}{5} =$ _______ **6.** $1\frac{6}{13} + 1\frac{2}{3} =$ _______

7. $1\frac{1}{2} + 3\frac{3}{4} + 2\frac{3}{8} =$ _______ **8.** $4\frac{3}{11} + 2\frac{1}{2} =$ _______ **9.** $2\frac{2}{3} + 3\frac{7}{9} =$ _______

10. $1\frac{3}{10} + 4\frac{2}{5} + \frac{2}{3} =$ _______ **11.** $3\frac{1}{2} + 2\frac{5}{6} + 2\frac{2}{3} =$ _______ **12.** $5\frac{5}{6} + 2\frac{2}{5} =$ _______

Directions: Subtract and reduce fractions to lowest terms.

1. $\frac{2}{3} - \frac{3}{7} =$ _______ **2.** $\frac{7}{8} - \frac{5}{16} =$ _______ **3.** $\frac{9}{16} - \frac{5}{12} =$ _______

4. $1\frac{1}{3} - \frac{5}{6} =$ _______ **5.** $2\frac{17}{20} - 1\frac{3}{4} =$ _______ **6.** $5\frac{1}{4} - 3\frac{5}{16} =$ _______

7. $5\frac{3}{8} - 4\frac{3}{4} =$ _______ 8. $3\frac{1}{4} - 1\frac{11}{12} =$ _______ 9. $6\frac{1}{2} - 3\frac{7}{8} =$ _______

10. $4\frac{1}{6} - 2\frac{3}{4} =$ _______ 11. $5\frac{2}{3} - 3\frac{7}{8} =$ _______ 12. $2\frac{5}{16} - 1\frac{3}{8} =$ _______

Directions: Multiply and reduce fractions to lowest terms.

1. $\frac{1}{3} \times \frac{4}{5} =$ _______ 2. $\frac{7}{8} \times \frac{2}{3} =$ _______ 3. $6 \times \frac{2}{3} =$ _______

4. $\frac{3}{8} \times 4 =$ _______ 5. $2\frac{1}{3} \times 3\frac{3}{4} =$ _______ 6. $4\frac{3}{8} \times 2\frac{5}{7} =$ _______

7. $2\frac{5}{12} \times 5\frac{1}{4} =$ _______ 8. $\frac{3}{4} \times 2\frac{3}{8} =$ _______ 9. $\frac{3}{8} \times \frac{4}{5} \times \frac{2}{3} =$ _______

10. $\frac{1}{10} \times \frac{3}{100} =$ _______ 11. $3\frac{1}{2} \times 1\frac{5}{6} =$ _______ 12. $2\frac{4}{9} \times 1\frac{3}{11} =$ _______

Directions: Divide and reduce fractions to lowest terms.

1. $1\frac{2}{3} \div 3\frac{1}{2} =$ ______ **2.** $5\frac{1}{2} \div 2\frac{1}{2} =$ ______ **3.** $3\frac{1}{2} \div 2\frac{1}{4} =$ ______

4. $4\frac{3}{8} \div 1\frac{3}{4} =$ ______ **5.** $3\frac{1}{2} \div 1\frac{6}{7} =$ ______ **6.** $\frac{9}{10} \div \frac{2}{3} =$ ______

7. $3 \div 1\frac{5}{6} =$ ______ **8.** $6\frac{2}{3} \div 1\frac{7}{10} =$ ______ **9.** $\frac{7}{8}/\frac{1}{4} =$ ______

10. $6\frac{1}{2}/2\frac{5}{6} =$ ______ **11.** $5\frac{1}{2}/2\frac{2}{3} =$ ______ **12.** $2\frac{2}{3}/1\frac{7}{9} =$ ______

Answers on p. 426.

Name ________________________________

Date ________________________________

ACCEPTABLE SCORE 27

YOUR SCORE ______

POSTTEST 1

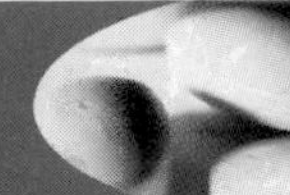

Directions: Perform the indicated calculations and reduce fractions to lowest terms.

1. $\frac{2}{3} + \frac{4}{9} =$ ______ **2.** $\frac{3}{8} + \frac{1}{3} =$ ______ **3.** $2\frac{3}{4} + 2\frac{1}{3} =$ ______

4. $2\frac{2}{3} + \frac{3}{7} =$ ______ **5.** $\frac{3}{4} + \frac{3}{100} =$ ______ **6.** $4\frac{2}{5} + 3\frac{3}{4} =$ ______

7. $4\frac{1}{6} + \frac{2}{3} + 2\frac{3}{4} =$ ______ **8.** $1\frac{3}{10} - \frac{2}{5} =$ ______ **9.** $2\frac{1}{2} - 1\frac{2}{3} =$ ______

10. $\frac{5}{7} - \frac{1}{2} =$ ______ **11.** $3\frac{1}{2} - 1\frac{9}{16} =$ ______ **12.** $2\frac{5}{7} - 1\frac{2}{9} =$ ______

13. $9\frac{1}{5} - 3\frac{1}{2} =$ ______ **14.** $2\frac{1}{4} - \frac{7}{9}/\frac{2}{3} =$ ______ **15.** $\frac{3}{4} \times \frac{6}{7} =$ ______

16. $3 \times 4/5 =$ _______

17. $2/9 \times 9 =$ _______

18. $2\,3/4 \times 1\,1/6 =$ _______

19. $1\,1/4 \times 2\,2/3 =$ _______

20. $10\,1/2 \times 1\,2/5 =$ _______

21. $5\,6/7 \times 3/5 =$ _______

22. $1/4 \times 3\,1/2 =$ _______

23. $2/3 \div 5/8 =$ _______

24. $1/5 \div 1/50 =$ _______

25. $1/3 \div 1/2 =$ _______

26. $5/6 \div 2/3 =$ _______

27. $\frac{1}{5} \big/ \frac{1}{3} =$ _______

28. $1\frac{1}{5} \big/ \frac{8}{9} =$ _______

29. $\frac{3}{4} \big/ \frac{1}{6} =$ _______

30. $3\frac{1}{8} \big/ 2\frac{3}{4} =$ _______

Answers on p. 426.

Name ____________________

Date ____________________

ACCEPTABLE SCORE 27

YOUR SCORE ______

POSTTEST 2

Directions: Perform the indicated calculations and reduce fractions to lowest terms.

1. $\frac{1}{4} + \frac{5}{6} =$ ______
2. $2\frac{3}{5} + 1\frac{1}{2} =$ ______
3. $\frac{2}{3} + 2\frac{3}{7} =$ ______
4. $1\frac{7}{8} + 3\frac{2}{5} =$ ______
5. $1\frac{3}{4} + \frac{5}{8} + 2\frac{5}{12} =$ ______
6. $10\frac{1}{2} + 1\frac{3}{10} =$ ______
7. $1\frac{5}{14} + 2\frac{3}{21} =$ ______
8. $\frac{4}{9} - \frac{1}{3} =$ ______
9. $2\frac{3}{4} - \frac{7}{8} =$ ______
10. $3\frac{1}{2} - 1\frac{2}{3} =$ ______
11. $3\frac{5}{8} - 1\frac{5}{16} =$ ______
12. $7\frac{1}{3} - 5\frac{5}{6} =$ ______
13. $7\frac{7}{10} - 3\frac{4}{5} =$ ______
14. $3\frac{4}{15} - 2\frac{2}{3} =$ ______
15. $\frac{2}{7} \times \frac{2}{3} =$ ______
16. $3\frac{4}{9} \times 1\frac{4}{5} =$ ______
17. $2 \times \frac{2}{3} =$ ______
18. $\frac{5}{6} \times 2\frac{1}{3} =$ ______

19. $1/100 \times 1/10 =$ _______

20. $6\frac{3}{4} \times 5\frac{1}{3} =$ _______

21. $2\frac{5}{8} \times 1\frac{1}{3} =$ _______

22. $3\frac{1}{2} \times 3\frac{3}{14} =$ _______

23. $3/4 \div 8/9 =$ _______

24. $1\frac{1}{2} \div 1\frac{6}{7} =$ _______

25. $2\frac{1}{3} \div 3/8 =$ _______

26. $1/7 \div 7 =$ _______

27. $5/6 / 1\frac{1}{3} =$ _______

28. $1\frac{1}{2} / 2\frac{2}{7} =$ _______

29. $2\frac{1}{4} / 1\frac{1}{3} =$ _______

30. $3/8 / 3/9 =$ _______

Answers on p. 427.

Name ______________________________

Date ______________________________

ACCEPTABLE SCORE 36

YOUR SCORE ______

PRETEST

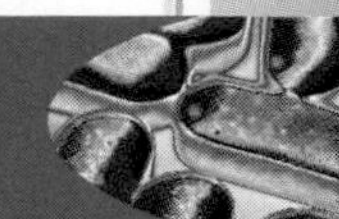

Complete the Decimals Pretest. A score of 36 out of 40 indicates an acceptable understanding and competency of basic calculations involving decimals. You may skip to the Percents Pretest on p. 51. However, if you score 35 or below, completion of Chapter 2, Decimals, will be helpful for your continued success in the calculation of drug dosages.

Directions: Write the following numbers in words.

1. 0.04 ______________________________
2. 1.6 ______________________________
3. 16.06734 ______________________________

   ____
4. 1.015 ______________________________
5. 0.009 ______________________________

Directions: Circle the decimal with the *least value.*

6. 0.2, 0.25, 0.025, 0.02
7. 0.4, 0.48, 0.04, 0.004
8. 1.6, 1.64, 1.682, 1.69
9. 2.8, 2.82, 2.082, 2.822
10. 0.3, 0.33, 0.003, 0.033

Directions: Perform the indicated calculations.

11. 6.8 + 2.986 + 14.7 + 0.89 = ______
12. 141.71 + 84.98 + 9.98 + 87.63 = ______
13. 1006.48 + 0.008 + 6.2 + 0.179 = ______
14. 47.21 + 48.496 + 0.2976 + 54.67 = ______
15. 5.971 + 63.1 + 8.264 + 7.23 = ______
16. 2.176 − 1.098 = ______

17. 2.006 − 0.998 = _______ **18.** 836.2 − 76.8 = _______ **19.** 100.3 − 98.6 = _______

20. 12.6 − 1.654 = _______ **21.** 0.63 × 0.09 = _______ **22.** 41.545 × 0.16 = _______

23. 5.25 × 0.37 = _______ **24.** 44.08 × 0.67 = _______ **25.** 56.7 × 3.29 = _______

26. 0.89 ÷ 4.32 = _______ **27.** 1.436 ÷ 0.08 = _______ **28.** 0.689 ÷ 62.8 = _______

29. 12.54 ÷ 0.02 = _______ **30.** 23 ÷ 1236 = _______

Directions: Change the following decimal fractions to proper fractions.

31. 0.008 = _______ **32.** 0.25 = _______ **33.** 0.322 = _______ **34.** 0.004 = _______

35. 0.34 = _______

Directions: Change the following proper fractions to decimal fractions.

36. $3/5$ = _______ **37.** $2/3$ = _______ **38.** $3/500$ = _______ **39.** $7/20$ = _______

40. $5/8$ = _______

Answers on p. 427.

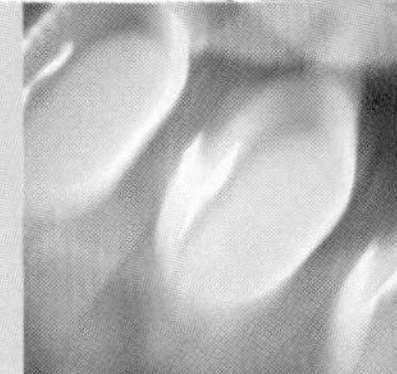

CHAPTER

2

Decimals

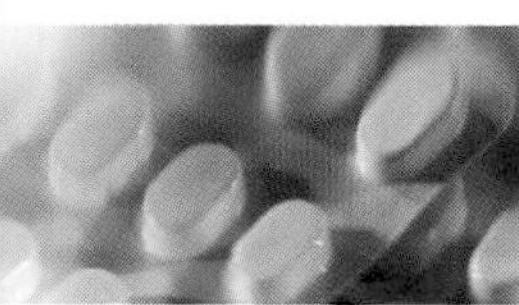

LEARNING OBJECTIVES

On completion of the materials provided in this chapter, you will be able to perform computations accurately by mastering the following mathematical concepts:

1. Reading and writing decimal numbers
2. Determining the value of decimal fractions
3. Adding, subtracting, multiplying, and dividing decimals
4. Rounding decimal fractions to an indicated place value
5. Multiplying and dividing decimals by 10 or a power of 10
6. Multiplying and dividing decimals by 0.1 or a multiple of 0.1
7. Converting a decimal fraction to a proper fraction
8. Converting a proper fraction to a decimal fraction

Study the introductory material for decimals. The processes for the calculation of decimal problems are listed in steps. Memorize the steps for each calculation before beginning the work sheet. Complete the work sheet, at the end of this chapter, which provides for extensive practice in the manipulation of decimals. Check your answers. If you have difficulties, go back and review the steps for that type of calculation. When you feel ready to evaluate your learning, take the first posttest. Check your answers. An acceptable score as indicated on the posttest signifies that you are ready for the next chapter. An unacceptable score signifies a need for further study before you take the second posttest.

Decimals are used in the metric system of measurement. The nurse uses the metric system in the calculation of drug dosages. Therefore it is essential for the nurse to be able to manipulate decimals easily and accurately.

Each **decimal fraction** consists of a numerator that is expressed in numerals, a decimal point placed so that it designates the value of the denominator, and the denominator, which is understood to be 10 or some power of 10. **In writing a decimal fraction, always place a zero to the left**

of the decimal point so that the decimal point can readily be seen. The omission of the zero may result in a critical medication error. Some examples are as follows:

Fraction	Decimal fraction
$\frac{7}{10}$	0.7
$\frac{13}{100}$	0.13
$\frac{227}{1000}$	0.227

Decimal numbers include an integer, a decimal point, and a decimal fraction. The value of the combined integer and decimal fraction is determined by the placement of the decimal point. Whole numbers are written to the *left* of the decimal point, and decimal fractions, to the *right*. The diagram in Figure 2-1 illustrates the place occupied by the numeral that has the value indicated.

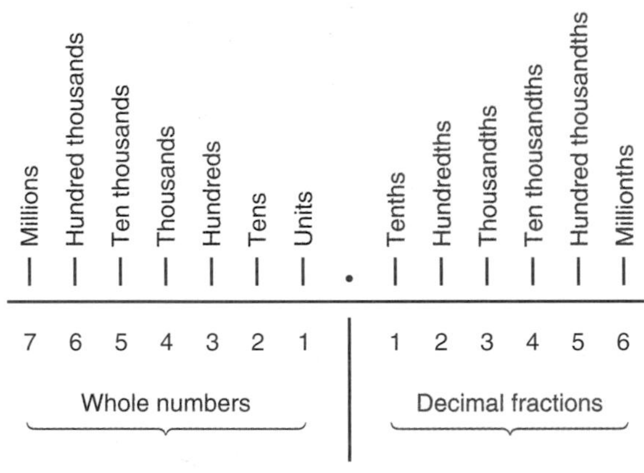

FIGURE 2-1 Decimal place values.

Reading Decimal Numbers

The reading of a decimal number is determined by the place value of the integers and decimal fractions.

1. Read the whole number.
2. Read the decimal point as "and."
3. Read the decimal fraction.

Examples:

0.4	four tenths
0.86	eighty-six hundredths
3.659	three and six hundred fifty-nine thousandths
182.0012	one hundred eighty-two and twelve ten-thousandths
9.47735	nine and forty-seven thousand seven hundred thirty-five one hundred-thousandths

Determining the Values of Decimal Fractions

1. Place the numbers in a vertical column with the decimal points in a vertical line.
2. Add zeros on the right in the decimal fractions to make columns even.

3. The largest number in a column to the right of the decimal point has the *greatest* value.
4. If two numbers in a column are of equal value, examine the next column to the right and so on.
5. The smallest number in the column to the right of the decimal point has the *least* value. If two numbers in the first column are of equal value, examine the second column to the right and so on.

Example 1: Of the following fractions (0.623, 0.841, 0.0096, 0.432), which has the greatest value? the least value?

0.6320

0.8410

0.0096

0.4320

0.841 has the greatest value; 0.0096 has the least value.

Note: In mixed numbers the values of both the integer and the fraction are considered.

Example 2: Which decimal number (0.4, 0.25, 1.2, 1.002) has the greatest value? the least value?

0.400

0.250

1.200

1.002

1.2 has the greatest value; 0.25 has the least value.

ADDITION AND SUBTRACTION OF DECIMALS

1. Write the numerals in a vertical column with the decimal points in a straight line.
2. Add zeros as needed to complete the columns.
3. Add or subtract each column as indicated by the symbol.
4. Place the decimal point in the sum or difference directly below the decimal points in the column.
5. Place a zero to the left of the decimal point in a decimal fraction.

Example 1: Add: 14.8 + 6.29 + 3.028

$$\begin{array}{r} 14.800 \\ 6.290 \\ +\ 3.028 \\ \hline 24.118 \end{array}$$

Example 2: Subtract: 5.163 – 4.98

$$\begin{array}{r} 5.163 \\ -\ 4.980 \\ \hline 0.183 \end{array}$$

MULTIPLICATION OF DECIMALS

1. Place the smaller group of numbers under the larger group of numbers.
2. Multiply.
3. Add the number of places to the right of the decimal point in the multiplicand and the multiplier (i.e., the numbers being multiplied). The sum determines the placement of the decimal point within the product.
4. Count from right to left the value of the sum and place the decimal point.

Example 1: 0.19 × 0.24

```
   0.19   two place values
×  0.24   two place values
   076
  038
 000
 0.0456   four place values
```

Example 2: 0.459 × 0.52

```
   0.459   three place values
×   0.52   two place values
    0918
   2295
  0000
 0.23868   five place values
```

Example 3: 8.265 × 4.36

```
     8.265   three place values
×     4.36   two place values
     49590
    24795
   33060
  36.03540   five place values
```

Example 4: 160.41 × 3.527

```
    160.41   two place values
×    3.527   three place values
    112287
    32082
   80205
  48123
 565.76607   five place values
```

Multiplying a Decimal by 10 or a Power of 10 (100, 1000, 10,000, 100,000)

1. Move the decimal point to the right the same number of places as there are zeros in the multiplier.
2. Zeros may be added as indicated.

Example 1: 0.132 × 10 = 1.32

Example 2: 0.053 × 100 = 5.3

Example 3: 2.64 × 1000 = 2640

Example 4: 49.6 × 10,000 = 496,000

Multiplying a Whole Number or Decimal by 0.1 or a Multiple of 0.1 (0.01, 0.001, 0.0001, or 0.00001)

1. Move the decimal point to the left the same number of spaces as there are numbers to the right of the decimal point in the multiplier.
2. Zeros may be added as indicated.

Example 1: 354.86 × 0.0001 = 0.035486

Example 2: 0.729 × 0.1 = 0.0729

Example 3: 12.73 × 0.01 = 0.1273

Example 4: 5.752 × 0.001 = 0.005752

ROUNDING A DECIMAL FRACTION

1. Find the number to the right of the place value desired.
2. If the number is 5, 6, 7, 8, or 9, add one to the number in the place value desired and drop the rest of the numbers.
3. If the number is 0, 1, 2, 3, or 4, remove all numbers to the right of the desired place value.

Example 1: Round the following decimal fractions to the nearest tenth.

A. 0.268

0.2)68 — 6 is the number to the right of the tenth place. Therefore 1 should be added to the number 2 and the 68 dropped.

0.3 — correct answer

B. 4.374
4.3)74 — 7 is the number to the right of the tenth place. Therefore 1 should be added to the number 3 and the 74 dropped.

4.4 — correct answer

C. 5.723
5.7)23 — 2 is the number to the right of the tenth place. Therefore all numbers to the right of the tenth place should be removed.

5.7 — correct answer

Example 2: Round the following decimal fractions to the nearest hundredth.

A. 0.876
0.87)6 — 6 is the number to the right of the hundredths place. Therefore 1 should be added to the number 7 and the 6 dropped.

0.88 — correct answer

B. 2.3249
2.32)49 — 4 is the number to the right of the hundredths place. Therefore all numbers to the right of the hundredths place should be removed.

2.32 — correct answer

Example 3: Round the following decimal fractions to the nearest thousandth.

A. 3.1325
3.132)5 — 5 is the number to the right of the thousandths place. Therefore 1 should be added to the number 2 and the 5 dropped.

3.133 — correct answer

B. 0.4674
0.467)4 — 4 is the number to the right of the thousandths place. Therefore all numbers to the right of the thousandths place should be removed.

0.467 — correct answer

Rounding numbers helps to estimate values, compare values, have more realistic and workable numbers, and spot errors. Decimal fractions may be rounded to any designated place value.

DIVISION OF DECIMALS

1. Place a caret (‸) to the right of the last number in the divisor, signifying the movement of the decimal point that will make the divisor a whole number.
2. Count the number of spaces that the decimal point is moved in the divisor.
3. Count to the right an equal number of spaces in the dividend and place a caret to signify the movement of the decimal.
4. Place a decimal point on the quotient line directly above the caret.
5. Divide, extending the decimal fraction three places to the right of the decimal point.
6. Zeros may be added as indicated to extend the decimal fraction dividend.
7. Round the quotient to the nearest hundredth.

Example 1: 8.326 ÷ 1.062

```
                7.839 or 7.84
1.062^)8.326^000
       7 434
       892 0
       849 6
        42 40
        31 86
        10 540
         9 558
```

Example 2: 386 ÷ 719

```
      0.536 or 0.54
719)386.000
    359 5
     26 50
     21 57
      4 930
      4 314
```

Note: The decimal fraction is emphasized by the placement of a zero to the left of the decimal point.

Dividing a Decimal by 10 or a Multiple of 10 (100, 1000, 10,000, 100,000)

1. Move the decimal point to the left the same number of places as there are zeros in the divisor.
2. Zeros may be added as indicated.

Example 1: 6.41 ÷ 10 = 0.641

Example 2: 358.0 ÷ 100 = 3.58

Dividing a Whole Number or a Decimal Fraction by 0.1 or a Multiple of 0.1 (0.01, 0.001, 0.0001, 0.00001)

1. Move the decimal point to the right as many places as there are numbers in the divisor.
2. Zeros may be added as indicated.

Example 1: 5.897 ÷ 0.01 = 589.7

Example 2: 46.31 ÷ 0.001 = 46,310

CONVERSION

Converting a Decimal Fraction to a Proper Fraction

1. Remove the decimal point and the zero preceding it.
2. The numerals are the numerator.
3. The placement of the decimal point has indicated what the denominator will be.
4. Reduce to lowest terms.

Example 1: 0.3

$$\frac{3}{10}$$

Example 2: 0.86

$$\frac{86}{100} = \frac{43}{50}$$

Example 3: 0.375

$$\frac{375}{1000} = \frac{3}{8}$$

Converting a Proper Fraction to a Decimal Fraction

1. Divide the numerator by the denominator.
2. Extend the decimal the desired number of places (often three).
3. Place a zero to the left of the decimal point in a decimal fraction.

Example 1: $\frac{4}{5}$

$$\begin{array}{r} 0.8 \\ 5\overline{)4.0} \\ \underline{4\ 0} \end{array}$$

$\frac{4}{5} = 0.8$

Example 2: $\frac{7}{8}$

$$\begin{array}{r} 0.875 \\ 8\overline{)7.000} \\ \underline{6\ 4} \\ 60 \\ \underline{56} \\ 40 \\ \underline{40} \end{array}$$

$\frac{7}{8} = 0.875$

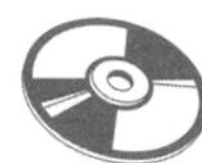

Refer to Mathematics Review: Decimals on the CD for additional help and practice problems.

WORK SHEET

Directions: Write the following numbers in words.

1. 0.2 ______________________________
2. 9.68 ______________________________
3. 0.0003 ______________________________
4. 1,968.342 ______________________________

   ____
5. 0.02 ______________________________

Directions: Circle the decimal numbers with the *greatest value*.

6. 0.2, 0.15, 0.1, 0.25
7. 0.4, 0.45, 0.04, 0.042
8. 0.9, 0.09, 0.95, 0.98
9. 0.5, 0.065, 0.58, 0.68
10. 1.8, 1.08, 1.18, 1.468
11. 7.4, 7.42, 7.423, 7.44

Directions: Circle the decimal numbers with the *least value*.

12. 0.6, 0.66, 0.666, 0.6666
13. 0.3, 0.03, 0.003, 0.0003
14. 1.2, 1.22, 1.022, 1.0022
15. 0.8, 0.08, 0.868, 0.859
16. 0.75, 0.07, 0.007, 0.0075
17. 3.015, 3.1, 3.006, 3.02

Directions: Add the following decimal problems.

1. 1.080 + 31.2 + 0.065 + 9.41 = ______
2. 2.2 + 355.6 + 8.125 + 6.75 = ______
3. 24.684 + 5.3697 + 8.025 + 2.9 = ______
4. 18.95 + 1.903 + 8.82 + 9.4 = ______
5. 56.93 + 765.7 + 64.882 + 7.33 = ______
6. 0.3 + 0.874 + 2.763 + 63.2 = ______

7. 13.5 + 1.023 + 8.83 + 3.267 = _______

8. 3.6 + 8.25 + 2.05 + 24 = _______

9. 0.6 + 0.985 + 1.432 + 52.1 = _______

10. 3.75 + 0.718 + 136.95 + 0.8 = _______

Directions: Subtract the following decimal problems.

1. 1321.52 – 63.65 = _______
2. 4.745 – 2.896 = _______
3. 1.8 – 1.09 = _______
4. 250.7 – 75.896 = _______
5. 24.186 – 16.768 = _______
6. 6.33 – 2.186 = _______
7. 0.486 – 0.025 = _______
8. 1 – 0.012 = _______
9. 63 – 0.978 = _______
10. 300 – 12.629 = _______

Directions: Multiply the following decimal problems.

1. 1.3 × 12.5 = _______
2. 127 × 4.8 = _______
3. 1.69 × 30.8 = _______
4. 9.08 × 6.18 = _______
5. 52.4 × 0.8 = _______
6. 420 × 0.08 = _______
7. 2.3 × 45.21 = _______
8. 7.46 × 54.83 = _______
9. 1.19 × 0.127 = _______
10. 7.85 × 3.006 = _______

Directions: Multiply the following numbers by 10 by moving the decimal point.

1. 0.09 _______
2. 0.2 _______
3. 0.18 _______
4. 0.3 _______
5. 0.625 _______
6. 2.33 _______

Directions: Multiply the following numbers by 100 by moving the decimal point.

1. 0.023 _______
2. 1.5 _______
3. 0.004 _______
4. 0.125 _______
5. 8.65 _______
6. 76.4 _______

Directions: Multiply the following numbers by 1000 by moving the decimal point.

1. 0.2 _______
2. 0.005 _______
3. 0.187 _______
4. 9.65 _______
5. 0.46 _______
6. 0.489 _______

Directions: Multiply the following numbers by 0.1 by moving the decimal point.

1. 30.0 ______ **2.** 0.69 ______ **3.** 1.7 ______

4. 0.95 ______ **5.** 0.138 ______ **6.** 5.67 ______

Directions: Multiply the following numbers by 0.01 by moving the decimal point.

1. 0.26 ______ **2.** 90.8 ______ **3.** 5.5 ______

4. 11.2 ______ **5.** 0.875 ______ **6.** 63.3 ______

Directions: Multiply the following numbers by 0.001 by moving the decimal point.

1. 56.0 ______ **2.** 12.55 ______ **3.** 126.5 ______

4. 33.3 ______ **5.** 9.684 ______ **6.** 241 ______

Directions: Round the following decimal fractions to the nearest tenth.

1. 0.33 ______ **2.** 0.913______ **3.** 2.359 ______

4. 0.66 ______ **5.** 58.36 ______ **6.** 8.092 ______

Directions: Round the following decimal fractions to the nearest hundredth.

1. 2.555 ______ **2.** 4.275 ______ **3.** 0.284 ______

4. 3.923 ______ **5.** 6.534 ______ **6.** 2.988 ______

Directions: Round the following decimal fractions to the nearest thousandth.

1. 27.86314 ______ **2.** 5.9246 ______ **3.** 2.1574 ______

4. 0.8493 ______ **5.** 321.0869 ______ **6.** 455.7682 ______

Directions: Divide. Round the quotient to the nearest hundredth.

1. $7.02 \div 6 =$ ______ **2.** $124.2 \div 0.03 =$ ______ **3.** $5.46 \div 0.7 =$ ______

4. $24 \div 0.06 =$ ______ **5.** $24 \div 1500 =$ ______ **6.** $4.6 \div 35.362 =$ ______

7. $4.13 \div 0.05 =$ _______

8. $9.08 \div 2.006 =$ _______

9. $63 \div 132.3 =$ _______

10. $21.25 \div 8.43 =$ _______

Directions: Divide the following numbers by 10 by moving the decimal point.

1. 6.0 _______
2. 0.2 _______
3. 9.8 _______
4. 0.05 _______
5. 0.375 _______
6. 0.99 _______

Directions: Divide the following numbers by 100 by moving the decimal point.

1. 0.7 _______
2. 8.11 _______
3. 700.0 _______
4. 0.19 _______
5. 12.0 _______
6. 30.2 _______

Directions: Divide the following numbers by 1000 by moving the decimal point.

1. 1.8 _______
2. 360.0 _______
3. 0.25 _______
4. 54.6 _______
5. 7.5 _______
6. 7140 _______

Directions: Divide the following numbers by 0.1 by moving the decimal point.

1. 2.8 _______
2. 0.1 _______
3. 0.65 _______
4. 0.987 _______
5. 15.0 _______
6. 8.25 _______

Directions: Divide the following numbers by 0.01 by moving the decimal point.

1. 36.0 _______
2. 0.16 _______
3. 0.48 _______
4. 9.59 _______
5. 0.8 _______
6. 0.097 _______

Directions: Divide the following numbers by 0.001 by moving the decimal point.

1. 6.2 _______
2. 839.0 _______
3. 5.0 _______
4. 0.86 _______
5. 13.8 _______
6. 0.0156 _______

Directions: Change the following decimal fractions to proper fractions.

1. 0.06 ______
2. 0.8 ______
3. 0.68 ______
4. 0.0025 ______
5. 0.625 ______
6. 0.25 ______
7. 0.64 ______
8. 0.005 ______
9. 0.01 ______
10. 0.044 ______

Directions: Change the following proper fractions to decimal fractions.

1. $\frac{1}{8}$ ______
2. $\frac{2}{3}$ ______
3. $\frac{16}{25}$ ______
4. $\frac{3}{5}$ ______
5. $\frac{8}{200}$ ______
6. $\frac{1}{3}$ ______
7. $\frac{4}{5}$ ______
8. $\frac{7}{8}$ ______
9. $\frac{1}{200}$ ______
10. $\frac{5}{6}$ ______

Answers on pp. 427-429.

Name ______________________________

Date ______________________________

ACCEPTABLE SCORE 32

YOUR SCORE ______

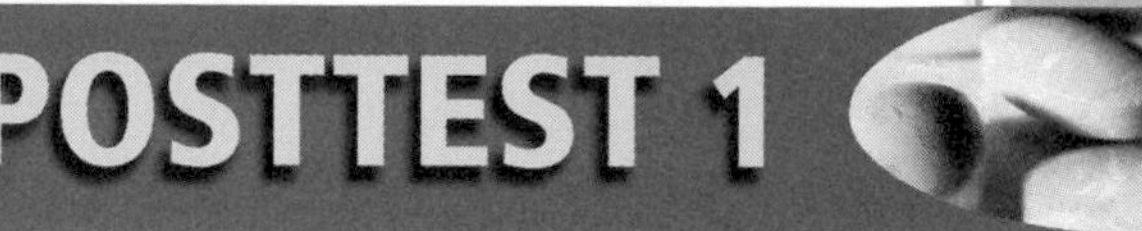

Directions: Write the following numbers in words.

1. 634.18 ______________________________

2. 0.9 ______________________________

3. 64.231 ______________________________

Directions: Circle the decimal fractions with the *greatest value*.

4. 0.1, 0.01, 0.15, 0.015

5. 0.666, 0.068, 0.006, 0.66

Directions: Perform the indicated calculations.

6. 1.342 + 0.987 + 8.062 + 44.269 = ______

7. 0.6 + 0.45 + 2.9 + 4.94 = ______

8. 3.004 + 0.848 + 0.9 + 1.6 = ______

9. 2.875 + 0.75 + 0.094 + 2.385 = ______

10. 1981.62 + 4.876 + 146.35 + 19.78 = ______

11. 1 – 0.661 = ______

12. 2.46 – 1.0068 = ______

13. 844.6 – 521.52 = ______

14. 43.69 – 0.0823 = ______

15. 0.9 – 0.689 = ______

16. 72.8 × 9.649 = ______

17. 1.58 × 0.088 = ______

18. 360 × 0.45 = _______ **19.** 26.2 × 1.69 = _______ **20.** 1.5 × 0.39 = _______

21. 268.8 ÷ 16 = _______ **22.** 8.89 ÷ 0.006 = _______ **23.** 12.54 ÷ 0.02 = _______

24. 56.4 ÷ 40 = _______ **25.** 165.9 ÷ 3.006 = _______

Directions: Change the following decimal fractions to proper fractions.

26. 0.09 _______ **27.** 0.0025 _______ **28.** 0.375 _______ **29.** 0.4 _______

30. 0.006 _______

Directions: Change the following proper fractions to decimal fractions.

31. $\frac{5}{7}$ _______ **32.** $\frac{1}{100}$ _______ **33.** $\frac{1}{250}$ _______ **34.** $\frac{1}{8}$ _______

35. $\frac{3}{32}$ _______

Answers on p. 429.

Name ______________________

Date ______________________

ACCEPTABLE SCORE 32

YOUR SCORE ______

POSTTEST 2

Directions: Write the following numbers in words.

1. 0.516 ______________________

2. 4.0002 ______________________

3. 123.69 ______________________

Directions: Circle the decimal with the *greatest value.*

4. 0.04, 0.45, 0.8, 0.86

5. 1.202, 1.22, 1.2, 1.222

Directions: Perform the indicated calculations.

6. 1.2791 + 327.8 + 123.07 + 4.67 = ______

7. 6.95 + 0.8 + 0.625 + 7.68 = ______

8. 19.29 + 3.5 + 5.869 + 4.55 = ______

9. 1.5 + 6.3 + 10.46 + 29.465 = ______

10. 322 + 0.95 + 6.45 + 9.6 = ______

11. 632.838 − 19.869 = ______

12. 1.572 − 0.985 = ______

13. 6.4 − 3.634 = ______

14. 2.6 − 0.087 = ______

15. 4.819 − 3.734 = ______

16. 57.6 × 2.9 = ______

17. 149.36 × 700 = ______

18. $56.43 \times 0.018 =$ _______ 19. $12.8 \times 6.5 =$ _______ 20. $27.5 \times 5.89 =$ _______

21. $5.9 \div 5.3 =$ _______ 22. $0.295 \div 0.059 =$ _______ 23. $124 \div 0.008 =$ _______

24. $0.7 \div 2.3 =$ _______ 25. $5.928 \div 2.4 =$ _______

Directions: Change the following decimal fractions to proper fractions.

26. 0.005 _______ 27. 0.35 _______ 28. 0.125 _______ 29. 0.85 _______

30. 0.6 _______

Directions: Change the following proper fractions to decimal fractions.

31. $\frac{1}{6}$ _______ 32. $\frac{1}{400}$ _______ 33. $\frac{7}{8}$ _______ 34. $\frac{1}{150}$ _______

35. $\frac{1}{125}$ _______

Answers on p. 429.

Name ________________________________

Date ________________________________

ACCEPTABLE SCORE 36

YOUR SCORE ______

PRETEST

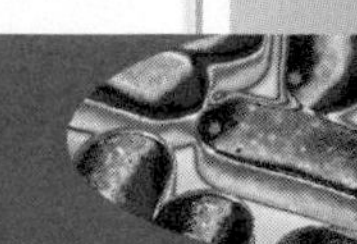

Complete the Percents Pretest. A score of 36 out of 40 indicates an acceptable understanding and competency of basic calculations involving percents. You may skip to the Ratios Pretest on p. 69. However, if you score 35 or below, completion of Chapter 3, Percents, will be helpful for your continued success in the calculation of drug dosages.

Directions: Change the following fractions to percents.

1. $\frac{1}{60}$ ______ **2.** $\frac{5}{7}$ ______ **3.** $\frac{1}{8}$ ______

4. $\frac{3}{10}$ ______ **5.** $\frac{4}{3}$ ______

Directions: Change the following decimals to percents.

6. 0.006 ______ **7.** 0.35 ______ **8.** 0.427 ______

9. 3.821 ______ **10.** 0.7 ______

Directions: Change the following percents to proper fractions.

11. 0.5% ______ **12.** 75% ______ **13.** 9½% ______

14. 24.8% ______ **15.** ⅜% ______

Directions: Change the following percents to decimals.

16. 1⅙% ______ **17.** 7.5% ______ **18.** 13$\frac{3}{10}$% ______

19. $\frac{8}{9}$% ______ **20.** 63% ______

Directions: What percent of

21. 1.60 is 6 ______ **22.** ¾ is ⅛ ______ **23.** 100 is 65 ______

24. 500 is 1 ______ **25.** 4.5 is 1.5 ______ **26.** 37.8 is 4.6 ______

27. $1\frac{4}{9}$ is $\frac{5}{8}$ _______

28. 1000 is 100 _______

29. $3\frac{1}{2}$ is $\frac{1}{4}$ _______

30. 9.7 is $\frac{1}{6}$ _______

Directions: What is

31. 3% of 60 _______

32. $\frac{1}{4}$% of 60_______

33. 4.5% of 57 _______

34. $2\frac{1}{8}$% of 32 _______

35. 4% of 77 _______

36. 9.3% of 46 _______

37. $\frac{3}{7}$% of 14 _______

38. 22% of 88 _______

39. 7.6% of 156 _______

40. 5% of 300 _______

Answers on pp. 429-430.

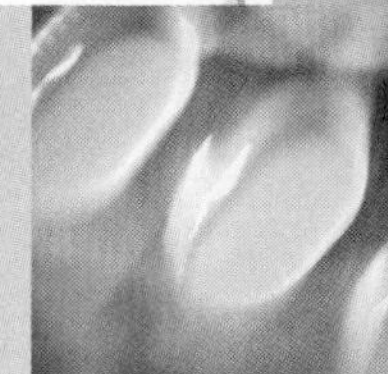

CHAPTER 3

Percents

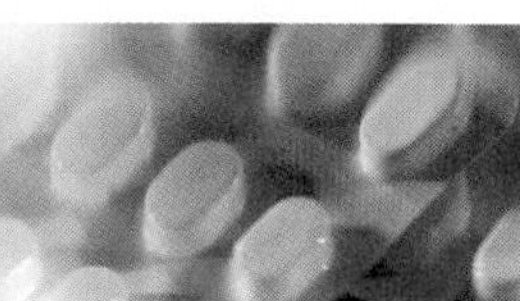

LEARNING OBJECTIVES

On completion of the materials provided in this chapter, you will be able to perform computations accurately by mastering the following mathematical concepts:

1. Changing a fraction or decimal to a percent
2. Changing a percent to a fraction or decimal
3. Changing a percent containing a fraction to a decimal
4. Finding what percent one number is of another
5. Finding the given percent of a number

Study the introductory material on percents. The processes for the calculation of percent problems are listed in steps. Memorize the steps for each calculation before beginning the work sheet. Complete the work sheet at the end of this chapter, which provides for extensive practice in the manipulation of percents. Check your answers. If you have any difficulty, go back and review the steps for that type of calculation. When you feel ready to evaluate your learning, take the first posttest. Check your answers. An acceptable score as indicated on the posttest signifies that you are ready for the next chapter. An unacceptable score signifies a need for further study before taking the second posttest.

A **percent** is a third way of showing a fractional relationship. Fractions, decimals, and percents can all be converted from one form to the others. Conversions of fractions and decimals are discussed in Chapter 2. A percent indicates a value equal to the number of hundredths. Therefore when a percent is written as a fraction, the denominator is *always* 100. The number beside the percent sign (%) becomes the numerator.

Changing a Fraction to a Percent

1. Multiply by 100.
2. Add the percent sign (%).

Example 1: 2/5

$$\frac{2}{\cancel{5}_{1}} \times \frac{\cancel{100}^{20}}{1} =$$

$$\frac{2 \times 20}{1 \times 1} = 40$$

40%

Example 2: 3/10

$$\frac{3}{\cancel{10}_{1}} \times \frac{\cancel{100}^{10}}{1} =$$

$$\frac{3 \times 10}{1 \times 1} = 30$$

30%

Example 3: 1¼

$$\frac{5}{\cancel{4}_{1}} \times \frac{\cancel{100}^{25}}{1} =$$

$$\frac{5 \times 25}{1 \times 1} = 125$$

125%

Example 4: 1/3

$$\frac{1}{3} \times \frac{100}{1} =$$

$$\frac{1 \times 100}{3 \times 1} = \frac{100}{3} = 33\frac{1}{3}$$

33⅓%

Changing a Decimal to a Percent

1. Multiply by 100 (by moving the decimal point two places to the right).
2. Add the percent sign (%).

Example 1: 0.421

0.421 × 100 = 42.1

42.1%

Example 2: 0.98

0.98 × 100 = 98

98%

Example 3: 0.2

0.2 × 100 = 20

20%

Example 4: 1.1212

1.1212 × 100 = 112.12

112.12%

Changing a Percent to a Fraction

1. Drop the % sign.
2. Write the remaining number as the fraction's numerator.
3. Write 100 as the denominator. (The denominator will *always* be 100.)
4. Reduce to lowest terms.

Example 1: 45%

$$\frac{45}{100} = \frac{9}{20}$$ (reduced to lowest terms)

Example 2: 0.3%

$$\frac{0.3}{100} =$$

$$\frac{\frac{3}{10}}{100}$$

$$\frac{3}{10} \div \frac{100}{1} =$$

$$\frac{3}{10} \times \frac{1}{100} = \frac{3}{1000}$$

Example 3: 3½%

$$\frac{3\frac{1}{2}}{100} = \frac{7/2}{100}$$

$$\frac{7}{2} \div \frac{100}{1} =$$

$$\frac{7}{2} \times \frac{1}{100} = \frac{7}{200}$$

Changing a Percent to a Decimal

1. Drop the % sign.
2. Divide the remaining number by 100 (by moving the decimal point two places to the left).
3. Express the quotient as a decimal. Place a zero before the decimal if there are no whole numbers.

Example 1: 32%

0.32

Example 2: 125%

1.25

Changing a Percent Containing a Fraction to a Decimal

1. Drop the % sign.
2. Change the mixed number to an improper fraction.
3. Divide by 100. Remember, the denominator of all whole numbers is 1.
4. Reduce to lowest terms.
5. Divide the numerator by the denominator, expressing the quotient as a decimal.

Example 1: 12½%

$$\frac{25}{2} \div \frac{100}{1} =$$

$$\frac{\overset{1}{\cancel{25}}}{2} \times \frac{1}{\underset{4}{\cancel{100}}} = \frac{1}{8}$$

$$\begin{array}{r} 0.125 \\ 8\overline{)1.000} \\ \underline{8} \\ 20 \\ \underline{16} \\ 40 \\ \underline{40} \end{array}$$

12½% = 0.125

Example 2: 3¾%

$$\frac{15}{4} \div \frac{100}{1} =$$

$$\frac{\overset{3}{\cancel{15}}}{4} \times \frac{1}{\underset{20}{\cancel{100}}} = \frac{3}{80}$$

$$\begin{array}{r} 0.0375 \\ 80\overline{)3.0000} \\ \underline{2\ 40} \\ 600 \\ \underline{560} \\ 400 \\ \underline{400} \end{array}$$

3¾% = 0.0375

Finding What Percent One Number Is of Another

1. Write the number following the word *of* as the denominator of a fraction.
2. Write the other number as the numerator of the fraction.
3. Divide the numerator by the denominator, extending the decimal fraction four places to the right of the decimal point.
4. Multiply by 100.
5. Add the % sign.

Example 1: What percent of 24 is 9?

$$\frac{9}{24} = \frac{3}{8}$$

```
   0.375
8)3.000
  2 4
    60
    56
     40
     40
```

$0.375 \times 100 = 37.5$

$37.5 + \%$ sign $= 37.5\%$

Example 2: What percent of 5.4 is 1.2?

```
                0.2222
1.2/5.4 = 5.4 )1.2 0000
               1 0 8
                 1 20
                 1 08
                   120
                   108
                    120
                    108
```

$0.2222 \times 100 = 22.22$

$22.22 + \%$ sign $= 22.22\%$

Example 3: What percent of 2 is ¼?

¼/2

$$\frac{1}{4} \div 2 =$$

$$\frac{1}{4} \div \frac{2}{1} =$$

$$\frac{1}{4} \times \frac{1}{2} = \frac{1}{8}$$

$$\frac{1}{\cancel{8}_{2}} \times \frac{\cancel{100}^{25}}{1} = \frac{25}{2} = 12.5$$

$12.5 + \%$ sign $= 12.5\%$

Example 4: What percent of 8.7 is 3½?

$$\frac{3\frac{1}{2}}{8.7} = \frac{3.5}{8.7}$$

```
        0.402
8.7 )3.5 000
      3 4 8
         20
         00
         200
         174
```

$0.402 \times 100 = 40.2$

$40.2 + \%$ sign $= 40.2\%$

Finding the Given Percent of a Number

1. Write the percent as a decimal number.
2. Multiply by the other number.

Example 1: What is 40% of 180?

$$\frac{40}{100} = 100\overline{)40.0}\quad 0.4$$

$$\begin{array}{r} 0.4 \\ 100\overline{)40.0} \\ \underline{40\ 0} \end{array}$$

$$\begin{array}{r} 180 \\ \times\ 0.4 \\ \hline 72.0 \end{array}$$

40% of 180 = 72

Example 2: What is 3⁄10% of 52?

$$\frac{\frac{3}{10}}{100} = \frac{3}{10} \div \frac{100}{1} =$$

$$\frac{3}{10} \times \frac{1}{100} = \frac{3}{1000}$$

$$\frac{3}{1000} = 0.003$$

$$\begin{array}{r} 0.003 \\ \times\quad 52 \\ \hline 0\ 006 \\ 00\ 15 \\ \hline 00.156 \end{array}$$

3⁄10% of 52 = 0.156

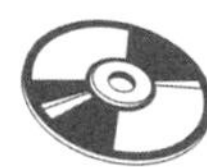

Refer to Mathematics Review: Percents on the CD for additional help and practice problems.

WORK SHEET

Directions: Change each of the following proper fractions to a percent.

1. $3/4$ _______
2. $3/8$ _______
3. $4/5$ _______
4. $8/25$ _______
5. $3/1000$ _______
6. $7/200$ _______
7. $9/400$ _______
8. $3/20$ _______
9. $9/150$ _______
10. $11/16$ _______
11. $5/6$ _______
12. $75/10{,}000$ _______

Directions: Change each of the following decimals to a percent.

1. 0.402 _______
2. 0.0367 _______
3. 0.163 _______
4. 0.98 _______
5. 0.3 _______
6. 0.145 _______
7. 0.7 _______
8. 0.42 _______
9. 0.159 _______
10. 0.673 _______
11. 0.3712 _______
12. 2.2 _______

Directions: Change each of the following percents to a mixed number or a proper fraction.

1. 3.5% ______ **2.** $\frac{3}{4}$% ______ **3.** 0.125% ______ **4.** 10% ______

5. $\frac{2}{3}$% ______ **6.** 20.2% ______ **7.** 12% ______ **8.** 0.25% ______

9. $2\frac{3}{8}$% ______ **10.** $6\frac{1}{4}$% ______ **11.** 2.1% ______ **12.** $66\frac{2}{3}$% ______

Directions: Change each of the following percents to a decimal.

1. 37.5% ______ **2.** 3% ______ **3.** $6\frac{3}{4}$% ______ **4.** 0.42% ______

5. $\frac{1}{4}$% ______ **6.** $2\frac{1}{2}$% ______ **7.** 0.23% ______ **8.** 72.6% ______

9. 16% ______ **10.** $\frac{5}{16}$% ______ **11.** $\frac{1}{2}$% ______ **12.** $\frac{7}{12}$% ______

Directions: What percent of

1. 40 is 22 ______ 2. 80 is 6.3 ______ 3. 200 is 4 ______ 4. 500 is 60 ______

5. 20 is 1 ______ 6. 24 is 3.6 ______ 7. 275 is 55 ______ 8. 1000 is 100 ______

9. 800 is 360 ______ 10. 25 is $\frac{1}{4}$ ______ 11. 250 is 5.2 ______ 12. 35 is 7 ______

Directions: What is

1. 25% of 478 ______ 2. 10% of 34 ______ 3. 2.8% of 510 ______

4. $\frac{1}{2}$% of 28 ______ 5. 33$\frac{1}{3}$% of 3000 ______ 6. $\frac{1}{5}$% of 65 ______

7. 2$\frac{1}{4}$% of 26 ______ 8. $\frac{3}{8}$% of 32 ______ 9. 62% of 871 ______

10. $\frac{1}{4}$% of 68 ______ 11. 41% of 27 ______ 12. 8.4% of 128 ______

Answers on p. 430.

Name ______________________

Date ______________________

ACCEPTABLE SCORE 27

YOUR SCORE ______

POSTTEST 1

Directions: Change the following fractions to percents.

1. $\frac{7}{8}$ ______
2. $\frac{11}{20}$ ______
3. $\frac{3}{1000}$ ______

Directions: Change the following decimals to percents.

4. 0.256 ______
5. 0.004 ______
6. 0.9 ______

Directions: Change the following percents to proper fractions.

7. 85% ______
8. 0.3% ______
9. $3\frac{1}{2}$% ______

Directions: Change the following percents to decimals.

10. 86.3% ______
11. $4\frac{5}{8}$% ______
12. 0.36% ______

Directions: What percent of

13. 70 is 7 ______
14. 24 is 1.2 ______
15. 300 is 1 ______

16. $66\frac{2}{3}$ is 8 ______

17. 3.5 is 1.5 ______

18. 2.5 is 0.5 ______

19. $\frac{3}{4}$ is $\frac{3}{8}$ ______

20. 160 is 12 ______

21. 250 is 20 ______

Directions: What is

22. 65% of 800 ______

23. 90% of 40 ______

24. $\frac{1}{8}$% of 72 ______

25. 8.5% of 2000 ______

26. $4\frac{1}{2}$% of 940 ______

27. 65% of 450 ______

28. $\frac{1}{4}$% of 60 ______

29. 4.3% of 56 ______

30. 0.52% of 88 ______

Answers on pp. 430-431.

Name ______________________________

Date ______________________________

ACCEPTABLE SCORE 36

YOUR SCORE ______

POSTTEST 2

Directions: Change the following fractions to percents.

1. $\frac{1}{8}$ ______ **2.** $\frac{2}{5}$ ______ **3.** $\frac{1}{6}$ ______

Directions: Change the following decimals to percents.

4. 0.065 ______ **5.** 0.005 ______ **6.** 0.2 ______

Directions: Change the following percents to proper fractions.

7. 0.3% ______ **8.** $16\frac{1}{2}$% ______ **9.** 0.25% ______

Directions: Change the following percents to decimals.

10. $3\frac{3}{4}$% ______ **11.** 7% ______ **12.** 5.55% ______

Directions: What percent of

13. 5.4 is 1.2 ______ **14.** $\frac{1}{4}$ is $\frac{1}{8}$ ______ **15.** 250 is 6 ______

16. 40 is 32 _______

17. 160 is 12 _______

18. 500 is 50 _______

19. 5¾ is 2⅜ _______

20. 120 is 15 _______

21. 9/16 is 5/7 _______

Directions: What is

22. 35% of 650 _______

23. ¼% of 116 _______

24. 4½% of 940 _______

25. 11% of 88 _______

26. 16% of 90 _______

27. 7.5% of 261 _______

28. 45% of 24.27 _______

29. ⅞% of 64 _______

30. 82.4% of 118 _______

Answers on p. 431.

Name ________________________________

Date ________________________________

ACCEPTABLE SCORE 27

YOUR SCORE ______

PRETEST

Complete the Ratios Pretest. A score of 27 out of 30 indicates an acceptable understanding and competency of basic calculations involving ratios. You may skip to the Proportions Pretest on p. 83. However, if you score 26 or below, completion of Chapter 4, Ratios, will be helpful for your continued success in the calculation of drug dosages.

Directions: Convert to equivalents.

	Ratio	Fraction	Decimal	Percent
1.	17 : 51			
2.			0.715	
3.		8/20		
4.				12 1/2%
5.	21 : 420			
6.		5/32		
7.			0.286	
8.				71 3/7%
9.				16 1/4%
10.			0.462	

Answers on p. 431.

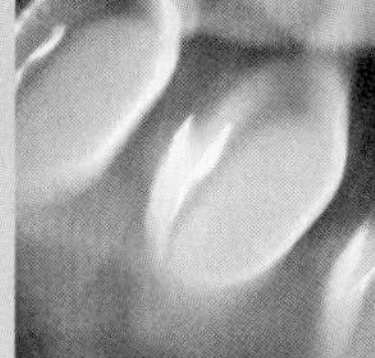

CHAPTER

4

Ratios

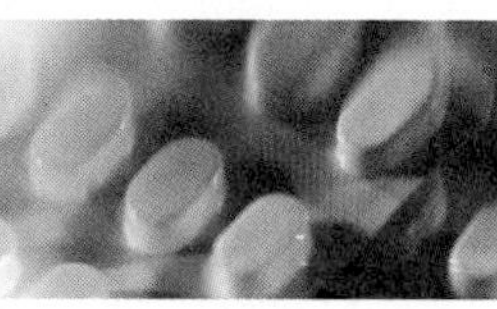

LEARNING OBJECTIVES

On the completion of the materials provided in this chapter, you will be able to perform computations by mastering the following mathematical concepts:

1. Changing a proper fraction, decimal fraction, and percent to a ratio reduced to lowest terms
2. Changing a ratio to a proper fraction, a decimal fraction, and a percent

Study the introductory material on ratios. The processes for the calculation of ratio problems are listed in steps. Memorize the steps for each calculation before beginning the work sheet. Review previous chapters on fractions, decimals, and percents as necessary. Complete the work sheet at the end of this chapter, which provides for extensive practice in the manipulation of ratios. Check your answers. If you have difficulties, go back and review the steps for that type of calculation. When you feel ready to evaluate your learning, take the first posttest. Check your answers. An acceptable score as indicated on the posttest signifies that you are ready for the next chapter. An unacceptable score signifies a need for further study before taking the second posttest.

A **ratio** is another way of indicating a relationship between two numbers. In other words, it is another way to express a fraction. A ratio indicates *division.*

Example 1: $\frac{3}{4}$ written as a ratio is 3 : 4
In reading a ratio the colon is read as "is to." The example would then be read as "three is to four."

Example 2: 7 written as a ratio is 7 : 1
To express any whole number as a ratio, the number following the colon is *always* 1. The example would be read as "seven is to one."

Changing a Proper Fraction to a Ratio Reduced to Lowest Terms

1. Reduce to lowest terms.
2. Write the numerator of the fraction as the first number of the ratio.
3. Place a colon after the first number.
4. Write the denominator of the fraction as the second number of the ratio.

Example 1: $\frac{4}{12}$

$\frac{4}{12}$ reduced to lowest terms equals $\frac{1}{3}$

$\frac{1}{3}$ written as a ratio would be 1 : 3

Example 2: $\frac{1}{1000}/\frac{1}{10}$

$$\frac{1}{1000} \div \frac{1}{10} =$$

$$\frac{1}{\cancelto{100}{1000}} \times \frac{\cancelto{1}{10}}{1} = \frac{1}{100}$$

$\frac{1}{1000}/\frac{1}{10}$ reduced to lowest terms equals $\frac{1}{100}$

$\frac{1}{100}$ written as a ratio would be 1 : 100

Changing a Decimal Fraction to a Ratio Reduced to Lowest Terms

1. Express the decimal fraction as a proper fraction reduced to lowest terms.
2. Write the numerator of the fraction as the first number of the ratio.
3. Place a colon after the first number.
4. Write the denominator of the fraction as the second number of the ratio.

Example 1: 0.85

$\frac{85}{100} = \frac{17}{20}$ (reduced to lowest terms)

$\frac{17}{20}$ written as a ratio would be 17 : 20

Example 2: 0.125

$\frac{125}{1000} = \frac{1}{8}$ (reduced to lowest terms)

$\frac{1}{8}$ written as a ratio would be 1 : 8

Changing a Percent to a Ratio Reduced to Lowest Terms

1. Express the percent as a proper fraction reduced to lowest terms.
2. Write the numerator of the fraction as the first number of the ratio.
3. Place a colon after the first number.
4. Write the denominator of the fraction as the second number of the ratio.

Example 1: 30%

$\frac{30}{100} = \frac{3}{10}$ (reduced to lowest terms)

$\frac{3}{10}$ written as a ratio would be 3 : 10

Example 2: ½%

$$\frac{\frac{1}{2}}{100} =$$

$$\frac{1}{2} \div \frac{100}{1} =$$

$$\frac{1}{2} \times \frac{1}{100} = \frac{1}{200}$$

$\frac{1}{200}$ written as a ratio would be 1 : 200

Example 3: 3⁹⁄₁₀%

$$\frac{3\frac{9}{10}}{100} =$$

$$\frac{39}{10} \div \frac{100}{1} =$$

$$\frac{39}{10} \times \frac{1}{100} = \frac{39}{1000}$$

$\frac{39}{1000}$ written as a ratio would be 39 : 1000

Changing a Ratio to a Proper Fraction Reduced to Lowest Terms

1. Write the first number of the ratio as a numerator.
2. Write the second number of the ratio as the denominator.
3. Reduce to lowest terms.

Example 1: 9 : 15

$\frac{9}{15} = \frac{3}{5}$ (reduced to lowest terms)

Example 2: 11 : 22

$\frac{11}{22} = \frac{1}{2}$ (reduced to lowest terms)

Changing a Ratio to a Decimal Fraction

Divide the first number of the ratio by the second number of the ratio, using long division.

Example 1: 4 : 5

$$\begin{array}{r} 0.8 \\ 5\overline{)4.0} \\ \underline{4\,0} \end{array}$$

4 : 5 written as a decimal is 0.8

Example 2: 3½ : 2¼

3.5 : 2.25

```
           1. 555
2.25^)3.50^ 000
      2 25
      1 25  0
      1 12  5
        12  50
        11  25
         1  250
         1  125
```

3½ : 2¼ written as a decimal is 1.555

Changing a Ratio to a Percent

1. Express the ratio as a proper fraction or a decimal fraction, whichever you prefer to work with.
2. Multiply by 100.
3. Add the percent sign (%).

Example 1: 3 : 5

Changing to a proper fraction:

$$\frac{3}{\cancel{5}_1} \times \frac{\cancel{100}^{20}}{1} = \frac{60}{1}$$

60 + % = 60%

Changing to a decimal fraction:

```
  0.6
5)3.0
  3 0
```

0.6 × 100 = 60

60 + % = 60%

Example 2: 60 : 180

Changing to a proper fraction:

$$\frac{60}{180} = \frac{1}{3}$$

$$\frac{1}{3} \times \frac{100}{1} = \frac{100}{3} = 33\tfrac{1}{3}$$

33⅓ + % = 33⅓%

Changing to a decimal fraction:

```
      0.333
180)60.000
     54 0
      6 00
      5 40
        600
        540
         600
         540
          60
```

0.333 × 100 = 33.3

33.3 + % = 33.3%

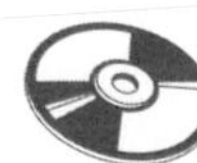

Refer to Mathematics Review: Ratios on the CD for additional help and practice problems.

WORK SHEET

Directions: Change the following fractions to ratios reduced to lowest terms.

1. $\frac{9}{12}$ _______
2. $\frac{4}{6}$ _______
3. $\frac{11}{22}$ _______
4. $\frac{56}{100}$ _______
5. $\frac{20}{50}$ _______
6. $\frac{310}{1000}$ _______
7. $\frac{10}{16}$ _______
8. $\frac{5}{6}/3\frac{1}{3}$ _______
9. $1\frac{3}{5}/2\frac{7}{10}$ _______
10. $\frac{1}{10}/\frac{1}{100}$ _______
11. $\frac{14}{30}/2$ _______
12. $3\frac{1}{3}/3\frac{1}{3}$ _______

Directions: Change the following decimal fractions to ratios reduced to lowest terms.

1. 0.896 _______
2. 0.96 _______
3. 0.06 _______
4. 0.6 _______
5. 0.4032 _______
6. 0.74 _______

7. 0.166 ______ 8. 0.26 ______ 9. 0.492 ______

10. 0.95 ______ 11. 0.235 ______ 12. 0.172 ______

Directions: Change the following percents to ratios reduced to lowest terms.

1. 10% ______ 2. $33\frac{1}{3}$% ______ 3. $\frac{3}{8}$% ______

4. $2\frac{7}{10}$% ______ 5. 44% ______ 6. 15.7% ______

7. $7\frac{3}{4}$% ______ 8. 0.44% ______ 9. 7.8% ______

10. 1% ______ 11. $\frac{3}{5}$% ______ 12. $3\frac{3}{7}$% ______

Directions: Change the following ratios to fractions reduced to lowest terms.

1. 4 : 64 _______ 2. 4 : 800 _______ 3. 3 : 150 _______

4. $\frac{3}{8} : \frac{1}{4}$ _______ 5. $\frac{8}{12} : \frac{2}{3}$ _______ 6. $2\frac{1}{2} : 7\frac{1}{2}$ _______

7. $\frac{4}{5} : \frac{1}{4}$ _______ 8. $\frac{1}{10} : \frac{4}{20}$ _______ 9. $\frac{4}{75} : \frac{3}{10}$ _______

10. 0.68 : 0.44 _______ 11. 1.85 : 3.35 _______ 12. 1.64 : 2.54 _______

Directions: Change the following ratios to decimal numbers.

1. 7 : 14 _______ 2. 5 : 20 _______ 3. 3 : 8 _______

4. 11 : 33 _______ 5. $\frac{5}{8} : \frac{1}{10}$ _______ 6. $\frac{1}{1000} : \frac{1}{500}$ _______

7. $\frac{3}{4} : \frac{1}{2}$ _______

8. $\frac{3}{1000} : \frac{3}{100}$ _______

9. 2 : 5 _______

10. $\frac{1}{2} : \frac{5}{9}$ _______

11. 7 : 259 _______

12. $1\frac{2}{5} : \frac{12}{30}$ _______

Directions: Change the following ratios to percents.

1. 2 : 4 _______

2. 7 : 231 _______

3. 25 : 250 _______

4. 30 : 150 _______

5. $1\frac{1}{4} : 3\frac{3}{8}$ _______

6. 1 : 1000 _______

7. 0.15 : 0.6 _______

8. $\frac{5}{16} : \frac{3}{5}$ _______

9. 1 : 500 _______

10. $1\frac{8}{12} : 2\frac{3}{6}$ _______

11. 2.5 : 4.5 _______

12. $4 : \frac{3}{16}$ _______

Answers on pp. 431-432.

Name ______________________

Date ______________________

ACCEPTABLE SCORE 27

YOUR SCORE ______

POSTTEST 1

Directions: Convert to equivalents.

	Ratio	Fraction	Decimal	Percent
1.	42 : 48			
2.			0.004	
3.		13/20		
4.				$2\frac{1}{4}\%$
5.			0.35	
6.		6/25		
7.	3/8 : 5/9			
8.				0.3%
9.			0.205	
10.		4/11		

Answers on p. 432.

Name ______________________

Date ______________________

ACCEPTABLE SCORE 27

YOUR SCORE ______

POSTTEST 2

Directions: Convert to equivalents.

	Ratio	Fraction	Decimal	Percent
1.	7 : 10			
2.		5/16		
3.			0.075	
4.				6%
5.				3/8%
6.		1/150		
7.			0.007	
8.	6 : 21			
9.			0.322	
10.				18.2%

Answers on p. 432.

Proportions

Name ______________________________

Date ______________________________

ACCEPTABLE SCORE 18

YOUR SCORE ______

PRETEST

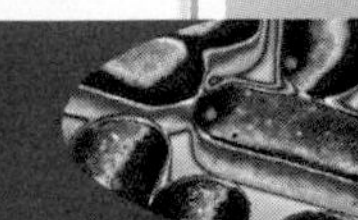

Complete the Proportions Pretest. A score of 18 out of 20 indicates an acceptable understanding and competency of basic calculations involving proportions. You may skip to the Mathematics Review Posttest on p. 97. However, if you score 17 or below, completion of Chapter 5, Proportions, will be helpful for your continued success in the calculation of drug dosages.

Directions: Find the value of x. Show your work.

1. $25 : 75 :: x : 300$ ______

2. $450 : 15 :: 225 : x$ ______

3. $x : \frac{1}{4}\% :: 8 : 12$ ______

4. $12 : 3 :: x : 0.8$ ______

5. $0.6 : 2.4 :: 32 : x$ ______

6. $150 : x :: 75 : 2$ ______

7. $\frac{1}{8} : \frac{2}{3} :: 75 : x$ ______

8. $\frac{1}{200} : 8 :: x : 800$ ______

9. $x : \frac{1}{2} :: \frac{3}{4} : \frac{7}{8}$ ______

10. $16 : x :: 24 : 12$ ______

11. $\frac{2}{3} : \frac{1}{5} :: x : 24$ ______

12. $x : 9 :: \frac{2}{3} : 36$ ______

13. $\frac{1}{7} : x :: \frac{1}{2} : 49$ ______

14. $0.8 : 4 :: 9.6 : x$ ______

15. $\frac{4}{5} : x :: \frac{2}{3} : \frac{1}{4}$ ______

16. 40 : 80 :: x : 160 _______ **17.** 2.5 : x :: 4 : 16 _______ **18.** 8 : 72 :: 14 : x _______

19. x : $\frac{1}{15}$ :: 50 : 500 _______ **20.** 5 : 100 :: x : 325 _______

Answers on p. 432.

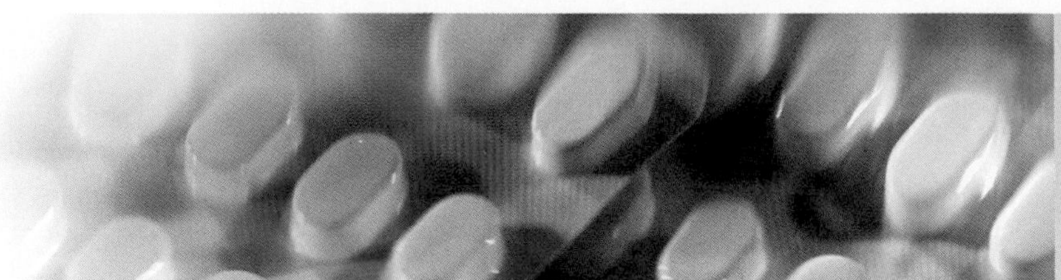

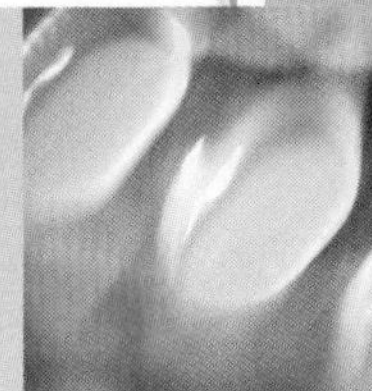

CHAPTER
5

Proportions

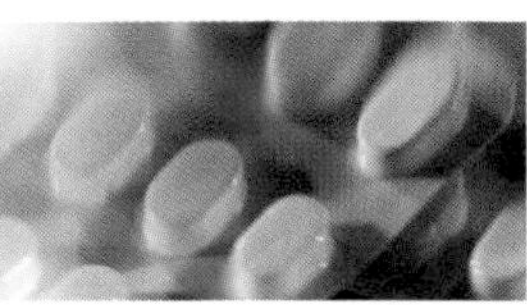

LEARNING OBJECTIVES

On completion of the materials provided in this chapter, you will be able to perform computations accurately by mastering the following mathematical concepts:

1. Solving simple proportion problems
2. Solving proportion problems involving fractions, decimals, and percents

Most problems concerning drug dosage can be solved by a proportion problem, whether it involves fractions, decimals, or percents. If a proportion problem contains any combination of fractions, decimals, or percents, all forms within the problem must be converted to either fractions or decimals.

Study the introductory material on proportions. The process for the calculation of proportion problems is listed in steps. Memorize the steps before beginning the work sheet. Complete the work sheet at the end of this chapter, which provides for extensive practice in the manipulation of proportions. Check your answers. If you have difficulties, go back and review the necessary steps. When you feel ready to evaluate your learning, take the first posttest. Check your answers. An acceptable score as indicated on the posttest signifies that you are ready for the next chapter. An unacceptable score signifies a need for further study before taking the second posttest.

A **proportion** consists of two ratios of equal value. The ratios are connected by a double colon (::) which symbolizes the word *as.*

$$2 : 3 :: 4 : 6$$

Read the above proportion : "Two is to three as four is to six."

The first and fourth terms of the proportion are the **extremes.** The second and third terms are the **means.**

$$2 : 3 :: 4 : 6$$

2 and 6 are the extremes
3 and 4 are the means

In a proportion the product of the means equals the product of the extremes because the ratios are of equal value. This principle may be used to verify your answer in a proportion problem.

$$3 \times 4 = 12, \text{ product of the means}$$
$$2 \times 6 = 12, \text{ product of the extremes}$$

If three terms in the proportions are known and one term is unknown, an *x* is inserted in the space for the unknown term.

$$2 : 3 :: 4 : x$$

SOLVING A SIMPLE PROPORTION PROBLEM

1. Multiply the means.
2. Multiply the extremes.
3. Place the product including the x on the *left* and the product of the known terms on the *right*.
4. Divide the product of the known terms by the number next to x. The quotient will be the value of x.

Proportion Problem Involving Whole Numbers

Example: $2 : 3 :: 4 : x$

$$2x = 3 \times 4$$
$$2x = 12$$
$$x = 12 \div 2$$
$$x = \frac{12}{2}$$
$$x = 6$$

Proportion Problem Involving Fractions

Example: $\frac{1}{150} : \frac{1}{100} :: x : 60$

$$\frac{1}{100}x = \frac{1}{150} \times 60$$
$$\frac{1}{100}x = \frac{2}{5}$$
$$x = \frac{2}{5} \div \frac{1}{100}$$
$$x = \frac{2}{\cancel{5}_{1}} \times \frac{\cancel{100}^{20}}{1}$$
$$x = 40$$

Proportion Problem Involving Decimals

Example: $0.4 : 0.8 :: 0.25 : x$

$0.4x = 0.8 \times 0.25$

$0.4x = 0.2$

$x = 0.2 \div 0.4$

$x = 0.5$

Proportion Problem Involving Fractions and Percents

Example: $x : \frac{1}{4}\% :: 9\frac{3}{5} : \frac{1}{200}$

Convert $\frac{1}{4}\%$ to a proper fraction and $9\frac{3}{5}$ to an improper fraction. Then rewrite the proportion using these fractions.

$$x : \frac{1}{400} :: \frac{48}{5} : \frac{1}{200}$$

$$\frac{1}{200}x = \frac{1}{400} \times \frac{48}{5}$$

$$\frac{1}{200}x = \frac{1}{\underset{25}{\cancel{400}}} \times \frac{\overset{3}{\cancel{48}}}{5}$$

$$\frac{1}{200}x = \frac{3}{125}$$

$$x = \frac{3}{125} \div \frac{1}{200}$$

$$x = \frac{3}{\underset{5}{\cancel{125}}} \times \frac{\overset{8}{\cancel{200}}}{1}$$

$$x = \frac{24}{5}$$

$$x = 4\frac{4}{5}$$

Proportion Problem Involving Decimals and Percents

Example: $0.3\% : 1.8 :: x : 14.4$

Convert 0.3% to a decimal

$0.003 : 1.8 = x : 14.4$

$1.8x = 0.003 \times 14.4$

$1.8x = 0.0432$

$x = 0.0432 \div 1.8$

$x = 0.024$

Proportion Problem Involving Numerous Zeros

Example: $250{,}000 : x :: 500{,}000 : 4$

$$500{,}000x = 250{,}000 \times 4$$

$$500{,}000x = 1{,}000{,}000$$

$$x = 1{,}000{,}000 \div 500{,}000$$

$$x = \frac{1{,}000{,}000}{500{,}000}$$

$$x = 2$$

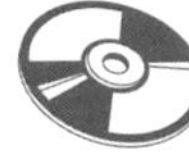

Refer to Mathematics Review: Proportions on the CD for additional help and practice problems.

WORK SHEET

Directions: Find the value of x. Show your work.

1. $20 : 400 :: x : 1680$ _______

2. $0.9 : 2.4 :: x : 75$ _______

3. $\frac{5}{6} : x :: \frac{5}{9} : \frac{4}{5}$ _______

4. $3 : 90 :: 1\frac{3}{4} : x$ _______

5. $75 : x :: 100 : 2$ _______

6. $\frac{1}{6} : 1 :: \frac{1}{8} : x$ _______

7. $200{,}000 : x :: 1{,}000{,}000 : 5$ _______

8. $x : \frac{3}{4}\% :: 3\frac{1}{5} : \frac{1}{200}$ _______

9. $\frac{1}{150} : 1 :: \frac{1}{100} : x$ _______

10. $3 : 150 :: 40 : x$ _______

11. $\frac{1}{8} : x :: 7 : 56$ _______

12. $\frac{1}{200} : 40 :: \frac{1}{100} : x$ _______

13. $12\frac{1}{2} : x :: 50 : 2400$ _______

14. $\frac{1}{2}\% : \frac{1}{100} :: x : 80$ _______

15. $x : 6.4 :: 0.03 : 6$ _______

16. $0.25 : 1 :: 0.05 : x$ _______

17. $\frac{1}{120} : 2 :: 4 : x$ _______

18. $x : \frac{1}{1000} :: 5 : \frac{1}{5000}$ _______

19. $6 : 15 :: 8 : x$ _______

20. $x : 3 :: 9 : 54$ _______

21. $1.4 : 0.4 :: 4.2 : x$ _______

22. $x : 0.65 :: 9 : 5$ _______

23. $12\frac{1}{2}\% : 5 :: x : 120$ _______

24. $\frac{1}{300} : 6 :: \frac{1}{120} : x$ _______

25. $25 : 75 :: 16 : x$ _______

26. $0.3 : x :: 7 : 21$ _______

27. $4 : x :: 12 : 48$ _______

28. $x : 12 :: 2 : 4$ _______

29. $\frac{4}{5} : x :: \frac{1}{3} : \frac{5}{9}$ _______

30. $0.6 : x :: 7 : 42$ _______

31. $15 : x :: 20 : 600$ _______

32. $9\% : x :: 11 : 73$ _______

33. $500{,}000 : 1 :: 300{,}000 : x$ _______

34. $\frac{1}{6} : \frac{9}{10} :: \frac{1}{2} : x$ _______

35. 2.8 : 12 :: 40 : x _______

36. 8 : 8⁄100 :: x : 5 _______

37. 1⁄8% : 1⁄200 :: x : 40 _______

38. x : 25 :: 18 : 36 _______

39. 0.15 : 0.25 :: x : 400 _______

40. 1⁄20 : 1⁄15 :: x : 25 _______

41. 800,000 : 5 :: 960,000 : x _______

42. 27 : x :: 9 : 60 _______

43. 1⁄20 : 1⁄5 :: x : 50 _______

44. 1⁄150 : 1⁄200 :: x : 60 _______

45. 1⁄2% : 4 :: x : 25 _______

46. 500 : 2.5 :: x : 8.1 _______

Answers on p. 433.

Name ________________

Date ________________

ACCEPTABLE SCORE 18

YOUR SCORE ______

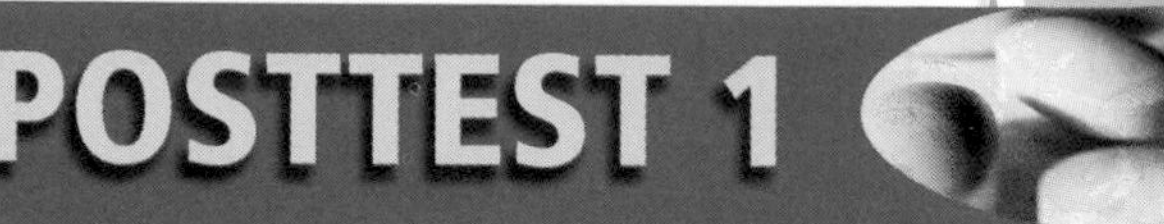

Directions: Find the value of x. Show your work.

1. $x : 2.5 :: 4 : 5$ ______
2. $7/8 : x :: 4/5 : 2/3$ ______
3. $30 : 90 :: 2 : x$ ______
4. $x : 3.5 :: 25 : 14$ ______
5. $2/7 : 1/2 :: x : 56$ ______
6. $1/4 : x :: 160 : 320$ ______
7. $x : 7 :: 5 : 14$ ______
8. $3 : x :: 18 : 12$ ______
9. $1/5 : 90 :: x : 250$ ______
10. $1.8 : 4.8 :: x : 96$ ______
11. $x : 8 :: 10 : 20$ ______
12. $2/3 : x :: 4.5 : 27$ ______
13. $1/150 : x :: 1/200 : 6$ ______
14. $2/3\% : 1/5 :: 50 : x$ ______
15. $14 : x :: 6 : 18$ ______

16. $x : \frac{2}{3} :: 12 : 18$ _______ **17.** $50 : 250 :: \frac{4}{5} : x$ _______ **18.** $50 : 3 :: x : 6$ _______

19. $\frac{1}{2} : x :: 40 : 80$ _______ **20.** $0.8 : 10 :: x : 40$ _______

Answers on p. 433.

Name ______________________________

Date ______________________________

ACCEPTABLE SCORE 18

YOUR SCORE ______

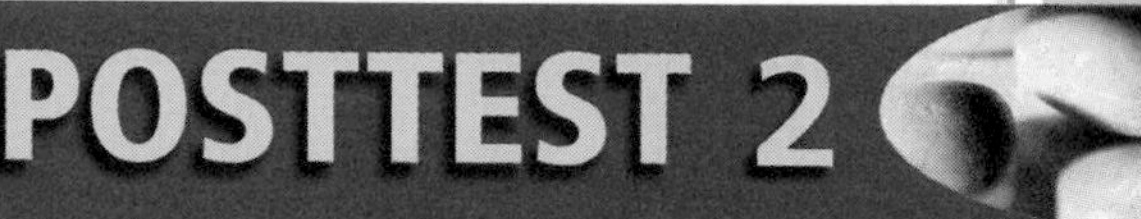

Directions: Find the value of x. Show your work.

1. $x : 300 :: 9 : 12$ ______

2. $4 : 32\% :: 16 : x$ ______

3. $18 : x :: 6 : 40$ ______

4. $1.8 : 2.5 :: x : 9.5$ ______

5. $x : 30 :: \frac{1}{3} : \frac{3}{4}$ ______

6. $\frac{7}{8} : x :: \frac{5}{8} : 40$ ______

7. $400 : 500 :: \frac{4}{5} : x$ ______

8. $x : 7.6 :: 3 : 6$ ______

9. $\frac{1}{4} : x :: \frac{2}{3} : \frac{2}{5}$ ______

10. $\frac{1}{150} : \frac{1}{100} :: x : 60$ ______

11. $0.6 : x :: 15 : 90$ ______

12. $3.5 : 12 :: x : 360$ ______

13. $\frac{2}{9} : \frac{4}{5} :: \frac{3}{4} : x$ ______

14. $\frac{1}{8} : x :: \frac{1}{7} : \frac{5}{9}$ ______

15. $x : 2.5 :: 16 : 4$ ______

16. $0.6 : 3 :: 72 : x$ _______ **17.** $20 : x :: 6 : 4.5$ _______ **18.** $x : \frac{1}{4} :: 96 : \frac{1}{3}$ _______

19. $300 : 5000 :: x : 18$ _______ **20.** $\frac{1}{3} : x :: \frac{1}{5} : 90$ _______

Answers on p. 433.

Name ______________________

Date ______________________

ACCEPTABLE SCORE ___90___

YOUR SCORE ______

POSTTEST

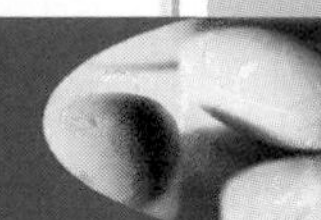

After your successful completion of Chapters 1 through 5, complete the Review of Mathematics Posttest. A score of 90 out of 100 indicates an acceptable understanding and competency of basic mathematics. You are now ready to begin Part II, Units and Measurements for the Calculation of Drug Dosages. However, if you score 89 or below, an additional review of previous chapter content may be helpful before beginning Part II.

Directions: Complete the following definitions and exercises.

1. *Improper fractions* can be reduced to a __________ number or a __________ number.

2. In the following fractions, circle only those that are *improper fractions.*

4/12 7/6 6/3 4/7 9/9 14/21

3. A *complex fraction* contains a __________ in its numerator, its denominator, or both.

4. In the following examples, circle only the *complex fractions.*

1 2/3 1/2/4 12/4 3/7/4/2 21 9/6 21/2/3

5-6. A *ratio* is the __________ between __________ numbers.

Write each of the following numbers as a *ratio.*

7. 4/12 __________

8. 24% __________

9. 0.03 __________

10. 13/8 __________

11. 2.2% __________

12. 1.24 __________

13. The *divisor* of a fraction is known as the __________ .

Division problems can be expressed in different ways. Circle the *divisor* in each of the following examples.

14. 2/3 **15.** 4 ÷ 8 **16.** 10 : 5 **17.** 4)12 **18.** 14/8 **19.** 6 ÷ 24 **20.** 42)7 **21.** 7 : 10

22-24. The number shown in a decimal is the __________ of a fraction. The denominator of this fraction is implied by the number of decimal places shown and is ______ or some power of ______.

Write the fraction values for the following *decimal fraction* numbers.

25. 0.436 ______ **26.** 0.051 ______ **27.** 1.0042 ______

28. 0.9684 ______ **29.** 0.0019 ______ **30.** 1.02064 ______

Directions: Add and reduce fractions to lowest terms.

31. $\frac{5}{9} + \frac{2}{5} + \frac{2}{3} =$ ______

32. $4\frac{1}{4} + 2\frac{5}{6} =$ ______

33. $5\frac{1}{2} + \frac{3}{9} =$ ______

34. $\frac{3}{4}/\frac{5}{6} + 4\frac{3}{5} =$ ______

Directions: Add and round answers to hundredths.

35. $4.02 + 3.4 + 1.099 =$ ______

36. $45.009 + 0.076 + 1.2 =$ ______

37. $0.0082 + 0.923 + 234 =$ ______

38. $456 + 3.56 + 0.0029 =$ ______

Directions: Subtract and reduce fractions to lowest terms.

39. $\frac{2}{4} - \frac{3}{9} =$ ______

40. $\frac{4}{7}/\frac{2}{8} - \frac{2}{3} =$ ______

41. $3\frac{4}{5} - 2\frac{8}{9} =$ ______

42. $6\frac{1}{2} - \frac{8}{9} =$ ______

Directions: Subtract and round answers to tenths.

43. $23.98 - 0.0987 =$ ______

44. $23.191 - 23.099 =$ ______

45. $9.002 - 4.9089 =$ ______

46. $2.009 - 0.9834 =$ ______

Directions: Multiply and reduce fractions to lowest terms.

47. $9 \times \frac{5}{8} =$ _______

48. $\frac{3}{4} \times \frac{8}{9} =$ _______

49. $4\frac{8}{9} \times 1\frac{5}{6} =$ _______

50. $3\frac{4}{5} \times 7 =$ _______

Directions: Multiply and round answers to hundredths.

51. $3.45 \times 0.56 =$ _______

52. $21.4 \times 0.092 =$ _______

53. $0.0452 \times 99.1 =$ _______

54. $739 \times 0.246 =$ _______

Directions: Divide and reduce fractions to lowest terms.

55. $\frac{7}{8} \div \frac{4}{9} =$ _______

56. $\frac{2}{5} \div \frac{7}{9} =$ _______

57. $\frac{1}{300} \div \frac{3}{4} =$ _______

58. $4\frac{7}{9} \div 5\frac{9}{11} =$ _______

Directions: Divide and round answers to thousandths.

59. $52.014 \div 9.2 =$ _______

60. $0.0982 \div 75 =$ _______

61. $3200 \div 0.04 =$ _______

62. $78.09 \div 4.501 =$ _______

Directions: Number the following decimal numbers in order from *lesser to greater value.*

63. 0.45 _______ 1.46 _______ 0.407 _______ 2.401 _______ 0.048 _______ 0.014 _______

64. 0.15 _______ 0.015 _______ 1.015 _______ 1.15 _______ 0.155 _______ 1.0015 _______

65. 9.09 _______ 0.99 _______ 0.090 _______ 0.90 _______ 90.90 _______ 9.009 _______

66. 0.6 _______ 0.4 _______ 0.7 _______ 0.52 _______ 0.44 _______ 0.24 _______

67. 0.21 _______ 0.191 _______ 0.021 _______ 0.1091 _______ 0.201 _______ 0.2 _______

Directions: Change the following fractions to decimals and round the answers to hundredths.

68. $\frac{5}{6}$ _______

69. $\frac{5}{9}$ _______

70. $\frac{9}{16}$ _______

71. $\frac{1}{150}$ _______

Directions: Change the following decimals to fractions and reduce to lowest terms.

72. 0.225 _______

73. 0.465 _______

74. 0.06 _______

75. 0.372 _______

Directions: Make the following calculations.

76. Express 0.275 as a percent. _______

77. Express $\frac{3}{8}$ as a percent. _______

78. Express 42% as a proper fraction and reduce to lowest terms. _______

79. Express 0.62% as a ratio. _______

80. What percent of 3.2 is 0.4? _______

81. What percent of $\frac{5}{7}$ is $\frac{5}{28}$? _______

82. What percent of 240 is 36? _______

83. What is $\frac{1}{2}$% of 48? _______

84. What is $6\frac{1}{2}$% of 840? _______

85. What is 46% of 325? _______

Directions: Change the following fractions and decimals to ratios reduced to lowest terms.

86. $\frac{10}{45}$ _______

87. $1\frac{3}{4}/4\frac{2}{3}$ _______

88. 0.584 _______

89. $\frac{250}{375}$ _______

90. 0.48 _______

Directions: Find the value of x and round decimal answers to hundredths.

91. $8 : \frac{4}{45} :: x : 3$ _______

92. $x : 34 :: 4 : 81$ _______

93. $4.6 : 3 :: 20 : x$ _______

94. $x : \frac{1}{2}\% :: 4.5 : \frac{1}{50}$ _______

95. $\frac{1}{300} : \frac{1}{150} :: x : 300$ _______

96. $22 : x :: 4 : 88$ _______

97. $0.35 : 0.75 :: x : 425$ _______

98. $400 : x :: \frac{1}{300} : \frac{1}{225}$ _______

99. $x : 54 :: 4 : 8$ _______

100. $\frac{1}{2}/\frac{3}{4} : 8 :: x : 45$ _______

Answers on pp. 433-434.

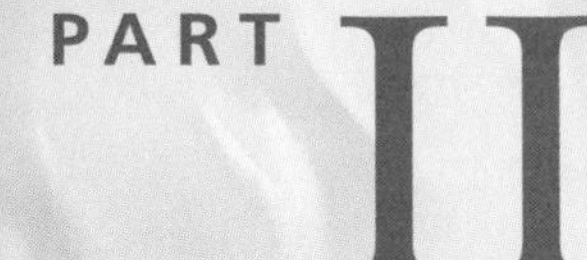

Units and Measurements for the Calculation of Drug Dosages

CHAPTERS

Part II is designed in the same way as Part I, Review of Mathematics. After completing Part I, you have validated that you do have the basic mathematical skills required to progress with Part II. A pretest precedes each of the three chapters in Part II. For some of you who have had experience in nursing and the administration of medications (such as an LPN, LVN, or ADN), these pretests will allow you to assess your need for a more extensive review of the material. After completion of the test, check your answers with the key provided. A score of 90% correct as indicated on each test indicates a mastery of the material covered in that chapter. You may then skip to the next pretest and follow the same exercises until Part II has been completed.

For those of you who have *not* had experience in nursing and the administration of medications, the following chapters of Part II should be worked as written *without utilizing the pretests preceding Chapters 6, 7, and 8.*

You are now ready to follow the path that matches your experience to complete the mastery of the following three chapters. Begin now, and good luck!

Metric and Household Measurements

Name ____________________

Date ____________________

ACCEPTABLE SCORE 27

YOUR SCORE ______

PRETEST

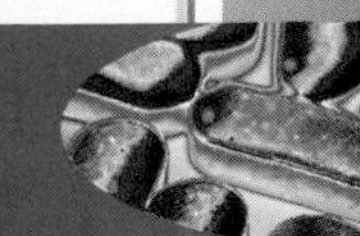

Directions: Change to equivalent metric measurements. Solve each problem by using a proportion. Show your work.

1. 800,000 mcg = ______ g

2. 3 mg = ______ mcg

3. 255 mg = ______ g

4. 46 mg = ______ mcg

5. 3000 mcg = ______ mg

6. 0.68 g = ______ mg

7. 326 mL = ______ L

8. 33 kg = ______ lb

9. 2.1 g = ______ mg

10. 3000 g = ______ kg

11. 0.1 L = ______ mL

12. 53 kg = ______ lb

13. 5 mL = ______ cc

14. 0.8 kg = ______ g

15. 250 mcg = ______ mg

16. 1¼ glass = _______ mL

17. 22 lb = _______ g

18. 0.63 L = _______ mL

19. 733 g = _______ kg

20. 1.25 g = _______ mcg

21. 60 mg = _______ g

22. 0.25 mg = _______ mcg

23. 0.25 L = _______ mL

24. 45 lb = _______ kg

25. 10,000 mcg = _______ g

26. 1.2 kg = _______ g

27. 1⅔ c = _______ mL

28. 0.71 g = _______ mg

29. 480 mL = _______ L

30. 650 g = _______ lb

Answers on p. 434.

CHAPTER 6

Metric and Household Measurements

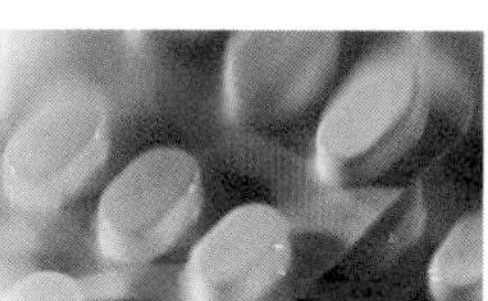

LEARNING OBJECTIVES

On completion of the materials provided in this chapter, you will be able to perform computations accurately by mastering the following mathematical concepts:

1. Recalling the metric measures of weight, volume, and length
2. Computing equivalents within the metric system by using a proportion
3. Recalling approximate equivalents between metric and household measures
4. Computing equivalents between the metric and household systems of measure by using a proportion

METRIC MEASUREMENTS

The metric system has become the system of choice for dealing with the weights and measures involved in the calculation of drug dosages. This is a result of its accuracy and simplicity because it is based on the decimal system. The use of decimals tends to eliminate errors made when working with fractions. Therefore all answers within the metric system need to be expressed as decimals, not as fractions.

Examples: 0.5, not ½
0.75, not ¾
0.007, not 7/1000

Certain prefixes identify the multiples of 10 that are being used. The four most commonly used prefixes of the metric system involved with the calculation of drug dosages are the following:

micro = 0.000001 or one millionth

milli = 0.001 or one thousandth

centi = 0.01 or one hundredth

kilo = 1000 or one thousand

These prefixes may be used with any of the base units of weight (gram), volume (liter), or length (meter). The nurse most often uses the following list of metric measures (Box 6-1). Memorize all the entries in the list.

BOX 6-1 ■ COMMON METRIC MEASURES

Metric Measure of Weight

1,000,000 micrograms (mcg) = 1 gram (g)
1000 micrograms (mcg) = 1 milligram (mg)
1000 milligrams (mg) = 1 gram (g)
1000 grams (g) = 1 kilogram (kg)

Metric Measure of Volume

1000 milliliters (mL) = 1 liter (L)
1 cubic centimeter (cc) = 1 milliliter (mL)*

Metric Measure of Length

1 meter (m) = 1000 mm or 100 cm
1 centimeter (cm) = 10 mm or 0.01 m
1 millimeter (mm) = 0.1 cm or 0.001 m

*The abbreviations cc and mL are used interchangeably. However, in this book, mL is used exclusively. Milliliter (mL) should be used only for liquids, whereas cubic centimeter (cc) should be used only for solids and gases.

Sometimes, to compute drug dosages, the nurse must convert a metric measure to an equivalent measure within the system. This may be done easily by using a proportion.

Example: 300 mg equals how many grams?

a. On the left side of the proportion, place what you know to be an equivalent between milligrams and grams. From the preceding chart we know that there are 1000 mg in 1 g. Therefore the left side of the proportion would be

1000 mg : 1 g ::

b. The right side of the proportion is determined by the problem and by the abbreviations used on the left side of the proportion. Only *two* different abbreviations may be used in a single proportion. The abbreviations must also be in the same position on the right as they are on the left.

1000 mg : 1 g :: ______ mg : ______ g

From the problem we know we have 300 mg

1000 mg : 1 g :: 300 mg : ______ g

We need to find the number of grams 300 mg equals, so we use the symbol x to represent the unknown. Therefore the full proportion would be

$$1000 \text{ mg} : 1 \text{ g} :: 300 \text{ mg} : x \text{ g}$$

c. Rewrite the proportion without using the abbreviations.

$$1000 : 1 :: 300 : x$$

d. Solve for x by multiplying the means and extremes. Write the answer as a decimal, since the metric system is based on decimals.

$$1000 : 1 :: 300 : x$$

$$1000x = 300$$

$$x = \frac{300}{1000}$$

$$x = 0.3$$

e. Label your answer, as determined by the abbreviation placed next to x in the original proportion.

$$300 \text{ mg} = 0.3 \text{ g}$$

Example 1: 2.5 L equals how many milliliters?

a. 1000 mL : 1 L ::
b. 1000 mL : 1 L :: _______ mL : _______ L
   1000 mL : 1 L :: x mL : 2.5 L
c. 1000 : 1 :: x : 2.5
d. $1x = 2500$
   $x = 2500$
e. 2.5 L equals 2500 mL

Example 2: 180 mcg equals how many grams?

a. 1,000,000 mcg : 1 g ::
b. 1,000,000 mcg : 1 g :: _______ mcg : _______ g
   1,000,000 mcg : 1 g :: 180 mcg : x g
c. 1,000,000 : 1 :: 180 : x
d. $1{,}000{,}000x = 180$
   $x = \frac{180}{1{,}000{,}000}$
   $x = 0.00018$
e. 180 mcg equals 0.00018 g

Example 3: 15 mm equals how many centimeters?

a. 1 cm : 10 mm
b. 1 cm : 10 mm :: _______ cm : _______ mm
   1 cm : 10 mm :: x cm : 15 mm
c. 1 : 10 :: x : 15
d. $10x = 1 \times 15$
   $10x = 15$
   $x = \frac{15}{10}$
   $x = 1.5$
e. 15 mm equals 1.5 cm

HOUSEHOLD MEASUREMENTS

Household measures are not accurate enough for the nurse to use in the calculation of drug dosages in the hospital. However, their metric equivalents are used in keeping a written record of a patient's "I" and "O," or intake and output. Always use your institution's conversions when documenting intake. For example, one cup of coffee at one institution may be 250 mL and at another institution, it may be 300 mL. The sample equivalents for a cup and glass allow the student to practice calculating these types of conversions.

Memorize the following list of approximate equivalents between metric and household measurements (Box 6-2).

BOX 6-2 ■ METRIC HOUSEHOLD EQUIVALENTS

Metric Measure	=	*Household Measure*
1 milliliter (mL)	=	15 drops (gtt)
5 milliliters	=	1 teaspoon (tsp)
15 milliliters	=	1 tablespoon (Tbsp)
180 milliliters	=	1 cup (c)
240 milliliters	=	1 glass
1 kilogram (kg) or 1000 grams (g)	=	2.2 pounds (lb)
2.5 cm	=	1 inch
1 foot	=	12 inches

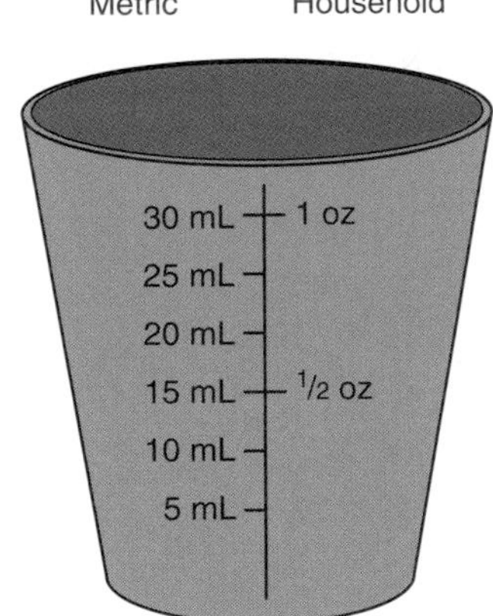

Conversion of measures between the metric and household systems of measure may also be done by using a proportion, as has been illustrated.

Example 1: 1½ c equals how many milliliters?

a. 1 c : 180 mL ::

b. 1 c : 180 mL :: ______ c : ______ mL

1 c : 180 mL :: 1½ c : x mL

c. 1 : 180 :: 1½ : x

d. $x = \dfrac{180}{1} \times \dfrac{3}{2}$

$x = \dfrac{540}{2} = 270$ mL

e. 1½ c equals 270 mL

Example 2: 35 kg equals how many pounds?

a. 1 kg : 2.2 lb ::
b. 1 kg : 2.2 lb :: _______ kg : _______ lb
   1 kg : 2.2 lb :: 35 kg : x lb
c. 1 : 2.2 :: 35 : x
d. $1x = 2.2 \times 35$
   $x = 77$
e. 35 kg equals 77 lb

Example 3: 18 inches equals how many centimeters?

a. 2.5 cm : 1 inch ::
b. 2.5 cm : 1 inch :: _______ cm : _______ inch
   2.5 cm : 1 inch :: _______ cm : 18 inches
c. 2.5 : 1 :: x : 18
d. $x = 2.5 \times 18$
   $x = 45$ cm
e. 18 inches equals 45 cm

Memorize the tables of metric and household measurements. Study the material on forming proportions for the calculation of problems relating to the metric and household systems of measure. Complete the following work sheet, which provides for extensive practice in the manipulation of measurements within the metric and household systems. Check your answers. If you have difficulties, go back and review the necessary material. When you feel ready to evaluate your learning, take the first posttest. Check your answers. An acceptable score as indicated on the posttest signifies that you are ready for the next chapter. An unacceptable score signifies a need for further study before taking the second posttest.

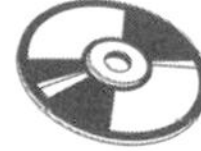

Refer to Introducing Drug Measures: Systems of Measurement on the CD for additional help and practice problems.

CHAPTER 6 Metric and Household Measurements

WORK SHEET

Directions: Change to equivalents within the metric system. Solve the problems by using a proportion. Show your work.

1. 230 mcg = _______ g

2. 5 mg = _______ mcg

3. 2.5 g = _______ mcg

4. 4000 mcg = _______ mg

5. 0.33 g = _______ mg

6. 6 kg = _______ g

7. 725 mL = _______ L

8. 2000 mcg = _______ g

9. 3 cm = _______ mm

10. 620 g = _______ kg

11. 36 cc = _______ mL

12. 460 mL = _______ L

13. 0.66 mg = _______ mcg

14. 0.5 g = _______ mcg

15. 18 inches = _______ feet

16. 350,000 mcg = _______ g

17. 25 mg = _______ g

18. 1.46 L = _______ mL

19. 2.5 kg = _______ g

20. 12 mg = _______ mcg

21. 3.4 kg = _______ g

22. 920 mcg = _______ g

23. 25 mm = _______ cm

24. 300 mcg = _______ mg

25. 0.16 L = _______ mL

26. 0.01 g = _______ mg

27. 500 mcg = _______ mg

28. 360 mg = _______ g

29. 1.7 L = _______ mL

30. 0.45 g = _______ mg

31. 240 mL = _______ L

32. 10 cc = _______ mL

Directions: Change the following household measurements into the approximate equivalents within the metric system. Solve the problems by using a proportion. Show your work.

33. 3 inches = _______ cm

34. $2\frac{1}{4}$ c = _______ mL

35. $1\frac{1}{3}$ glass = _______ mL

36. $\frac{2}{3}$ glass = _______ mL

37. $1\frac{1}{2}$ c = _______ mL

38. 8 kg = _______ lb

39. 3825 g = _______ lb

40. 7 inches = _______ cm

41. 3 lb = _______ kg

42. 12 kg = _______ lb

43. 1400 g = _______ lb

44. $2\frac{1}{2}$ feet = _______ inches

45. 150 lb = _______ kg

Answers on p. 434.

CHAPTER 6 **Metric and Household Measurements**

Name ______________________________

Date ______________________________

ACCEPTABLE SCORE 27

YOUR SCORE ______

POSTTEST 1

Directions: Change to equivalent metric measurements. Solve each problem by using a proportion. Show your work.

1. 5000 mcg = ______ g

2. 10 mg = ______ mcg

3. 0.81 L = ______ mL

4. 35 mg = ______ g

5. 2½ feet = ______ inches

6. 0.12 g = ______ mcg

7. 16 kg = ______ lb

8. 280 mL = ______ L

9. 0.4 kg = ______ g

10. 42 inches = ______ feet

11. 28 lb = ______ g

12. 4 inches = ______ cm

13. 500,000 mcg = _______ g

14. 37 mL = _______ L

15. 20 mL = _______ cc

16. $1\frac{1}{5}$ c = _______ mL

17. 2.5 g = _______ mg

18. 12 cc = _______ mL

19. 6700 g = _______ kg

20. 0.3 L = _______ mL

21. 4 mg = _______ mcg

22. 2600 g = _______ lb

23. $1\frac{1}{2}$ glass = _______ mL

24. 0.2 L = _______ mL

25. 533 mL = _______ L

26. 1.5 g = _______ mcg

27. 620 mg = _______ g

28. 2.3 kg = _______ g

29. 15 inches = _______ feet

30. 7 lb = _______ kg

Answers on p. 435.

CHAPTER 6 **Metric and Household Measurements**

Name ____________________

Date ____________________

ACCEPTABLE SCORE 27

YOUR SCORE ______

POSTTEST 2

Directions: Change to equivalent metric measurements. Solve each problem by using a proportion. Show your work.

1. 4000 mcg = ______ mg

2. 150 g = ______ kg

3. 2½ c = ______ mL

4. 800 g = ______ lb

5. 44 kg = ______ lb

6. 760 mg = ______ g

7. 0.55 L = ______ mL

8. 35 mm = ______ cm

9. ⅓ glass = ______ mL

10. 2⅛ lb = ______ g

11. 0.1 L = ______ mL

12. 32 mg = ______ mcg

13. 618 mL = ______ L

14. 100,000 mcg = ______ g

15. 28 inches = ______ feet

16. 714 mL = _______ L

17. 350 mg = _______ g

18. 250,000 mcg = _______ g

19. 0.87 g = _______ mg

20. 7 mg = _______ mcg

21. 37 mcg = _______ mg

22. 1.4 L = _______ mL

23. 0.78 g = _______ mg

24. 225 mcg = _______ mg

25. 4500 g = _______ kg

26. 0.2 L = _______ mL

27. $3\frac{1}{3}$ feet = _______ inches

28. 40 cc = _______ mL

29. 2.6 g = _______ mcg

30. 73 lb = _______ kg

Answers on p. 435.

Apothecary and Household Measurements

PRETEST

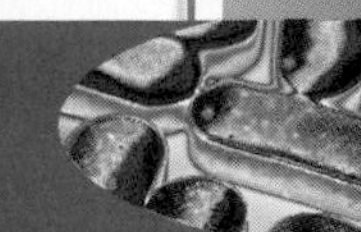

Name ______________________

Date ______________________

ACCEPTABLE SCORE 9

YOUR SCORE ______

Directions: Change to equivalents within the apothecary system. Solve by using proportions. Show your work.

1-2. 20 fl oz = ______ pt = ______ qt

3-4. 5 pt = ______ fl oz = ______ qt

5-6. 7 qt = ______ gal = ______ pt

Directions: Change the following household measurements into approximate equivalents within the apothecary system. Solve the problems by using proportions. Show your work.

7. 3 medium size glasses = ______ fl oz

8. 4 coffee c = ______ pt

9. 1½ medium size glasses = ______ fl oz

10. 2½ coffee c = ______ fl oz

Answers on p. 435.

CHAPTER

7

Apothecary and Household Measurements

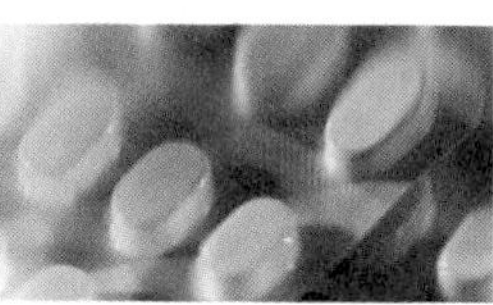

LEARNING OBJECTIVES

On completion of the materials provided in this chapter, you will be able to perform computations accurately by mastering the following mathematical concepts:

1. Adding and subtracting Roman numerals
2. Converting Roman numerals to Arabic numerals
3. Converting Arabic numerals to Roman numerals
4. Recalling the apothecary measures of weights and liquids
5. Computing equivalents within the apothecary system by using a proportion
6. Recalling approximate equivalents between apothecary and household measures
7. Computing equivalents between the apothecary and household measurement systems by the use of a proportion

The apothecary system of measure is a very old English system. It has slowly been replaced by the metric system. When writing orders in the apothecary system, physicians often use Roman numerals. All parts of a whole are expressed as a fraction except the fraction one half, which is commonly represented as $\overline{ss}$ or ss.

On the next page is a list of the more commonly used Roman numerals and their Arabic equivalents. Memorize the list.

Roman numeral	Arabic numeral
i	1
v	5
x	10
l	50
c	100

Only addition and subtraction may be performed in the Roman numeral system.

Addition of Roman Numerals

1. Addition is performed when a smaller numeral follows a larger numeral.

Examples: xi = 11 xv = 15 li = 51

2. Addition is performed when a numeral is repeated. However, a numeral is *never* repeated more than three times.

Examples: viii = 8 xii = 12 ccxi = 211

Subtraction of Roman Numerals

1. Subtraction is performed when a smaller numeral is placed before a larger numeral.

Examples: ix = 9 iv = 4 ic = 99

2. Subtraction is performed when a smaller numeral is placed between two larger numerals. The smaller numeral is subtracted from the larger numeral following the smaller numeral.

Examples: xiv = 14 xxiv = 24 cxc = 190

Apothecary Measurements

It is still important for a nurse to be knowledgeable about the apothecary system. Some of the older medications are still ordered with the apothecary unit of measure.

Example: aspirin gr x*

Some pharmaceutical companies label a drug using both the apothecary system and the metric system of measure.

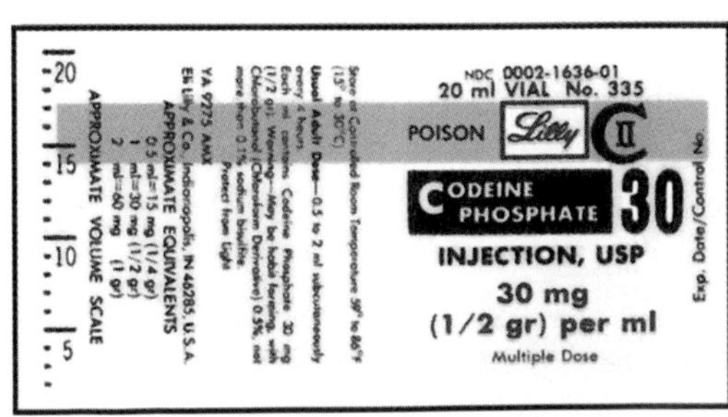

*Note: In the apothecary system, the symbol of measure precedes the number.

A nurse is already familiar with many of the units of measure in the apothecary system because they are used every day. A nurse most commonly uses the following list of apothecary system units of measure (Box 7-1). Memorize all entries in the list.

BOX 7-1 ■ COMMON APOTHECARY SYSTEM UNITS OF MEASURE

Apothecary Measure of Liquid

16 fluid ounces (fl oz) = 1 pint (pt)
32 fluid ounces (fl oz) = 2 pints (pt) or 1 quart (qt)
4 quarts (qt) = 1 gallon (gal)

Apothecary

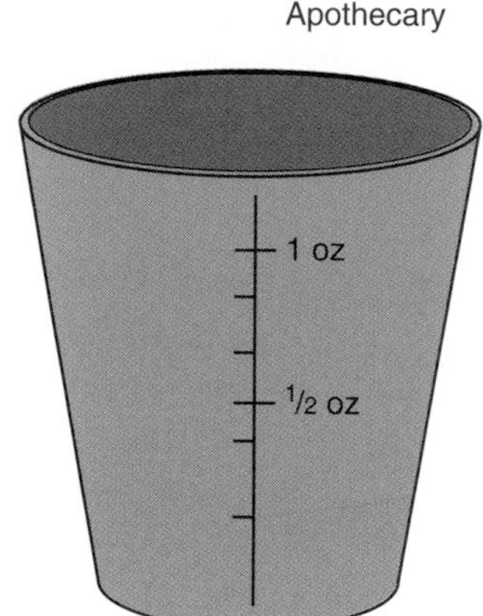

Sometimes, to compute drug dosages, the nurse must convert an apothecary measure to an equivalent measure within the same system. This may be done easily by using a proportion.

Example: 12 fl oz cquals how many pints?

a. 16 fl oz : 1 pt ::
b. 16 fl oz : 1 pt :: ______ fl oz : ______ pt
   16 fl oz : 1 pt :: 12 fl oz : x pt
c. 16 : 1 :: 12 : x
d. $16x = 12$

$$x = \frac{12}{16} = \frac{3}{4}$$

e. 12 fl oz equals ¾ pt

Note that fractions (not decimals) are used when working with the apothecary system.

Household Measurements

Household measures are not accurate enough to be used by nurses in the calculation of drug dosages in the hospital. It is sometimes necessary to compute their approximate equivalents with the apothecary system of measure, especially when sending medicines home from the hospital.

Memorize the following list of approximate equivalents (Box 7-2).

BOX 7-2 ■ APOTHECARY/HOUSEHOLD EQUIVALENTS
Apothecary Measure = Household Measure
6 fluid ounces (fl oz) = 1 coffee cup (c)
8 fluid ounces (fl oz) = 1 medium size glass

Conversion of measures between the apothecary and household systems of measure may also be made by using a proportion, as has been illustrated.

Example: 1½ coffee cup equals how many fl oz?

a. 6 fl oz : 1 c ::
b. 6 fl oz : 1 c :: ______ fl oz : ______ c
   6 fl oz : 1 c :: x fl oz : 1½ coffee c
c. 6 : 1 :: x : 1½
d. $x = 6 \times 1\frac{1}{2}$

$$x = \frac{\overset{3}{\cancel{6}}}{1} \times \frac{3}{\underset{1}{\cancel{2}}}$$

$$x = \frac{9}{1} = 9$$

e. 1½ c = 9 fl oz

Memorize the tables for the apothecary and household measurements. Study the material on forming proportions for the calculation of problems relating to the apothecary and household systems of measure. Complete the following work sheet, which provides for extensive practice in the manipulation of measurements within the apothecary and household systems. Check your answers. If you have difficulties, go back and review the necessary material. When you feel ready to evaluate your learning, take the first posttest. Check your answers. An acceptable score as indicated on the posttest signifies that you are ready for the next chapter. An unacceptable score signifies a need for further study before you take the second posttest.

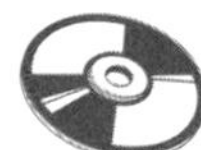

Refer to Introducing Drug Measures: Systems of Measurement on the CD for additional help and practice problems.

CHAPTER 7 **Apothecary and Household Measurements**

WORK SHEET

Directions: Express the following Arabic numerals as Roman numerals.

1. 22 _______ **2.** 9 _______ **3.** 3 _______ **4.** 30 _______

5. 14 _______ **6.** 6 _______ **7.** 15 _______ **8.** 12 _______

Directions: Express the following Roman numerals as Arabic numerals.

1. xxix _______ **2.** vii _______ **3.** xx _______ **4.** vi _______

5. xvi _______ **6.** iv _______ **7.** xxv _______ **8.** ccxl _______

Directions: Change to equivalents within the apothecary system. Solve by using proportions. Show your work.

1. 2½ fl oz = _______ pt

2. 15 fl oz = _______ pt

3. 4 pt = _______ fl oz = _______ qt

4. 2½ pt = _______ fl oz

5. 8 pt = _______ qt = _______ gal

6. ½ pt = _______ fl oz

7. 3 qt = _______ gal = _______ pt

8. 10 qt = _______ pt = _______ gal

Directions: Change the following household measurements into appropriate equivalents within the apothecary system. Solve the problems by using proportions. Show your work.

9. 2 medium size glasses = _______ fl oz

10. ½ coffee c = _______ fl oz

11. 3¼ medium size glasses = _______ fl oz

12. 2 coffee c = _______ fl oz

Answers on p. 435.

Name ______________________________

Date ______________________________

ACCEPTABLE SCORE 9

YOUR SCORE ______

POSTTEST 1

Directions: Change to equivalents within the apothecary system. Solve by using proportions. Show your work.

1-2. 24 fl oz = _______ qt = _______ pt

3-4. 48 fl oz = _______ pt = _______ qt

5-6. 5 qt = _______ gal = _______ pt

7-8. $1\frac{3}{4}$ gal = _______ qt = _______ fl oz

Directions: Change the following household measurements into approximate equivalents within the apothecary system. Solve the problems by using proportions. Show your work.

9. $1\frac{1}{2}$ medium size glasses = _______ fl oz
= _______ pt

10. $\frac{3}{4}$ coffee c = _______ fl oz

Answers on p. 436.

CHAPTER 7 Apothecary and Household Measurements

Name ________________________

Date ________________________

ACCEPTABLE SCORE 9

YOUR SCORE ______

POSTTEST 2

Directions: Change to equivalents within the apothecary system. Solve by using proportions. Show your work.

1-2. 48 fl oz = ______ pt = ______ qt

3-4. $4\frac{1}{2}$ pt = ______ fl oz = ______ qt

5-6. 6 qt = ______ gal = ______ fl oz

7-8. $2\frac{1}{2}$ gal = ______ qt = ______ pt

Directions: Change the following household measurements into approximate equivalents within the apothecary system. Solve the problems by using proportions. Show your work.

9. $2\frac{1}{4}$ coffee c = ______ fl oz
= ______ pt

10. $\frac{1}{2}$ medium size glass = ______ fl oz

Answers on p. 436.

Equivalents between Apothecary and Metric Measurements

Name ______________________________

Date ______________________________

ACCEPTABLE SCORE 32

YOUR SCORE ______

PRETEST

Directions: Change to approximate equivalents as indicated. Solve the problems by using proportions. Show your work.

1. 110 lb = _______ kg

2. 500 mL = _______ L

3. 36 kg = _______ lb

4. 5¼ qt = _______ mL

5. 90 mL = _______ fl oz

6. 1¾ qt = _______ L

7. 90 gr = _______ g

8. 8.2 kg = _______ lb

9. 8⅗ lb = _______ g

10. 2¼ pt = _______ mL

11. 7 fl oz = _______ mL

12. 10 gr = _______ g

13. 5.5 L = _______ qt

14. 1.6 kg = _______ lb

15. 4 gr = _______ mg

16. 360 mL = _______ fl oz **17.** 600 mL = _______ pt **18.** 5500 g = _______ lb

19. 20 mL = _______ fl oz **20.** 12 mg = _______ gr **21.** 1/300 gr = _______ mg

22. 85 lb = _______ kg **23.** 0.4 mg = _______ gr **24.** 12¼ lb = _______ kg

25. 4200 mL = _______ qt **26.** 1½ fl oz = _______ mL **27.** 1/5 gr = _______ mg

28. 4.6 g = _______ gr **29.** 98.8° F = _______ ° C **30.** 41° C = _______ ° F

31. 97.6° F = _______ ° C **32.** 38.5° C = _______ ° F **33.** 99.8° F = _______ ° C

34. 39.6° C = _______ ° F **35.** 102.6° F = _______ ° C **36.** 40.2° C = _______ ° F

Answers on p. 436.

CHAPTER

8

Equivalents between Apothecary and Metric Measurements

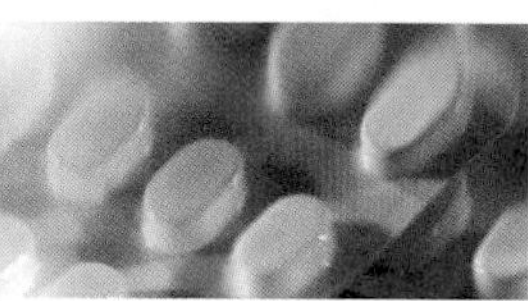

LEARNING OBJECTIVES

On completion of the materials provided in this chapter, you will be able to perform computations accurately by mastering the following mathematical concepts:

1. Recalling equivalent apothecary and metric measures
2. Computing equivalents between the apothecary and metric systems by using a proportion
3. Converting from the Fahrenheit scale to the Celsius scale
4. Converting from the Celsius scale to the Fahrenheit scale

One of a nurse's many responsibilities is the administration of medication. Historically, two different systems of measurements were used in the calculation of drug dosages: the apothecary system and the metric system. Currently, the majority of hospitals and physicians use the metric system. However, a few physicians continue to write orders using the apothecary system of measure. Nurses must therefore be able to use both systems and know the approximate equivalents between the two systems. This brief chapter is devoted to the parts of the apothecary and metric systems that are found most often in physician orders.

Approximate Equivalents between Apothecary and Metric Measurements

A list of the most commonly used equivalents between apothecary and metric systems of measure is provided in Box 8-1. Memorize these equivalents.

Sometimes a nurse will have to convert a medication order from one system to the other. This can be done by using a proportion, as shown in the examples on pp. 135-136.

BOX 8-1 ■ APOTHECARY/METRIC EQUIVALENTS

Apothecary Measure	=	Metric Measure
1 fluid ounce (fl oz)	=	30 mL
6 fluid ounces (fl oz)	=	180 mL
8 fluid ounces (fl oz)	=	240 mL
16 fluid ounces (fl oz) or 1 pint (pt)	=	500 mL
32 fluid ounces (fl oz) or 1 quart (qt)	=	1000 mL or 1 liter (L)
1 grain (gr)	=	60 or 65 milligrams (mg)
15 grains (gr)	=	1 gram (g)
2.2 pounds (lb)	=	1000 grams (g) or 1 kilogram (kg)

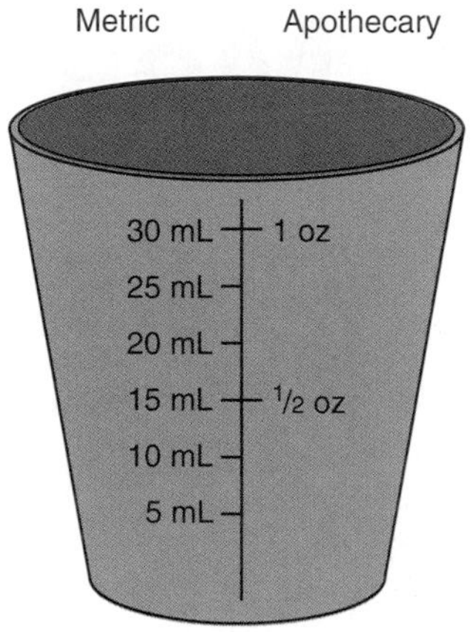

Example 1: 150 mL equals how many fluid ounces?

a. On the left side of the proportion, place what you know to be an equivalent between milliliters and fluid ounces. In this example the most appropriate equivalent is 30 mL = 1 fl oz. So the left side of the proportion would be

30 mL : 1 fl oz ::

b. The right side of the proportion is determined by the problem and by the abbreviations used on the left side. Only *two* different abbreviations may be used in a single proportion. The abbreviations must be in the same position on the right as they are on the left.

30 mL : 1 fl oz :: ______ mL : ______ fl oz

From the problem we know we have 150 mL.

30 mL : 1 fl oz :: 150 mL : ______ fl oz

We need to find the number of fluid ounces in 150 mL, so we use the symbol x to represent the unknown. Therefore the full proportion would be

30 mL : 1 fl oz :: 150 mL : x fl oz

c. Rewrite the proportion without using the abbreviations.

30 : 1 :: 150 : x

d. Solve for x.

$$30x = 150$$

$$x = \frac{150}{30} = 5$$

e. Label your answer, as determined by the abbreviation placed next to x in the original proportion.

150 mL = 5 fl oz

Example 2: 45 mg equals how many grains?

a. 1 gr : 60 mg ::
b. 1 gr : 60 mg :: _______ gr : _______ mg
   1 gr : 60 mg :: x gr : 45 mg
c. 1 : 60 :: x : 45
d. $60x = 1 \times 45$
   $60x = 45$
   $x = \frac{45}{60}$
   $x = \frac{3}{4}$
e. 45 mg equals ¾ gr

Approximate Equivalents between Celsius and Fahrenheit Measurements

Many hospitals and health care centers use the metric system of measurement, including thermometers calibrated in the Celsius scale. It may be necessary for the nurse to convert the Celsius, or centigrade, scale to the Fahrenheit scale for patient or family information. Because not everyone concerned with patient care uses the same scale, it is also important for the nurse to be able to convert the Fahrenheit scale to the Celsius scale.

Most hospitals now use digital thermometers rather than mercury thermometers. The following thermometers are included for illustration purposes only. Digital thermometers are available in the Fahrenheit or Celsius scale. Patients frequently ask for conversion charts at the time of discharge so they can understand the readings when they take their hospital thermometers home. The conversion charts are helpful for the nurse as well. However, the nurse should be able to convert from one scale to the other if necessary.

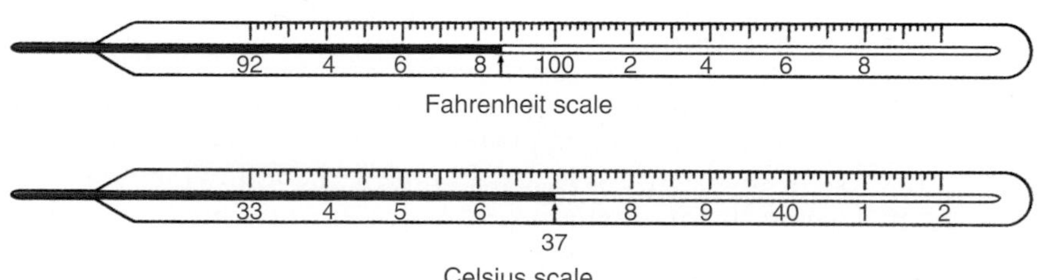

For conversion from one scale to another, the following proportion may be used:

Celsius : Fahrenheit – 32 :: 5 : 9
C : F – 32 :: 5 : 9

C or F will be the unknown.

Extend the decimal to hundredths; round to tenths.

Another means of converting Celsius and Fahrenheit temperatures to equivalents is to follow the rules listed in Box 8-2.

BOX 8-2 ■ CONVERTING CELSIUS AND FAHRENHEIT TEMPERATURES

Fahrenheit to Celsius	*Celsius to Fahrenheit*
Subtract 32	Multiply by 1.8
Divide by 1.8	Add 32

The following examples illustrate each method.

Example 1: 100.6° F equals _______ ° C.

$C : F - 32 :: 5 : 9$

$C : 100.6 - 32 :: 5 : 9$

$9C = (100.6 - 32) \times 5$
$9C = 68.6 \times 5$
$9C = 343$
$C = \frac{343}{9}$
$C = 38.11$

100.6° F equals 38.1° C.

$100.6 - 32 = 68.6$

$68.6 \div 1.8 = 38.111\ldots$
or 38.1° C

Example 2: 37.6° C equals _______ ° F.

$C : F - 32 :: 5 : 9$

$37.6 : F - 32 :: 5 : 9$
$5(F - 32) = 9 \times 37.6$
$5F - 160 = 338.4$

$5F - 160 + 160 = 338.4 + 160$

$5F = 498.4$
$F = \frac{498.4}{5}$
$F = 99.68$

37.8° C equals 99.7° F.

$37.6 \times 1.8 = 67.68$

$67.68 + 32 = 99.68$
or 99.7° F

Memorize the table of approximate equivalents between the apothecary and the metric systems of measure. Study the material on forming proportions for the calculations of problems converting between the apothecary and metric systems. Complete the following work sheet, which provides for extensive practice in the manipulation of measurements between the apothecary and metric systems. Check your answers. If you have difficulties, go back and review the necessary material. When you feel ready to evaluate your learning, take the first posttest. Check your answers. An acceptable score as indicated on the posttest signifies that you are ready for the next chapter. An unacceptable score signifies a need for further study before you take the second posttest.

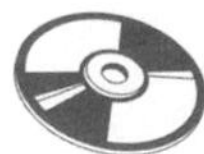

Refer to Introducing Drug Measures: Systems of Measurement on the CD for additional help and practice problems.

Equivalents between Apothecary and Metric Measurements

WORK SHEET

Directions: Change to approximate equivalents as indicated. Solve the problems by using a proportion. Show your work.

1. 200 mg = ______ gr
2. 22 lb = ______ kg
3. 150 gr = ______ g
4. 1¾ qt = ______ mL
5. 210 mL = ______ fl oz
6. 10 kg = ______ lb
7. 1750 mL = ______ pt
8. ½ fl oz = ______ mL
9. 4½ gr = ______ mg
10. 4200 g = ______ lb
11. 420 mg = ______ gr
12. 6 pt = ______ mL
13. 3500 mL = ______ qt
14. 5 gr = ______ mg
15. 150 mL = ______ fl oz

16. 3.3 kg = _______ lb

17. $6\frac{4}{5}$ lb = _______ g

18. $\frac{3}{8}$ fl oz = _______ mL

19. $2\frac{3}{4}$ gr = _______ mg

20. 5 lb = _______ kg

21. 2700 mL = _______ pt

22. 340 mg = _______ gr

23. $2\frac{1}{2}$ qt = _______ L

24. 3650 g = _______ lb

25. 4 fl oz = _______ mL

26. 12 lb = _______ g

27. 75 lb = _______ kg

28. $2\frac{1}{8}$ qt = _______ mL

29. 100 mg = _______ gr

30. 3.5 L = _______ qt

31. $1\frac{1}{2}$ gr = _______ mg

32. 25 kg = _______ lb

33. 99.6° F = _______ ° C

34. 101.8° F = _______ ° C **35.** 104.2° F = _______ ° C **36.** 97.4° F = _______ ° C

37. 40.4° C = _______ ° F **38.** 35.4° C = _______ ° F **39.** 36.8° C = _______ ° F

40. 39.2° C = _______ ° F **41.** 33° C = _______ ° F **42.** 98.4° F = _______ ° C

43. 41.2° C = _______ ° F **44.** 103.6° F = _______ ° C **45.** 40.6° C = _______ ° F

46. 102.2° F = _______ ° C **47.** 37.4° C = _______ ° F **48.** 100.4° F = _______ ° C

Answers on p. 436.

CHAPTER 8 **Equivalents between Apothecary and Metric Measurements**

Name ______________________________

Date ______________________________

ACCEPTABLE SCORE 27

YOUR SCORE ______

POSTTEST 1

Directions: Change to approximate equivalents as indicated. Solve the problems by using proportions. Show your work.

1. 3 gr = ______ mg

2. 75 gr = ______ g

3. 3 fl oz = ______ mL

4. 1½ pt = ______ mL

5. 15 mg = ______ gr

6. 1500 mL = ______ qt

7. 7½ lb = ______ g

8. 1.7 L = ______ qt

9. 5 gr = ______ g

10. 20 lb = ______ kg

11. ⅙ gr = ______ mg

12. 1000 mL = ______ pt

13. 0.3 mg = ______ gr

14. 3 g = ______ gr

15. 60 mL = ______ fl oz

16. 2700 g = _______ lb

17. 5 fl oz = _______ mL

18. 32 kg = _______ lb

19. 0.5 mg = _______ gr

20. 80 gr = _______ g

21. 2¾ qt = _______ L

22. 540 mL = _______ fl oz

23. 95.4° F = _______ ° C

24. 35.6° C = _______ ° F

25. 103.2° F = _______ ° C

26. 40.8° C = _______ ° F

27. 104.2° F = _______ ° C

28. 37.2° C = _______ ° F

29. 99.4° F = _______ ° C

30. 33.8° C = _______ ° F

Answers on p. 437.

CHAPTER 8 **Equivalents between Apothecary and Metric Measurements**

POSTTEST 2

Name ______________________

Date ______________________

ACCEPTABLE SCORE 27

YOUR SCORE ______

Directions: Change to approximate equivalents as indicated. Solve the problems by using proportions. Show your work.

1. 60 lb = ______ kg

2. 2500 mL = ______ qt

3. 1¼ pt = ______ mL

4. ¼ gr = ______ mg

5. 1.25 L = ______ qt

6. 20 mg = ______ gr

7. 20 lb = ______ kg

8. ¾ pt = ______ mL

9. 2⅜ qt = ______ mL

10. 3 g = ______ gr

11. 1/120 gr = ______ mg

12. 7 gr = ______ g

13. 3½ qt = ______ L

14. 1500 mL = ______ pt

15. 1200 g = ______ lb

16. 0.8 mg = _______ gr

17. 42 kg = _______ lb

18. 1/20 gr = _______ mg

19. 3 1/3 lb = _______ g

20. 7 kg = _______ lb

21. 1.3 g = _______ gr

22. 3 1/2 lb = _______ g

23. 96.2° F = _______ ° C

24. 38.2° C = _______ ° F

25. 36.8° C = _______ ° F

26. 97.8° F = _______ ° C

27. 40.4° C = _______ ° F

28. 100.8° F = _______ ° C

29. 41.4° C = _______ ° F

30. 103.2° F = _______ ° C

Answers on p. 437.

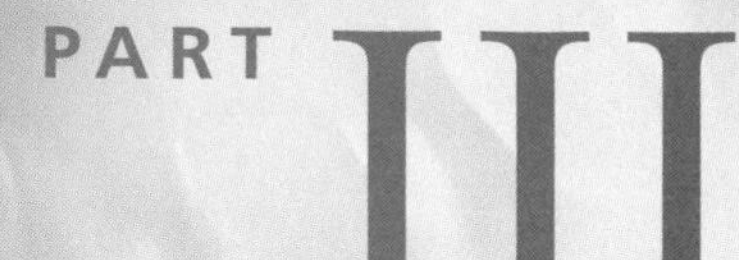

Calculation of Drug Dosages

CHAPTERS

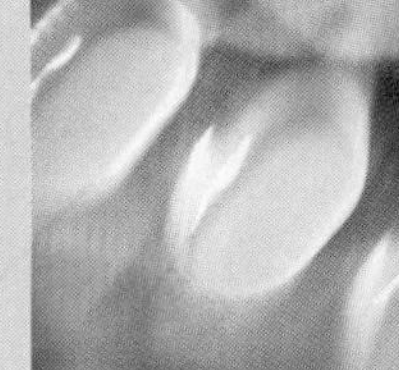

CHAPTER 9

Interpretation of the Physician's Orders

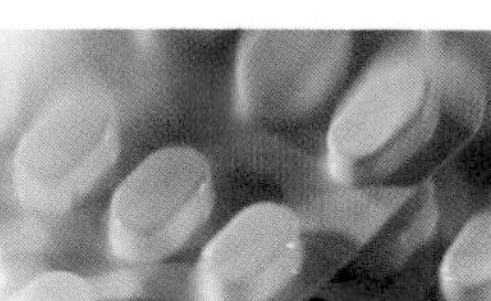

LEARNING OBJECTIVES

On completion of the materials provided in this chapter, you will be able to successfully complete a patient's medication administration record based on a physician's order.

Administration of medications is one of the most important responsibilities of the nurse. For medications to be administered safely and effectively, the nurse must know how to interpret the physician's medication orders.

Written Orders

The physician prescribes medications. In hospitals and health care centers, the physician uses a physician's order sheet, which is part of the patient's hospital chart or record. The orders are written for a drug to be given until a stated date and time, until a certain amount of the medication has been given, or until the order is changed or discontinued.

The physician's order requires the date the order was written, the name and dosage of the drug, the route and frequency of administration, and any special instructions. For drugs ordered as needed (prn), the purpose for administration is also added. The physician's signature is required each time orders are written. In many institutions the time that the order is written is also encouraged. However, if the time is not included, the order is still valid.

The nurse should review the policy and procedure for medication administration at each facility where he or she is employed to determine the appropriate schedule.

To interpret the medication order, the nurse must know the terminology, abbreviations, and symbols used in writing medical prescriptions and orders for medications. A list of the most frequently used abbreviations and symbols relating to medications can be found in Table 9-1. Memorize this list. Refer to the Glossary for help with unfamiliar terms.

In many states, other health care providers are legally authorized to prescribe medications. These may include a dentist, nurse practitioner, physician's assistant, or chiropractor. The nurse should always be knowledgeable of the laws governing practice in his or her own state and facility.

Verbal Orders

Although verbal orders are discouraged as routine policy, certain situations or emergencies may require telephone orders. Such orders are generally initiated by the nurse. The order must include the same information as the written order: the date the order is recorded, the name and dosage of the drug, the route and frequency of administration, and any special instructions. After the nurse has recorded the orders on the patient's chart, the orders must be repeated to the physician for verification. The physician's name, a notation that this is a telephone order, and the nurse's signature are required. The physician should sign the verbal orders as soon as possible. The nurse should follow her institution's policy.

Example: 1/18/07 Demerol 100 mg IM q 4 h prn for pain
1400 T.O. Dr. James T. Smith/Helen Alexander, RN

Scheduling the Administration of Medications

The physician's orders provide guidelines for the nurse in planning when each medication will be given to the patient. The purpose for prescribing the medication, drug interactions, absorption of the drug, or side effects caused by the drug may determine when the drug is given. The prescribed order may be very specific or may give the nurse latitude in scheduling.

Most hospitals and health care centers have routine times for administering medications. These times may differ from one hospital to another. The nurse should review the policy and procedure for medication administration at each facility where he or she is employed to determine the appropriate schedule. The guidelines assist the nurse in planning a medication routine that is safe for the patient. Table 9-1 provides examples of planning times for administering each medication at one institution.

The majority of hospitals use military time rather than ante meridiem (AM) and post merid-

TABLE 9-1 ■ Examples of Times for Administering Medications

Abbreviations	Definition	Example Times of Administration
ac*	Before meals	7:30-11:30-5:30
AM	Morning, before noon	9 AM
bid	Twice a day	9-9
hs	At bedtime	9 PM
pc*	After meals	8:30-12:30-6:30
PM	Evening, before midnight	9 PM
prn	As needed	
qd	Once a day	9 AM
qh	Every hour	8-9-10-etc
q2 h	Every 2 hours	8-10-12-etc
q3 h	Every 3 hours	9-12-3-etc
q4 h	Every 4 hours	8-12-4-etc
q6 h	Every 6 hours	9-3-9-3
q8 h	Every 8 hours	8-4-12
q12 h	Every 12 hours	9-9
qid	Four times a day	8-12-4-8
qod	Every other day	
qoh	Every other hour	8-10-12-2-4-6-etc
STAT	Immediately	
tid	Three times a day	9-1-5

*Providing that meals are served at 8:00 AM, 12:00 noon, and 6:00 PM.

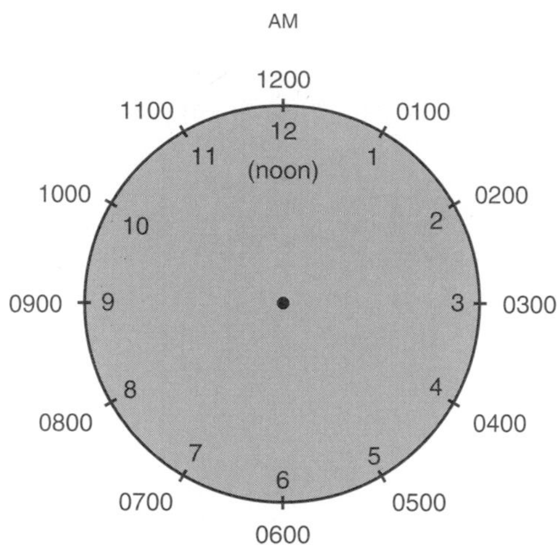

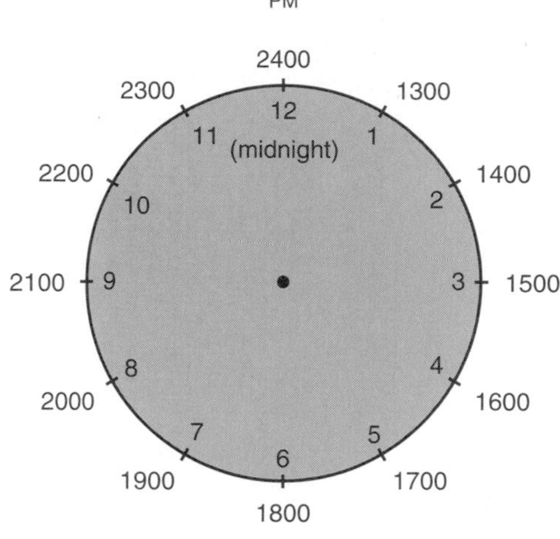

TABLE 9-2 ■ Conversion from Military Time to AM–PM Time

0100—1:00 AM	0900—9:00 AM	1700—5:00 PM
0200—2:00 AM	1000—10:00 AM	1800—6:00 PM
0300—3:00 AM	1100—11:00 AM	1900—7:00 PM
0400—4:00 AM	1200—12:00 noon	2000—8:00 PM
0500—5:00 AM	1300—1:00 PM	2100—9:00 PM
0600—6:00 AM	1400—2:00 PM	2200—10:00 PM
0700—7:00 AM	1500—3:00 PM	2300—11:00 PM
0800—8:00 AM	1600—4:00 PM	2400—12:00 midnight

iem (PM) time. Table 9-2 will assist in conversion from military time. Military time can be computed quickly by adding 12 to PM time—for example, 12 + 3 = 1500 hours.

Introduction to Drug Dosages

The nurse obtains the medication from the pharmacy or from an available supply in the clinical unit, prepares the dosage, and administers the medication. Unit dosages are prepared in individual doses by the manufacturer or hospital pharmacy and are ready for the nurse to administer.

Most medications are secured in the required dosage. However, problems of drug calculation arise when a drug is not manufactured in the strength required by the patient, the drug is not available in the strength ordered, or the drug is ordered in one system of measurement but is available only in another system of measurement.

When you change from one system of measurement to another, you have an equivalent measure that may or may not be exact. Therefore the answer to your problem may vary according to the system of measurement used. For example, if you change the required dosage to the available dosage, the equivalent dosage may be different than if you changed the available dosage to the required dosage. All problems in this book are calculated by changing the required dosage to the available dosage. The answers reflect this method of calculation. This is good practice because you have the medication on hand in the dosage provided.

The nurse is ethically and legally responsible for the medications administered to the patient. Even though the physician writes the order for the medication to be given to the patient, or even if the pharmacy prepares the wrong medication, the nurse who administers the medication is responsible for the error. Before preparing the drug, the nurse *must know* the maximum and minimum dosages and the actions of and contraindications for each administered drug. In addition, the nurse should consult the patient and the patient's medical record for any known allergies.

The Six Rights of Medication Administration

Because the nurse is legally responsible for ensuring that medications are correctly administered, the following six rights of medication administration listed in Box 9-1 must be diligently checked.

BOX 9-1 ■ SIX RIGHTS OF MEDICATION ADMINISTRATION

1. Drug
2. Dose
3. Patient
4. Route
5. Time
6. Documentation

Anytime these rights are not checked in the preparation and administration of medications, an error may occur for which the nurse is legally responsible.

When medications are prepared for administration, the information on the medication profile sheet or drug card should be checked *three* times:

1. As the medicine is taken from the drawer or shelf
2. As the medicine is prepared
3. As the medicine is replaced

If unit doses are used, the label should be checked three times. It is critical that all calculations be done accurately and checked. It is especially important to check computations involving fractions and decimals. Many nurses use calculators. In some institutions certain medications (for example, heparin and insulin) are to be checked by another nurse before the medicine is administered to the patient. Always use the appropriate measuring devices.

When administering the medication, *ALWAYS* ask the patient his or her name and *ALWAYS* check the patient's identification armband.

Medications can be ordered to be administered by various routes. However, they must be administered only by the route included in the physician's order. Never assume the route by which the medication is to be given. If the route has not been included in the order, the physician must be notified and asked to clarify the route requested.

Timing is very important—both the time of day and the interval between doses. With all medications, judgment and assessment by the nurse are required as to whether the medication should be given or withheld.

Medication Administration Record. Documentation has become more and more important for legal purposes. Remember that documentation of medications administered must include the five components of drug, dose, patient, route, and time. It is also necessary to document whether a medication has been withheld or refused. Each facility has its own policy concerning the full documentation of medications. The official medication administration record (commonly called *the patient's MAR*) varies in format from one institution to another but contains the same information. It is mandatory that all documentation be legible, and it usually is written in blue or black ink or printed out from a computer.

In most institutions, personnel other than nurses perform the transcription of the physician's orders to the patient's MAR. Nurses are then required to verify the transcription against the physician's order and to place their initials on the form indicating the transcription was correctly completed.

Figure 9-1 represents examples of *A,* a physician's order, and *B,* a patient's MAR. Notice that the appropriate drug interpretations for the MAR include the patient's name, the medication name, the date, the drug dosage, the medication route, and the medication schedule.

PHYSICIAN'S ORDERS

1. ADDRESSOGRAPH BEFORE PLACING IN PATIENT'S CHART ▶
2. INITIAL AND DETACH COPY EACH TIME PHYSICIAN WRITES ORDERS
3. TRANSMIT COPY TO PHARMACY
4. ORDERS MUST BE DATED AND TIMED

Patient, James A.

DATE	ORDERS			TRANS BY
	Diagnosis:	Weight:	Height:	
	Sensitivities/Drug Allergies:			
1/12/07	0900 Lasix 80 mg. p.o. b.i.d.			
	Digoxin 0.125 mg. p.o. q.d.			
	Slow-K 10 mEq. p.o. b.i.d.			
	A. Physician, M.D.			

MEDICAL RECORDS COPY **PHYSICIAN'S ORDERS** **T-5**

B-CLIN. NOTES	E-LAB	G-X-RAY	K-DIAGNOSTIC	M-SURGERY	Q-THERAPY	T-ORDERS	W-NURSING	Y-MISC.

A

Transcription of Med Sheet by: ________

Reviewed by: ________ Page ___ of ___

Patient, James A.

Initials	Signature
NJ	N. Jones R.N.
AN	A. Nurse R.N.

Allergies: ☑ NKDA

Injection Sites: A = RUE, B = LUE, C = RLE, D = LLE, E = Abdomen, F = R Glut, G = L Glut

Special Notes:

☐ Inpatient ☐ Outpatient

See Legend on Back

DATE	DRUG			08 09 10 11	12 13 14 15	16 17 18 19	20 21 22 23	24 01 02 03	04 05 06 07	1/12/07		1/13/07		1/14/07		1/15/07		1/16/07	
1 1/12	Lasix									09 AN	21 NJ	09 AN	21 NJ						
	80 mg dose	p.o. route	b.i.d. interval	09			21												
2 1/12	Digoxin									09 AN		09 AN							
	0.125 mg dose	p.o. route	q.d. interval	09															
3 1/12	Slow-K									09 AN	21 NJ	09 AN	21 NJ						
	10 mEq dose	p.o. route	b.i.d. interval	09			21												
4																			
	dose	route	interval																
5																			
	dose	route	interval																

MEDICATION PROFILE

B-CLIN. NOTES	E-LAB	G-X-RAY	K-DIAGNOSTIC	M-SURGERY	Q-THERAPY	T-ORDERS	W-NURSING	Y-MISC.

B

FIGURE 9-1 Examples of physician's orders **(A)** and patient's medication administration record **(B)** with appropriate drug interpretations. (Forms courtesy Clarian Health, Indianapolis, Indiana.)

CHAPTER 9 **Interpretation of the Physician's Orders**

Name ____________________

Date ____________________

ACCEPTABLE SCORE 17

YOUR SCORE ______

POSTTEST

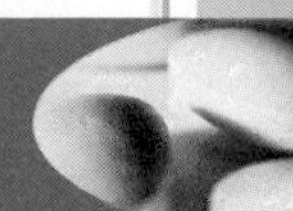

Directions: Copy the following physician's orders onto the medication administration record sheet below. Be sure to schedule the times for each drug administration.

PHYSICIAN'S ORDERS

1. ADDRESSOGRAPH BEFORE PLACING IN PATIENT'S CHART ▶
2. INITIAL AND DETACH COPY EACH TIME PHYSICIAN WRITES ORDERS
3. TRANSMIT COPY TO PHARMACY
4. ORDERS MUST BE DATED AND TIMED

Patient, James A.

DATE	ORDERS	TRANS BY
	Diagnosis: Weight: Height:	
	Sensitivities/Drug Allergies:	
1/12/07	0800 Cefuroxime 1 g IV q 8 hours	
	Lasix 40 mg p.o. b.i.d.	
	Slow-K 10 mEq. p.o. b.i.d.	
	A. Physician, M.D.	

Transcription of Med Sheet by: ____________

Reviewed by: ____________ Page ____ of ____

Initials Signature

Allergies: ☐ NKDA

Injection Sites: A = RUE B = LUE C = RLE D = LLE E = Abdomen F = R Glut G = L Glut

Special Notes:

See Legend on Back

Patient, James A.

☐ Inpatient ☐ Outpatient

DATE	DRUG	08 09 10 11	12 13 14 15	16 17 18 19	20 21 22 23	24 01 02 03	04 05 06 07	DATES				
1												
	dose / route / interval											
2												
	dose / route / interval											
3												
	dose / route / interval											
4												
	dose / route / interval											
5												
	dose / route / interval											

Answers on p. 437.

CHAPTER

10

How to Read Drug Labels

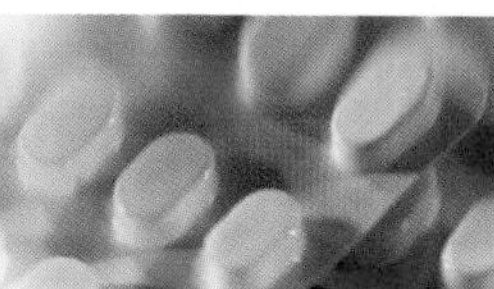

LEARNING OBJECTIVES

On completion of the materials provided in this chapter, you will be able to identify the following parts of each drug label:

1. Trade name of the medication
2. Generic name of the medication
3. Strength of the medication dosage
4. Form in which the medication is provided
5. Route of administration
6. Total amount or volume of the medication provided in the container
7. Directions for mixing of the medication if required

The safe administration of medications to patients begins with the nurse accurately reading and interpreting the drug label. Thus it is important for the nurse to be familiar and comfortable with the information that is found on the drug label.

Parts of a Drug Label

1. TRADE NAME. The trade name is usually capitalized and written in bold print. It is the first name written on the label. The trade name is always followed by the ® registration symbol. Different manufacturers market the same medication under different trade names.

2. GENERIC NAME. The generic name is the official name of the drug. Each drug has only *one* generic name. This name appears directly under the trade name, usually in smaller or different type letters. Physicians may order a patient's medication by generic or trade name. Nurses need to be familiar with both names and cross-check references as needed. Occasionally, only the generic name will appear on the label.

3. DOSAGE STRENGTH. The strength indicates the amount or weight of the medication that is supplied in the specific unit of measure. This amount may be per capsule, tablet, or milliliter.

4. FORM. The form indicates how the drug is supplied. Examples of various forms are tablets, capsules, liquids, suppositories, and ointments.

5. ROUTE. The label will indicate how the drug is to be administered. The route can be oral, topical, injection (subcutaneous, intradermal, intramuscular), or intravenous.

6. AMOUNT. The total amount or volume of the medication may be indicated. Some examples are 250 milliliters of oral suspension and a bottle that contains 50 capsules.

7. DIRECTIONS. Some medications must be mixed before use. The amounts and types of diluent required will be listed along with the resulting strengths of the medication. This information may also be found on package inserts.

Other information may be found on drug labels: the name of the manufacturer, expiration date, special instructions for storage, and an NDC (National Drug Code) number.

Examples for Practice in Reading Drug Labels

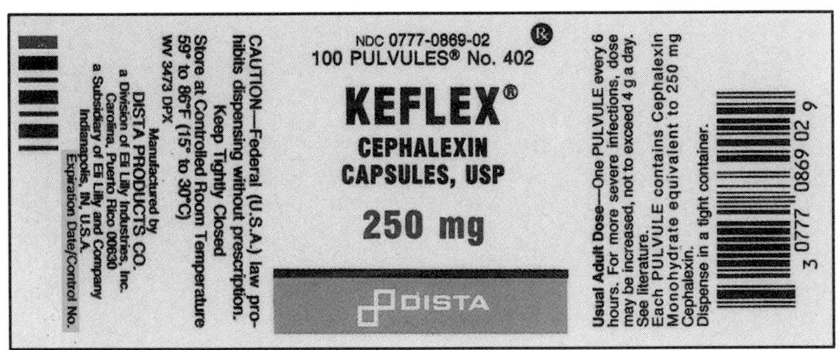

1. Trade name ....Keflex
2. Generic name ....cephalexin
3. Dosage strength.......................250 mg
4. Form ....Capsules
5. Amount...................................100
6. Directions...............................Keep tightly closed. Store at controlled room temperature 59° to 86° F (15° to 30° C).
7. NDC number 0777-0869-02
8. Manufacturer ....DISTA
9. Expiration date........................(Yellow highlight)

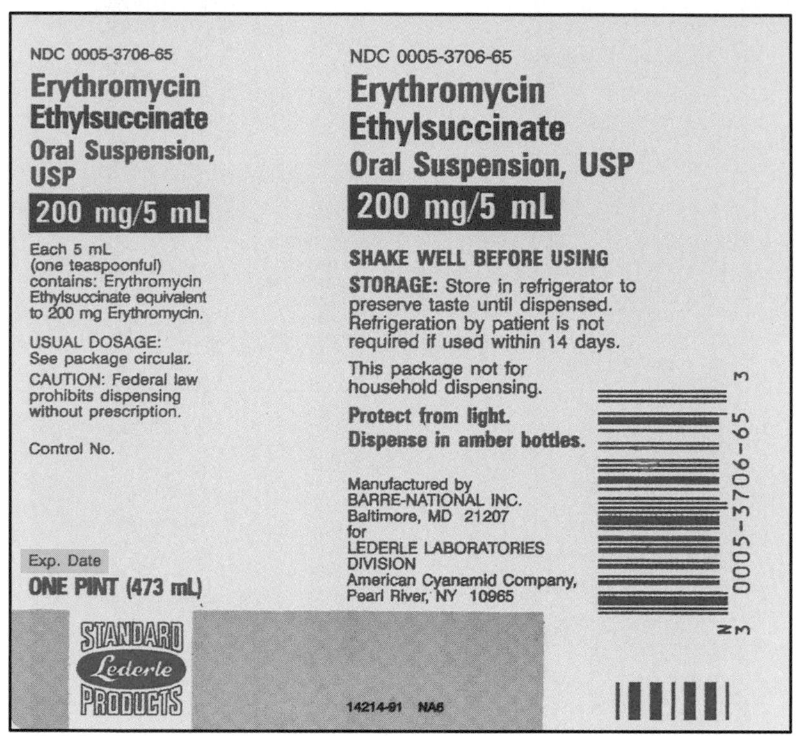

1. Trade name....................Erythromycin
2. Generic name.................erythromycin ethylsuccinate
3. Dosage strength ....200 mg/5 mL
4. Form..............................Suspension
5. Route.............................Oral
6. Amount ....1 pint or 473 mL
7. Directions ....Shake well before using. Storage: Store in refrigerator to preserve taste until dispensed. Refrigeration by patient is not required if used within 14 days. Protect from light. Dispense in amber bottles.
8. NDC number.................0005-3706-65
9. Manufacturer.................Barre-National Inc. for Lederle Laboratories Division
10. Expiration date..............(Green highlight)

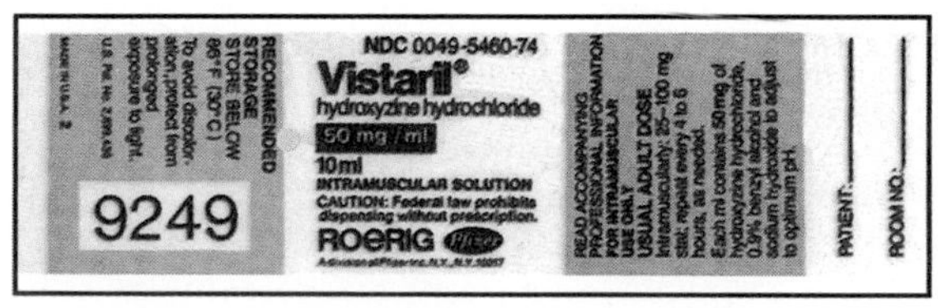

1. Trade name...............................Vistaril
2. Generic name............................hydroxyzine hydrochloride
3. Dosage strength ....50 mg/mL
4. Form...Intramuscular solution
5. Route.......................................Intramuscular injection
6. Amount ....Total amount of 10 mL in vial
7. Directions ....Storage: Store below 86° F (30° C). To avoid discoloration, protect from prolonged exposure to light.
8. NDC...0049-5460-74

Occasionally, a drug label will only have one name listed. The one name is the generic name. These are drugs that have been in use for many years and are very well known. The drug companies do not market them under different trade names. They all simply use the generic name.

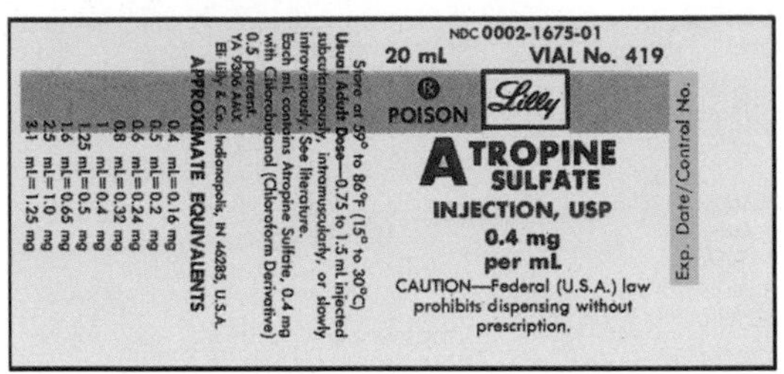

1. Trade name ....None
2. Generic name ....atropine sulfate
3. Dosage strength ....0.4 mg per mL
4. Form ....Solution
5. Route ....Injection
6. Amount............................20 mL
7. NDC number 0002-1675-01
8. Expiration date ....(Yellow highlight)

Study the material and examples for practice in reading drug labels. When you feel ready to evaluate your learning, take the first posttest. Check your answers. An acceptable score as indicated on the posttest signifies that you are ready for the next chapter. An unacceptable score signifies a need for further study before you take the second posttest.

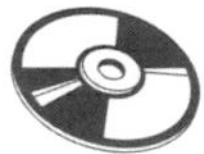

Refer to How to Read a Drug Label on the CD for additional help and practice problems.

Name ______________________

Date ______________________

ACCEPTABLE SCORE 18

YOUR SCORE ______

POSTTEST 1

Directions: Identify the requested parts of each of the following medication labels.

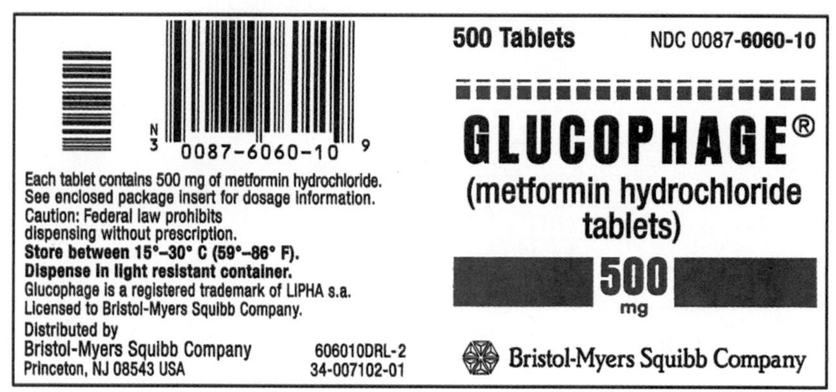

1. Trade name ______________
   Generic name ______________
   Dosage strength ______________
   Form ______________
   Amount ______________

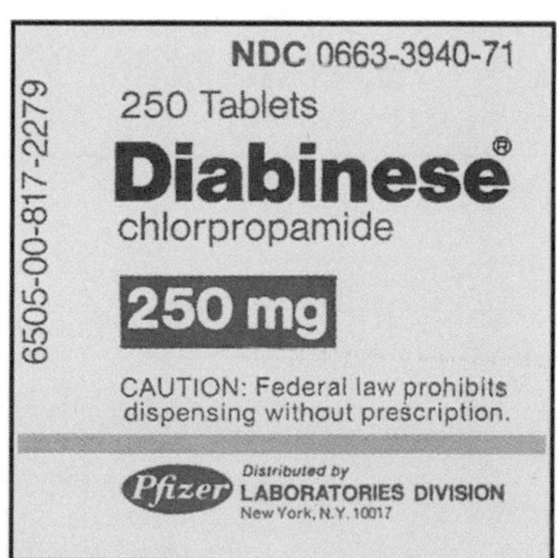

2. Trade name ______________
   Generic name ______________
   Dosage strength ______________
   Form ______________
   Amount ______________

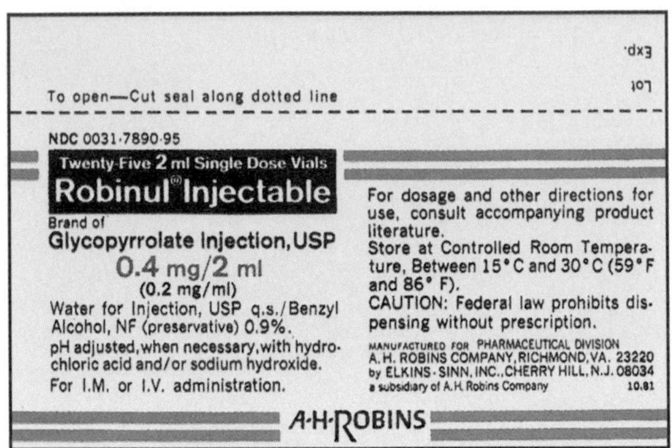

3. Trade name ____________________
Generic name ____________________
Dosage strength ____________________
Form ____________________
Route ____________________

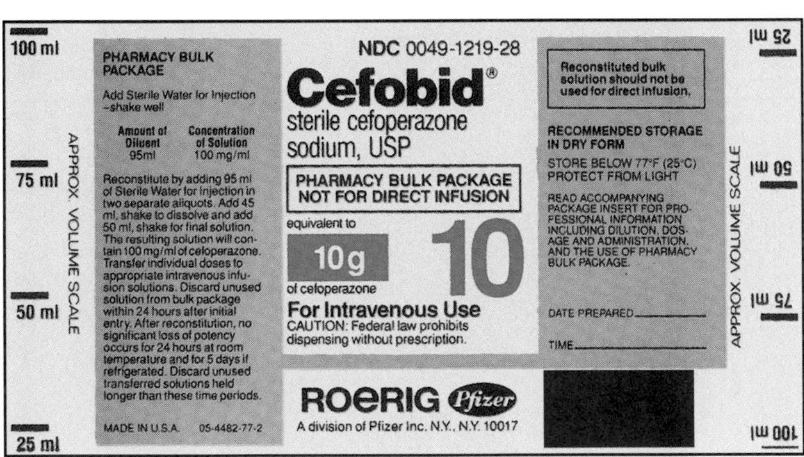

4. Trade name ____________________
Generic name ____________________
Dosage strength ____________________
Form ____________________
Route ____________________

Answers on p. 437.

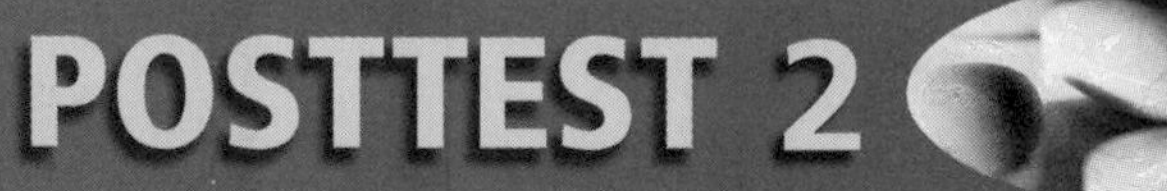

Name ______________________________

Date ______________________________

ACCEPTABLE SCORE 18

YOUR SCORE ______

Directions: Identify the requested parts of each of the following medication labels.

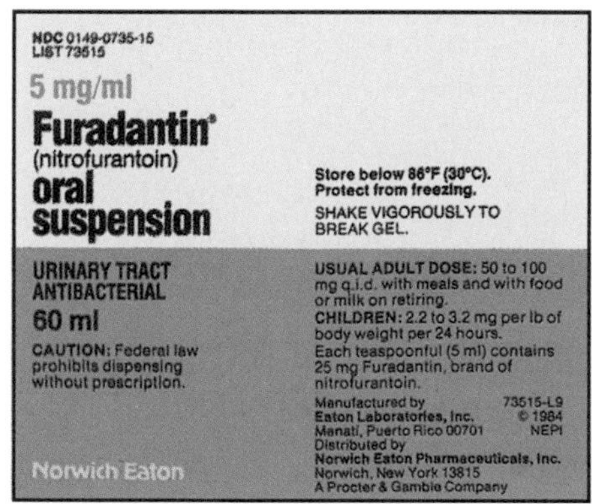

1. Trade name ______________________
   Generic name ______________________
   Dosage strength ______________________
   Form ______________________
   Route ______________________
   Amount ______________________

USUAL ADULT DOSAGE: See accompanying circular.
Dispense in a well-closed container.
CAUTION: Federal (USA) law prohibits dispensing without prescription.
50 | No. 7638 7605309
MSD
NDC 0006-0095-50
50 TABLETS
Decadron®
(Dexamethasone, MSD)
1.5 mg
MERCK SHARP & DOHME
DIVISION OF MERCK & CO., INC.
WEST POINT, PA 19486, USA
DECADRON
Lot
Exp.

2. Trade name ______________________
   Generic name ______________________
   Dosage strength ______________________
   Form ______________________

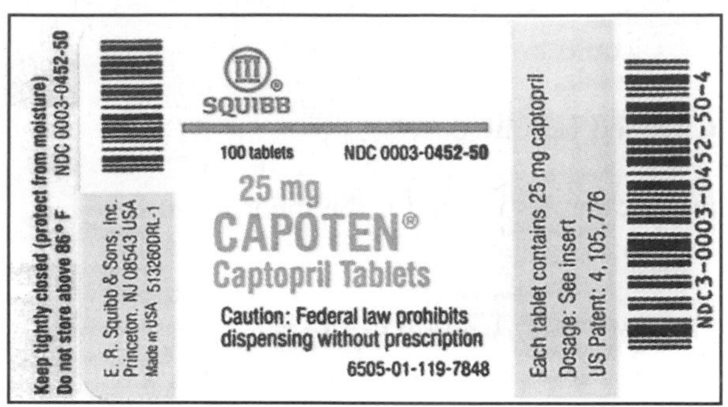

3. Trade name ____________________
Generic name ____________________
Dosage strength ____________________
Form ____________________
Amount ____________________

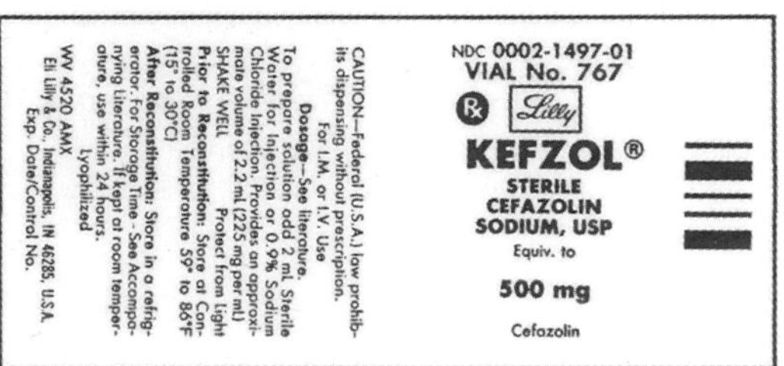

4. Trade name ____________________
Generic name ____________________
Dosage strength ____________________
Form ____________________
Route ____________________

Answers on p. 438.

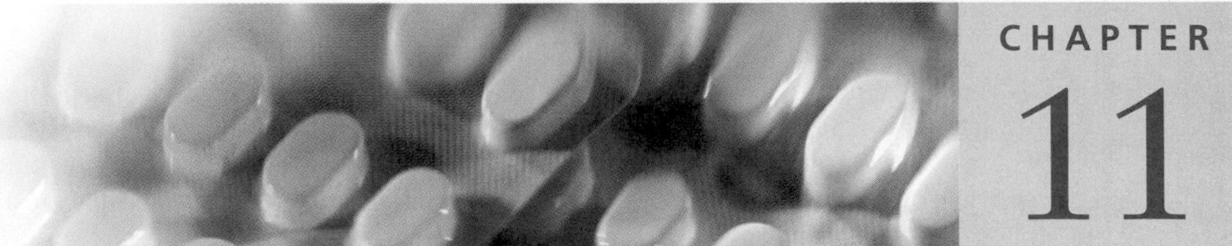

CHAPTER

11

Dimensional Analysis and the Calculation of Drug Dosages*

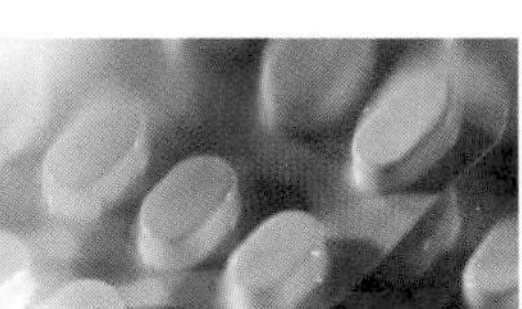

LEARNING OBJECTIVES

On completion of the materials provided in this chapter, you will be able to perform computations accurately by mastering the following mathematical concepts:

1. Using the dimensional analysis format to solve oral dosage problems
2. Using the dimensional analysis format to solve parenteral dosage problems
3. Using the dimensional analysis format to solve problems of intravenous flow rate in drops per minute
4. Using the dimensional analysis format to solve problems involving administration of medications in units per hour

Dimensional analysis is another format for setting up problems to calculate drug dosages. The advantage of dimensional analysis is that only one equation is needed. This is true even if the information supplied indicates a need to convert to like units before setting up the proportion to perform the actual calculation of the amount of medication to be given to the patient.

Example: The order states ampicillin 500 mg po qid. The drug is supplied in 250-mg capsules. How many capsules will the nurse administer? ______ .

a. On the left side of the equation, place the name or abbreviation of the drug form of x, or what you are solving for.

$$x \text{ capsule} =$$

*Linda Fluharty, MSN, RN, contributed to this chapter.

b. On the right side of the equation, place the available information related to the measurement or abbreviation that was placed on the left side. In this example, that is *capsule*. This information is placed in the equation as a common fraction; match the appropriate abbreviation or measurement. Thus the abbreviation that matches the x quantity must be placed in the numerator. We also know from the problem that each capsule contains 250 mg of ampicillin. This information is the denominator of our fraction.

$$x \textit{ capsule} = \frac{\textit{1 capsule}}{\text{250 mg}}$$

c. Next, find the information that matches the measurement or abbreviation used in the denominator of the fraction you created. In this example *mg* is in the denominator and our order is for 500 mg. Therefore the full proportion is

$$x \text{ capsule} = \frac{\text{1 capsule}}{250\ mg} \times \frac{500\ mg}{1}$$

d. Now cancel out the like abbreviations on the right side of the equation. If you have set up the problem correctly, the remaining measurement or abbreviation should match that used on the left side of the equation. You are now ready to solve for x.

$$x \text{ capsule} = \frac{\text{1 capsule}}{250\ \cancel{mg}} \times \frac{500\ \cancel{mg}}{1}$$

$$x = \frac{1 \times 500}{250}$$

$$x = 2$$

The answer to the problem is 2 capsules.

As stated earlier, the advantage of this method is not having to convert into like systems of measurement as would be required if the usual proportion method were used. With dimensional analysis, remember that only one equation is necessary. Let's take a look at an example of this type.

Example: The order states Kantrex 400 mg IM q12 h. The drug is supplied 0.5 g per 2 mL. How many milliliters will the nurse administer? _______ .

a. On the left side of the equation, place the name or abbreviation of the drug form for which you are solving, or x.

$$x \text{ mL} =$$

b. On the right side of the equation, place the available information related to the measurement or abbreviation that was placed on the left side. In this example that is *mL*. This information is placed in the equation as part of a fraction; match the appropriate abbreviation. Remember that the abbreviation that matches the x quantity must be placed in the numerator. We know from the problem that each 2 mL contains 0.5 g of Kantrex.

$$x\ mL = \frac{2\ mL}{\text{0.5 g}}$$

c. Because the order is for 400 mg and the medication is supplied to us as 0.5 g, a conversion would normally be required. However, with the dimensional analysis method, an additional fraction is added on the right side of the equation. From information supplied in earlier chapters, we know that 1 g equals 1000 mg. This information is then placed in the equation next in the form of the fraction $\frac{1\ g}{1000\ mg}$. Note that the abbreviation or measurement in the *numerator* of this fraction must match the abbreviation or measurement in the *denominator* of the immediate previous fraction. The equation now looks like

$$x\ \text{mL} = \frac{2\ \text{mL}}{0.5\ g} \times \frac{1\ g}{1000\ \text{mg}}$$

d. Next, place the amount of drug ordered in the equation. Note that this will once again match the measurement or abbreviation of the denominator of the fraction immediately before. In this example, that is 400 mg. Therefore the full equation is

$$x\ \text{mL} = \frac{2\ \text{mL}}{0.5\ \text{g}} \times \frac{1\ \text{g}}{1000\ \text{mg}} \times \frac{400\ \text{mg}}{1}$$

e. For the final step, cancel out the like abbreviations on the right side of the equation. If the equation has been set up correctly, the remaining abbreviation should match that located on the left side. Now solve for x.

$$x\ \text{mL} = \frac{2\ \text{mL}}{0.5\ \cancel{g}} \times \frac{1\ \cancel{g}}{1000\ \cancel{\text{mg}}} \times \frac{400\ \cancel{\text{mg}}}{1}$$

$$x = \frac{2 \times 400}{0.5 \times 1000}$$

$$x = \frac{800}{500}$$

$$x = 1.6$$

The answer to the problem is 1.6 mL.

Using Dimensional Analysis to Calculate IV Flow Rates

The dimensional analysis method can also be used to calculate intravenous (IV) flow rates. The following formulas demonstrate how to calculate drops per minute (gtt/min) and milliliters per hour (mL/h). These formulas can be used to solve IV problems in chapters 15 and 16.

Example 1: A patient has an order for enalaprilat 0.625 mg qd IVPB. The enalaprilat is diluted in 50 mL of D5W and is to be infused over 20 minutes. The tubing drop factor is 60 gtt/mL. At what rate, in drops per minute, should the intravenous piggyback (IVPB) be programmed? _______ .

a. On the left side of the equation, place what you are solving for.

$$x\ \text{gtt/min} =$$

b. On the right side of the equation, place the available information related to the measurement that was placed on the left side of the equation. In this example, the measurement we are solving for is *gtt/min*. We will deal with the numerator portion of our answer first: the gtt. This information is placed in the equation as a common fraction; match the appropriate measurement. Thus the abbreviation that matches the x quantity must be placed in the numerator. We also know from the problem that each milliliter contains 60 gtt. This information is the denominator of our fraction.

$$x\ gtt/\text{min} = \frac{60\ gtt}{1\ \text{mL}}$$

c. Next, find the information that matches the measurement used in the denominator of the fraction you created. In this example *mL* is in the denominator and our order is for 50 mL. We also know that the enalaprilat should be infused over 20 minutes. The equation now looks like

$$x \text{ gtt}/min = \frac{60 \text{ gtt}}{1 \text{ mL}} \times \frac{50 \text{ mL}}{20 \; min}$$

d. Then cancel out the like abbreviations on the right side of the equation. If you have set up the problem correctly, the remaining measurement should match the measurement on the left side of the equation. Now solve for x.

$$x \text{ gtt/min} = \frac{60 \text{ gtt}}{1 \cancel{\text{mL}}} \times \frac{50 \cancel{\text{mL}}}{20 \text{ min}}$$

$$x \text{ gtt/min} = \frac{60 \text{ gtt} \times 50}{20 \text{ min}}$$

$$x = \frac{3000 \text{ gtt}}{20 \text{ min}}$$

$$x = 150 \text{ gtt/min}$$

Therefore the nurse will regulate the IVPB for 150 gtt/min, and the enalaprilat will be infused over 20 minutes.

Example 2: A postoperative patient has an order for 200 mL 0.9% normal saline solution (NS) over 2 hours. The tubing drop factor is 10 gtt/min. At what rate, in drops per minute, should the NS be infused? ________ .

a. On the left side of the equation, place what you are solving for.

$$x = \text{gtt/min}$$

b. On the right side of the equation, place the available information related to the measurement that was placed on the left side of the equation. In this example, the measurement we are solving for is *gtt/min.* We will deal with the numerator portion of our answer first: the gtt. This information is placed in the equation as a common fraction; match the appropriate measurement. Thus the abbreviation that matches the x quantity must be placed in the numerator on the right side of the equation. We know from the problem that each milliliter contains 10 gtt. This information is the denominator of our fraction.

$$x \; gtt/\text{min} = \frac{10 \; gtt}{1 \text{ mL}}$$

c. Next, find the information that matches the measurement used in the denominator of the fraction you created. In this example, mL is in the denominator and our order is for 200 mL. We also know that this 200 mL should be infused over 2 hours. The equation now looks like

$$x \text{ gtt/min} = \frac{10 \text{ gtt}}{1 \text{ mL}} \times \frac{200 \text{ mL}}{2\text{h}}$$

d. Now, we need to solve for minutes, but the order is for hours. So, the equivalent of *1 h : 60 min* must be added to the equation as a fraction. The equation would now look like this

$$x \text{ gtt}/min = \frac{10 \text{ gtt}}{1 \cancel{\text{mL}}} \times \frac{200 \cancel{\text{mL}}}{2 \text{ h}} \times \frac{1 \text{ h}}{60 \; min}$$

e. Then cancel out the abbreviations on the right side of the equation. If you have set up the problem correctly, the remaining measurement should match that used on the left side of the equation. Now solve for x.

$$x \text{ gtt/min} = \frac{10 \text{ gtt}}{1 \cancel{\text{mL}}} \times \frac{200 \cancel{\text{mL}}}{2 \cancel{\text{h}}} \times \frac{1 \cancel{\text{h}}}{60 \text{ min}}$$

$$x \text{ gtt/min} = \frac{10 \text{ gtt} \times 200}{2 \times 60 \text{ min}}$$

$$x = \frac{2000 \text{ gtt}}{120 \text{ min}}$$

$$x = 16.6 \text{ or } 17 \text{ gtt/min}$$

Therefore the nurse will regulate the IV for 17 gtt/min, and 200 mL of 0.9% NS will be infused over 2 hours.

Example 3: A patient has an order for regular insulin IV at a rate of 5 U/h. The concentration is insulin 100 U in 100 mL 0.9% NS. At what rate, in milliliters per hour, should the IV pump be programmed? _______ .

a. On the left side of the equation, place what you are solving for.

$$x \text{ mL/h} =$$

b. On the right side of the equation, place the available information related to the measurement that was placed on the left side of the equation. In this example the measurement we are solving for is mL/h. We will deal with the numerator portion of our answer first: the mL. This information is placed in the equation as a common fraction: match the appropriate measurement. Thus the abbreviation that matches the x quantity must be placed in the numerator on the right side of the equation. We know from the problem that there is 100 U of insulin diluted in the 100 mL; this information becomes the fraction of our equation.

$$x \text{ mL/h} = \frac{100 \text{ mL}}{100 \text{ U}}$$

c. Next, find the information that matches the measurement used in the denominator of the fraction you created. In this example, U is the denominator and our order is for 5 U/h. The equation now looks like

$$x \text{ mL/h} = \frac{100 \text{ mL}}{100 \text{ U}} \times \frac{5 \text{ U}}{1 \text{ h}}$$

d. Then cancel out the abbreviations on the right side of the equation. If you have set up the problem correctly, the remaining measurement should match the measurement on the left side of the equation. Now solve for x.

$$x \text{ mL/h} = \frac{100 \text{ mL}}{100 \cancel{\text{U}}} \times \frac{5 \cancel{\text{U}}}{1 \text{ h}}$$

$$x = \frac{500 \text{ mL}}{100 \text{ h}}$$

$$x = 5 \text{ mL/h}$$

Therefore the nurse will program the IV pump for 5 mL/h, and the insulin will be infused at a rate of 5 U/h.

Example 4: A patient with a femoral thrombus has an order for heparin IV at 1200 U/h. The concentration is heparin 20,000 U in 250 mL of D5W. At what rate, in milliliters per hour, should the IV pump be programmed? ______

a. On the left side of the equation, place what you are solving for.

$$x \text{ mL/h} =$$

b. On the right side of the equation, place the available information related to the measurement that was placed on the left side of the equation. In this example the measurement we are solving for is *mL/h*. We will deal with the numerator portion of our answer first: the mL. This information is placed in the equation as a common fraction; match the appropriate measurement. Thus the abbreviation that matches the *x* quantity must be placed in the numerator. We also know from the problem that there are 20,000 U of heparin in 250 mL. This information becomes the fraction of our equation.

$$x \text{ mL/h} = \frac{250 \text{ mL}}{20{,}000 \text{ U}}$$

c. Next, find the information that matches the measurement used in the denominator of the fraction you created. In this example, U is the denominator. The order is for 1200 U/h. The equation now looks like

$$x \text{ mL/h} = \frac{250 \text{ mL}}{20{,}000 \text{ U}} \times \frac{1200 \text{ U}}{1 \text{ h}}$$

d. Then cancel out the like abbreviations on the right side of the equation. If you have set up the problem correctly, the remaining measurement should match the measurement on the left side of the equation. Now solve for *x*.

$$x \text{ mL/h} = \frac{250 \text{ mL}}{20{,}000 \not{\text{U}}} \times \frac{1200 \not{\text{U}}}{1 \text{ h}}$$

$$x = \frac{250 \text{ mL} \times 1200}{20{,}000 \text{ h}}$$

$$x = \frac{300{,}000 \text{ mL}}{20{,}000 \text{ h}}$$

$$x = 15 \text{ mL/h}$$

Therefore the nurse will program the IV pump for 15 mL/h, and the heparin will be infused at a rate of 1200 U/h.

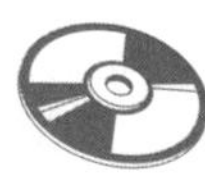

Refer to Calculating Dosages: Introduction (then go to Understanding the Dimensional Analysis Method) on the CD for additional help and practice problems.

CHAPTER 11 **Dimensional Analysis and the Calculation of Drug Dosages**

WORK SHEET

Directions: Calculate the following drug dosages by using the dimensional analysis method. Show your work and check your answers.

1. Your patient with diabetes receives glipizide 10 mg po qAM. The drug is supplied in 5-mg scored tablets. How many tablets will you administer? _______ .

2. Mr. Theson receives Vistaril 60 mg po q6 h for relief of nausea after his acoustic neuroma revision. Vistaril oral suspension, 25 mg per 5 mL, is supplied. How many milliliters will the nurse administer? _______ .

3. A patient who has undergone a lumbar laminectomy receives Demerol 0.025 g po q4 h prn for relief of pain. Demerol 50-mg tablets are available. How many tablets will the nurse administer? _______ .

4. Mrs. Fare receives codeine 30 mg po q3 h prn for pain relief after knee replacement surgery. You have codeine tablets, gr 1/4, available. How many tablets will you administer? _______ .

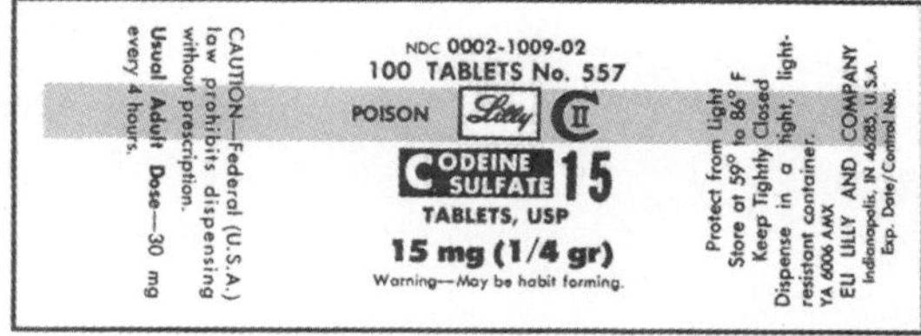

5. Your patient receives Keflex 0.5 g po qid. You have Keflex 250-mg capsules available. How many capsules will you administer? _______ .

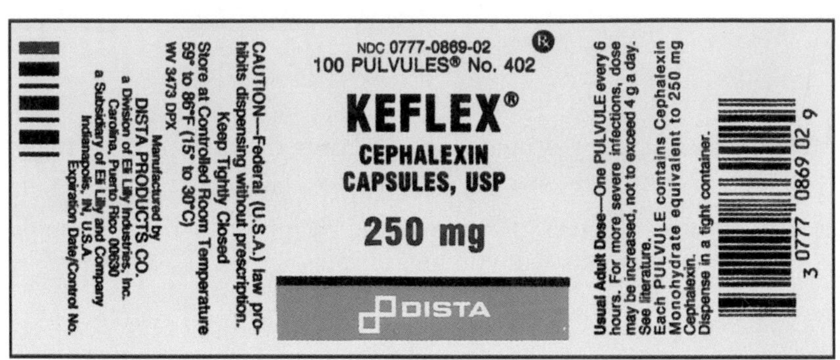

6. Your patient may receive Dilaudid 3 mg IM q3 h for relief of pain caused by a total hip replacement. Dilaudid is supplied in 1-ml ampules containing 4 mg. How many milliliters will you administer? _______ .

7. Mr. Grey receives Lanoxin 40 mcg po q12 h for treatment of cardiac dysrhythmias. Lanoxin, 0.05 mg per mL, is available. How many milliliters will the nurse administer? _______ .

60 mL NDC 0173-0264-27
LANOXIN®
(DIGOXIN)
ELIXIR
PEDIATRIC
Each mL contains
50 μg (0.05 mg)
PLEASANTLY FLAVORED
GlaxoWellcome
Glaxo Wellcome Inc.
Research Triangle Park, NC 27709
Made in U.S.A. Rev. 2/96 542404
Alcohol 10%, Methylparaben 0.1% (added as a preservative)
For indications, dosage, precautions, etc., see accompanying package insert.
Store at 15° to 25°C (59° to 77°F) and protect from light.
CAUTION: Federal law prohibits dispensing without prescription.
LOT
EXP

8. The physician prescribes Stadol 1 mg IV q4 h for a patient with a below-the-knee amputation. Stadol, 2 mg per mL, is available. How many milliliters will the nurse administer? _______ .

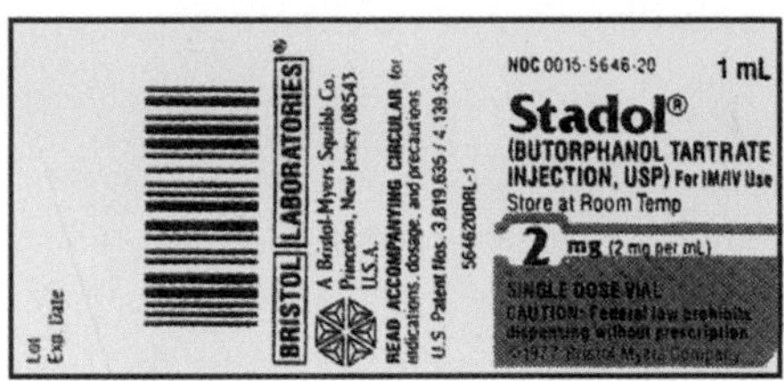

9. The physician orders heparin 2500 U SQ q12 h for your patient with a jejunostomy. You have heparin, 5000 U per mL, available. How many milliliters will you administer? _______ .

10. The physician has ordered Gantrisin 2 g po stat. Gantrisin is supplied in 500-mg tablets. How many tablets will the nurse administer? _______ .

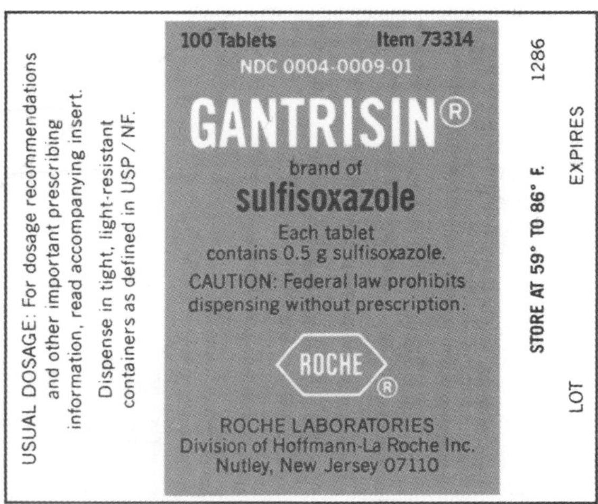

11. A patient with an infection has Timentin 3.1 g q6h IVPB ordered. The Timentin is dissolved in 100 mL of D5W and is to be infused over 1 hour. The tubing drop factor is 20 gtt/mL. At what rate, in drops per minute, should the IVPB be programmed? _______ .

12. A patient with anuria has an order for 500 mL of 0.9% NS over 2 hours. The tubing drop factor is 10 gtt/mL. At what rate, in drops per minute, should the IV pump be programmed? _______ .

13. A patient who takes Coumadin at home is admitted to the hospital before surgery to receive a regulated infusion of heparin. The heparin is ordered for 1400 U/h. The heparin bag concentration is heparin, 25,000 U in 250 mL of D5W. At what rate, in milliliters per hour, should the IV pump be programmed? _______ .

14. A patient with hyperglycemia has an order for regular insulin IV at a rate of 8 U/h. The concentration is insulin 50 U in 100 mL of 0.9% NS. At what rate, in milliliters per hour, will the IV pump be programmed? _______ .

Answers on pp. 438-439.

CHAPTER 12

Oral Dosages

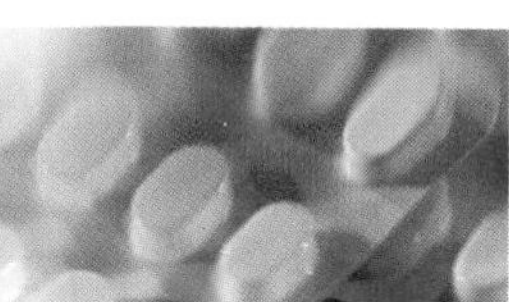

LEARNING OBJECTIVES

On completion of the materials provided in this chapter, you will be able to perform computations accurately by mastering the following mathematical concepts:

1. Converting all measures within the problem to equivalent measures in one system of measurement
2. Using a proportion to solve problems of oral dosage involving tablets, capsules, or liquid medications
3. Using a proportion to solve problems of oral dosages of medications measured in milliequivalents
4. Using the stated formula as an alternative method of solving oral-drug dosage problems

Oral drugs are preferred for administration of medications because they are easy to take and convenient for the patient. Oral medications are absorbed through the gastrointestinal tract; therefore the skin is not interrupted. Oral medications may be more economical because the production cost is usually lower than that for other forms of medication.

Oral medications are absorbed primarily in the small intestine. Because of the differences in absorption factors, they might not be as effective as other forms of medication. Some oral medications are irritating to the alimentary canal and must be given with meals or a snack. Others may be harmful to the teeth and should be taken through a straw or feeding tube.

Oral medications are supplied in a variety of forms (Figure 12-1). The most common form is a tablet. Tablets come in many colors, sizes, and shapes. A tablet is produced from a drug powder. The tablet may be grooved for ease in administering only a fraction of the whole tablet. Some tablets are scored into halves, and others are divided into fourths.

If a patient has difficulty swallowing pills, the pills may be crushed by using a mortar and pestle or a device that is specifically made for crushing pills (Figure 12-2).

Oral medications may also be supplied in capsule form. A capsule is a hard or soft gelatin that houses a powder, liquid, or granular form of a specific medicine(s). Capsules are produced in a variety of sizes and colors (Figure 12-3). Capsules cannot be divided or crushed.

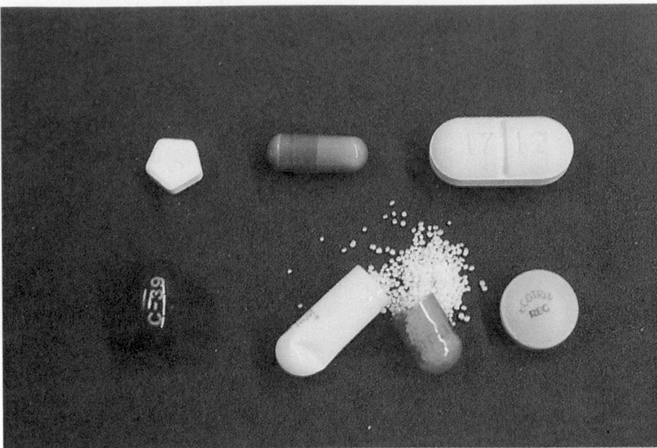

FIGURE 12-1 Forms of solid oral medication. (*Top row:* Uniquely shaped tablet, capsule, scored tablet. *Bottom row:* Gelatin-coated liquid, extended-release capsule, and enteric-coated tablet. (From Potter P, Perry A: *Fundamentals of nursing,* ed 5, St Louis, 2001, Mosby.)

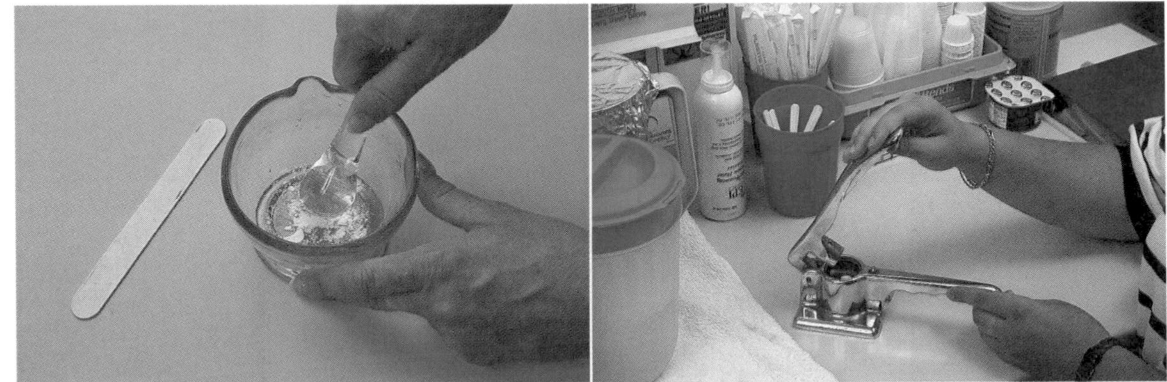

FIGURE 12-2 **A,** Mortar and pestle. **B,** Pill crusher. (From Elkin M, Perry P, Potter A: *Nursing interventions and clinical skills,* ed 2, St Louis, 2000, Mosby.)

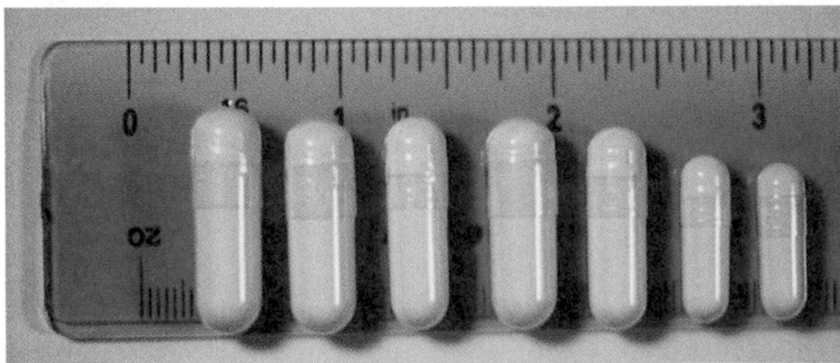

FIGURE 12-3 Various sizes and numbers of gelatin capsules (actual size).

Oral medications may also be administered in liquid form such as an elixir or an oral suspension. Oral liquid medications can be measured with a medication cup, syringe without the needle attached, or dropper (Figures 12-4, 12-5, and 12-6).

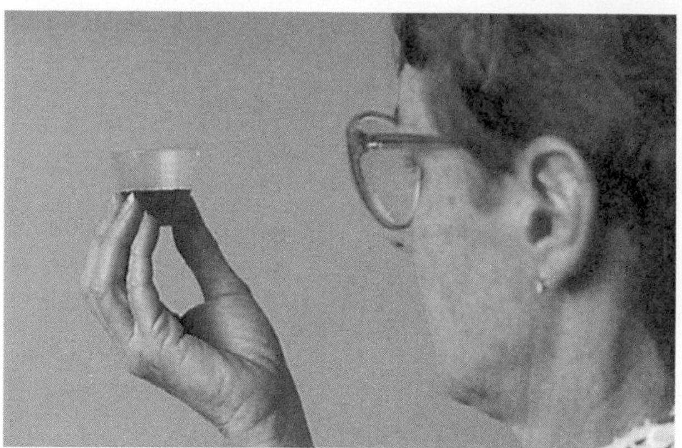

FIGURE 12-4 Oral liquid medication measured with a medication cup. (From Potter P, Perry A: *Fundamentals of nursing,* ed 5, St Louis, 2001, Mosby.)

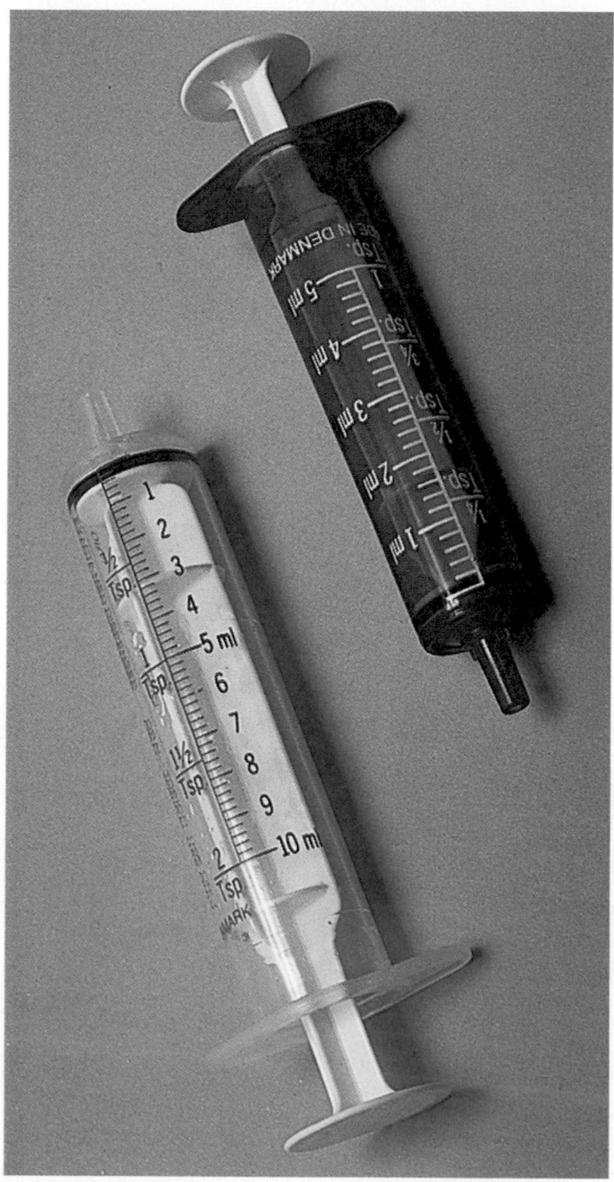

FIGURE 12-5 Plastic oral syringe. (From Clayton BD, Stock YN: *Basic pharmacology for nurses,* ed 12, St Louis, 2001, Mosby. Courtesy Chuck Dresner.)

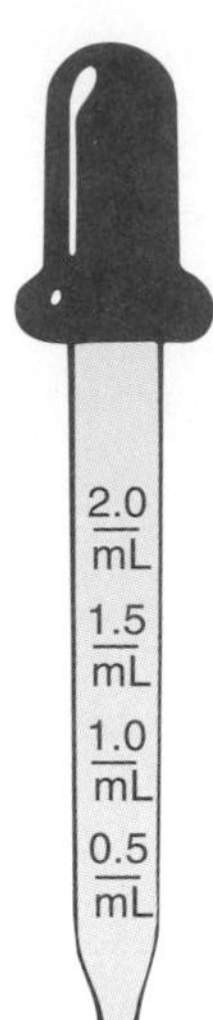

FIGURE 12-6 Medicine dropper. (From Clayton BD, Stock YN: *Basic pharmacology for nurses,* ed 12, St Louis, 2001, Mosby.)

Oral Dosages Involving Capsules and Tablets/Proportion Method

Sometimes the physician's order is in one system of measurement, and the drug is supplied in another system of measurement. It is therefore necessary to convert one of the measurements so that they are both in either the apothecary or the metric system of measurement. After this is done, another proportion will be written to calculate the actual drug dosage.

Example 1: Ordered ampicillin 0.5 g po qid. The drug is supplied in 250-mg capsules. How many capsules will the nurse administer? _______ .

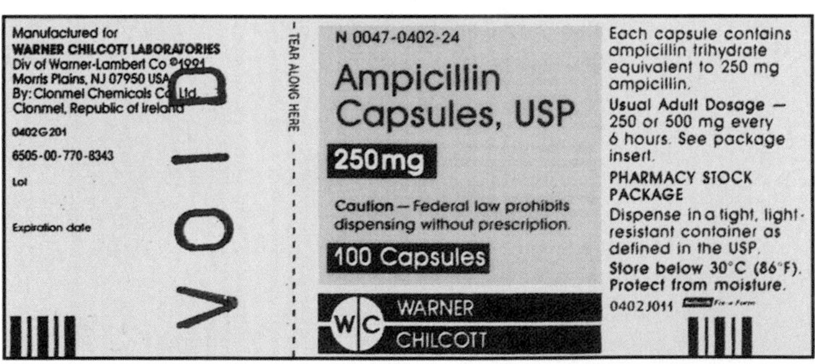

The physician's order is in grams and the drug is supplied in milligrams. The order and the supplied drug must be in the same metric measurement because only two different abbreviations can be used in each proportion. Therefore first convert 0.5 g to milligrams.

$$1000 \text{ mg} : 1 \text{ g} :: x \text{ mg} : 0.5 \text{ g}$$

$$1000 : 1 :: x : 0.5$$

$$1x = 1000 \times 0.5$$

$$x = 500 \text{ mg}$$

$$0.5 \text{ g} = 500 \text{ mg}$$

Now that the order and the supplied drug are in the same metric measurement, a proportion may be written to calculate the amount of the drug to be given.

a. 250 mg : 1 capsule ::
b. 250 mg : 1 capsule :: ______ mg : ______ capsule
   250 mg : 1 capsule :: 500 mg : x capsule
c. 250 : 1 :: 500 : x
d. $250x = 1 \times 500$

$$250x = 500$$

$$x = \frac{500}{250}$$

$$x = 2$$

e. $x = 2$ capsules. Therefore to give 0.5 g of the medication, the nurse will administer 2 capsules.

How many capsules will be given in 1 day? ______
The drug is to be given qid, or four times a day.

a. 2 capsules : 1 dose ::
b. 2 capsules : 1 dose :: ______ capsules : ______ dose
   2 capsules : 1 dose :: x capsules : 4 doses
c. 2 : 1 :: x : 4
d. $1x = 2 \times 4$
   $x = 8$
e. 8 capsules will be given each day.

Example 2: Ordered aspirin gr xx po qid. Aspirin tablets gr v are available. How many tablets will the nurse administer? ______ .

a. On the left side of the proportion place what you know or have available. In this example, each tablet contains 5 grains. So the left side of the proportion would be

1 tablet : 5 gr ::

b. The right side of the proportion is determined by the physician's order and the abbreviations used on the left side of the proportion. Only *two* different abbreviations may be used in a single proportion. The abbreviations must be in the same position on the right as they are on the left.

1 tablet : 5 gr :: ______ tablet : ______ gr

In the example, the physician has ordered gr xx or 20 grains.

1 tablet : 5 gr :: ______ tablet : 20 gr

We need to find the number of tablets to be given, so we use the symbol x to represent the unknown. Therefore the full proportion would be

1 tablet : 5 gr :: x tablet : 20 gr

c. Rewrite the proportion without using the abbreviations.

$$1 : 5 :: x : 20$$

d. Solve for x.

$$5x = 1 \times 20$$

$$5x = 20$$

$$x = \frac{20}{5}$$

$$x = 4$$

e. Label your answer, as determined by the abbreviation placed next to x in the original proportion.

20 gr = 4 tablets

Oral Dosages Involving Liquids/Proportion Method

Example 1: Ordered phenobarbital gr ¾ po bid. Phenobarbital elixir, 20 mg per 5 mL, is available. How many milliliters will the nurse administer? ______ .

Keep Tightly Closed
Store at Controlled Room Temperature 59° to 86° F (15° to 30° C)
WV 5931 AMX
Eli Lilly & Company, Indianapolis, IN 46285, U.S.A.
Expiration Date/Control No.
VOID

NDC **0002-2438-05**
16 fl oz (1 pt) (473 mL)
Lilly CIV
ELIXIR No. 227
PHENOBARBITAL ELIXIR, USP
Contains 20 mg Phenobarbital per 5 mL
WARNING—May be habit forming.
Contains Alcohol 14 Percent
CAUTION—Federal (U.S.A.) law prohibits dispensing without prescription.

Usual Adult Sedative Dose—60 mg (1 gr) (3 teaspoonfuls) two to four times a day.
Indiscriminate use may be harmful.
Dispense in a tight, light-resistant container.
3 0002 2438 05 9

The physician's order is in the apothecary system and the drug is available in the metric system. Both the order and the available drug must be in the same system of measurement. Therefore convert gr ¾ to milligrams.

$$60 \text{ mg} : 1 \text{ gr} :: x \text{ mg} : \tfrac{3}{4} \text{ gr}$$

$$60 : 1 :: x : \tfrac{3}{4}$$

$$x = \frac{\overset{15}{\cancel{60}}}{1} \times \frac{3}{\underset{1}{\cancel{4}}}$$

$$x = \frac{15 \times 3}{1 \times 1}$$

$$x = \frac{45}{1}$$

$$x = 45 \text{ mg}$$

$$\text{gr } \tfrac{3}{4} = 45 \text{ mg}$$

Now that the order and available drug are in the same system of measurement, a proportion may be written to calculate the actual amount of the drug to be administered.

a. 20 mg : 5 mL ::
b. 20 mg : 5 mL :: ______ mg : ______ mL
   20 mg : 5 mL :: 45 mg : x mL
c. 20 : 5 :: 45 : x
d. $20x = 5 \times 45$

$$20x = 225$$

$$x = \frac{225}{20}$$

$$x = 11.25$$

e. $x = 11.25$ mL. Therefore 11.25 mL is the amount of each individual dose bid.

Example 2: Ordered Thorazine 20 mg po q4 h. The drug is available in iv oz bottles of Thorazine syrup containing 10 mg per 5 mL. How many milliliters will the nurse administer? ______ . How many doses are available in iv oz? ______ .

1. a. 10 mg : 5 mL ::
   b. 10 mg : 5 mL :: ______ mg : ______ mL
      10 mg : 5 mL :: 20 mg : x mL
   c. 10 : 5 :: 20 : x
   d. $10x = 5 \times 20$

$$10x = 100$$

$$x = \frac{100}{10}$$

$$x = 10$$

   e. $x = 10$ mL. Therefore 10 mL is the amount of each individual dose q4 h.

2. The physician's order is in the metric system and the drug is supplied in the apothecary system. Both the order and the available drug must be in the same system of measurement. Therefore convert 10 mL to ounces, or the oz iv to milliliters, whichever is easier.

$$30 \text{ mL} : 1 \text{ fl oz} :: x \text{ mL} : 4 \text{ fl oz}$$

$$30 : 1 :: x : 4$$

$$x = 120$$

$$\text{iv oz bottle} = 120 \text{ mL}$$

Now that the order and available drug are in the same system of measurement, a proportion may be written to calculate the number of doses in a iv oz bottle.

a. 10 mL : 1 dose ::
b. 10 mL : 1 dose :: _______ mL : _______ dose
   10 mL : 1 dose :: 120 mL : x dose
c. 10 : 1 :: 120 : x
d. $10x = 120$

   $$x = \frac{120}{10}$$

   $$x = 12$$

e. $x = 12$ doses. Therefore each iv oz bottle contains 12 doses.

Oral Dosages Involving Milliequivalents/Proportion Method

Example: Ordered potassium chloride (KCl) 60 mEq tid with meals. KCl 40 mEq per 30 mL is available. How many milliliters will the nurse administer? _______ .

A **milliequivalent** is the number of grams of a solute contained in one milliliter of a normal solution. The milliequivalent is used in a drug dosage proportion, the same as a form of measurement in the apothecary or metric system.

a. 40 mEq : 30 mL ::
b. 40 mEq : 30 mL :: _______ mEq : _______ mL
   40 mEq : 30 mL :: 60 mEq : x mL
c. 40 : 30 :: 60 : x
d. $40x = 30 \times 60$

   $$40x = 1800$$

   $$x = \frac{1800}{40}$$

   $$x = 45$$

e. $x = 45$ mL. Therefore to give 60 mEq of the medication, the nurse will administer 45 mL.

Alternative Formula Method of Oral Drug Dosage Calculation

There is a formula that has been used for many years in the calculation of drug dosages by nurses. The formula method may be the method that some students learned first in an earlier nursing role (e.g., as a licensed practical nurse). If this is the case and the student accurately uses the formula method, I do not recommend changing to the proportion method. However, if calculations have frequently been difficult or incorrect, I recommend using the proportion method. Remember, choose the method that you feel is best for you and consistently use the chosen method. I do not recommend switching back and forth between the formula method and the proportion method. When you use the formula method, the desired and available amounts must be in the same units of measurement.

$$\text{Formula: } \frac{D}{A} \times Q = x$$

D represents the desired amount of the medication that has been ordered by the physician.

A represents the strength of the medication that is available.

Q represents the quantity or amount of the medication that contains the available strength. *(Note: When the medication is a solid such as a tablet, capsule, or caplet, the quantity will always be 1. If the medication is in liquid form, the number will vary. Remember from the math review, the denominator of a whole number is always one:* $\frac{1}{1}, \frac{2}{1}, \frac{3}{1}$, *etc.)*

x represents the dosage that is unknown.

This formula can be read as:

Desired over available multiplied by the quantity available equals x or the amount to be given to the patient.

Oral Dosages Involving Capsules and Tablets/Alternative Formula

If the physician's order is in one system of measurement and the drug is supplied in another system of measurement, it will still be necessary to convert one of the measurements so that both are expressed in the same system. After this is done, the formula may be used to calculate the drug dosage to be administered.

Example 1: Ordered ampicillin 0.5 g po qid. The drug is supplied in 250-mg capsules. How many capsules will the nurse administer? ______ .

The physician's order is expressed in grams and the drug is supplied in milligrams. Therefore convert the order to milligrams as outlined in Chapter 8.

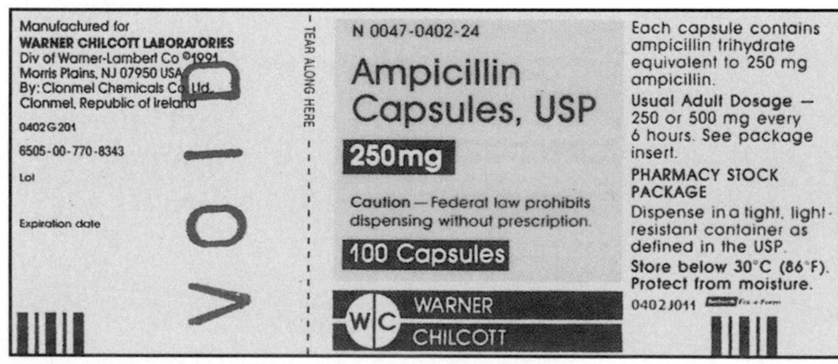

$$1000 \text{ mg} : 1 \text{ g} :: x \text{ mg} : 0.5 \text{ g}$$

$$1000 : 1 :: x : 0.5$$

$$1x = 1000 \times 0.5$$

$$x = 500 \text{ mg}$$

Now the numbers may be filled into the formula $\frac{D}{A} \times Q = x$.

a. The desired amount of ampicillin is 500 mg. The available amount or strength of ampicillin supplied is 250 mg.

$$\frac{500}{250}$$

b. The quantity available is in capsule form or 1.

$$\frac{500 \text{ mg}}{250 \text{ mg}} \times \frac{1 \text{ capsule}}{1 \text{ capsule}}$$

c. Rewrite the problem with the abbreviations cancelled.

$$\frac{500 \cancel{\text{mg}}}{250 \cancel{\text{mg}}} \times \frac{1 \cancel{\text{capsule}}}{1 \cancel{\text{capsule}}}$$

d. Solve for x.

$$x = \frac{500}{250} \times \frac{1}{1}$$

$$x = \frac{500 \times 1}{250 \times 1}$$

$$x = \frac{500}{250}$$

$$x = 2$$

e. Label your answer as determined by the quantity.

$$500 \text{ mg} = 2 \text{ capsules}$$

Example 2: Ordered aspirin gr xx po qid. Aspirin tablets gr v are available. How many tablets will the nurse administer? _______ .

$$\frac{D}{A} \times Q = x$$

a. The desired amount of aspirin is gr xx or 20 grains. The available amount or strength of the aspirin supplied is gr v or 5 grains.

$$\frac{20 \text{ gr}}{5 \text{ gr}}$$

b. The quantity of the medication for gr v is 1 tablet.

$$\frac{20 \text{ gr}}{5 \text{ gr}} \times \frac{1 \text{ tablet}}{1 \text{ tablet}}$$

c. Rewrite the problem with the abbreviations cancelled.

$$\frac{20 \cancel{\text{gr}}}{5 \cancel{\text{gr}}} \times \frac{1 \cancel{\text{tablet}}}{1 \cancel{\text{tablet}}}$$

d. We can now solve for x.

$$x = \frac{20}{5} \times \frac{1}{1}$$

$$x = \frac{20 \times 1}{5 \times 1}$$

$$x = \frac{20}{5}$$

$$x = 4$$

e. Label your answer as determined by the quantity.

20 grains = 4 tablets

Oral Dosages Involving Liquids/Alternative Formula

Example: Ordered phenobarbital gr ¾ po bid. Phenobarbital elixir 20 mg per 5 mL is available. How many milliliters will the nurse administer? _______ .

The physician's order is in the apothecary system and the drug is available in the metric system. Change the order to an equivalent within the metric system of measure as outlined in Chapter 8.

60 mg : 1 gr :: x mg : ¾ gr.

60 : 1 :: x : ¾

$$x = \frac{\overset{15}{\cancel{60}}}{1} \times \frac{3}{\underset{1}{\cancel{4}}}$$

$$x = 45$$

¾ gr = 45 mg

Now the numbers may be filled into the formula $\frac{D}{A} \times Q = x$.

a. The desired amount is 45 mg. The available amount or strength of phenobarbital is 20 mg.

$$\frac{45 \text{ mg}}{20 \text{ mg}}$$

b. The quantity available is 5 mL.

$$\frac{45 \text{ mg}}{20 \text{ mg}} \times \frac{5 \text{ mL}}{1 \text{ mL}}$$

c. Rewrite the problem with the abbreviations cancelled.

$$\frac{45 \cancel{\text{mg}}}{20 \cancel{\text{mg}}} \times \frac{5 \cancel{\text{mL}}}{1 \cancel{\text{mL}}}$$

d. Solve for x.

$$x = \frac{45}{20} \times \frac{5}{1}$$

$$x = \frac{45}{\underset{4}{\cancel{20}}} \times \frac{\overset{1}{\cancel{5}}}{1}$$

$$x = \frac{45 \times 1}{4 \times 1}$$

$$x = \frac{45}{4}$$

$$x = 11.25$$

e. Label your answer as determined by the quantity.

$$45 \text{ mg} = 11.25 \text{ mL}$$

Complete the following work sheet, which provides for extensive practice in the calculation of oral dosage problems. Use either the proportion or formula method. Check your answers. It is sometimes impossible to administer the exact amount ordered. All capsules and tablets that are not scored are impossible to divide accurately. If the exact answer contains a fraction less than one half, drop the fraction and give the number of capsules or tablets indicated by the whole number. If the fraction is one half or more and the capsule or tablet is not scored, round off to the nearest whole number to determine the number of tablets or capsules to be given. Note that in actual practice the physician would need to be notified and the order for the amount of medication changed to allow for giving more than the original prescribed amount. If you have difficulties, go back and review the necessary material. When you feel ready to evaluate your learning, take the first posttest. Check your answers. An acceptable score as indicated on the posttest signifies that you are ready for the next chapter. An unacceptable score signifies a need for further study before taking the second posttest.

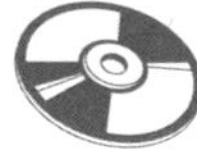

Refer to Calculating Dosages: Introduction and Oral Dosages for additional help and practice problems.

WORK SHEET

Directions: The medication order is listed at the beginning of each problem. Calculate the oral dosages. Show your work. Shade each medicine cup or plastic oral syringe when provided to indicate the correct dosage.

1. The physician orders Minipress 2 mg po bid for Mr. Shaw's high blood pressure. How many capsules will the nurse administer? _______ .

RECOMMENDED STORAGE
STORE BELOW 86° F (30° C)
Dispense in tight, light resistant containers (USP).
†Each capsule contains prazosin hydrochloride equivalent to 1 mg of prazosin.
Manufactured by Pfizer Pharmaceuticals, Inc., Barceloneta, P.R. 00617
4444
6505-01-039-6320
NDC0663-4310-71
250 Capsules
Minipress®
prazosin hydrochloride
1 mg†
CAUTION: Federal law prohibits dispensing without prescription.
Distributed by Pfizer LABORATORIES DIVISION New York, N.Y. 10017
READ ACCOMPANYING PROFESSIONAL INFORMATION
DOSAGE: See accompanying prescribing information.
IMPORTANT: This closure is not child-resistant.

2. Mrs. Taylor has a long history of seizures. Elixir of phenobarbital 30 mg po q12 h is ordered. How many milliliters will the nurse administer? _______ .

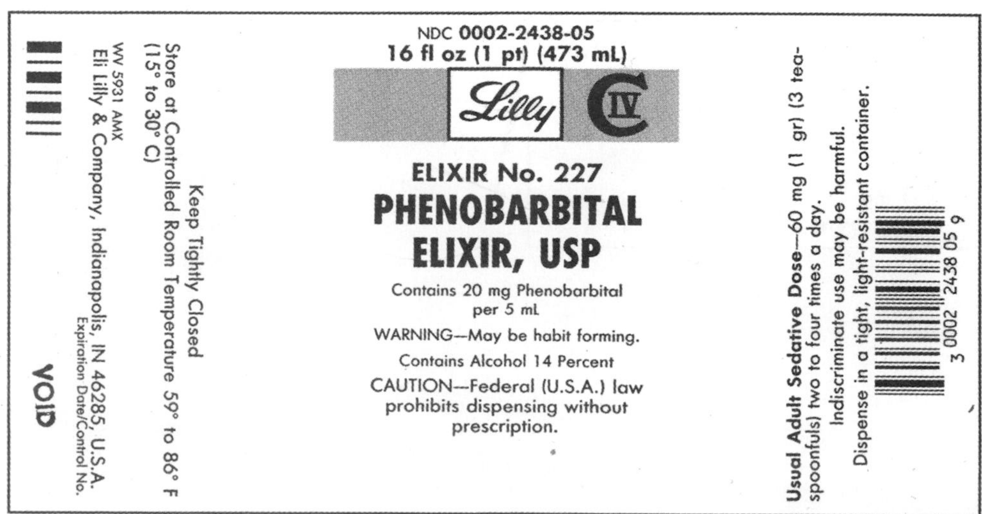

3. Ordered Crystodigin 0.2 mg po bid for 4 days, then 0.15 mg qd. You have Crystodigin 0.05-mg tablets available. How many tablets will you give for each dose the first 4 days? _______ . How many tablets will you give for each dose thereafter? _______ .

4. Mr. Davis has a diagnosis of acute maxillary sinusitis. His physician orders Biaxin 500 mg q12 h × 10 days. How many tablets will the nurse administer? _______ .

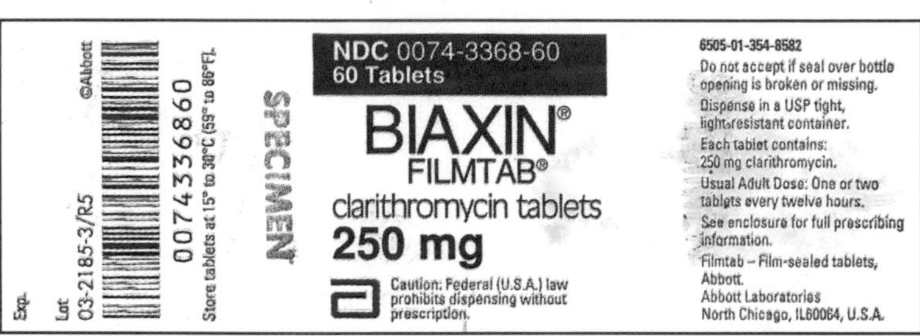

5. Mrs. Clay complains of nausea. Compazine 2.5 mg po tid is ordered. The stock supply is Compazine syrup 5 mg per 5 mL. How many milliliters will the nurse administer? _______ .

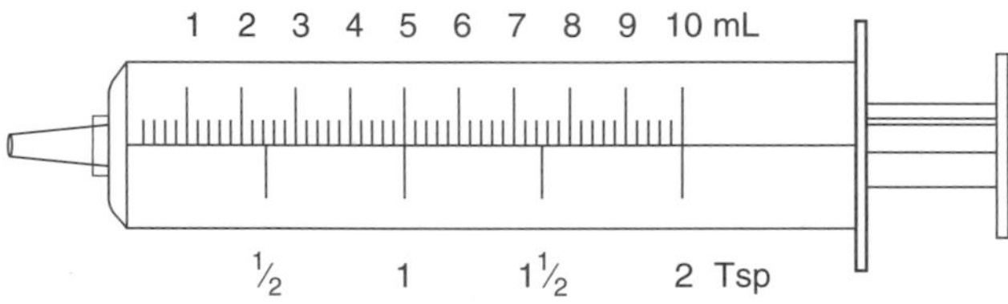

6. Ordered Ativan 2 mg hs. How many tablets will the nurse administer? _______ .

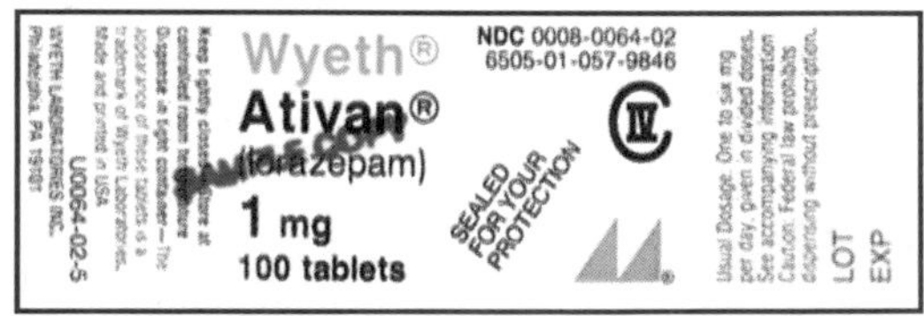

7. Ordered Pravachol 20 mg po qhs. How many tablets will the nurse administer? ______ .

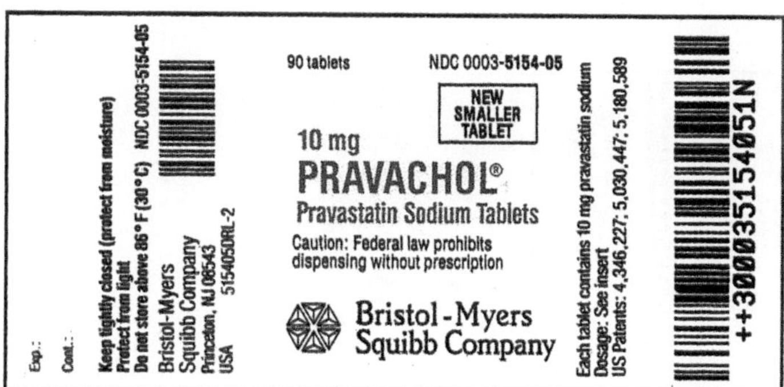

8. Mandelamine 1 g po qid is scheduled for Mr. Eaton to treat his urinary tract infection. You have 0.5-g tablets available. How many tablets will you administer? ______ .

9. Ordered Prozac 40 mg po qd in AM. How many milliliters will the nurse administer? ______ .

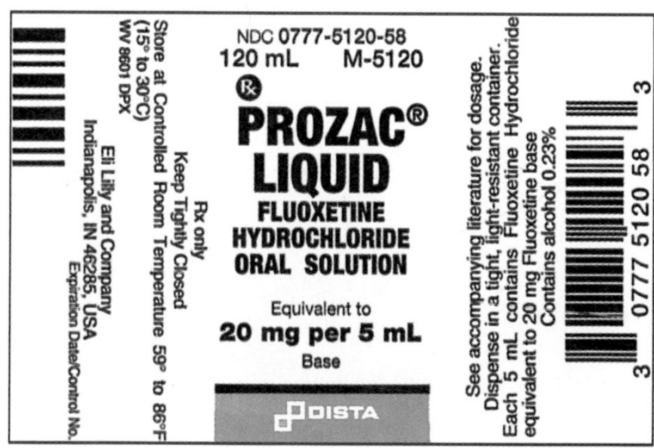

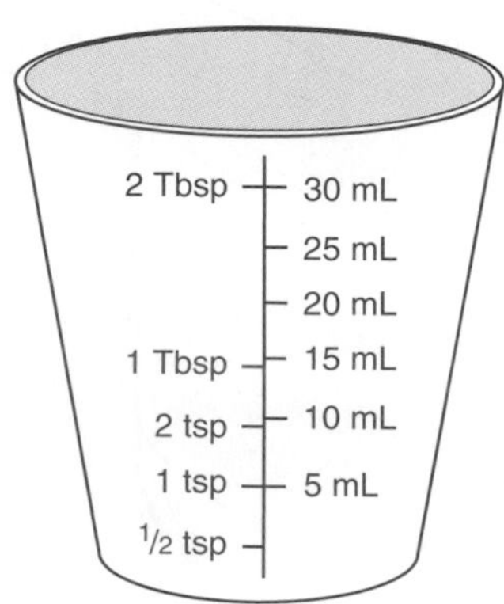

10. Mr. Scott has Parkinson's disease and is to receive Cogentin 1 mg po at 1900. How many tablets will the nurse administer? _______ .

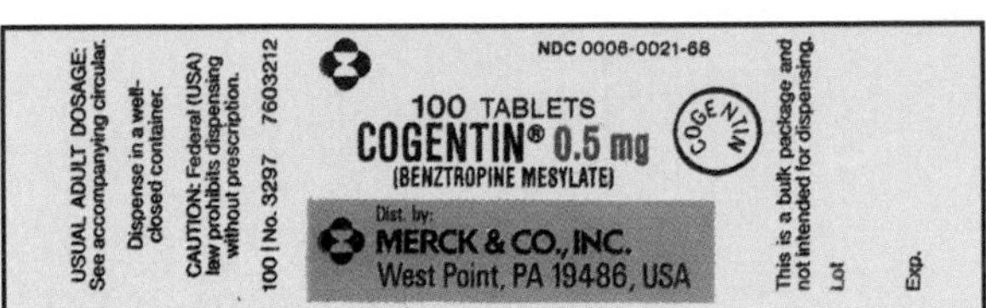

11. Mrs. Martin receives Motrin 300 mg po tid for arthritis pain. The drug is supplied in gr v tablets. How many tablets will the nurse administer? _______ .

12. Ordered lithium carbonate 0.6 g po bid. The drug is supplied in 300-mg scored tablets. How many tablets will the nurse administer? _______ . How many milligrams will be given each day? _______ .

13. Your patient has Naprosyn 0.25 g po bid ordered for relief of chronic back pain. You have Naprosyn 500-mg scored tablets available. How many tablets will you administer? _______ .

14. Mr. Hill is to receive Persantine 25 mg po bid after valve surgery. Persantine 50-mg tablets are available. How many tablets will the nurse administer? _______ .

15. The physician has ordered ferrous sulfate ($FeSO_4$) 300 mg po qd to treat Mrs. Basey's anemia. You have $FeSO_4$ gr v tablets available. How many tablets will you administer? _______ .

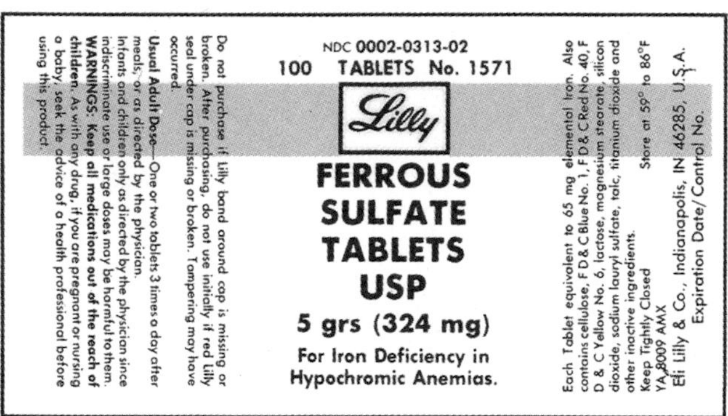

16. Ordered Gantrisin 4 g po stat, then 2 g q6 h. How many tablets will be given for the stat dose? _______ . How many tablets will be given for each of the 2-g doses? _______ .

100 Tablets Item 73314
NDC 0004-0009-01
GANTRISIN®
brand of
sulfisoxazole
Each tablet contains 0.5 g sulfisoxazole.
CAUTION: Federal law prohibits dispensing without prescription.
ROCHE®
ROCHE LABORATORIES
Division of Hoffmann-La Roche Inc.
Nutley, New Jersey 07110
USUAL DOSAGE: For dosage recommendations and other important prescribing information, read accompanying insert.
Dispense in tight, light-resistant containers as defined in USP/NF.
1286
STORE AT 59° TO 86° F.
EXPIRES
LOT

17. Ordered acyclovir 800 mg po q 4 hours while awake. Acyclovir 400-mg tablets are available. How many tablets will the nurse administer? _______ .

18. Ordered Gaviscon 30 mL po qid pc hs. Gaviscon is supplied in xii oz bottles. Each dose is equal to _______ oz. How many ounces will be given in 1 day? _______ .

19. Ms. Evans complains of a rash on her abdomen and has Benadryl 30 mg po tid ordered. How many milliliters will the nurse administer? _______ .

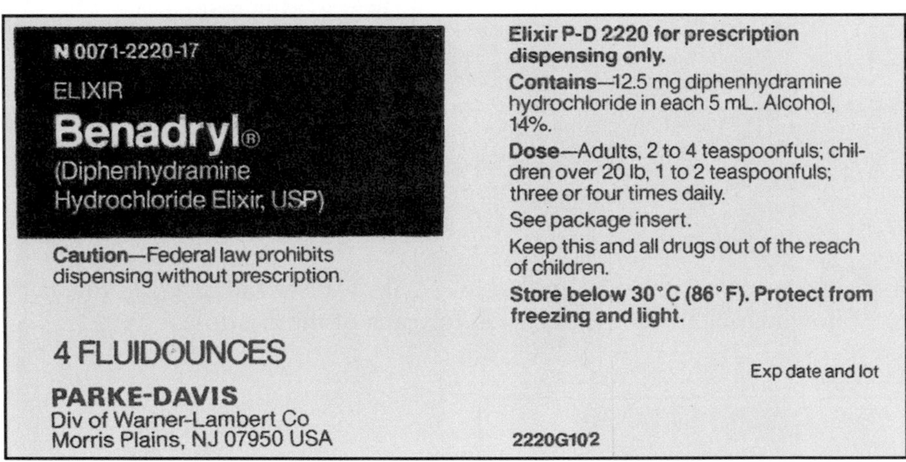

20. Mr. Gifford has had a lumbar laminectomy and requires pain medication. The patient has an order for codeine 60 mg po q3 h prn. How many tablets will the nurse administer? _______ .

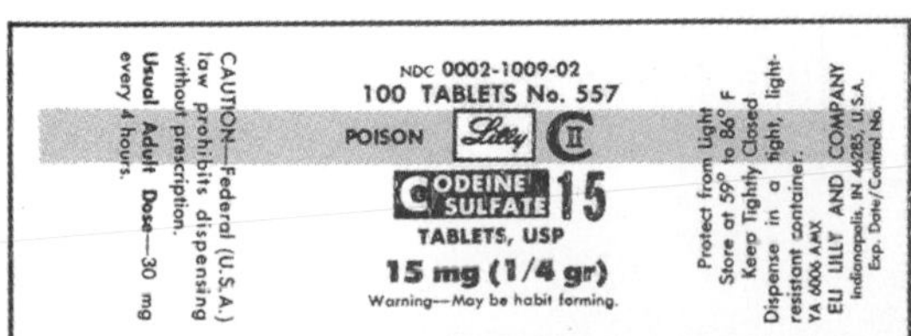

21. The physician orders Keflex suspension 5.5 mL po q6 h for your patient who had a tonsillectomy. How many milligrams will you administer every 6 hours? _______

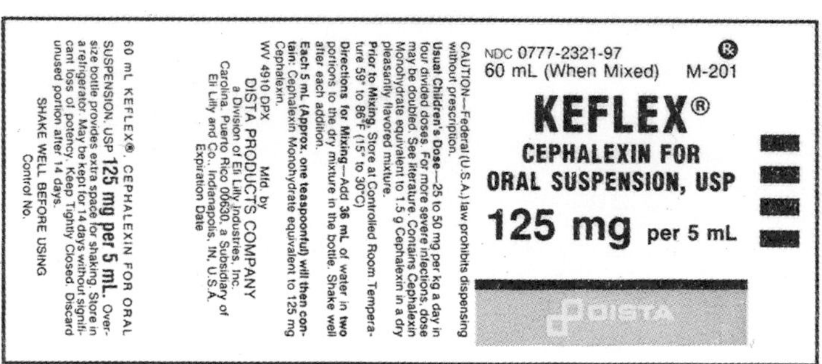

22. Mr. Sawyer is admitted with congestive heart failure. His orders require Lasix 80 mg po qd. How many tablets will the nurse administer? _______ .

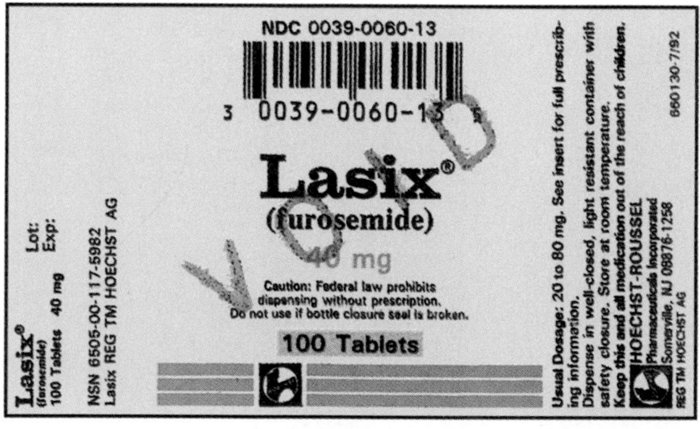

23. Ordered Nitroglycerin 1⁄150 gr SL prn for angina. Take no more than 3 tablets in 15 minutes. Mr. Cane took 2 tablets. How many milligrams did he receive? _______ .

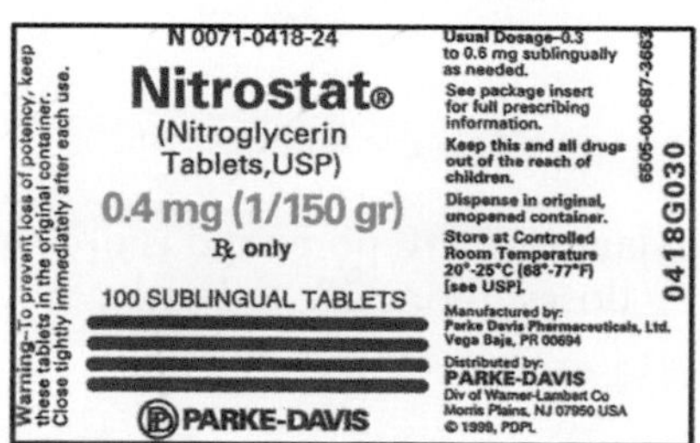

24. Mr. Koehler has rheumatoid arthritis and has Decadron 1.5 mg po q12 h ordered. You have Decadron elixir 0.5 mg per 5 mL. How many milliliters will you administer? _______ . How many ounces will you administer? _______ .

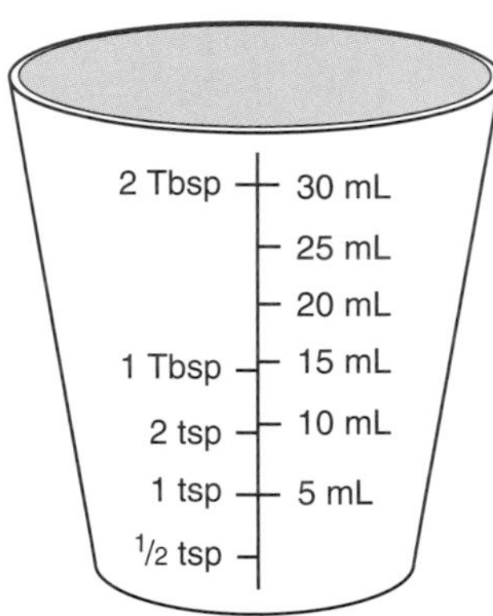

25. Your patient with chronic hiccups has Thorazine 15 mg po q4 h ordered. The drug is available in 4 oz bottles of Thorazine syrup containing 10 mg per 5 mL. How many milliliters will you administer? _______ .

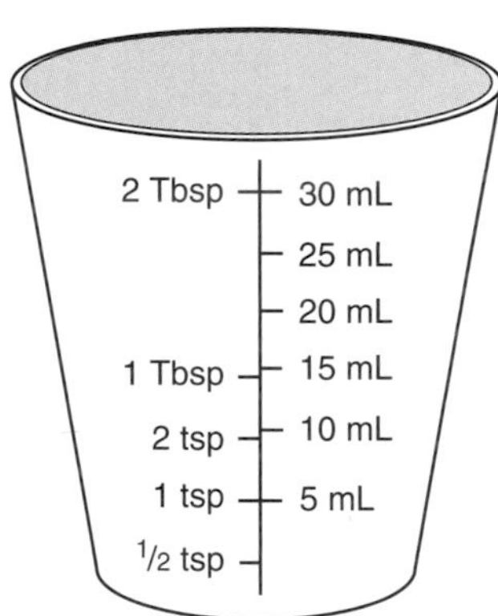

26. Mrs. Turner is admitted with hypertension. Apresoline 25 mg po qid is ordered. You have 50-mg scored tablets available. How many tablets will you administer? _______ .

27. Your patient complains of indigestion during meals. Mylanta 30 mL po pc qid is ordered. Mylanta is supplied in a 12-oz bottle. There are _______ doses in one 12-oz bottle. How many ounces will you administer? _______ .

28. Ordered Thorazine 200 mg po stat. The drug is available in 100-mg tablets. How many tablets will the nurse administer? _______ .

29. Mr. Bates has a history of seizure activity. Phenobarbital 15 mg po q3 h is ordered. How many tablets will the nurse administer? _______ .

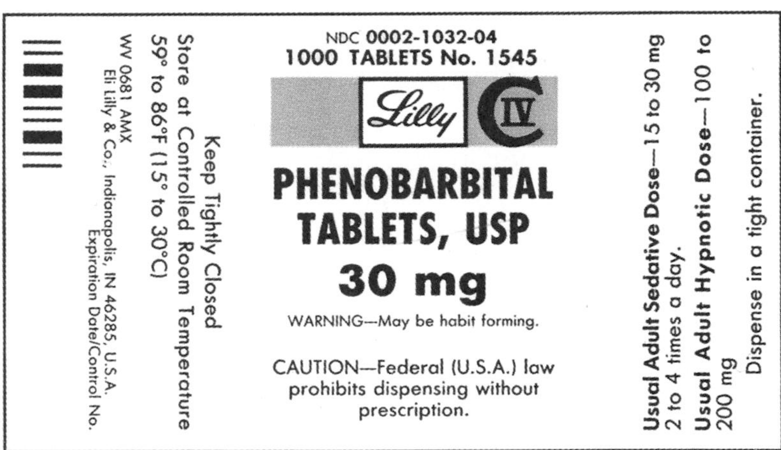

30. Mrs. Turner has chronic sinusitis. Her physician orders amoxicillin 125 mg po q8 h. How many milliliters will the nurse administer? _______ .

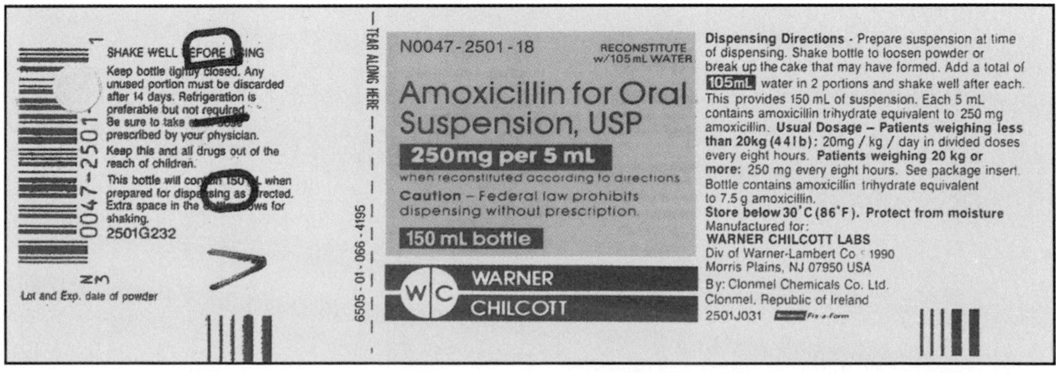

31. The physician prescribes Tenormin 25 mg po q4 h for Mr. Hutton's high blood pressure. You have Tenormin 50-mg scored tablets available. How many tablets will you administer? _______ .

32. Ordered Quinidine 0.6 g po q4 h. Quinidine is supplied in 200-mg tablets. How many tablets will you give for one dose? _______ . How many tablets will you give in 24 hours? _______ .

33. Mrs. Farmer has Phenergan 12.5 mg po tid ordered for relief of nausea. The drug is available in syrup containing 6.25 mg per 5 mL. How many milliliters will the nurse administer? _______ .

34. Your patient has Cipro 750 mg po q12 h ordered for a severe respiratory tract infection. You have Cipro oral suspension 500 mg/5 mL available. How many milliliters will you administer? _______ .

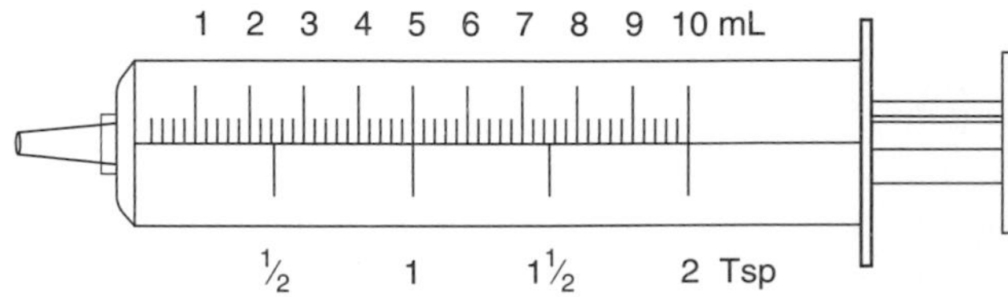

35. Mr. Golden, recovering from a left great toe amputation, has Colace elixir 100 mg po hs ordered for constipation. How many milliliters will the nurse administer? _______ .

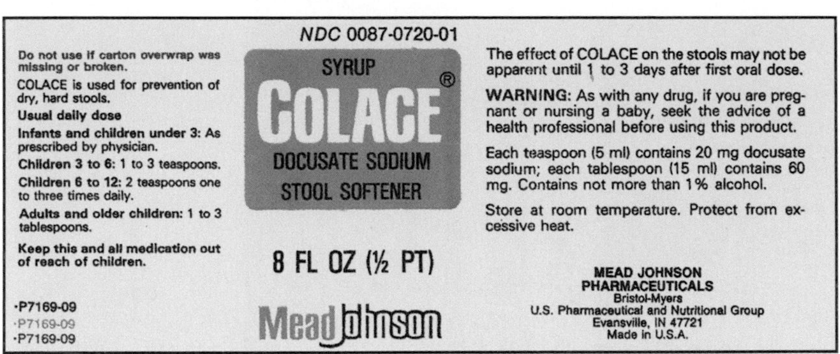

36. Your patient receives KCl 80 mEq po qd for hypokalemia. How many milliliters will you administer? _______ .

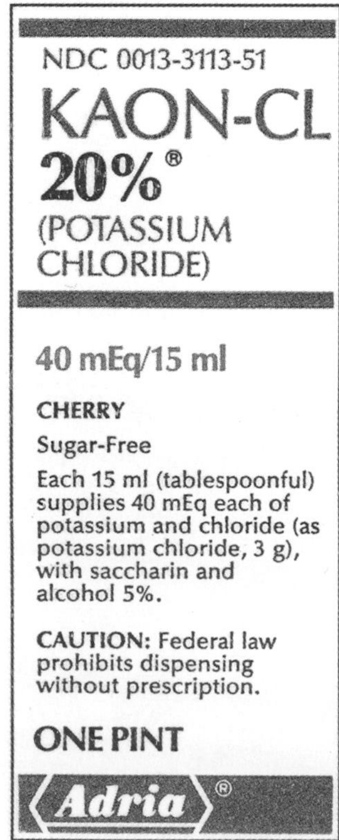

37. Mr. Mikal was admitted for treatment of leukemia and receives Deltasone 7.5 mg po tid as part of his chemotherapy. The drug is available in 2.5-mg tablets. How many tablets will the nurse administer? _______ .

38. The physician orders Tegretol 0.2 g po tid for Mr. Pine's epilepsy. How many tablets will the nurse administer? _______ .

Exp
Lot
NDC 0028-0052-01 FSC 1852 643322
Tegretol® 100 mg
carbamazepine USP
Chewable Tablets
100 tablets
Caution: Federal law prohibits dispensing without prescription.
Geigy
GEIGY Pharmaceuticals Div. of CIBA-GEIGY Corp. Ardsley, NY 10502
Dispense in tight container (USP).
Protect from moisture.
Dosage: See package insert.

39. Elixir of Tylenol gr v po tid is ordered for Mrs. Lindl's dysmenorrhea. You have the drug containing 160 mg per 5 mL. How many milliliters will you administer? _______ .

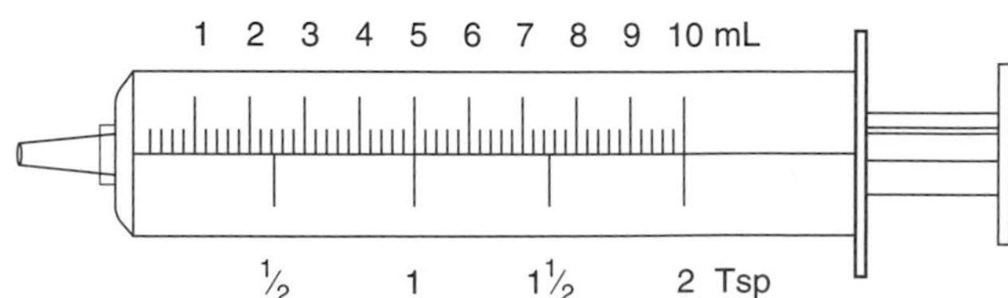

40. Mrs. Cross was admitted with a myasthenia crisis. Decadron 0.5 mg po q12 h is ordered. How many tablets will the nurse administer? _______ .

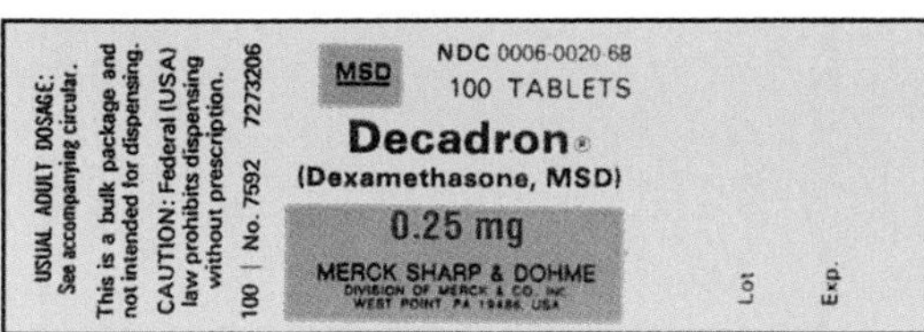

41. Mr. Cook requires medication for nausea. Compazine 10 mg po q4 h prn is ordered. You have Compazine 5-mg tablets available. How many tablets will you administer? _______ .

42. Mr. Pace receives Atarax 100 mg po hs prn to relieve anxiety. You have 50-mg tablets available. How many tablets will you administer? _______ .

43. The physician orders thyroid gr ss po qid for Mrs. Grass's hormone replacement. How many tablets will the nurse administer? _______ .

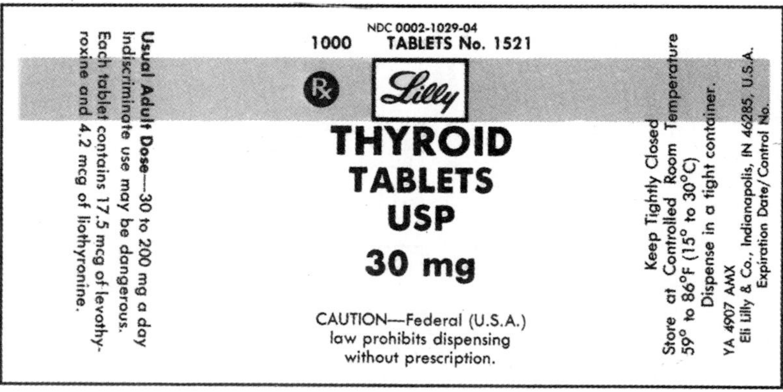

44. Mr. Day receives Lanoxin 0.25 mg po qd for atrial fibrillation. How many tablets will the nurse administer? _______ .

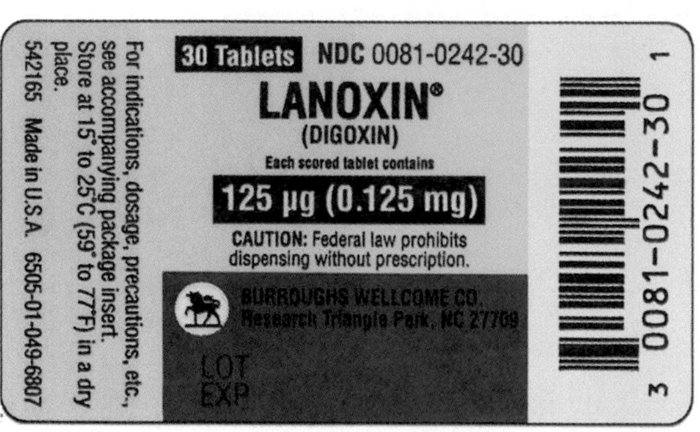

45. Mr. Payne receives Keflex 500 mg po qid before his dental extraction. How many capsules will the nurse administer in each dose? _______ . How many capsules will the nurse administer for 1 day? _______ .

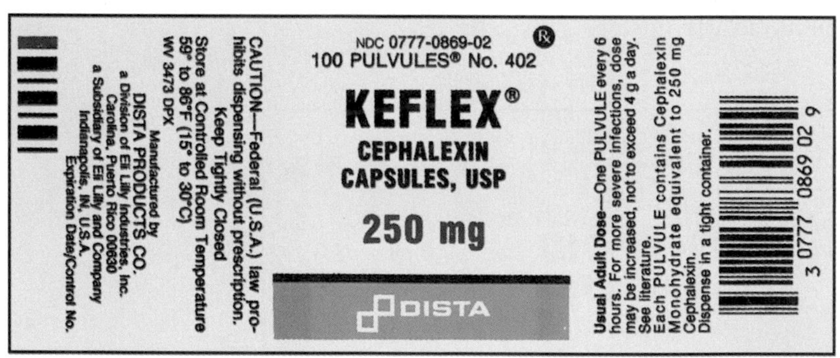

46. Mr. Tune is admitted with pancreatitis and receives Valium 5 mg po q6 h prn for anxiety. You have 10-mg tablets available. How many tablets will you administer? _______ .

47. Mrs. Graves receives phenobarbital tablets gr i ss po q3 h prn for seizure activity. How many tablets will the nurse administer? _______ .

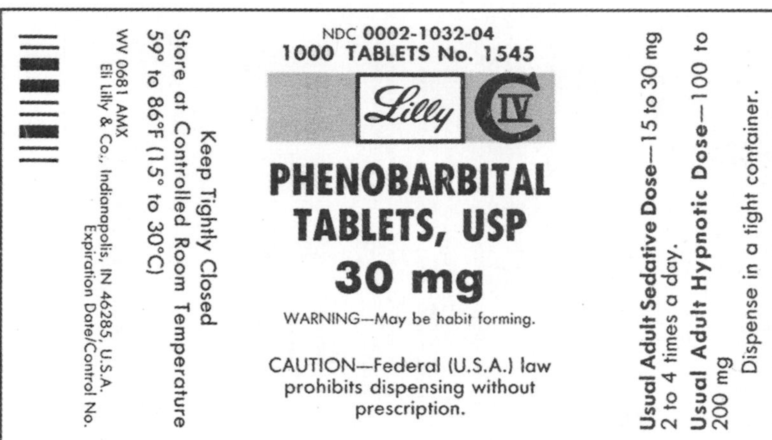

48. The physician prescribes a supplement of KCl 2 mEq po q8 h for Mr. Vee, admitted with chronic abdominal pain. How many milliliters will the nurse administer? _______ .

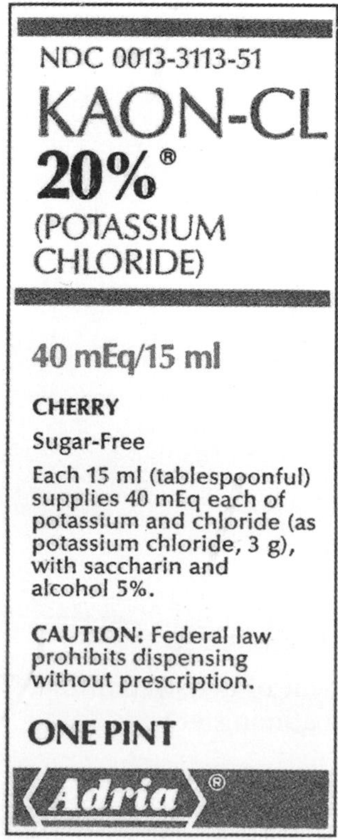

49. Mr. Sahl, recovering from a coronary artery bypass graft, receives aspirin gr x po q3 h. How many tablets will the nurse administer? _______ .

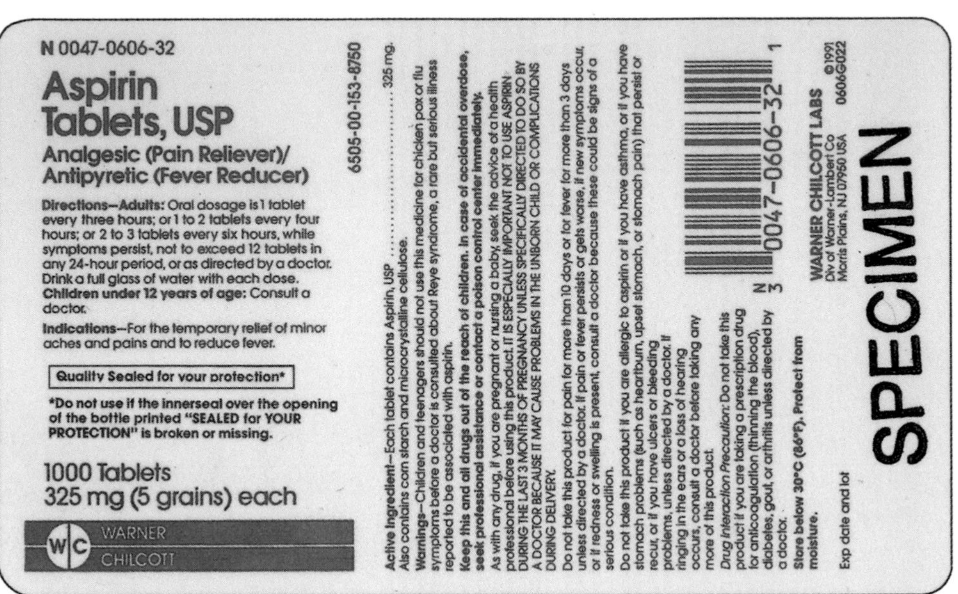

50. Mr. Dale has Zantac 150 mg bid as part of his treatment for esophagitis. How many milliliters will the nurse administer? _______ .

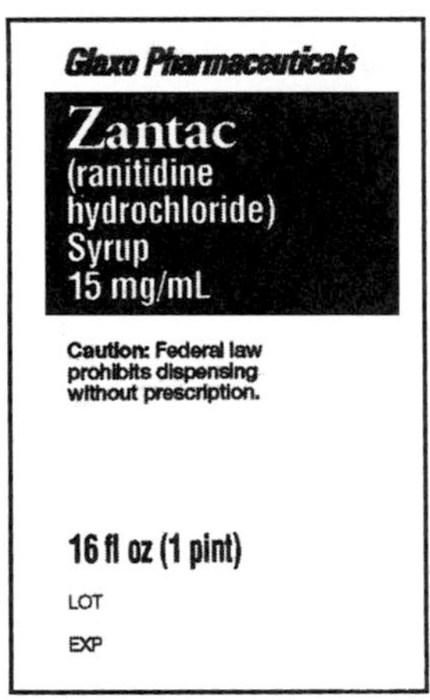

51. Mrs. Line has erythromycin prescribed 1 g po q6 h for treatment of her strep throat. You have 250-mg capsules available. How many capsules will you administer? _______ .

52. The physician prescribes $FeSO_4$ v gr po tid as a supplement for Mr. Bay, a patient who has undergone cardiac catheterization. How many tablets will the nurse administer? _______ . How many milligrams will be given? _______ .

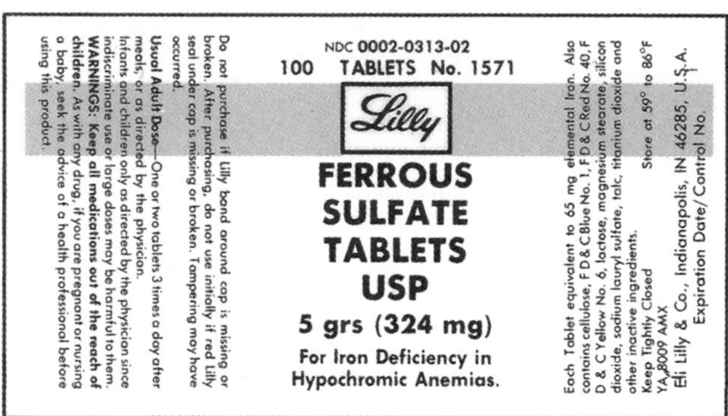

53. Mr. Jones, admitted with chronic obstructive lung disease, takes Bentyl 20 mg po tid ac. The drug is available in 10-mg capsules. How many capsules will the nurse administer? _______ .

54. Mrs. Tyth has pruritic dermatoses. The physician prescribes Atarax 30 mg po bid as part of her therapy. The drug is supplied in syrup containing 10 mg per 5 mL. How many milliliters will the nurse administer? _______ .

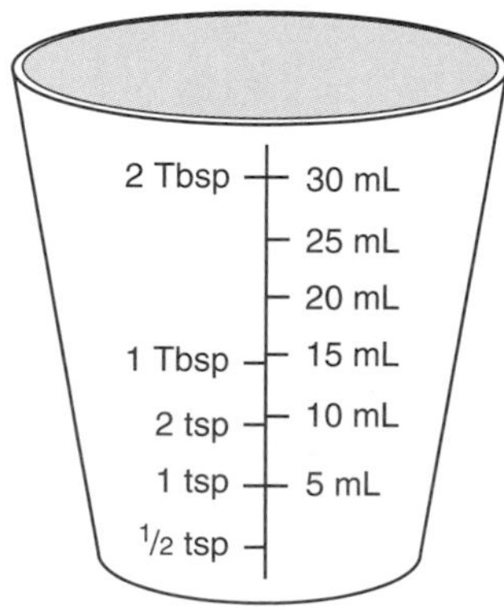

55. Mrs. Gale, admitted for alcohol abuse, has an order for ascorbic acid 0.75 g po daily while hospitalized. You have 250-mg tablets available. How many tablets will you administer? _______ .

56. Your patient with chronic pancreatitis has an order for Phenergan 25 mg po q4 h prn for relief of nausea. The drug is supplied in 12.5-mg tablets. How many tablets will the nurse administer? _______ .

57. Mr. Nade, hospitalized for a radical neck dissection, has Vistaril 15 mg po qid ordered to suppress nausea. You have Vistaril 25 mg per 5 mL available. How many milliliters will you administer? _______ .

58. Mrs. Snell requires Lopressor 100 mg bid. How many tablets will the nurse administer? _______ .

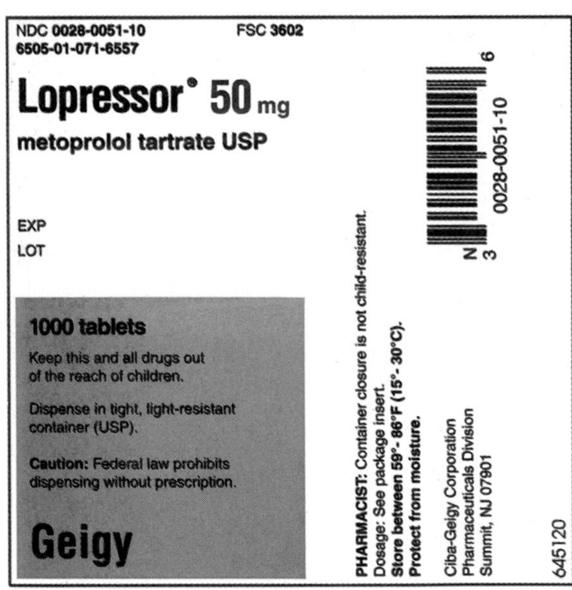

59. Your patient with acute rheumatoid arthritis receives Celebrex 200 mg bid. You have 100-mg capsules available. How many capsules will you administer? _______ .

60. Mr. Aden requires Chloromycetin 250 mg po q6 h for treatment of a *Salmonella* infection. You have Chloromycetin 150 mg per 5 mL available. How many milliliters will you administer? _______ .

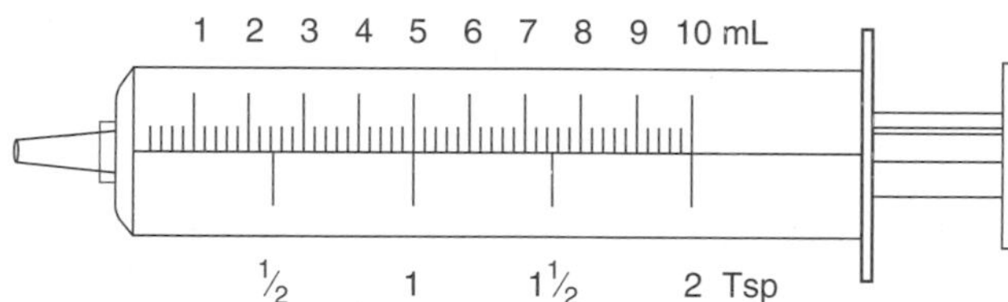

61. Mr. Scheottle receives Vibramycin 100 mg po q12 h for treatment of inclusion conjunctivitis. How many milliliters will the nurse administer? _______ .

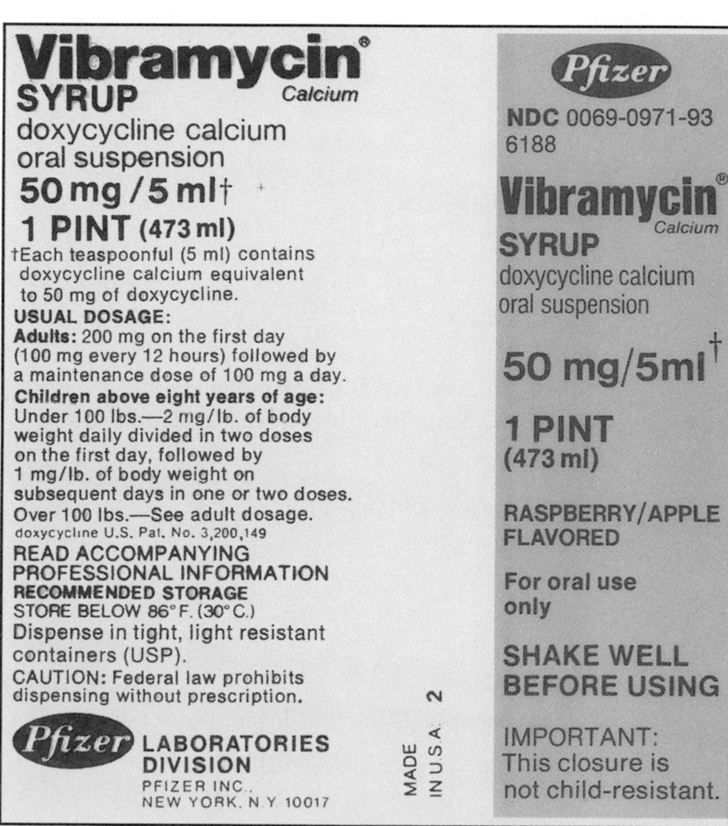

62. Your patient, admitted for cardiac catheterization, receives HydroDiuril 25 mg po bid for hypertension. You have 50-mg scored tablets available. How many tablets will you administer? _______ .

63. Tylenol 240 mg po q4 h is ordered for a temperature of 38.9° C. You have Tylenol 80-mg chewable tablets available. How many tablets will be required for each dose? _______ .

64. The physician prescribes Lanoxin elixir 90 mcg po bid for your patient with atrial fibrillation. How many milliliters will you administer? _______ .

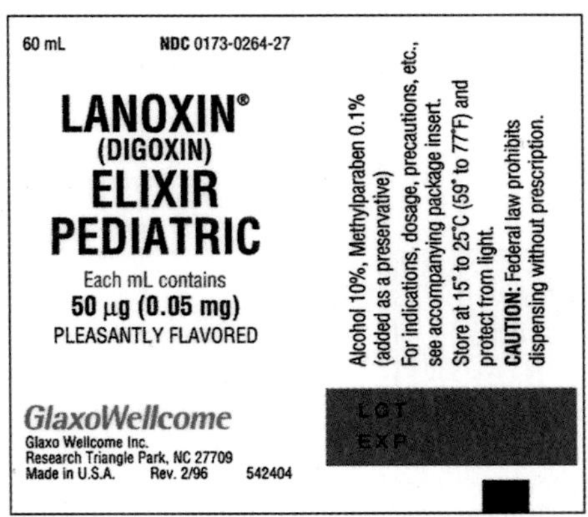

65. Mr. Ceney, admitted for contact dermatitis, receives elixir of Benadryl 10 mL po q6 h prn for relief of itching. The drug is supplied as 12.5 mg per 5 mL. This dose delivers _______ mg.

66. Ordered Orinase 0.5 g po tid. Orinase 500-mg tablets are available. How many tablets will the nurse administer? _______ .

67. Your patient receives Dilantin gr i ss po tid for past seizure activity. How many capsules will you administer? _______ .

Pediatric Dose—Initially, 5 mg/kg daily in two or three equally divided doses, with subsequent dosage individualized to a maximum of 300 mg daily.
See package insert for complete prescribing information.
Keep this and all drugs out of the reach of children.
0365G041

N 0071-0365-24
KAPSEALS®
Dilantin®
(Extended Phenytoin Sodium Capsules, USP)
30 mg
Caution—Federal law prohibits dispensing without prescription.
100 CAPSULES
PARKE-DAVIS
Div of Warner-Lambert Co
Morris Plains, NJ 07950 USA

Dispense in tight, light-resistant container as defined in the USP.
Store below 30°C (86°F). Protect from light and moisture.
NOTE TO PHARMACIST—Do not dispense capsules which are discolored.
Exp date and lot

68. Lipitor 40 mg po qd. You have available 10-mg, 20-mg, and 40-mg tablets. Which tablet would be most appropriate? _______ . How many tablets will you administer? _______ .

69. Your patient, admitted with a small-bowel obstruction, has KCl 10 mEq po qd ordered for his low potassium level. The drug is available as a liquid in KCl 20 mEq per 15 mL. How many milliliters will you administer? _______ .

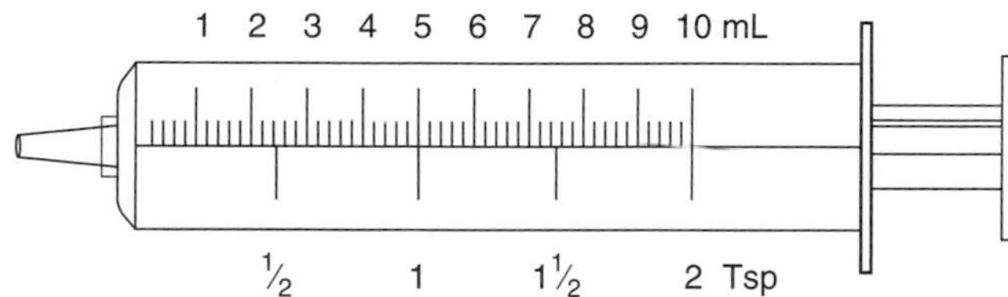

70. Mr. Brown receives Nalfon 300 mg po with meals or a snack for his osteoarthritis. How many tablets will the nurse administer? _______ .

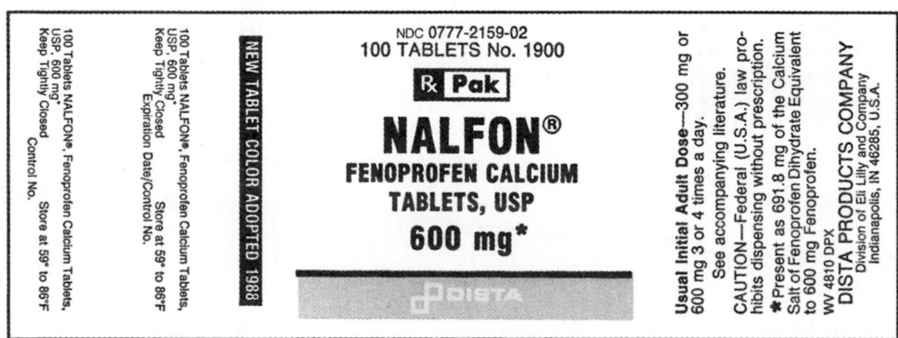

71. Mrs. Roget has been receiving digoxin 0.5 mg po qd for her cardiac dysrhythmia. The drug is available in 0.25-mg tablets. How many tablets will the nurse administer? _______ .

72. Acetaminophen 650 mg po q4 h is prescribed for a temperature of more than 38.5° C × 24 h. How many milliliters will the nurse administer every 4 hours? _______ .

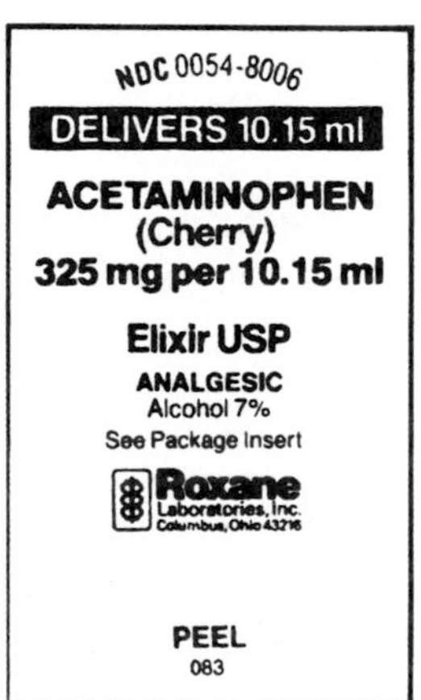

73. The physician prescribes Decadron 0.5 mg po q12 h for your patient's keratitis. How many tablets will you administer? _______ .

USUAL ADULT DOSAGE
See accompanying circular.
This is a bulk package and not intended for dispensing.
CAUTION: Federal (USA) law prohibits dispensing without prescription.
100 | No. 7592 7273206
MSD
NDC 0006-0020-68
100 TABLETS
Decadron®
(Dexamethasone, MSD)
0.25 mg
MERCK SHARP & DOHME
DIVISION OF MERCK & CO., Inc.
WEST POINT, PA 19486, USA
Lot
Exp.

74. Mr. Pein receives Keflex fl oz ss po q6 h after his thyroidectomy. How many milliliters will the nurse administer? _______ .

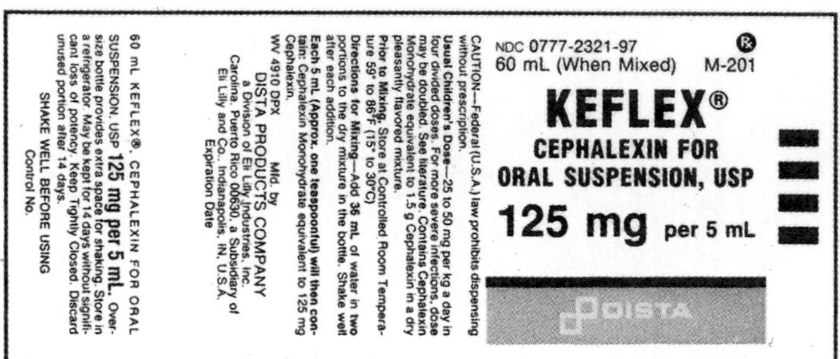

75. Your patient, who has undergone a lumbar laminectomy, receives Demerol 30 mg po q4 h prn for pain relief. The drug is supplied 50 mg per 5 mL. How many milliliters will you administer? _______ .

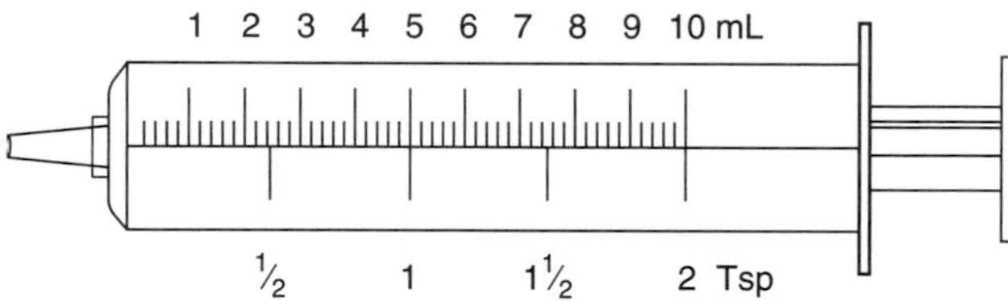

76. Ordered Crystodigin gr 1/200 po qd. You have Crystodigin in 0.05-mg, 0.15-mg, and 0.2-mg tablets. The best way to administer this drug is to give _______ tablets of _______ mg each.

77. Mr. Zeman has prednisone 7.5 mg po qd ordered for exfoliative dermatitis. Prednisone is supplied in 5-mg scored tablets. How many tablets will the nurse administer? _______ .

78. Your patient who has had a partial craniotomy has V-Cillin K suspension 250 mg po qid ordered. How many milliliters will you administer? _______ .

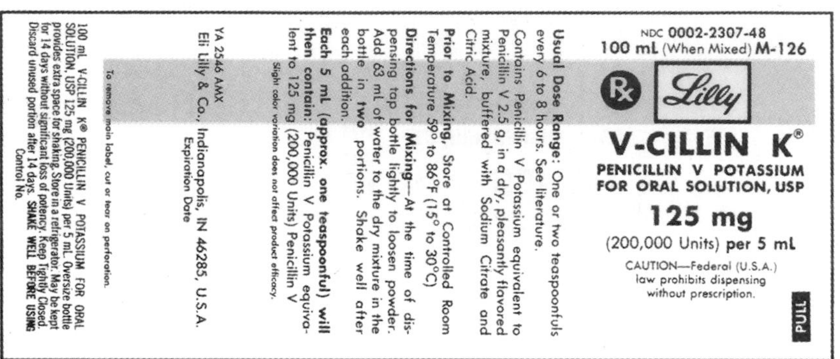

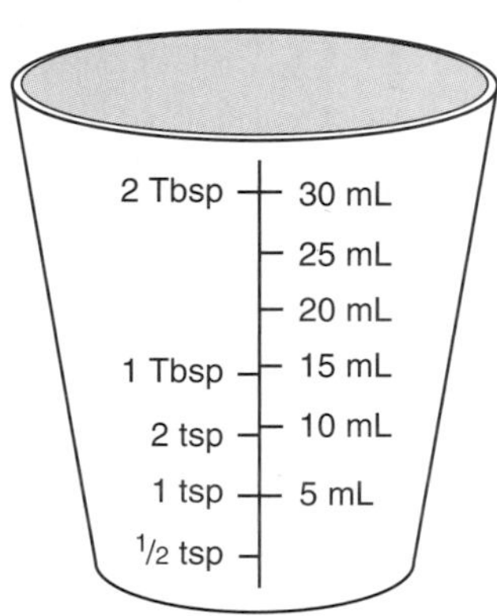

79. Your patient, who has undergone a coronary artery bypass graft, receives Surfak 250 mg po qd as a stool softener. How many capsules will you administer? _______ .

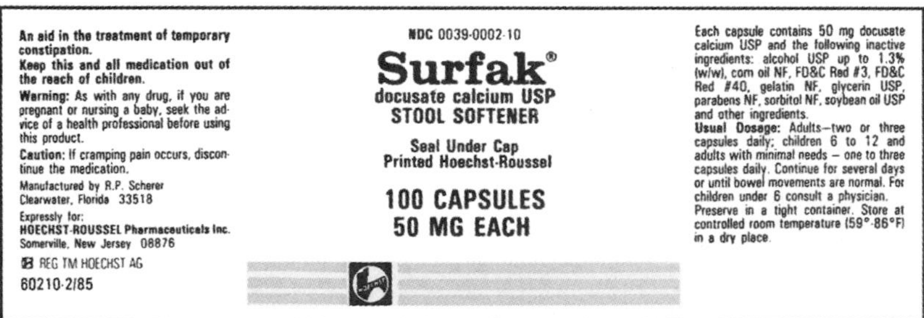

80. Ordered Elixir of KCl 15 mL po tid. Elixir of KCl 15 mEq per 11.25 mL is available. How many milliequivalents will be given? _______ .

81. Your patient with epilepsy receives phenobarbital 55 mg po bid. How many milliliters will you administer? _______ .

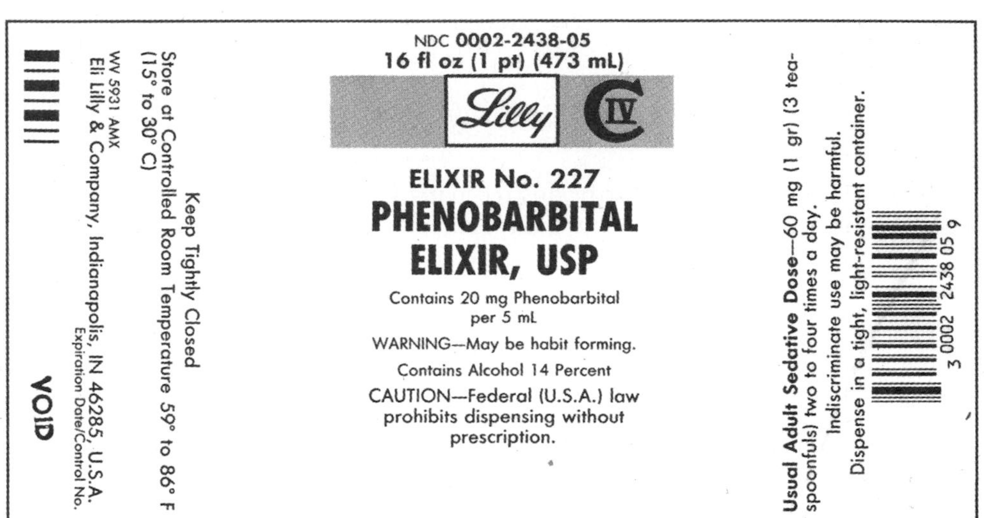

82. Ordered Aldomet 250 mg po bid. How many tablets will the nurse administer? _______ .

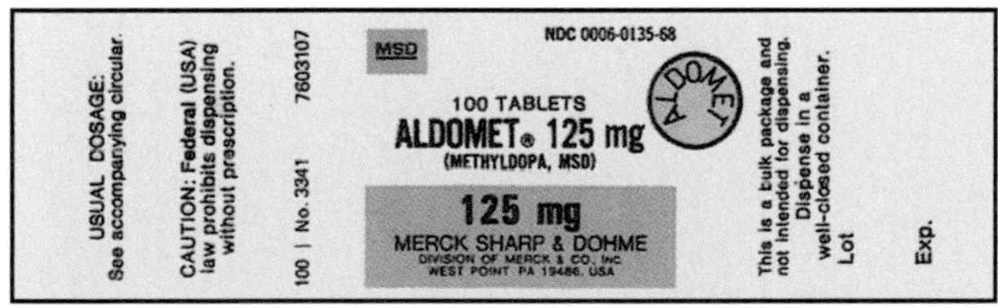

83. Mrs. Richardson, a patient who had a thyroidectomy, receives Synthroid 0.05 mg po qAM. How many tablets will the nurse administer? _______ .

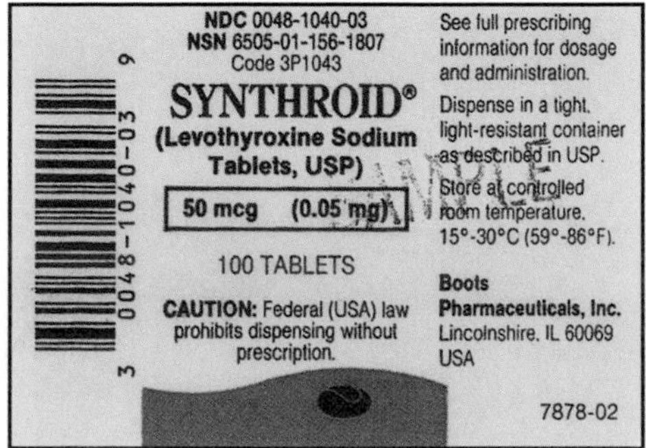

84. Ordered Theo-Dur 0.2 g po q8 h. Theo-Dur is supplied in 100-mg, 200-mg, and 300-mg sustained-action tablets. Give _______ tablets of _______ mg. How many milligrams will be given per day? _______ .

85. Your patient who had a valve repair begins receiving Coumadin 15 mg po stat. Coumadin 5-mg scored tablets are available. How many tablets will you administer? _______ .

86. Your patient, who has had angioplasty, receives cimetidine 300 mg po qid pc hs. How many milligrams will you administer each day? _______ .

87. The physician prescribes Restoril 30 mg po hs prn for a patient who has insomnia before surgery. How many capsules will the nurse administer at bedtime? _______ .

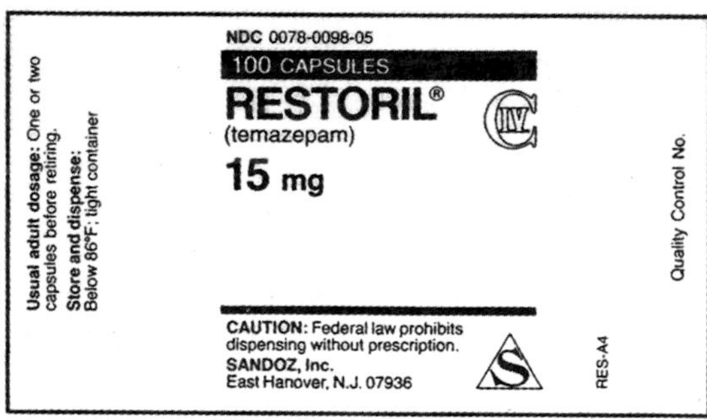

88. Ordered imipramine 50 mg po qAM and hs. The drug is supplied in 25-mg tablets. How many tablets will the nurse administer? _______ .

89. Your patient, admitted with schizophrenia, receives Mellaril 40 mg po bid. How many milliliters will you administer? _______ .

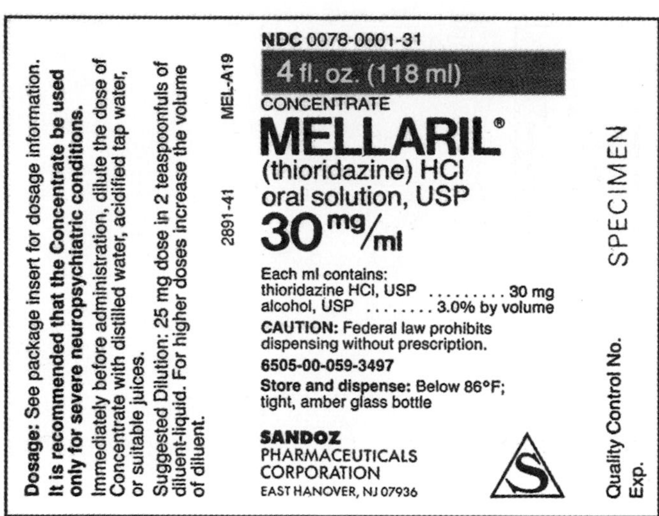

90. A patient receives Lasix 0.6 mL po bid with meals. Lasix is available in an oral solution of 10 mg per mL. How many milligrams will be given? _______ .

91. Mrs. Adams receives Cleocin 150 mg po q6 h for her upper respiratory tract infection. Cleocin is supplied in 75-mg capsules. How many capsules will the nurse administer? _______ .

92. Your patient receives Crystodigin 0.05 mg po qAM for congestive heart failure. How many tablets will you administer? _______ .

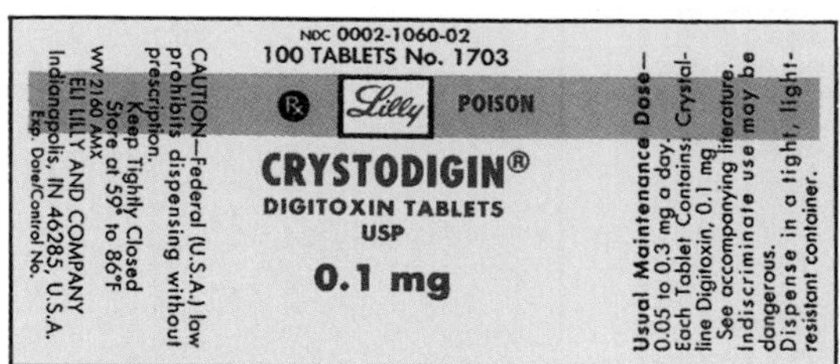

93. Coumadin 10 mg po at 6:00 PM today. How many tablets will the nurse administer? _______ .

COUMADIN® 2½ mg
(Warfarin Sodium Tablets, USP)
Crystalline
DuPont Pharma
Wilmington, Delaware 19880
LOT JJ275A
EXP 8/98

94. Your patient with diabetes receives Diabinese 0.25 g po qAM. How many tablets will you administer? _______ .

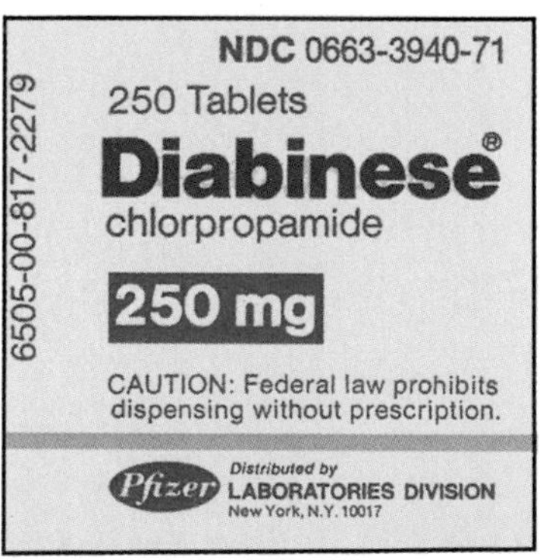

95. The physician prescribes Apresoline 25 mg po bid for Mr. Yu's hypertension. You have Apresoline scored tablets gr 1/6 available. How many tablets will you administer? _______ .

96. Ordered Flexeril 30 mg po hs. Flexeril 10-mg tablets are available. How many tablets will the nurse administer? _______ .

97. Your patient has begun receiving prednisone 15 mg po qd for asthma. Prednisone is available in 5-mg tablets. How many tablets will you administer? _______ .

98. Mr. Gray, who has undergone cervical discectomy, receives Restoril 0.015 g po hs for insomnia. How many capsules will the nurse administer? _______ .

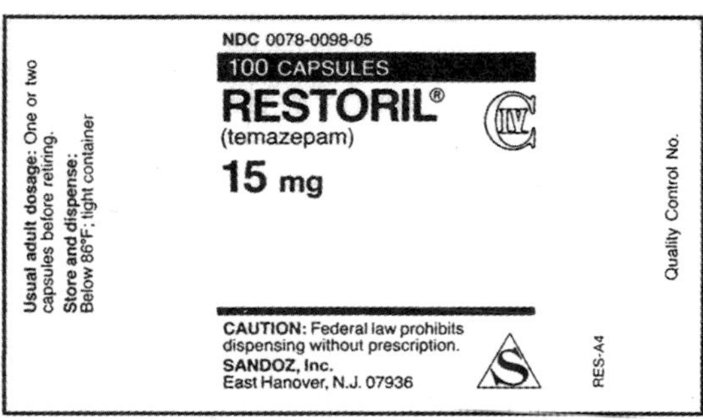

99. KCl elixir 40 mEq po qid c̄ juice. KCl 20 mEq per 15 mL is available. How many milliliters will the nurse administer? _______ .

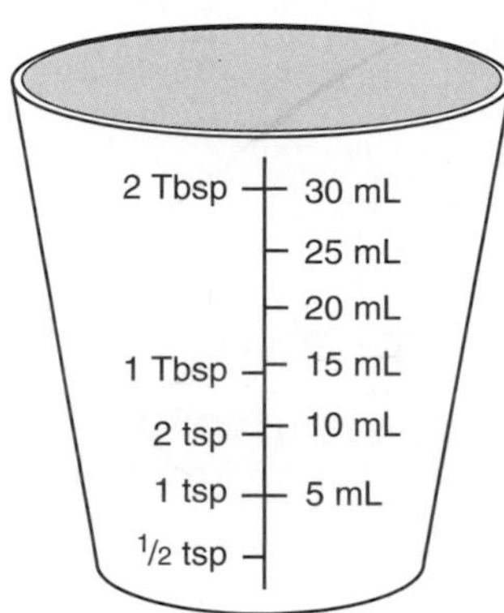

100. Mrs. Endres receives furosemide 20 mg po q8 h for congestive heart failure. How many tablets will the nurse administer? _______ .

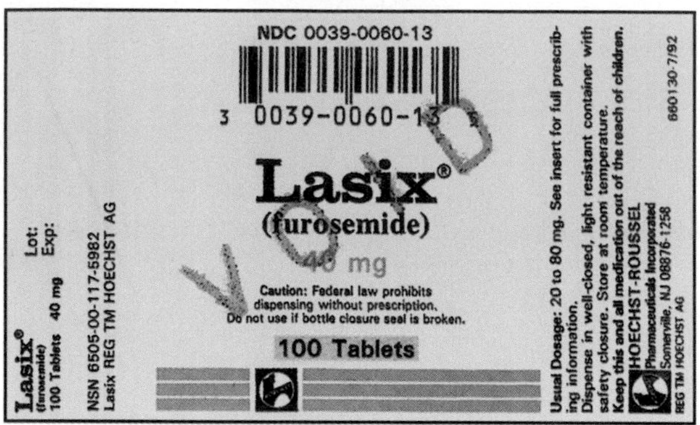

Answers on pp. 439-459.

CHAPTER 12 **Oral Dosages**

Name ______________________________

Date ______________________________

ACCEPTABLE SCORE <u>18</u>

YOUR SCORE ______

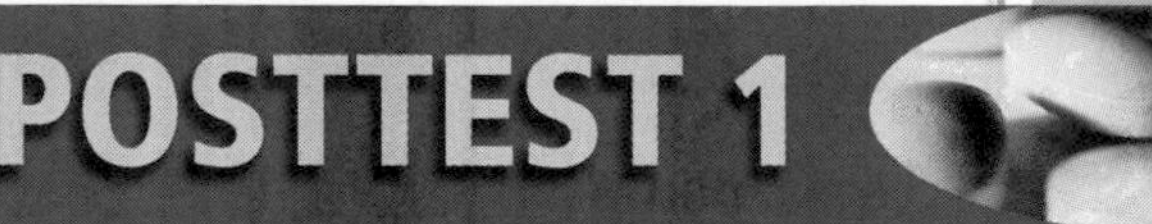

Directions: The medication order is listed at the beginning of each problem. Calculate the oral dosages. Show your work. Shade each medicine cup when provided to indicate the correct dosage.

1. The physician orders aspirin gr xv po qid for a patient who had a mitral valve repair. How many tablets will the nurse administer? ______ .

2. Mr. Clay receives tetracycline 0.5 g po qid for a gastrointestinal infection. The drug is supplied in 500-mg capsules. How many capsules will the nurse administer? ______ .

3. The physician orders ampicillin 1 g po q6 h for treatment of shigellosis. How many capsules will the nurse administer? _______ .

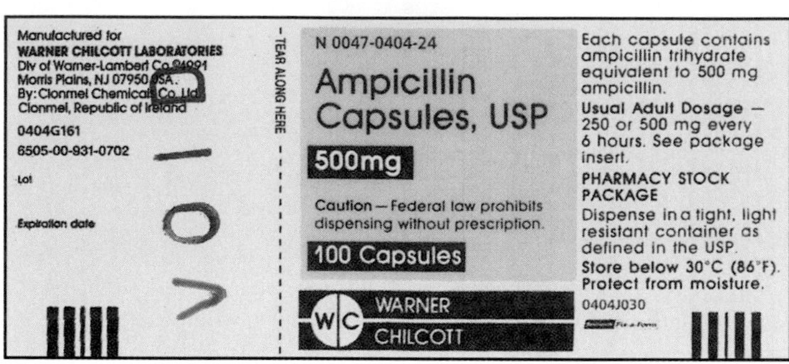

4. The physician prescribes Allegra 60 mg bid for your patient's complaints of allergic rhinitis. You have 0.03-g tablets available. How many tablets will you administer? _______ .

5. Ordered Orinase 500 mg po tid. You have 0.5-g tablets available. How many tablets will you administer? _______ .

6. Mr. Shen, admitted with a psychoneurotic disorder, receives Atarax 25 mg po qAM. You have Atarax 10 mg per 5 mL. How many milliliters will you administer? _______ .

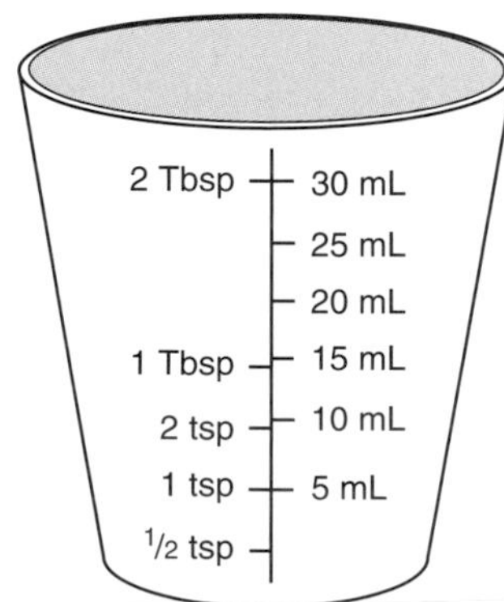

7. Your cardiac patient has Cardizem 60 mg qid ordered. How many tablets will you administer? _______ .

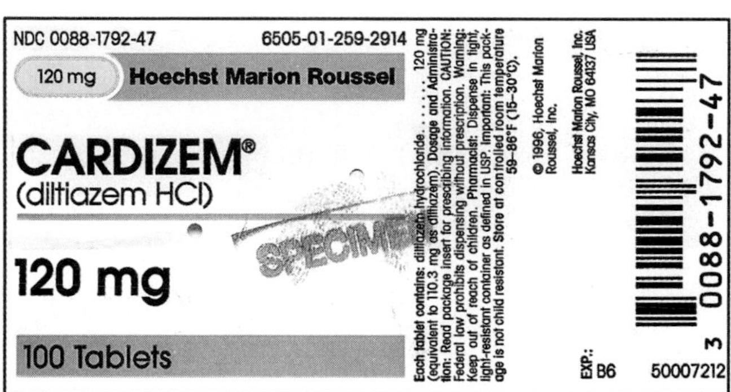

8. The physician prescribes codeine 30 mg po q3 h prn for pain relief for your patient with a total hip replacement. How many tablets will you administer? _______ .

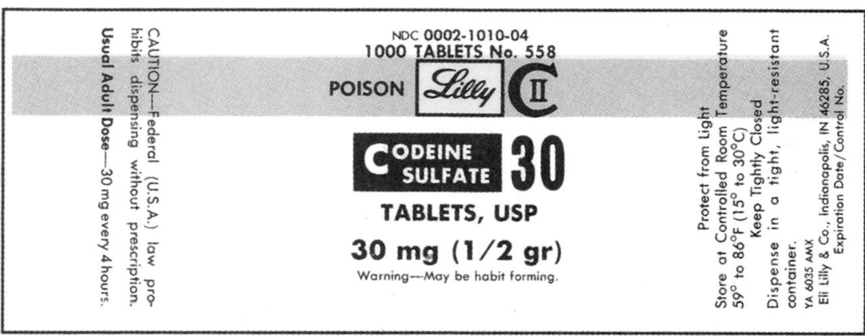

9. Your patient receives Vistaril 50 mg po tid for preoperative anxiety. Vistaril oral suspension 25 mg per 5 mL is available. How many milliliters will you administer? _______ .

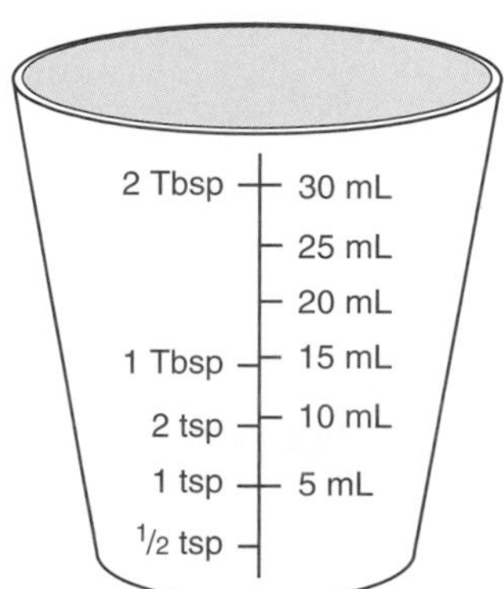

10. Ordered Naprosyn 0.25 g po bid. Naprosyn is supplied in 250-mg scored tablets. How many tablets will you give each day? _______ .

11. Your patient receives Crystodigin gr $\frac{1}{600}$ po qd for an atrial arrhythmia. Crystodigin tablets gr $\frac{1}{300}$ are available. How many tablets will you administer? _______ .

12. The physician prescribes KCl 20 mEq po bid for hypokalemia. KCl liquid is supplied 30 mEq per 22.5 mL. How many milliliters will the nurse administer? _______ .

13. Ordered Gantrisin 2 g po tid. How many tablets will the nurse administer? _______ .

USUAL DOSAGE: For dosage recommendations and other important prescribing information, read accompanying insert.
Dispense in tight, light-resistant containers as defined in USP / NF.
100 Tablets Item 73314
NDC 0004-0009-01
GANTRISIN®
brand of
sulfisoxazole
Each tablet contains 0.5 g sulfisoxazole.
CAUTION: Federal law prohibits dispensing without prescription.
ROCHE ®
ROCHE LABORATORIES
Division of Hoffmann-La Roche Inc.
Nutley, New Jersey 07110
1286
STORE AT 59° TO 86° F.
EXPIRES
LOT

14. Your patient with a lumbar laminectomy has Benadryl 100 mg po hs prn ordered for insomnia. How many capsules will you administer? ______ .

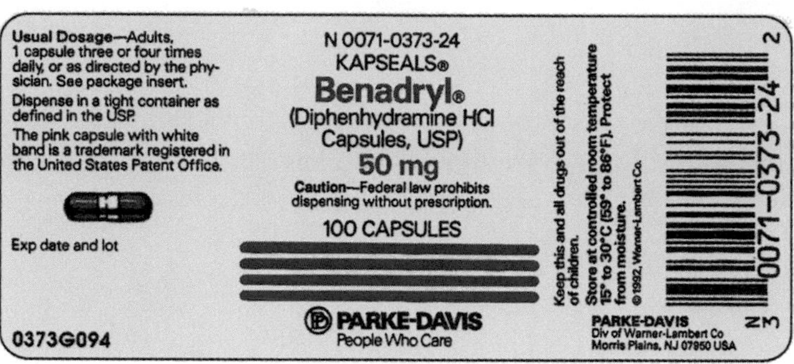

15. Your patient has Lasix 9 mg po q12 h ordered for hypercalcemia. You have Lasix 10 mg per mL. How many milliliters will you administer? ______ .

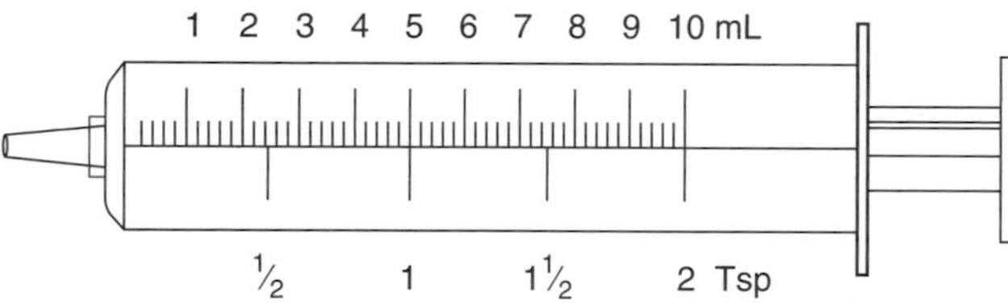

16. Mrs. Cook receives Keflex 100 mg po q6 h for a sinus infection. How many milliliters will the nurse administer? ______ .

NDC 0777-2321-97
60 mL (When Mixed) M-201
KEFLEX®
CEPHALEXIN FOR ORAL SUSPENSION, USP
125 mg per 5 mL
DISTA

17. The physician orders Mevacor 30 mg po qd to be given with evening meal. You have 10-mg tablets available. How many tablets will you administer? _______ .

18. Mr. Jones receives Inderal 80 mg po bid for a dysrhythmia. You have Inderal 40-mg scored tablets. How many tablets will you administer? _______ .

19. The physician prescribes Apresoline 20 mg po tid for your patient's hypertension. You have 10-mg tablets available. How many tablets will you administer? _______ .

20. Your patient with epilepsy receives phenobarbital gr i ss po tid. How many tablets will you administer in each dose? _______ . How many tablets will you administer in one day? _______ .

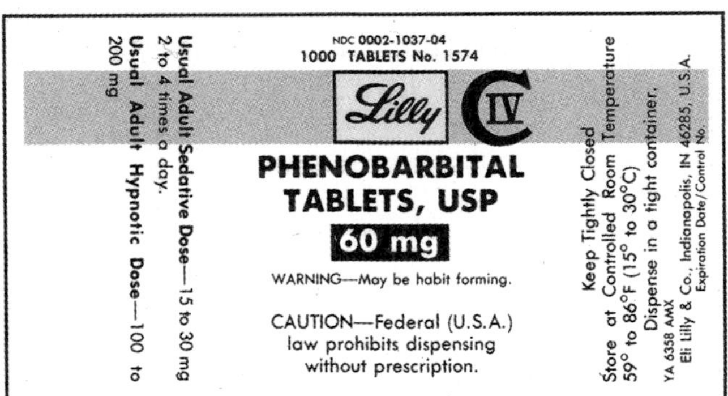

Answers on pp. 459-463.

Name ______________________

Date ______________________

ACCEPTABLE SCORE 18

YOUR SCORE ______

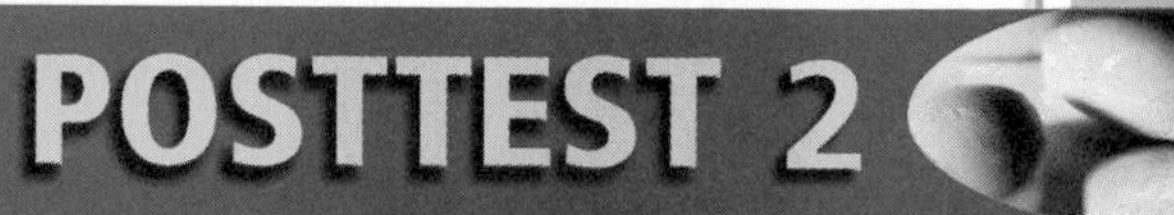

Directions: The medication order is listed at the beginning of each problem. Calculate the oral dosages. Show your work. Shade each medicine cup when provided to indicate correct dosage.

1. Your patient receives Feldene 20 mg po qd for gouty arthritis. Feldene 10-mg capsules are available. How many capsules will you administer? ______ .

2. Ordered Zofran 8 mg po before chemotherapy. How many milliliters will the nurse administer? ______ .

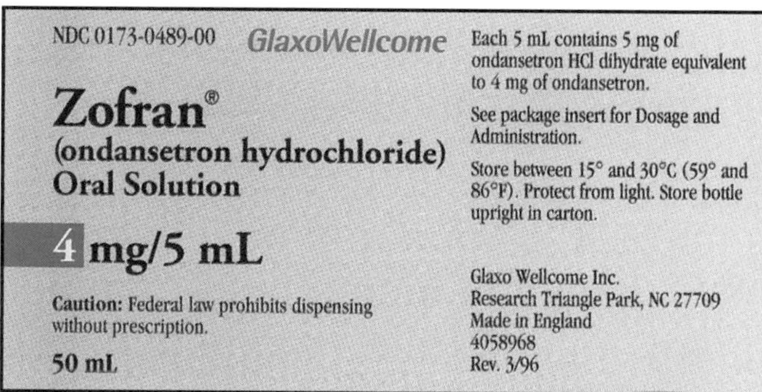

3. A patient who has undergone cleft palate revision requires Tylenol elixir 30 mg po stat. You have Children's Tylenol elixir 160 mg per 5 mL. How many milliliters will you administer? ______ .

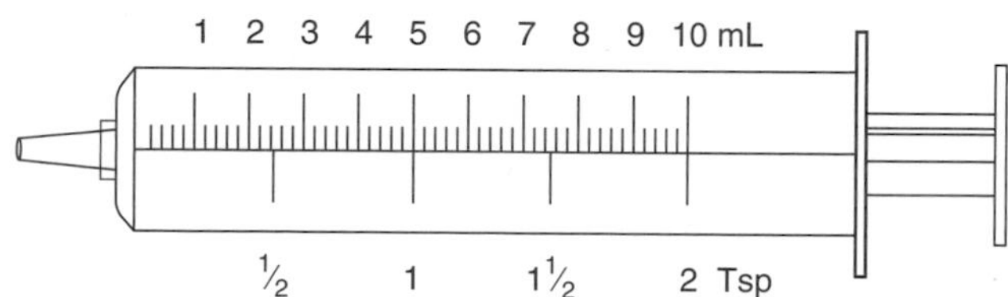

4. Ordered Glucotrol 15 mg qd. Glucotrol 10-mg scored tablets are available. How many tablets will the nurse administer? ______ .

5. Your patient who is being treated for congestive heart failure requires KCl 5 mEq po bid for hypokalemia. KCl 20 mEq per 30 mL is available. How many milliliters will you administer? ______ .

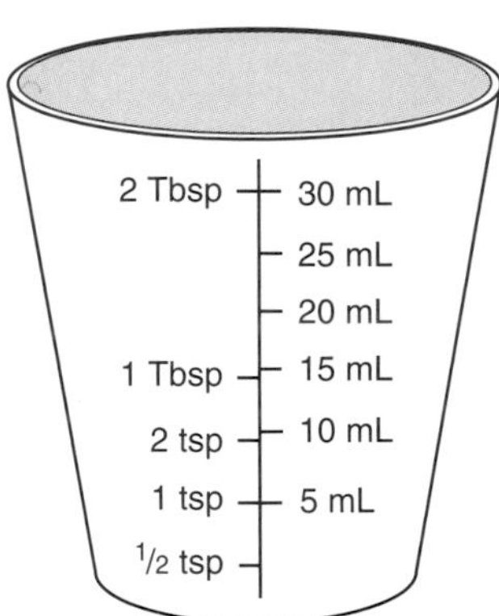

6. Your patient who has had a tonsillectomy receives Keflex 250 mg po qid. How many capsules will you administer? ______ .

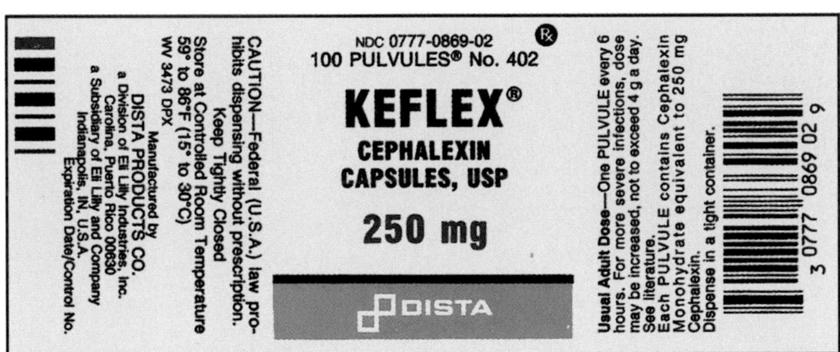

7. Mrs. Pace receives prednisone 7.5 mg po qid for asthma. Prednisone is supplied as 2.5-mg tablets. How many tablets will the nurse administer? ______ .

8. Your patient receives Lanoxin 0.05 mg po qd for cardiac arrhythmia. How many milliliters will you administer? _______ .

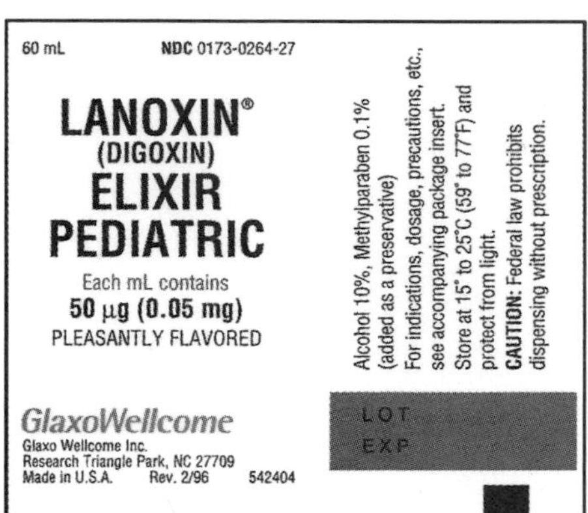

9. Ordered Macrodantin 0.1 g po qid. How many capsules will the nurse administer? _______ .

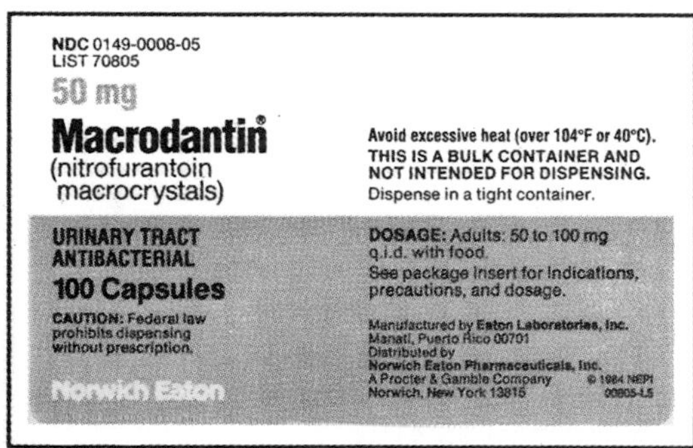

10. Your patient who had a bilateral turbinate reduction receives acetaminophen gr vi po q4 h for pain relief. Acetaminophen is supplied in 325-mg tablets. How many tablets will you administer? _______ .

11. The physician prescribes Dilantin gr ¾ po bid for seizure activity in your patient with epilepsy. Dilantin 50-mg Infatabs are available. How many tablets will you administer? _______ .

12. Mr. Bales requires Pen-Vee K 250 mg po q6 h for bacterial endocarditis. Pen-Vee K solution 125 mg per 5 mL is available. How many milliliters will the nurse administer? _______ .

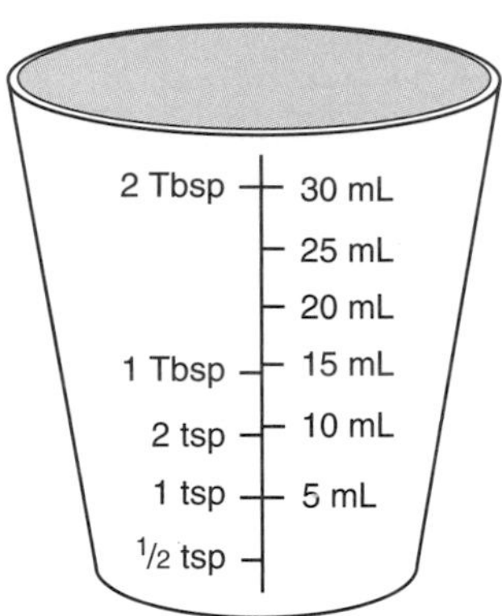

13. Ordered Deltasone 20 mg po qid. Deltasone is supplied in 2.5-mg, 5-mg, and 50-mg tablets. The nurse will give _______ tablets of _______ mg.

14. Mr. Cy, who has had mitral valve repair, receives Lanoxin 0.25 mg po qd. How many tablets will the nurse administer? _______ .

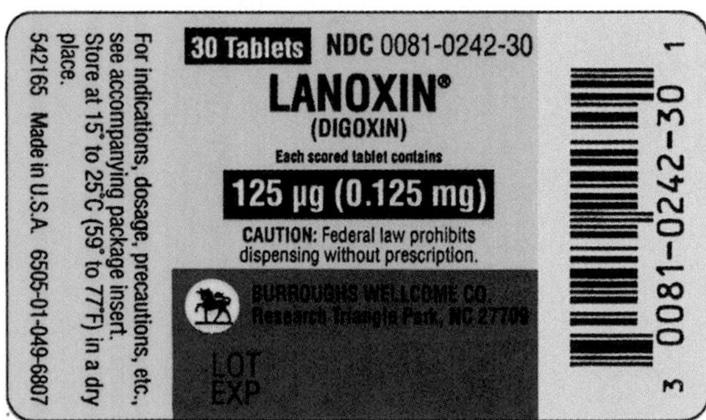

15. Colace elixir 25 mg po prn for constipation is ordered for your patient after an ethmoidectomy. How many milliliters will you administer? _______ .

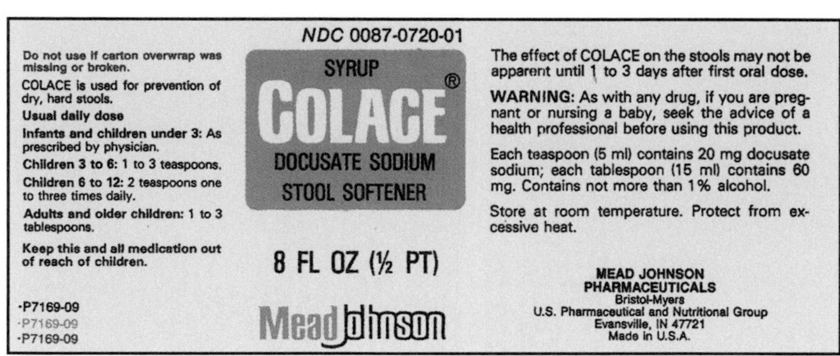

16. Mr. Tate, who has undergone left-leg debridement, receives aspirin 0.6 g po q3 h prn for relief of pain. How many tablets will the nurse administer? _______ .

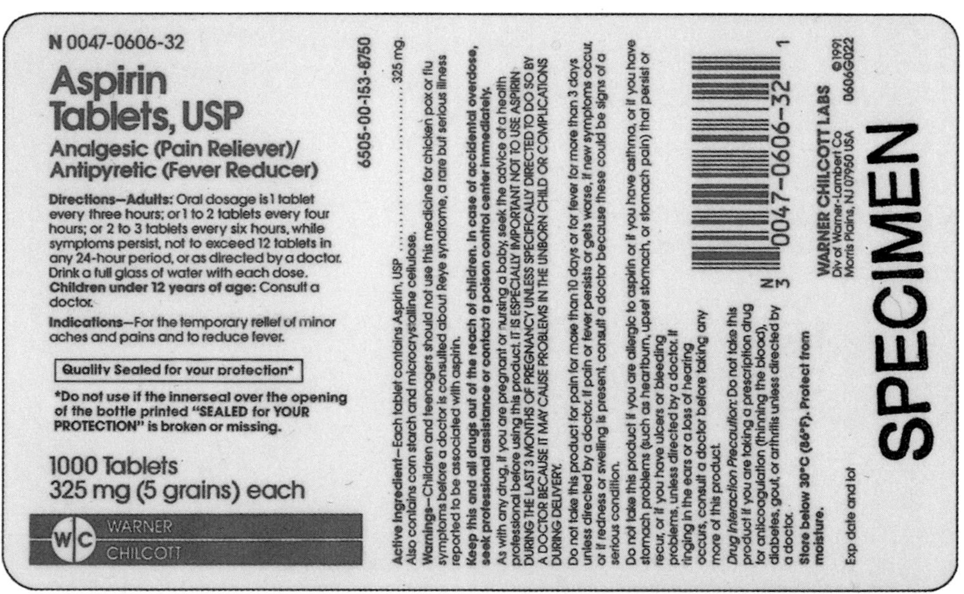

17. Your patient with hypertension has Verapamil 80 mg po tid ordered. You have 40-mg tablets. How many tablets will you administer? _______ .

18. Ordered Gantrisin tablets 1.5 g po qid. How many tablets will the nurse administer? _______ .

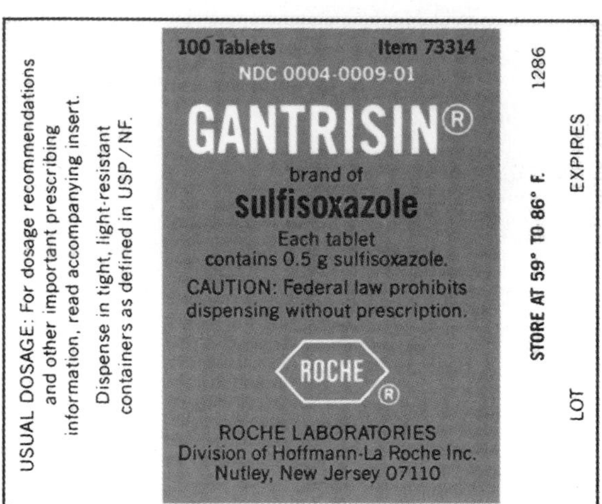

19. Your patient was admitted with seizure activity. The physician orders phenobarbital 30 mg po q8 h. How many tablets will you administer? _______ .

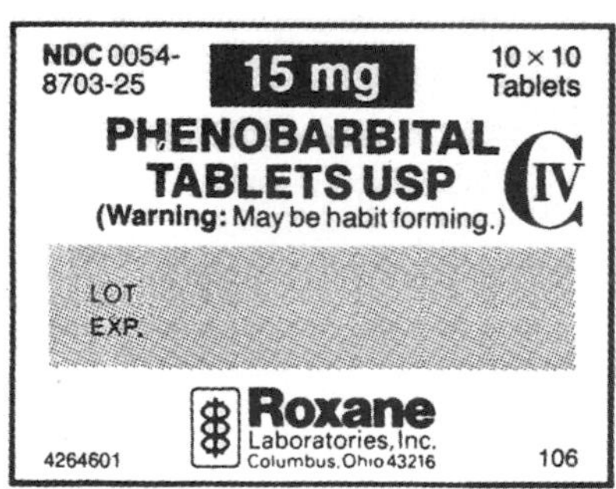

20. The physician orders Flagyl 750 mg po tid for 5 days for a yeast infection. Flagyl is supplied in 250-mg tablets. How many tablets will the nurse administer? _______ .

Answers on pp. 463-467.

CHAPTER 13

Parenteral Dosages

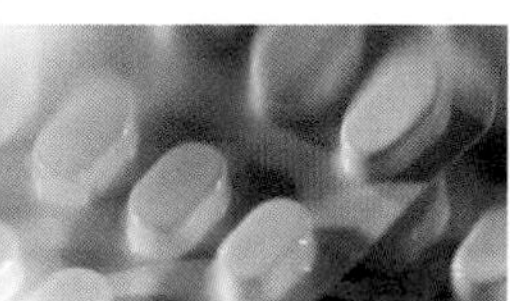

LEARNING OBJECTIVES

On completion of the materials provided in this chapter, you will be able to perform computations accurately by mastering the following mathematical concepts:

1. Converting the measure within the problem to equivalent measures in one system of measurement
2. Using a proportion to solve problems of parenteral dosages when medication is in liquid or reconstituted powder form
3. Using a proportion to solve problems of parenteral dosages of medications measured in milliequivalents
4. Using the stated formula as an alternative method of solving parenteral drug dosage problems

Parenteral refers to outside the alimentary canal or gastrointestinal tract. Medications may be given parenterally when they cannot be taken by mouth or when rapid action is desired. Parenteral medications are absorbed directly into the bloodstream; therefore the amount of drug needed can be determined more accurately. This type of administration of medications is necessary for the uncooperative or unconscious patient, or for a patient who has been designated *NPO* (nothing by mouth). An advantage of intravenous parenteral medications is that the patient does not have to endure the discomfort of multiple injections, especially when the medications are used for pain control.

Parenteral medications are administered by (1) subcutaneous injection—beneath the skin, (2) intramuscular injection—within the muscle, or (3) intradermal injection—within the skin (Figure 13-1). Parenteral medications may also be given intravenously—within the vein (Figure 13-2). Intravenous (IV) drugs may be diluted and administered by themselves, in conjunction with existing intravenous fluids, or in addition to IV fluids (Figure 13-3). Any time that the integrity of the skin—the body's prime defense against microorganisms—is threatened, infection may occur. Thus the nurse must use sterile technique when preparing and administering parenteral medications.

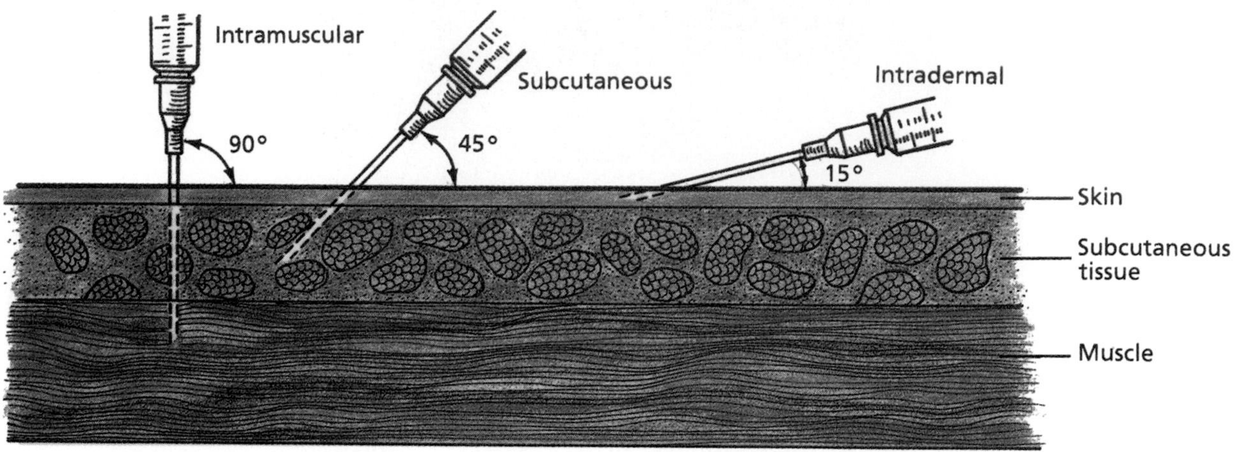

FIGURE 13-1 Intramuscular, subcutaneous, and intradermal injections, with comparison of the angles of insertion. (From Potter P, Perry A: *Fundamentals of nursing,* ed 5, St Louis, 2001, Mosby.)

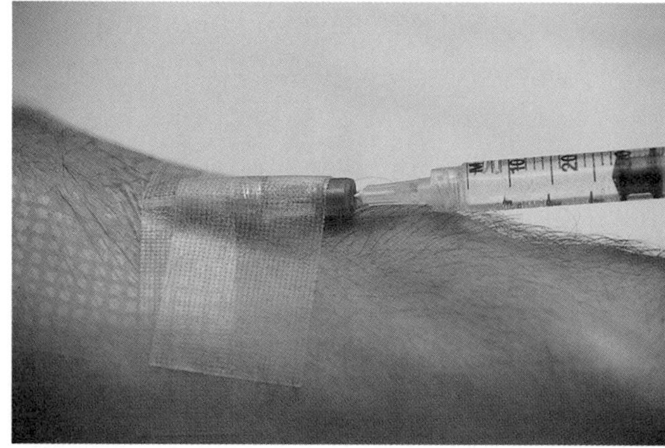

FIGURE 13-2 Intravenous injection. (From Potter P, Perry A: *Fundamentals of nursing,* ed 5, St Louis, 2001, Mosby.)

Drugs for parenteral use are supplied as liquids or powders. The medications are packaged in a variety of forms. A liquid may be contained in an ampule, which is a single-dose container that must be broken at the neck to withdraw the drug (Figures 13-4 and 13-5).

Vials are also used to package parenteral medications in liquid or powder form. A vial is a glass or plastic container that is sealed with a rubber stopper (Figure 13-6). Because vials usually contain more than one dose of a medication, the amount desired is withdrawn by inserting a needle through the rubber stopper and removing the required amount (Figure 13-7). If the medication is in powder form, the drug must be reconstituted before withdrawal and administration. The diluent in which to dissolve the powder is usually sterile water or normal saline solution. The amount of diluent recommended is normally printed on the vial; however, if it is not, no less than 1 mL is used for a single-dose vial. The powder must be completely dissolved. If the nurse is using a multiple-dose vial, the date and time of mixing should be noted on the vial's label.

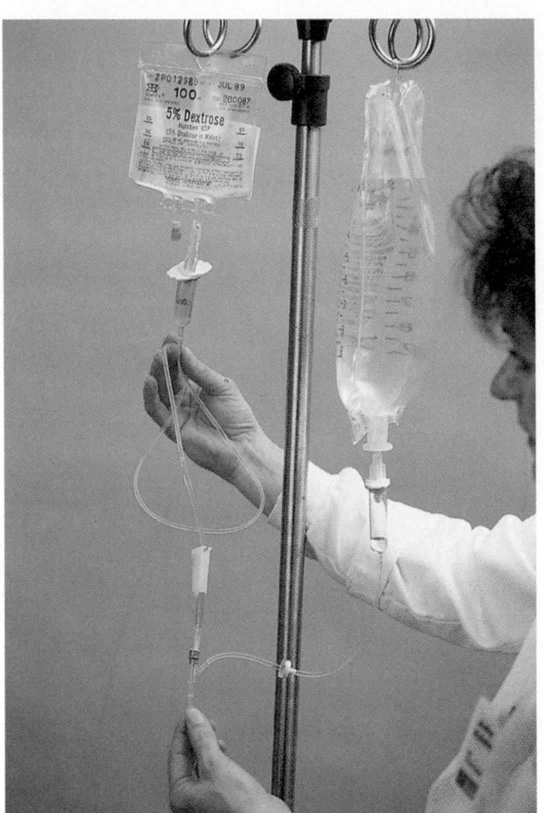

FIGURE 13-3 Intravenous drug administered with existing intravenous fluids. (From Potter P, Perry A: *Fundamentals of nursing,* ed 5, St Louis, 2001, Mosby.)

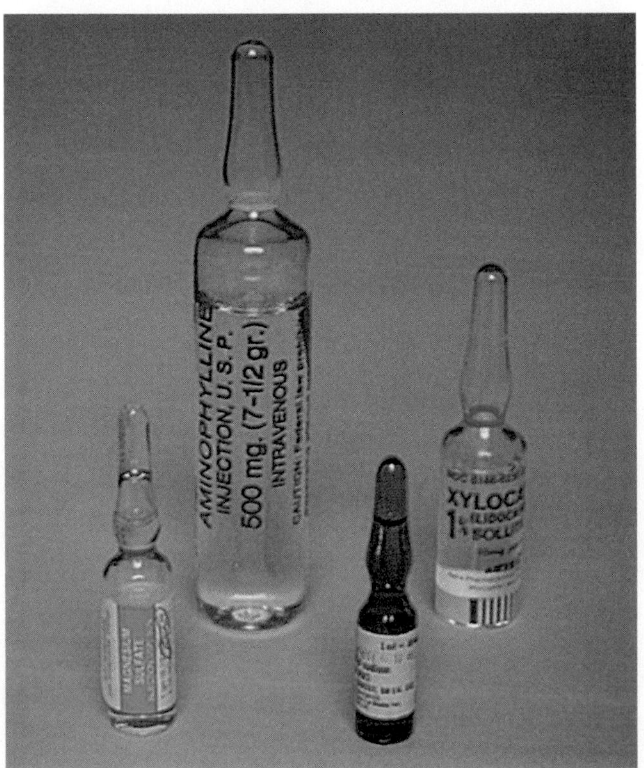

FIGURE 13-4 Examples of ampules. (From Potter P, Perry A: *Fundamentals of nursing,* ed 5, St Louis, 2001, Mosby.)

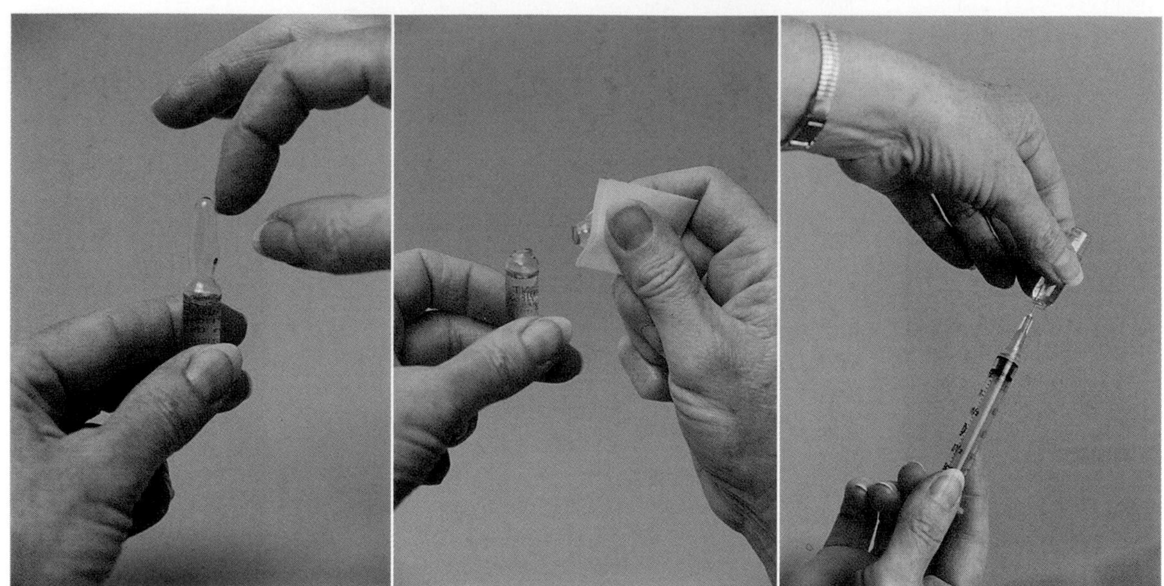

FIGURE 13-5 Breaking the ampule to withdraw the medication. (From Potter P, Perry A: *Fundamentals of nursing,* ed 5, St Louis, 2001, Mosby.)

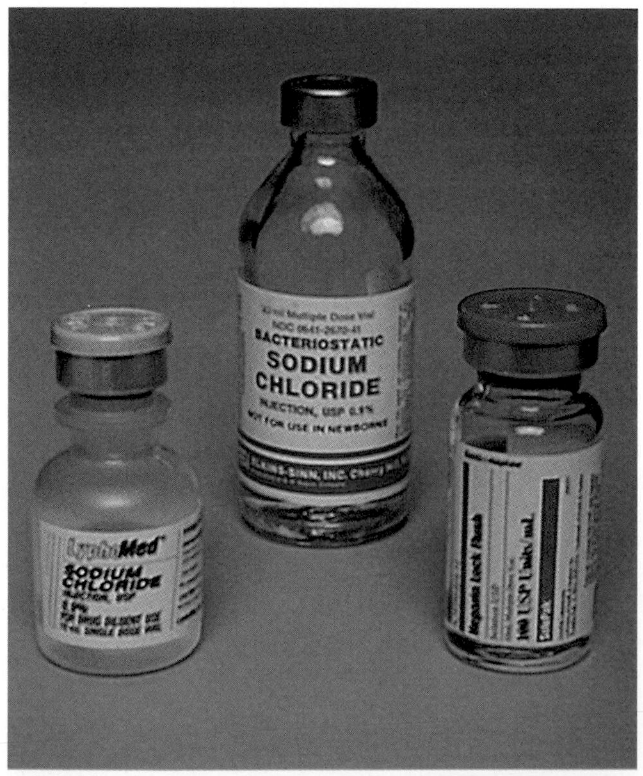

FIGURE 13-6 Examples of vials. (From Potter P, Perry A: *Fundamentals of nursing,* ed 5, St Louis, 2001, Mosby.)

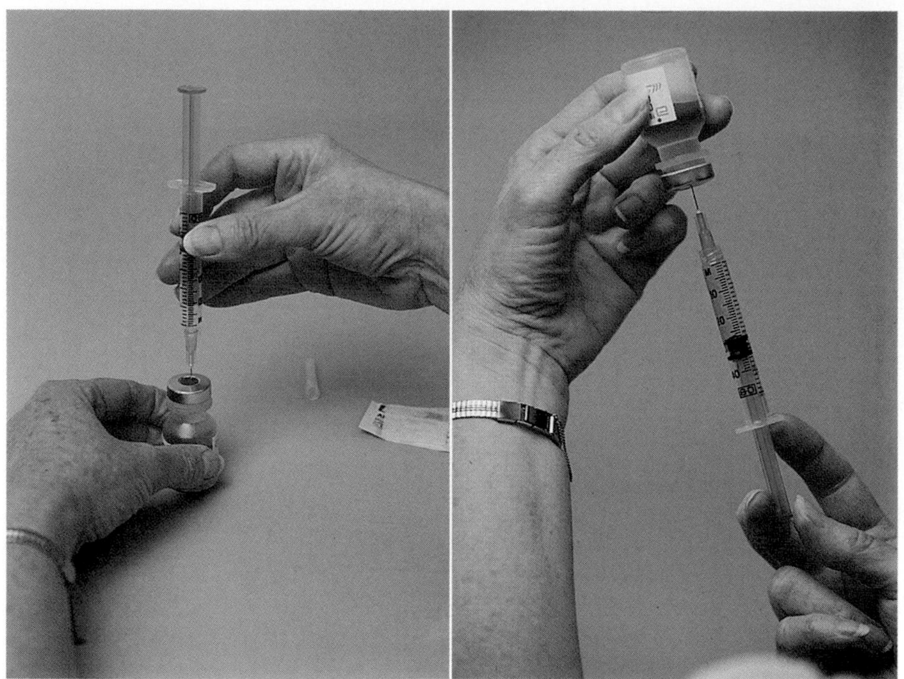

FIGURE 13-7 Withdrawing medication from a vial through the rubber stopper. (From Potter P, Perry A: *Fundamentals of nursing,* ed 5, St Louis, 2001, Mosby.)

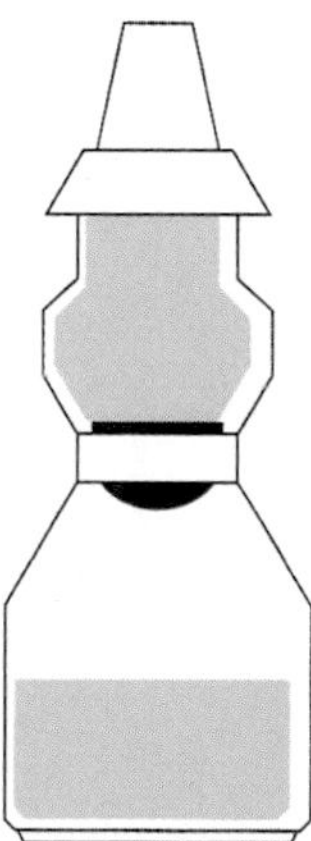

FIGURE 13-8 Example of a Mix-O-Vial.

Some of the more unstable drugs may be supplied in vials that have a compartment containing the liquid. Pressure applied to the top of the vial releases the stopper between the compartments and allows the drug to be dissolved. These are called *Mix-O-Vials* (Figure 13-8).

Medications may also be supplied in either prefilled disposable syringes or a plastic syringe with a disposable cartridge and a needle unit. Such units contain a specific amount of medication. If the medication order is less than the amount supplied, discard the unneeded portion before administering the medication to the patient.

Syringes

For accurate measurement of medications that are to be administered by the parenteral route, a syringe must be used. Each syringe is supplied in a sterile package. Although syringes may be made of glass or plastic, plastic syringes are more commonly used. They are designed to be used only once and then discarded. The syringe that is used to withdraw and measure the medication from its container may also be used to administer the medication to the patient.

Figure 13-9 shows the parts of a syringe.

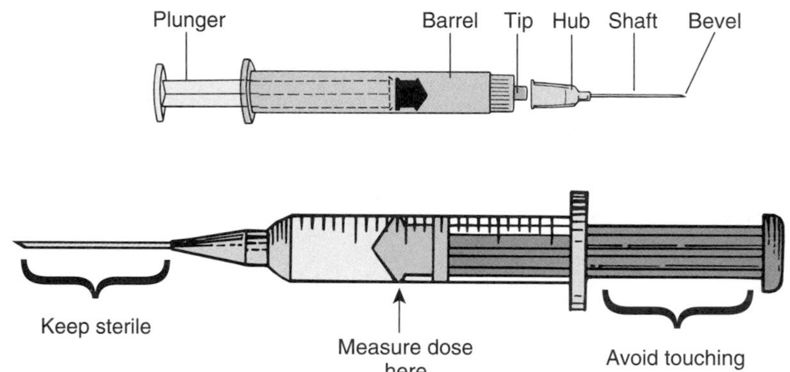

FIGURE 13-9 Parts of a syringe. (From Potter P, Perry A: *Fundamentals of nursing,* ed 5, St Louis, 2001, Mosby.)

1. TIP. The tip is located at the end of the syringe. This is the part that holds the needle.
2. BARREL. This is the outer part of the syringe that holds the medication. The various calibrations are printed on the outside of the barrel.
3. PLUNGER. This is the interior part of the syringe that slides within the barrel. The plunger is moved backward to withdraw and measure the medication. Then it is pushed forward to inject the medication into the patient.

Syringes come in a variety of sizes. The size used depends on the amount and type of medication to be administered. There are three types of syringes: hypodermic, tuberculin, and insulin syringes.

Hypodermic Syringes. Hypodermic syringes vary in size as to the amount of fluid they can measure. The most commonly used sizes are 2-, 2½-, 3-, and 5-cc syringes (Figure 13-10). Hypodermic syringes are also available in 10-, 20-, 30-, and 50-cc sizes. Remember that a cubic centimeter (cc) is equivalent to a milliliter and that syringes are labeled with both abbreviations. Small hypodermic syringes will also be calibrated in minims (♏). It is critical to use syringes with this calibration when the amount of medication to be administered has been calculated in minims.

Syringes that are smaller capacity may easily be used to measure decimal fractions of a cubic centimeter or milliliter. Longer lines mark the half and whole number cc/mL, and shorter lines mark the decimal fractions. Each line indicates one tenth of a cubic centimeter or milliliter. With larger-capacity syringes, each mark may represent a 0.2-cc increment, or whole cc increments. The larger-capacity syringes would not be appropriate for measuring smaller quantities of medication for administration.

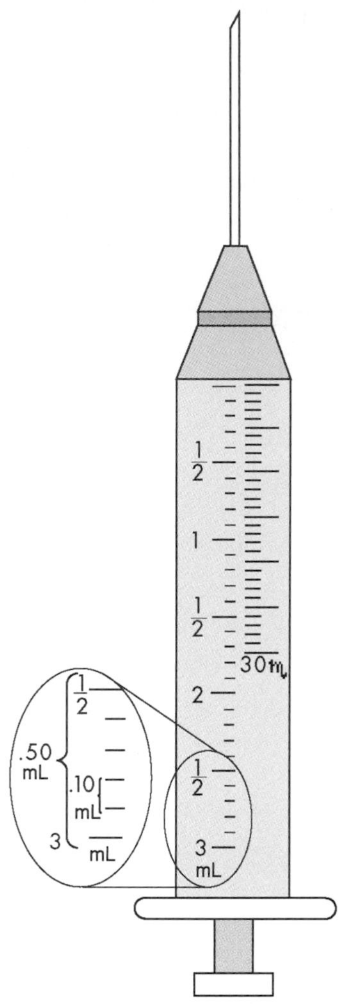

FIGURE 13-10 Calibrations on a 3-cc syringe. (From Clayton BD, Stock YN: *Basic pharmacology for nurses,* ed 12, St Louis, 2001, Mosby.)

Tuberculin Syringes. A tuberculin syringe is a thin, 1-cc/mL syringe (Figure 13-11). The cc/mL side of the syringe includes markings for hundredths of a cc/mL. The other side of the syringe is calibrated in minims. These syringes are commonly used in pediatrics and also to measure medications given in very small amounts, such as heparin.

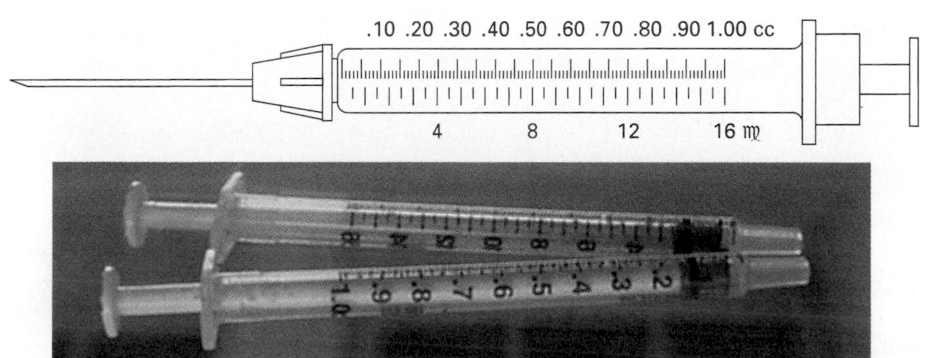

FIGURE 13-11 Tuberculin syringes. (From Brown M, Mulholland J: *Drug calculations, process and problems for clinical practice,* ed 5, St Louis, 1996, Mosby.)

Insulin Syringes. Insulin syringes were developed specifically for the administration of insulin. They are calibrated in units (U). These syringes were designed to be used with U-100 insulin. There are three types of insulin syringes.

1. The Lo-Dose syringe is used for administration of 50 units or less of insulin. The syringe is marked for each unit, with longer lines for each 5 units (Figure 13-12).

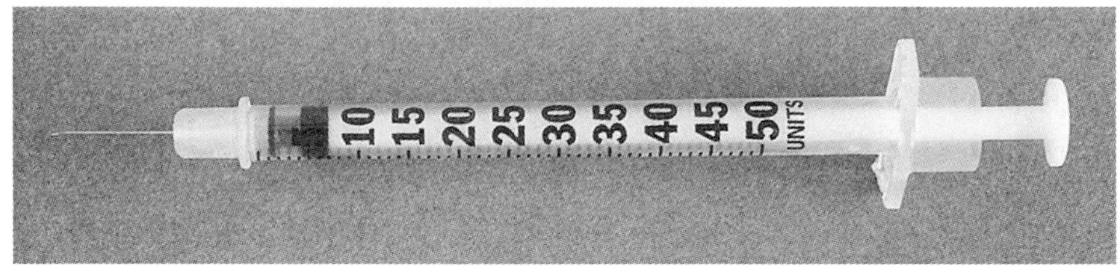

FIGURE 13-12 Lo-Dose insulin syringe. (From Brown M, Mulholland J: *Drug calculations, process and problems for clinical practice,* ed 6, St Louis, 2000, Mosby.)

2. The 30-U syringe is used for insulin doses that equal less than 30 units of U-100 insulin only (Figure 13-13).

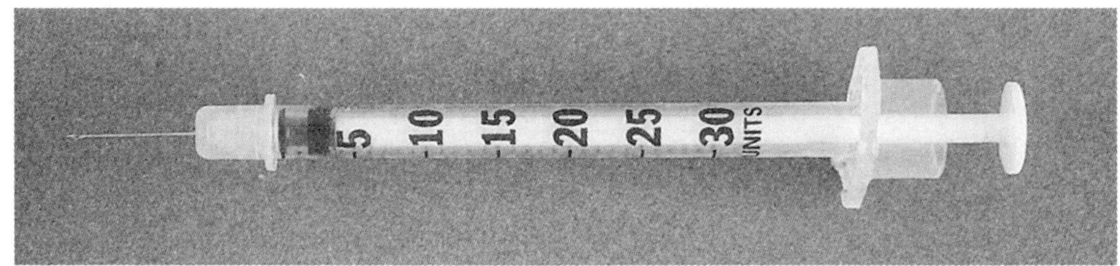

FIGURE 13-13 A 30-U syringe. (From Brown M, Mulholland J: *Drug calculations, process and problems for clinical practice,* ed 6, St Louis, 2000, Mosby.)

3. The U-100/1-mL syringe is used for the administration of up to 100 units of U-100 insulin (Figure 13-14).

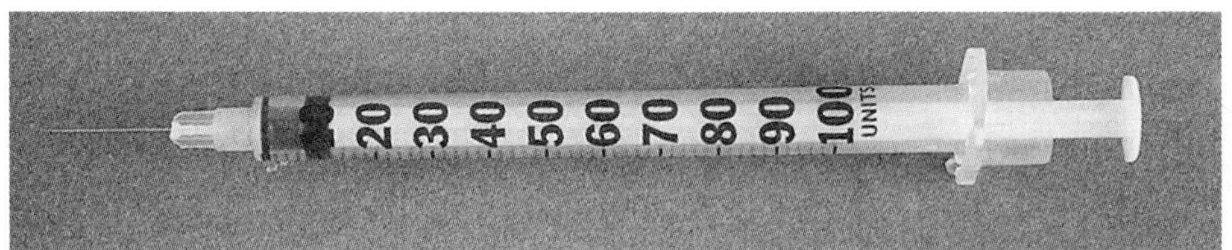

FIGURE 13-14 A 100-U (U-100) insulin syringe. (From Brown M, Mulholland J: *Drug calculations, process and problems for clinical practice,* ed 6, St Louis, 2000, Mosby.)

Remember, when preparing medication for administration, it is important to choose the correct size of syringe for accurate measurement of the medication.

Needleless System. The Occupational Safety and Health Administration (OSHA) has recommended administration of parenteral medications with the use of a needleless system. This recommendation is for the protection of both patients and nurses from needlesticks. Needleless systems provide a shield that protects the needle device (Figure 13-15).

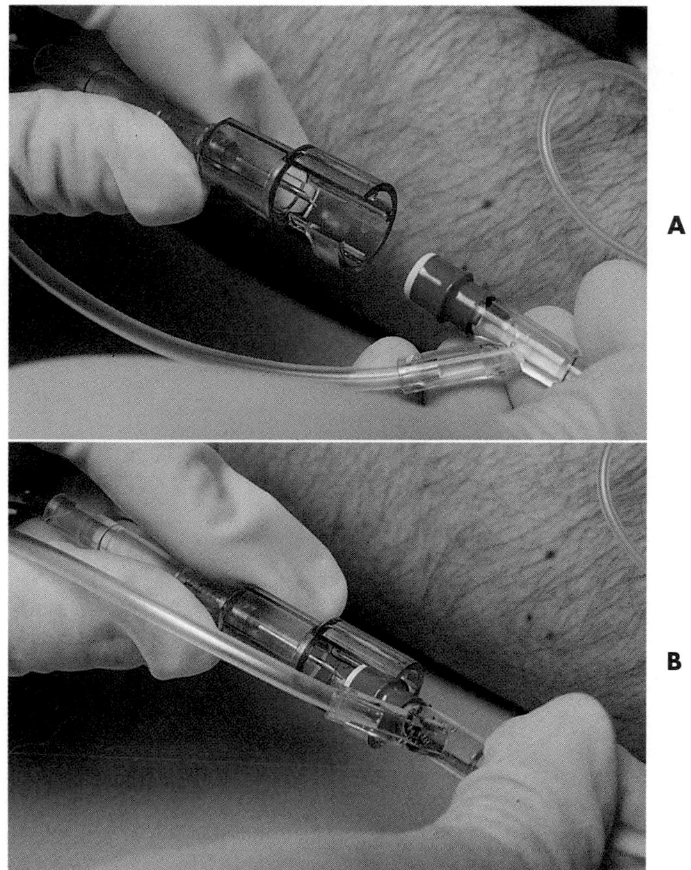

FIGURE 13-15 **A,** Needleless infusion system. **B,** Connection into an injection port. (From Elkin MK, Perry AG, Potter PA: *Nursing interventions & clinical skills,* ed 2, St Louis, 2000, Mosby.)

Calculation of Parenteral Drug Dosages/Proportion Method

Parenteral drug dosages may also be calculated by using a proportion. The physician's order and the available medication must be in the same system of measurement to write a proportion for the actual amount of medication to be administered. Examples of parenteral drug dosage problems follow.

Example 1: Ordered Apresoline 30 mg IM. Apresoline 20 mg per mL is available. How many milliliters will the nurse administer? _______ .

a. On the left side of the proportion, place what you know or have available. In this example, there are 20 mg per 1 mL. Therefore the left side of the proportion would be

20 mg : 1 mL ::

b. The right side of the proportion is determined by the physician's order and the abbreviations placed on the left side of the proportion. Remember, only *two* different abbreviations may be used in a single proportion.

20 mg : 1 mL :: ______ mg : ______ mL

The physician ordered 30 mg.

20 mg : 1 mL :: 30 mg : ______ mL

The symbol x is used to represent the unknown number of milliliters.

20 mg : 1 mL :: 30 mg : x mL

c. Rewrite the proportion without the abbreviations.

$$20 : 1 :: 30 : x$$

d. Solve for x.

$$20 : 1 :: 30 : x$$

$$20x = 30$$

$$x = \frac{30}{20}$$

$$x = 1.5$$

e. Label your answer as determined by the abbreviation placed next to x in the original proportion.

1.5 mL

The patient would receive 1.5 mL of Apresoline containing 30 mg.

Example 2: Ordered Demerol 30 mg IM q4 h prn. Demerol 25 mg per 0.5 mL is available. How many milliliters will the nurse administer? ______ .

a. On the left side of the proportion, place what you know or have available. In this example, each 0.5 mL contains 25 mg. So the left side of the proportion would be

25 mg : 0.5 mL ::

b. The right side of the proportion is determined by the physician's order and the abbreviations on the left side of the proportion. Only *two* different abbreviations may be used in a single proportion. The abbreviations must be in the same position on the right side as they are on the left.

25 mg : 0.5 mL :: ______ mg : ______ mL

In this example the physician ordered 30 mg.

25 mg : 0.5 mL :: 30 mg : ______ mL

We need to find the number of milliliters to be given, so we use the symbol x to represent the unknown.

25 mg : 0.5 mL :: 30 mg : x mL

c. Rewrite the proportion without using the abbreviations.

$$25 : 0.5 :: 30 : x$$

d. Solve for x.

$$25x = 0.5 \times 30$$
$$25x = 15$$
$$x = \frac{15}{25}$$
$$x = 0.6$$

e. Label your answer as determined by the abbreviation placed next to x in the original proportion.

0.6 mL would be measured in order to administer 30 mg of Demerol.

Example 3: Ordered gentamicin 9 mg IV q6 h. Gentamicin 20 mg per 2 mL is available. How many milliliters will the nurse administer? ______ .

a. 20 mg : 2 mL ::
b. 20 mg : 2 mL :: ______ mg : ______ mL
   20 mg : 2 mL :: 9 mg : x mL
c. 20 : 2 :: 9 : x
d. $20x = 18$

$$x = \frac{18}{20}$$
$$x = 0.9$$
$$x = 0.9 \text{ mL}$$

e. Label your answer as determined by the abbreviation placed next to x in the original proportion.

0.9 mL would be measured in order to administer 9 mg of gentamicin.

Parenteral Drug Dosage Calculation/Alternative Formula Method

In Chapter 12, the alternative formula was introduced as another method of calculating drug dosages. This formula also may be used when parenteral drug dosages are calculated.

Remember, the formula is

$$\frac{D}{A} \times Q = x$$

or

$$\frac{\text{Desired}}{\text{Available}} \times \text{Quantity available} = x \text{ (unknown)}$$

Example 1: Ordered Amikin 150 mg IM q8 h. Amikin 500 mg per 2 mL is available. How many milliliters will the nurse administer? ______ .

NDC 0015-3020-20 2 mL vial
EQUIVALENT TO
500 mg AMIKACIN per 2 mL
AMIKIN®
Amikacin Sulfate Injection, USP
FOR I.M. OR I.V. USE
CAUTION: Federal law prohibits dispensing without prescription.
0.66% sodium bisulfite added as an antioxidant; buffered with 2.5% sodium citrate, adjusted to pH 4.5 with H_2SO_4. • Store at controlled room temperature 15°-30°C (59°-86°F).
READ CIRCULAR
APOTHECON®
A Bristol-Myers Squibb Company
Princeton, NJ 08540 USA
3020200RL-3
Cont:
Exp. Date:

a. The desired amount of Amikin is 150 mg.

$$\frac{150 \text{ mg}}{}$$

b. The available amount of Amikin is 500 mg.

$$\frac{150 \text{ mg}}{500 \text{ mg}}$$

c. The quantity of the medication for 500 mg is 2 mL.

$$\frac{150 \text{ mg}}{500 \text{ mg}} \times \frac{2}{1} = x$$

d. We can now solve for x.

$$x = \frac{150 \text{ mg}}{500 \text{ mg}} \times \frac{2}{1}$$

$$x = \frac{150 \, \cancel{\text{mg}} \times \overset{1}{\cancel{2}}}{\underset{250}{\cancel{500}} \, \cancel{\text{mg}} \times 1} = \frac{150}{250}$$

$$x = \frac{150}{250}$$

$$x = \frac{3}{5} \text{ or } 0.6$$

e. Label your answer as determined by the quantity.

$$150 \text{ mg} = 0.6 \text{ mL of Amikin}$$

If the physician's order is in one system of measurement and the drug is supplied in another system of measurement, one of the measurements must be converted so they are both expressed in the same system. After this is done, the formula may be used to calculate the amount of medication to be administered.

Example 2: Mr. Davis is to receive atropine gr $\frac{1}{150}$ IM stat. Atropine 0.4 mg per mL is available. How many milliliters will the nurse administer? ______ .

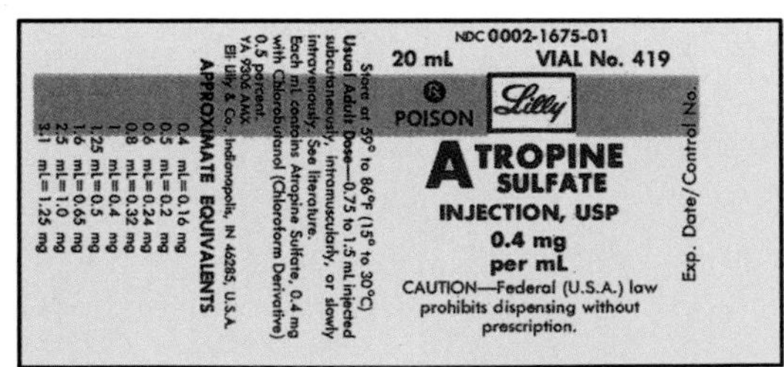

The physician's order is expressed in grains and the drug is supplied in milligrams. Convert the order to milligrams as outlined in Chapter 8.

$$60 \text{ mg} : 1 \text{ gr} :: x \text{ mg} : \tfrac{1}{150} \text{ gr}$$

$$60 : 1 :: x : \tfrac{1}{150}$$

$$x = \frac{60}{1} \times \frac{1}{150}$$

$$x = \frac{\overset{2}{\cancel{60}} \times 1}{1 \times \underset{5}{\cancel{150}}}$$

$$x = \frac{2}{5} \text{ or } 0.4$$

$$x = 0.4 \text{ mg}$$

$$\text{gr } \tfrac{1}{150} = 0.4 \text{ mg of atropine}$$

Now the numbers may be filled into the formula.

a. The desired amount is 0.4 mg.

$$\frac{0.4 \text{ mg}}{\phantom{0.4 \text{ mg}}}$$

b. The available amount or strength of atropine is 0.4 mg.

$$\frac{0.4 \text{ mg}}{0.4 \text{ mg}}$$

c. The quantity available is in 1 mL.

$$\frac{0.4 \cancel{\text{mg}}}{0.4 \cancel{\text{mg}}} \times \frac{1}{1}$$

d. Solve for x

$$x = \frac{0.4 \times 1}{0.4 \times 1}$$

$$x = 1$$

e. Label your answer as determined by the quantity.

$$0.4 \text{ mg} = 1 \text{ mL of atropine}$$

Example 3: Mr. Lewis's physician has ordered 60 mg of phenobarbital for treatment of agitation. Phenobarbital 120 mg per mL is available. How many milliliters will the nurse administer? ______ .

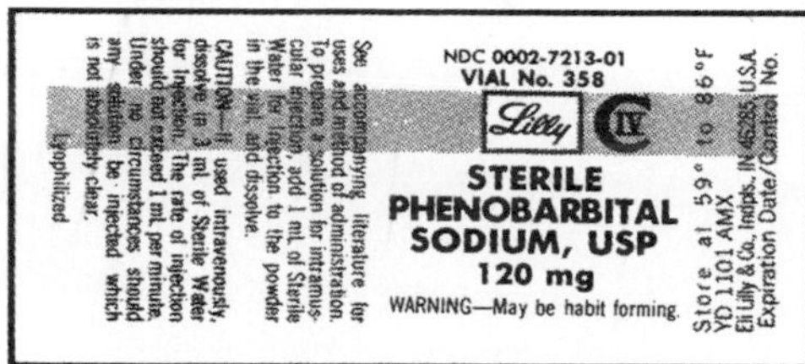

a. The desired amount of phenobarbital is 60 mg.

$$\frac{60 \text{ mg}}{}$$

b. The available amount or strength is 120 mg.

$$\frac{60 \text{ mg}}{120 \text{ mg}}$$

c. The quantity available is 1 mL.

$$\frac{60 \text{ mg}}{120 \text{ mg}} \times 1$$

d. Solve for x.

$$x = \frac{60 \text{ mg}}{120 \text{ mg}} \times \frac{1}{1}$$

$$x = \frac{60 \cancel{\text{mg}} \times 1}{120 \cancel{\text{mg}} \times 1}$$

$$x = \frac{1}{2}$$

$$x = 0.5$$

e. Label your answer as determined by the quantity.

60 mg = 0.5 mL of phenobarbital

Complete the following work sheet, which provides for extensive practice in the calculation of parenteral drug dosages. Check your answers. If you have difficulties, go back and review the necessary material. When you feel ready to evaluate your learning, take the first posttest. Check your answers. An acceptable score as indicated on the posttest signifies that you have successfully completed this chapter. An unacceptable score signifies a need for further study before taking the second posttest.

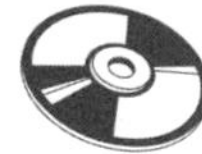

Refer to Calculating Dosages on the CD for additional help and practice problems.

WORK SHEET

Directions: The medication order is listed at the beginning of each problem. Calculate the parenteral dosages. Show your work. Shade the syringe when provided to indicate the correct dosage.

1. The physician orders gentamicin 30 mg IM q8 h for your patient with a central line infection. Gentamicin 10 mg per mL is available. How many milliliters will you administer? ______ .

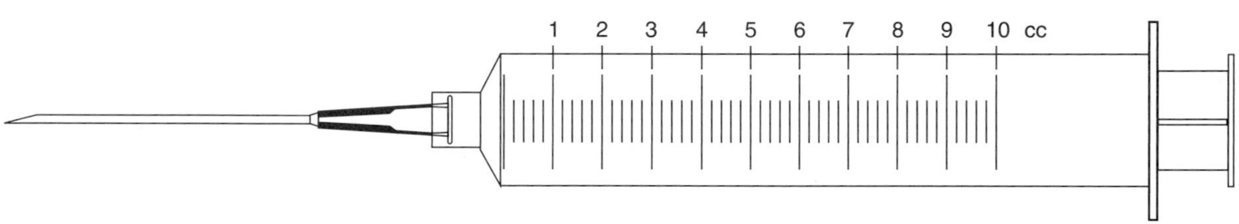

2. Your patient with an atrial valve repair has Lanoxin 110 mcg IV q12 h ordered. How many milliliters will you prepare? ______ .

2 mL
LANOXIN®
(DIGOXIN)
INJECTION
500 μg (0.5 mg)
in 2 mL
(250 μg [0.25 mg] per mL)
DILUTION NOT REQUIRED
PROPYLENE GLYCOL 40%
ALCOHOL 10%
Store at 15° to 25°C (59° to 77°F). Protect from light.
FOR I.V. OR I.M. USE
BURROUGHS WELLCOME CO.
Research Triangle Park, NC 27709
542282
LOT
EXP.

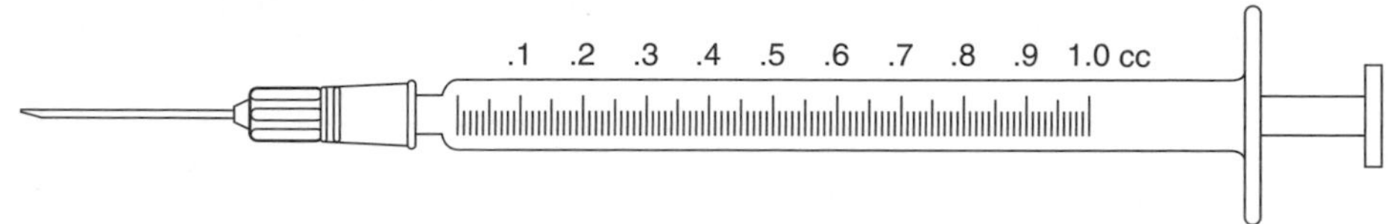

3. Ordered atropine gr 1⁄200 IM at 6:15 AM. How many milliliters will the nurse administer?______ .

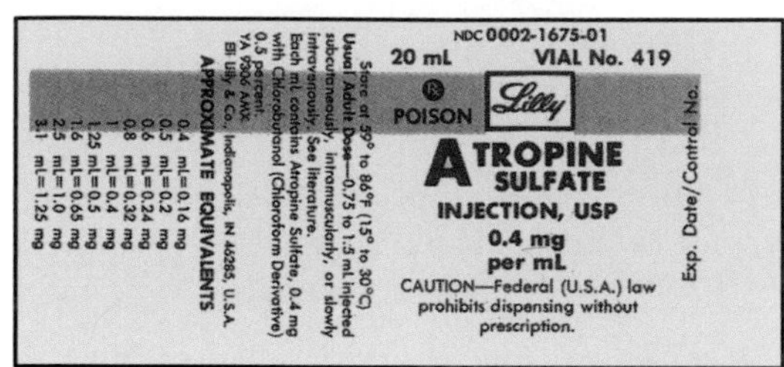

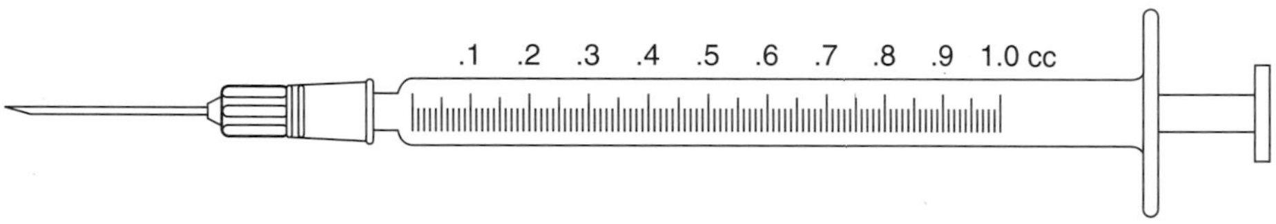

4. Your patient who has undergone pacemaker placement complains of nausea and has Compazine 10 mg IM q6 h ordered. How many milliliters will you administer? ______ .

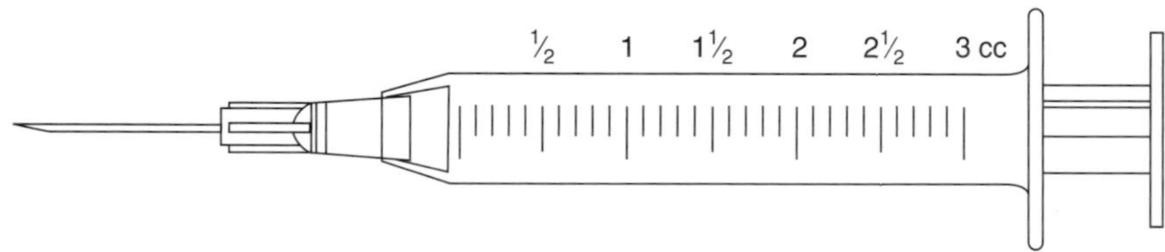

5. Ordered meperidine 45 mg IM q4 h. How many milliliters will the nurse administer? ______ .

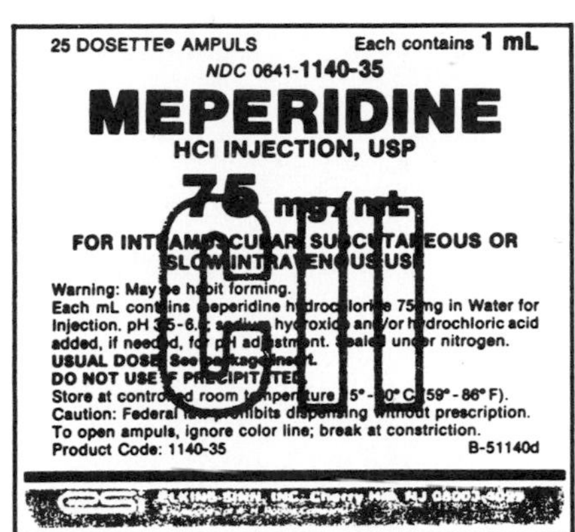

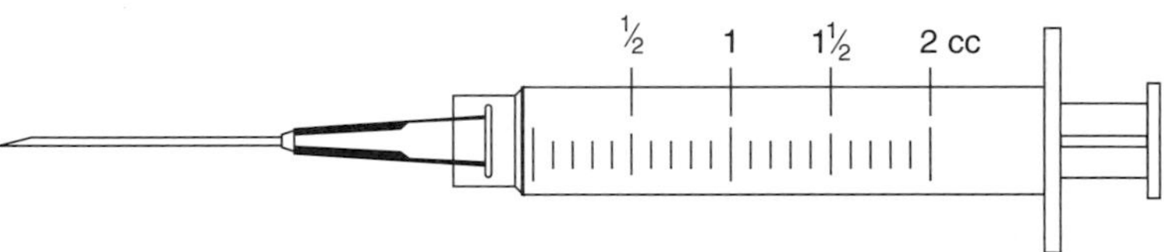

6. The physician orders piperacillin 3 g IV q8 h for your patient with sepsis. You have piperacillin 1 g per 2.5 mL available. How many milliliters will you prepare? ______ .

7. Ordered morphine 5 mg SQ q4 h. You have morphine gr ⅙ per mL available. How many milliliters will the nurse administer? ______ .

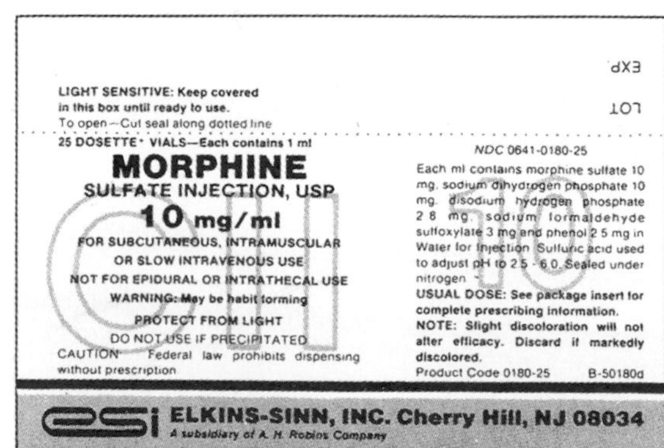

8. The physician orders vancomycin 1 g IV q12 h for your patient with a right-hand amputation. After reconstitution of the medication, you have vancomycin 500 mg per 6 mL. How many milliliters will you prepare? ______ .

9. Your patient with congestive heart failure requires furosemide 30 mg IM stat. How many milliliters will you administer? ______ .

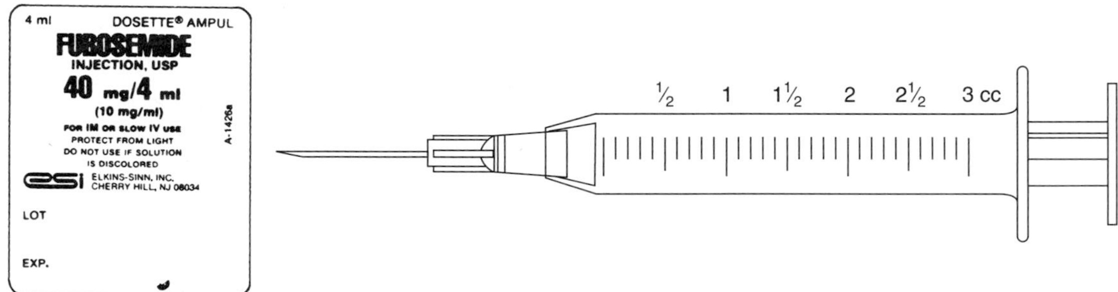

10. Your postoperative patient has Toradol 15 mg IM q6 h for 5 days ordered. You have 30 mg/mL prefilled syringes. How many milliliters will you administer? ______ .

11. Ordered D_5W 1000 mL plus sodium bicarbonate ($NaHCO_3$) 25.8 mEq at 12 mL per h IV. $NaHCO_3$ is supplied in a 50-mL ampule containing 44.6 mEq. How many milliliters of $NaHCO_3$ will be added to the 1000 mL of D_5W? _______ .

12. Your patient with asthma requires aminophylline 100 mg IV q6 h. How many milliliters will you prepare? _______ .

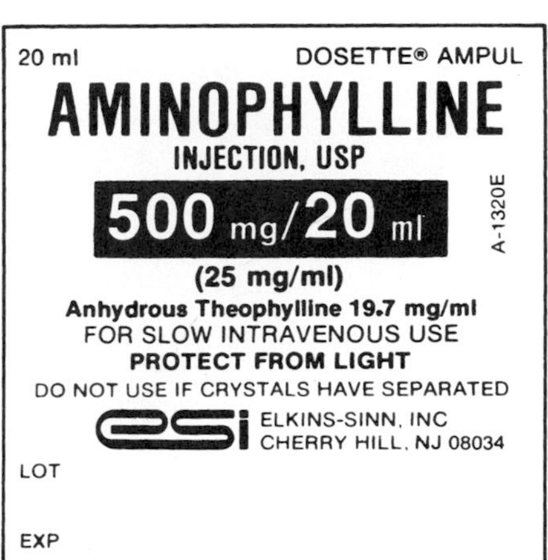

13. Ordered amphotericin B 350 mg IV qd. You have a 100-mg/20-mL vial. How many milliliters will you prepare? ______ .

14. Ordered Gantrisin gr xv IV stat. You have a 5-mL ampule containing 2 g. How many milliliters will you prepare? ______ .

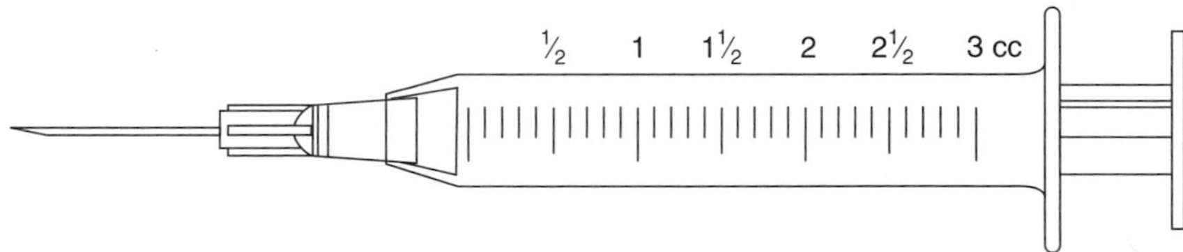

15. The physician orders Solu-Cortef 0.05 g IM q6 h for your patient with scleroderma. How many milliliters will you administer? ______ .

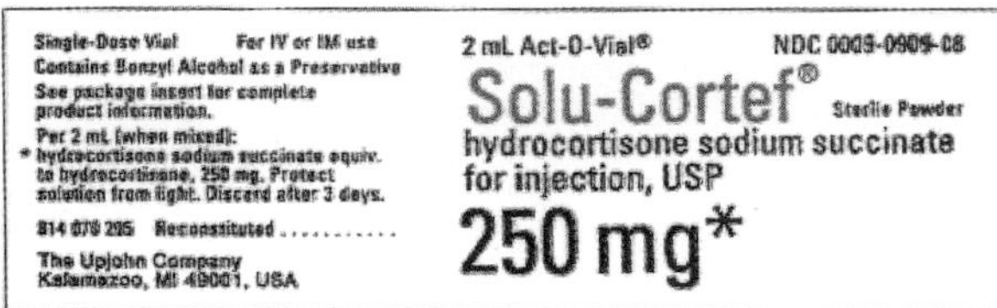

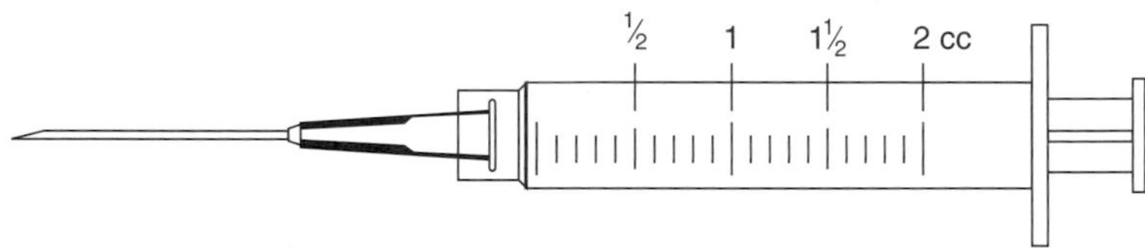

16. Your patient with epilepsy requires phenobarbital 0.3 g IM tid. How many milliliters will you administer? ______ .

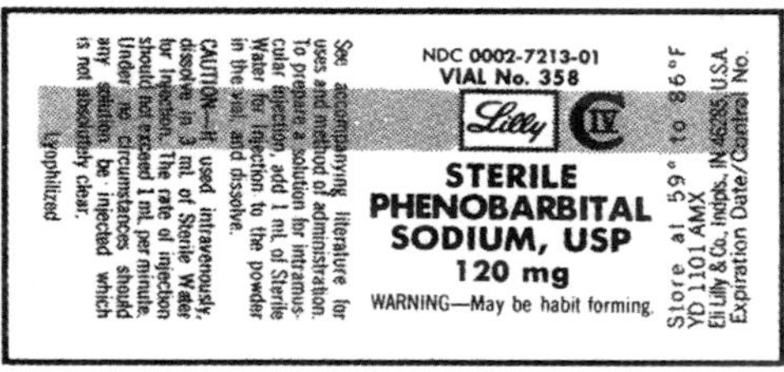

17. Ordered Tagamet 300 mg IV q6 h. How many milliliters will the nurse prepare? ______ .

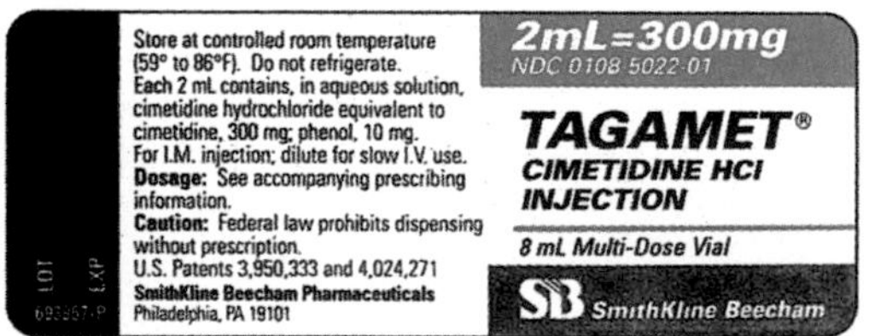

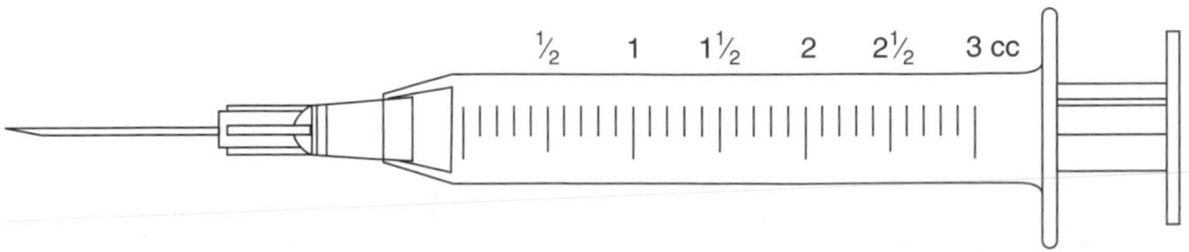

18. Mrs. Andis requires Reglan 10 mg IV q6 h. Reglan 5 mg/mL is available for injection. How many milliliters will the nurse administer? ______ .

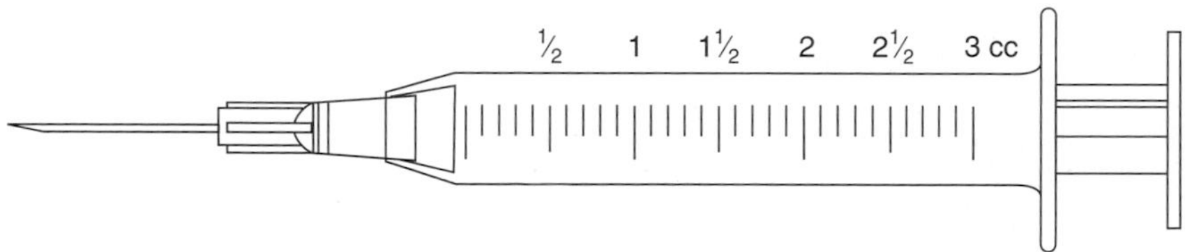

19. The physician orders Stadol 0.5 mg IM q4 h for Mrs. Switzer after childbirth. How many milliliters will the nurse administer? ______ .

20. Mr. Lewis requires Ativan 1 mg IM stat for severe agitation. How many milliliters will the nurse administer? ______ .

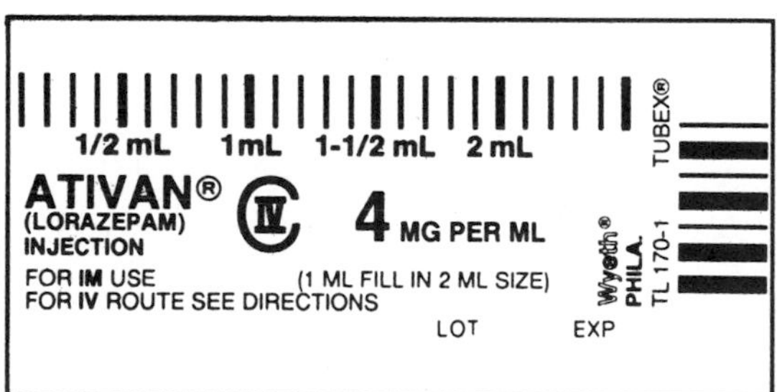

21. Mrs. Carroll requires Apresoline 10 mg IM q6 h for high blood pressure. Apresoline is supplied in 1-mL ampules containing 20 mg. How many milliliters will the nurse prepare? ______ .

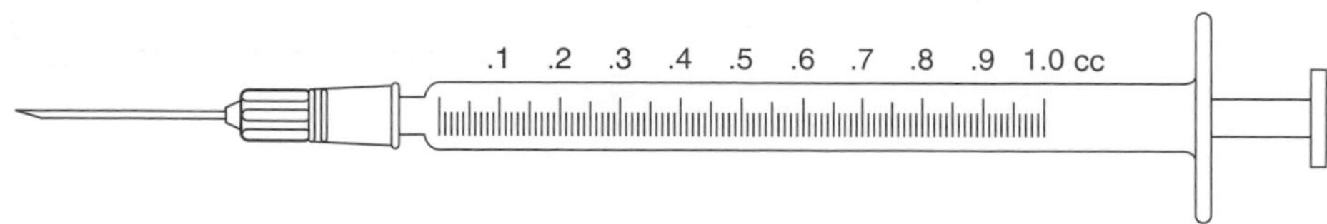

22. Ordered D_5W 1000 mL plus KCl 30 mEq at 60 mL IV per h. How many milliliters of KCl will be added to the 1000 mL of D_5W? ______ .

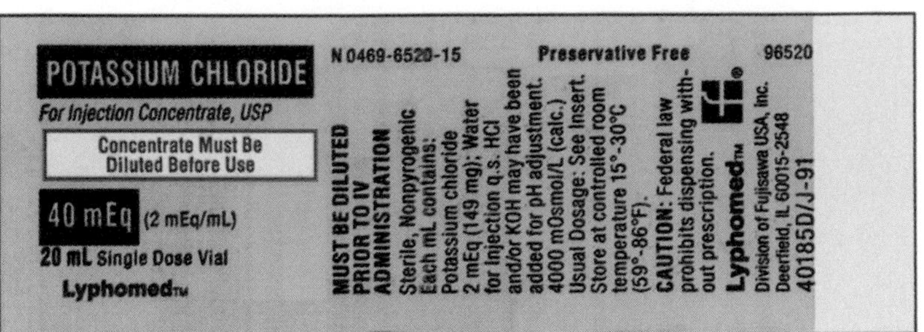

23. The physician orders Valium 10 mg IM q6 h for your anxious patient. You have Valium 5 mg per mL. How many milliliters will you administer? _____ .

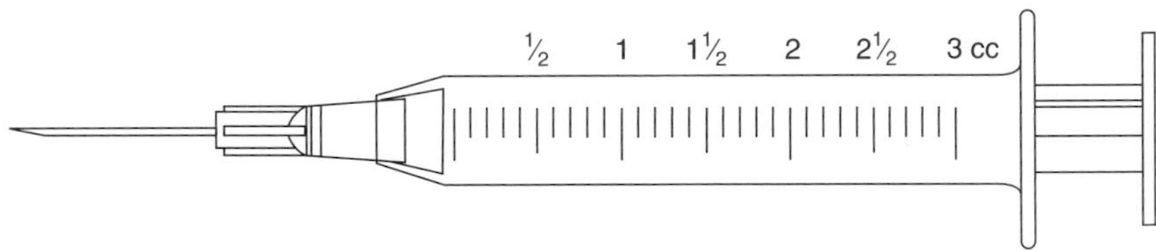

24. Mr. Keesling is diagnosed with an acoustic neuroma and complains of pain. He has codeine gr ¼ IM q3 h prn ordered. How many milliliters will the nurse administer? _____ .

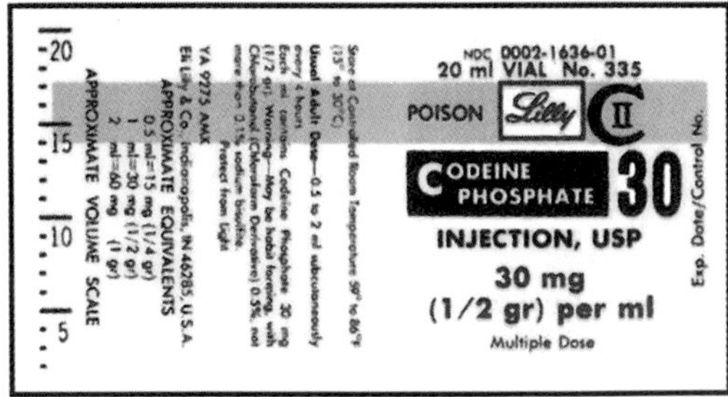

25. Ordered AquaMEPHYTON 0.01 g IM qAM. How many milliliters will the nurse administer? ______ .

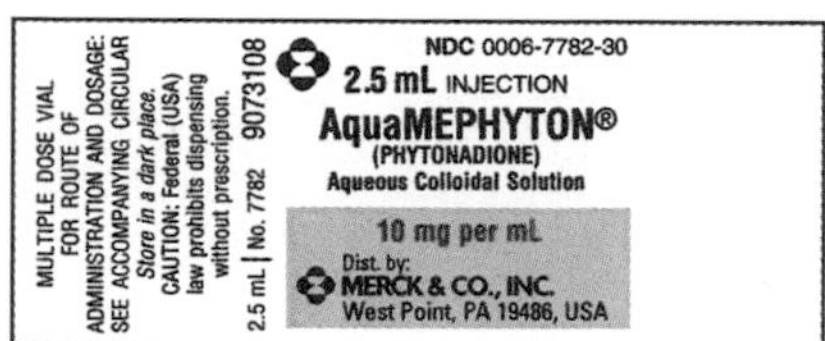

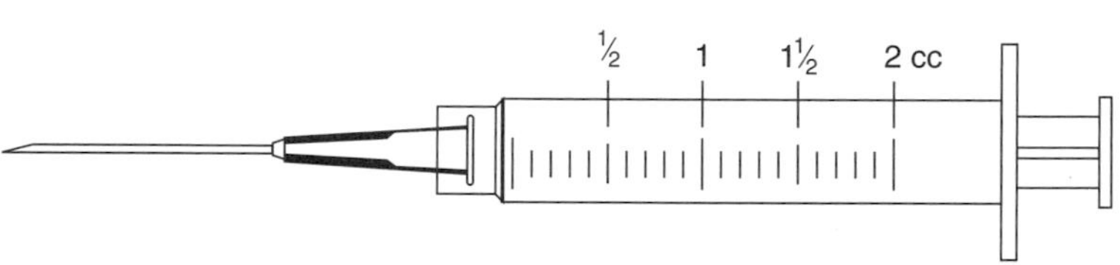

26. Ordered Cipro 0.3 g IV q12 h. How many milliliters will the nurse prepare? ______ .

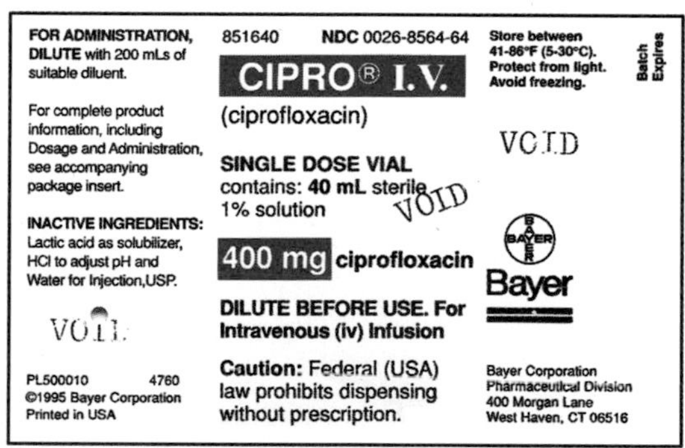

27. Mrs. Ring, who has undergone a hysterectomy, has morphine 12 mg IM q4 h prn ordered for pain relief. How many milliliters will the nurse administer? ______ .

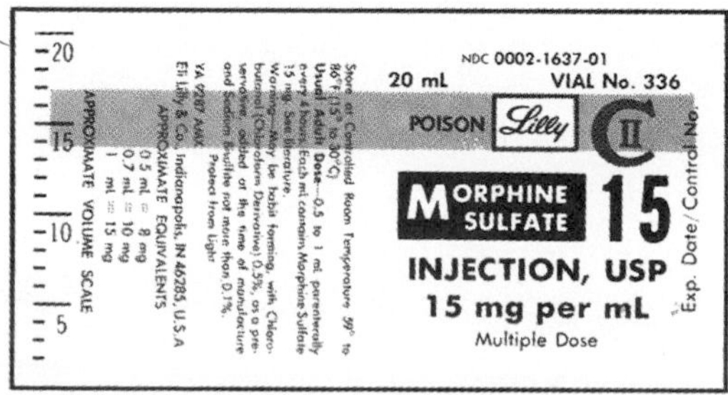

28. Ordered Benadryl 100 mg IM qid. The drug is supplied in ampules containing 50 mg per mL. How many milliliters will the nurse administer? ______ .

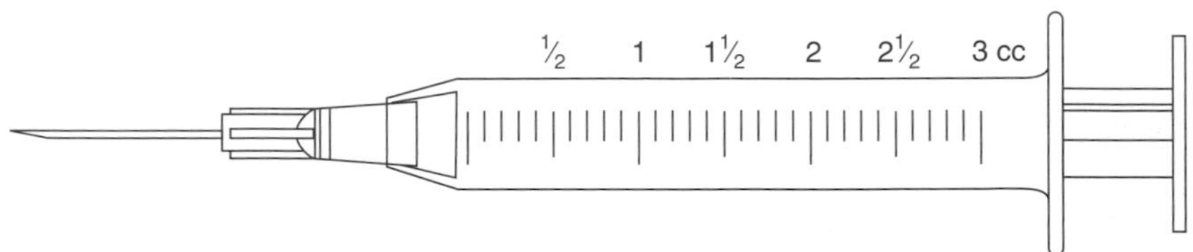

29. Mr. Fields requires digoxin 100 mcg IM qd for his cardiac dysrhythmia. How many milliliters will the nurse administer? ______ .

FOR I.V. OR I.M. USE
BURROUGHS WELLCOME CO.
Research Triangle Park, NC 27709 542282

2 mL
LANOXIN®
(DIGOXIN)
INJECTION
500 µg (0.5 mg)
in 2 mL
(250 µg [0.25 mg] per mL)
DILUTION NOT REQUIRED
PROPYLENE GLYCOL 40%
ALCOHOL 10%
Store at 15° to 25°C (59° to 77°F). Protect from light.

LOT
EXP.

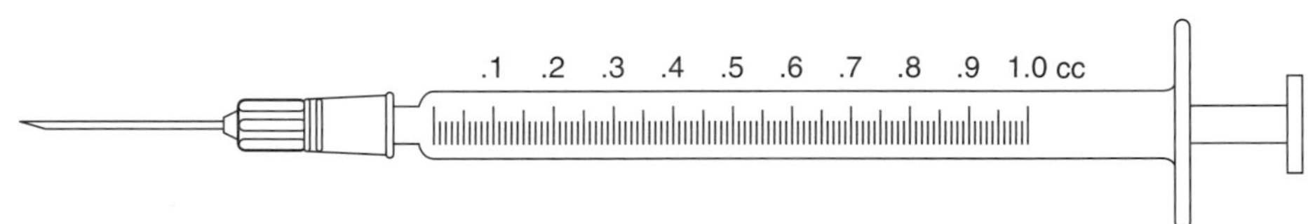

30. Ordered Kefzol 500 mg IV q6 h × 4 days. How many milliliters will the nurse prepare? ______ .

CAUTION—Federal (U.S.A.) law prohibits dispensing without prescription.
For I.M. or I.V. Use
Dosage—See literature.
To prepare solution add 2 ml Sterile Water for Injection or 0.9% Sodium Chloride Injection. Provides an approximate volume of 2.2 ml (225 mg per ml)
SHAKE WELL Protect from Light
Prior to Reconstitution: Store at Controlled Room Temperature 59° to 86°F (15° to 30°C)
After Reconstitution: Store in a refrigerator. For Storage Time - See Accompanying Literature. If kept at room temperature, use within 24 hours.
Lyophilized
WV 4520 AMX
Eli Lilly & Co., Indianapolis, IN 46285, U.S.A.
Exp. Date/Control No.

NDC 0002-1497-01
VIAL No. 767
℞ Lilly
KEFZOL®
STERILE
CEFAZOLIN
SODIUM, USP
Equiv. to
500 mg
Cefazolin

31. Your patient with epilepsy receives phenobarbital gr v IM q3 h. How many milliliters will you administer? ______ .

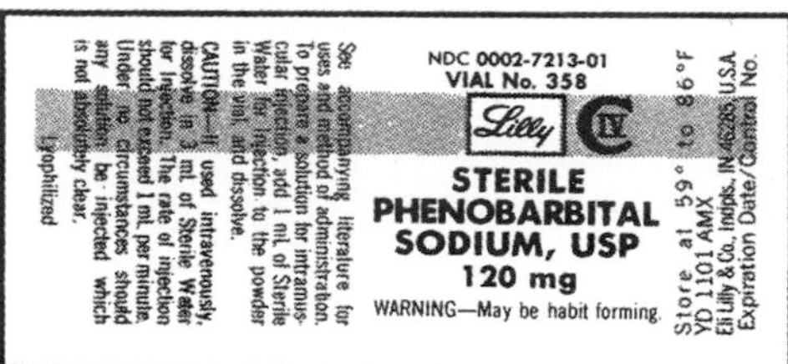

32. The physician orders Solu-Cortef 100 mg IM q8 h for your patient with severe contact dermatitis. How many milliliters will you administer? ______ .

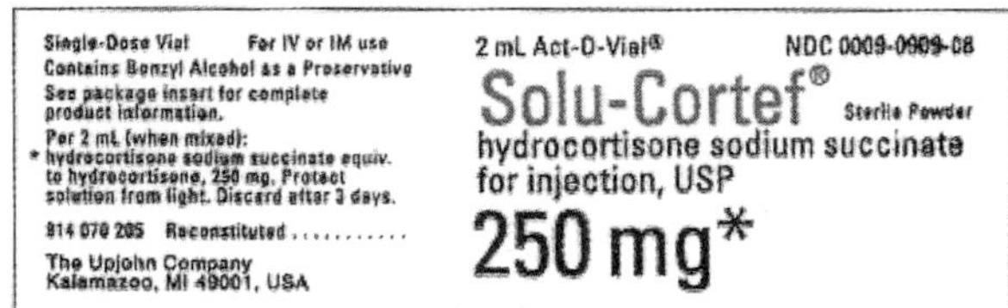

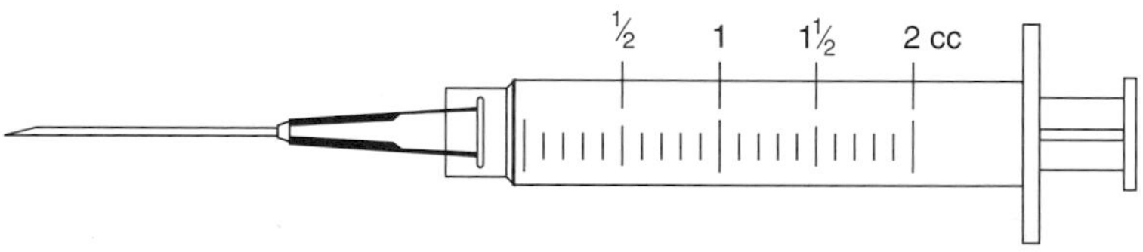

33. Ordered D_5W 250 mL plus NaCl 7.5 mEq at 2 mL IV per h. NaCl is supplied in a 40-mL vial containing 2.5 mEq per mL. How many milliliters of NaCl will be added to the 250 mL of D_5W? _______ .

34. Your patient with a lumbar laminectomy receives Vistaril 3 mL IM tid. How many milligrams does this patient receive in each dose? _______ .

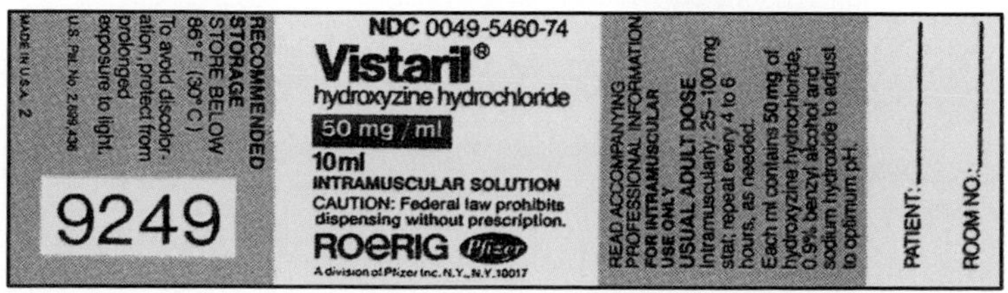

35. The physician orders atropine gr $\frac{1}{100}$ IM stat for your preop patient. How many milliliters will you administer? ______ .

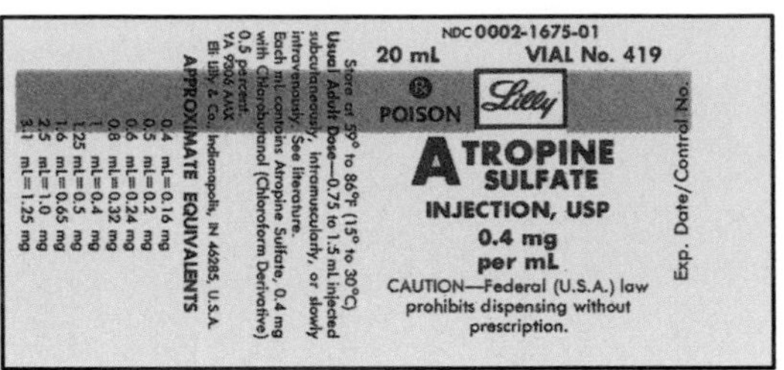

36. Your patient admitted with neuroleptic disorder has Seconal 50 mg IM hs prn ordered. How many milliliters will you administer? ______ .

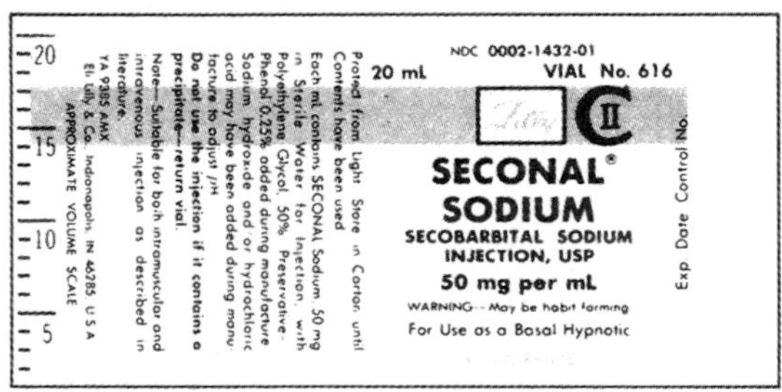

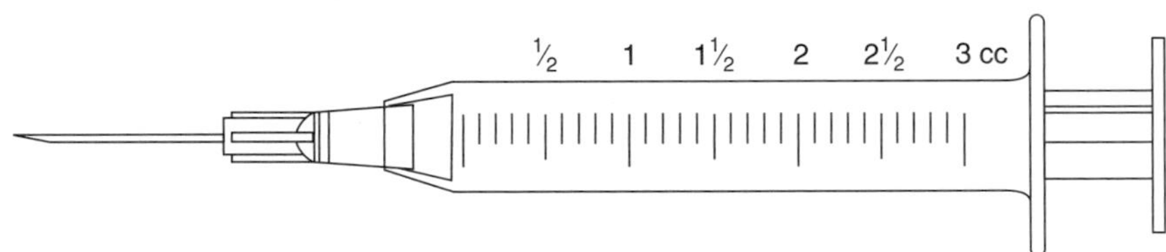

37. Ordered meperidine 75 mg IM q4 h prn. How many milliliters will the nurse administer? ______ .

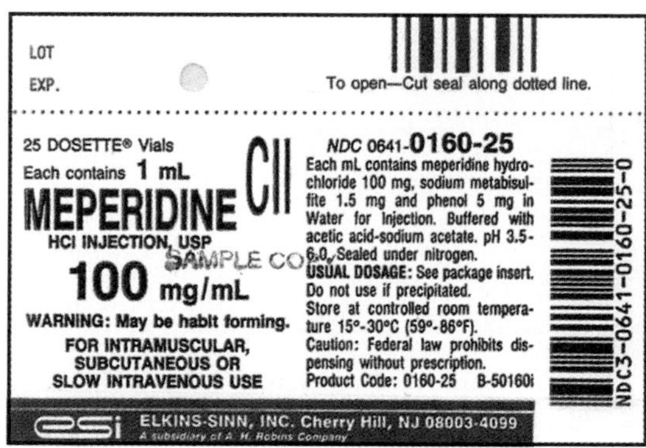

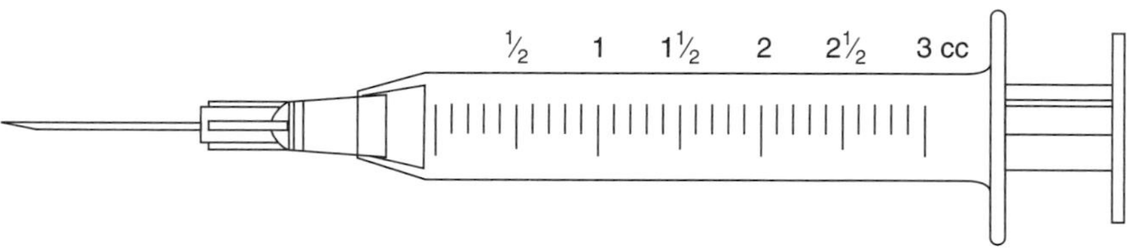

38. Your patient with chronic obstructive pulmonary disease (COPD) receives aminophylline 75 mg q 6 h. How many milliliters will you prepare? ______ .

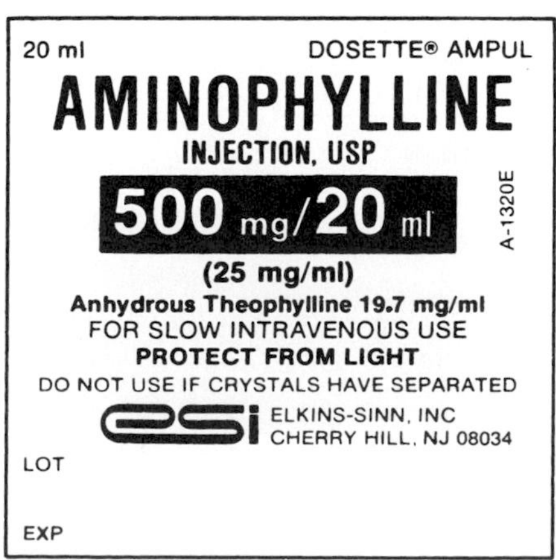

39. Ordered Naloxone 0.6 mg IM stat. How many milliliters will the nurse prepare? ______ .

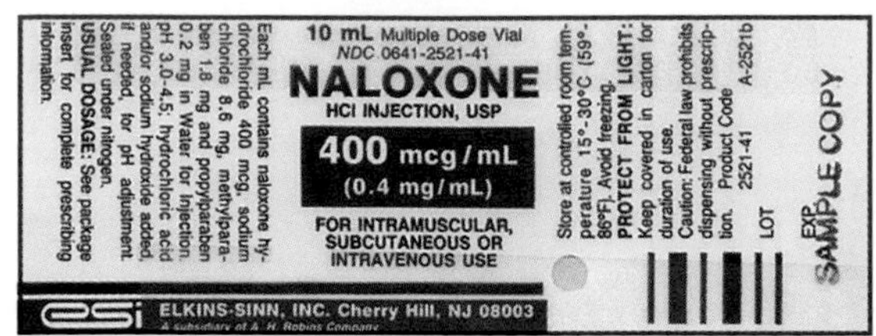

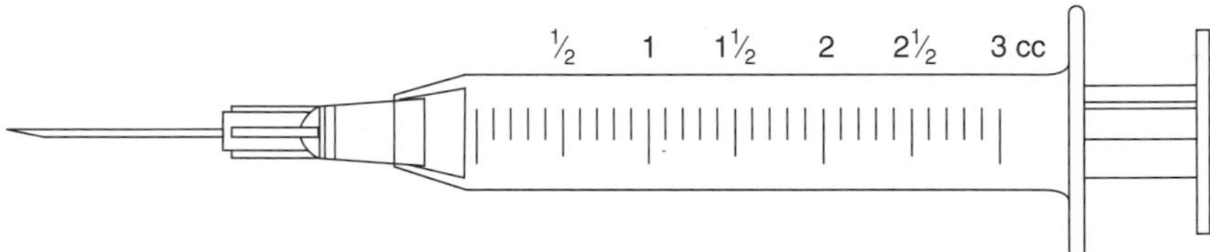

40. Ordered Valium 10 mg IV stat. Valium is supplied in a 10-mL vial containing 5 mg per mL. How many milliliters will the nurse prepare? ______ .

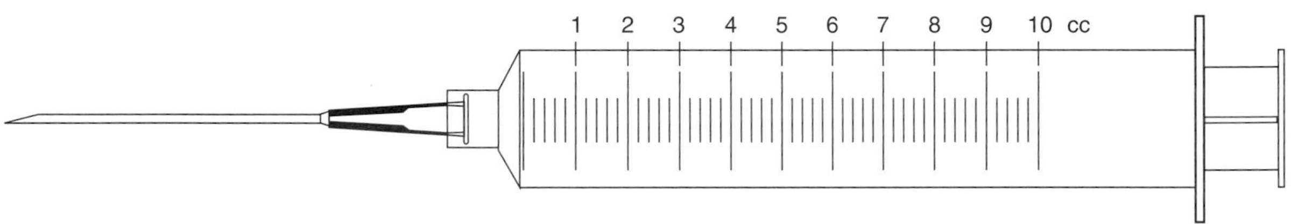

41. Mr. Norcross has psoriasis and requires hydrocortisone 25 mg IM qd. The drug is available at a concentration of 100 mg per 2 mL. How many milliliters will the nurse administer? ______ .

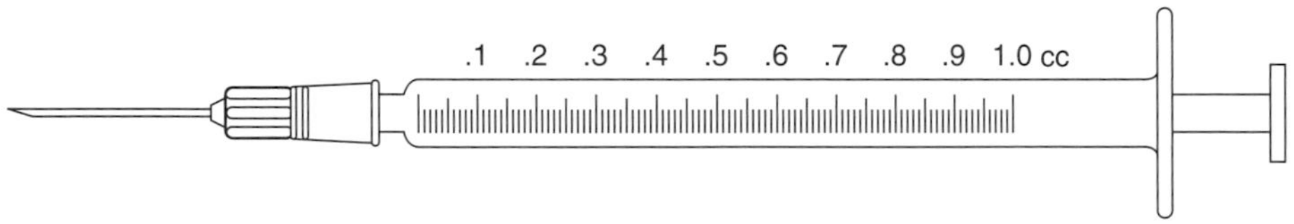

42. Your patient with a *Pseudomonas* infection receives Kantrex 400 mg IM q12 h. How many milliliters will you administer? ______ .

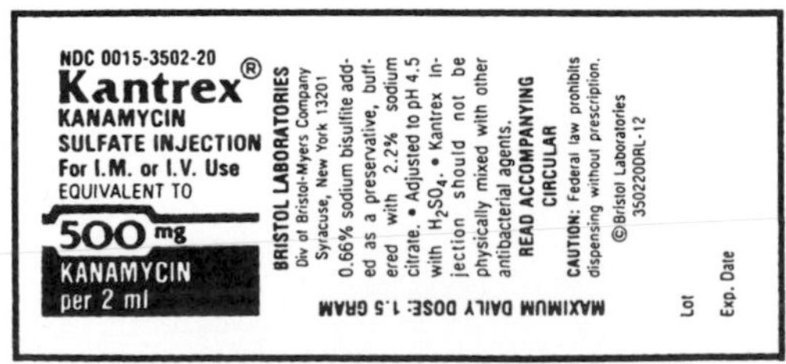

43. The physician orders ascorbic acid 0.25 g IM qd for your patient admitted with an alcohol abuse problem. You have ascorbic acid 500 mg per mL. How many milliliters will you administer? ______ .

44. Ordered D_5W 250 mL plus calcium chloride ($CaCl_2$) 5 mEq at 2 mL per h IV. $CaCl_2$ is supplied in a 10-mL ampule containing 13.6 mEq. How many milliliters of $CaCl_2$ will be added to the 250 mL of D_5W? _______ .

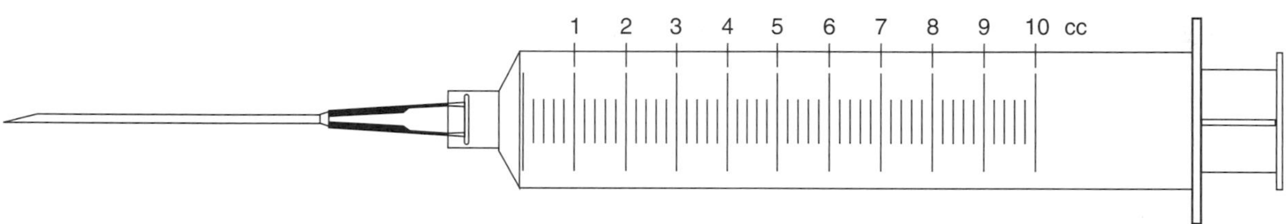

45. The physician orders phenobarbital 70 mg SQ q8 h for your patient with epilepsy. The drug is supplied in a 1-mL ampule containing 65 mg. How many milliliters will you administer? ______ .

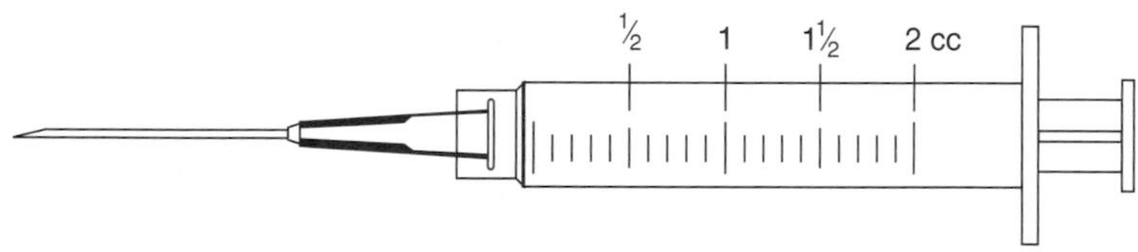

46. Ordered Vibramycin 200 mg IV qd. You have Vibramycin 10 mg per mL after reconstitution. How many milliliters will you prepare? ______ .

47. Ordered Dilaudid gr 1/30 IM q4 h prn. How many milliliters will the nurse administer? ______ .

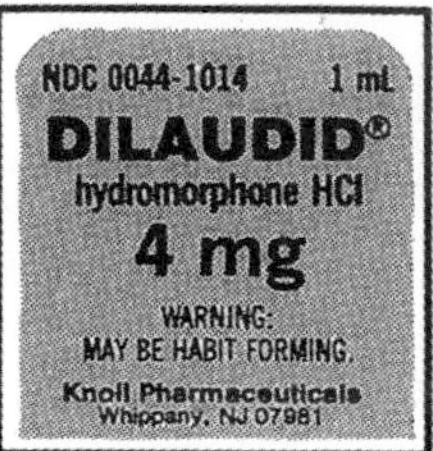

48. Your patient with atrial fibrillation has digoxin 0.2 mg IM qd ordered. How many milliliters will you administer? ______ .

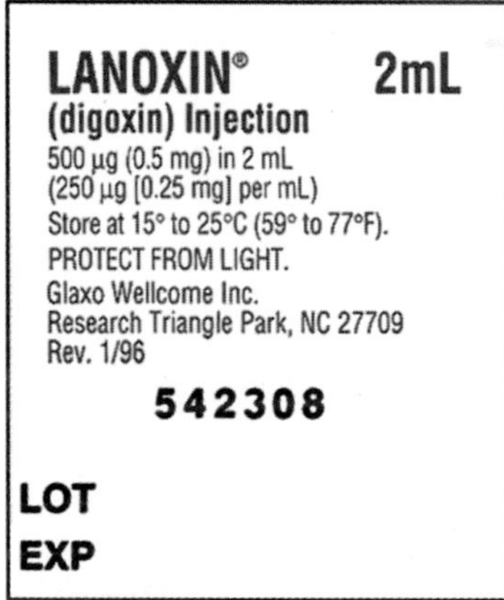

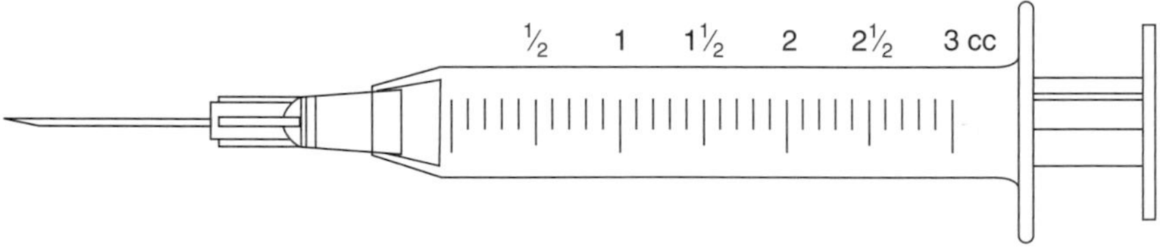

49. Ordered Morphine gr 1/6 SQ q3 h. How many milliliters will the nurse administer? ______ .

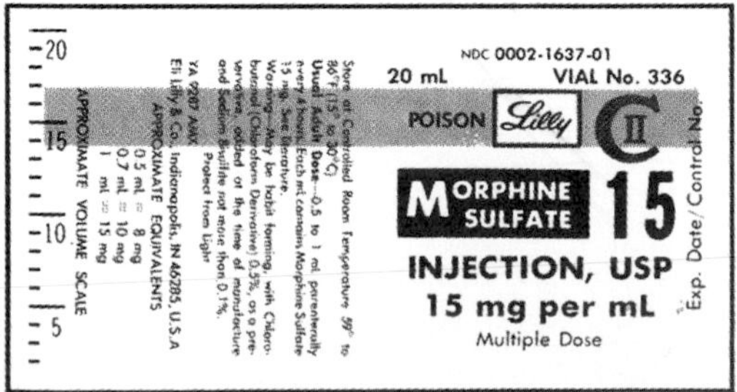

50. Your patient with bipolar disorder receives Haldol 3 mg IM qid. The drug is supplied in a 1-mL ampule containing 5 mg. How many milliliters will you administer? ______ .

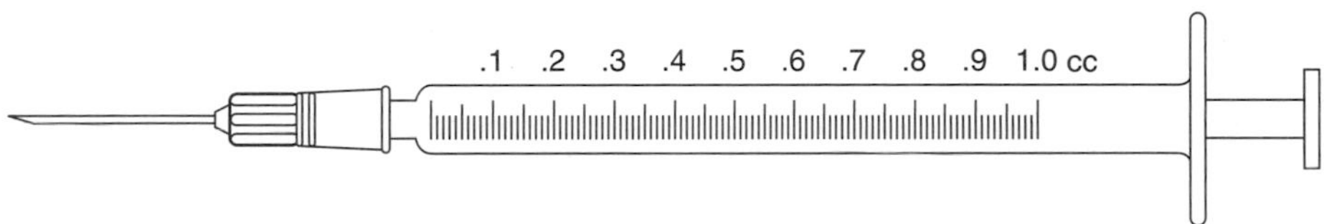

51. Ordered Cefadyl 600 mg IM q6 h. How many milliliters will the nurse administer? ______ .

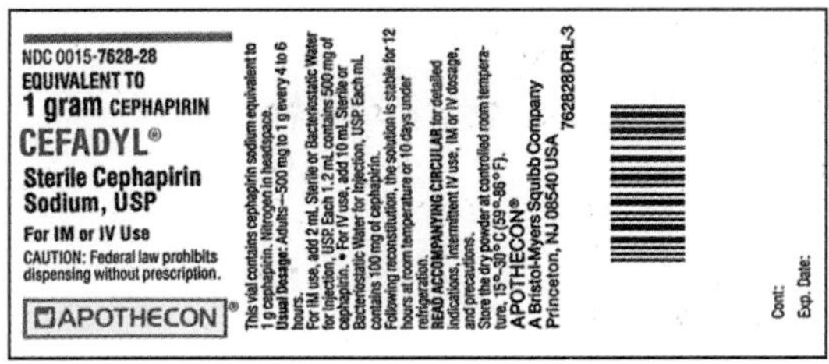

52. Your preop patient needs atropine 0.9 mg IM at 6:15 AM. How many milliliters will you administer? ______ .

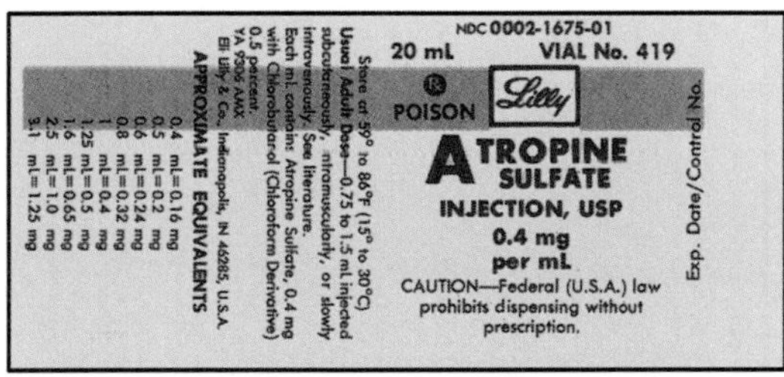

53. The physician orders codeine gr ss SQ q4 h for your patient after a lumbar laminectomy for pain relief. How many milliliters will you administer? ______ .

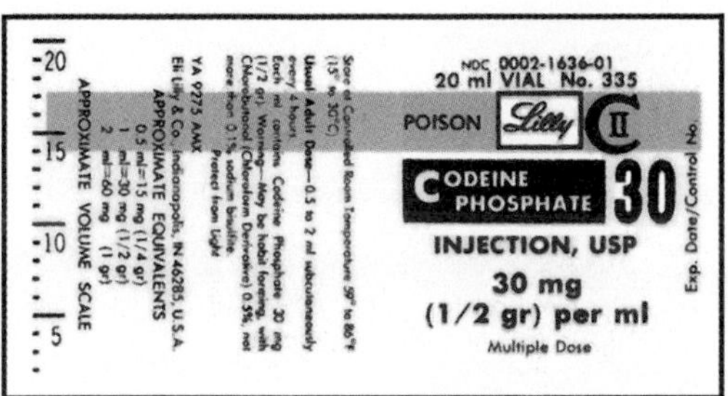

54. The physician orders phenobarbital gr ¼ SQ q3 h for your patient with head trauma. Phenobarbital is supplied in 1-mL ampules containing 65 mg. How many milliliters will you administer? ______ .

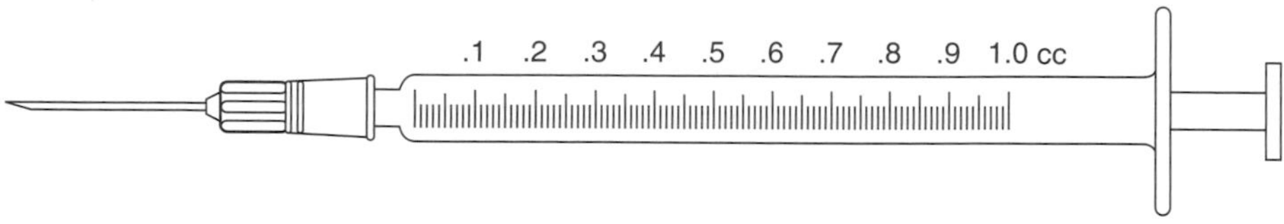

55. Ordered D_5W 500 mL plus 6 mEq of $NaHCO_3$ at 42 mL per h IV. $NaHCO_3$ is available in a 10-mL ampule containing 0.89 mEq per mL. How many milliliters of $NaHCO_3$ will be added to the 500 mL of D_5W? ______ .

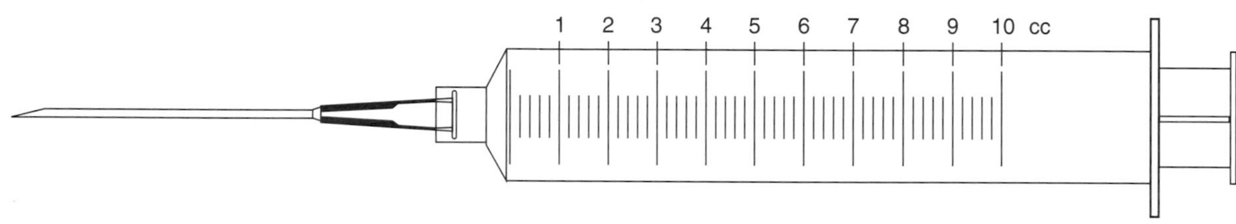

56. Mr. Grey, who has undergone cervical discectomy, has Garamycin 20 mg IM q8 h ordered. How many milliliters will the nurse administer? ______ .

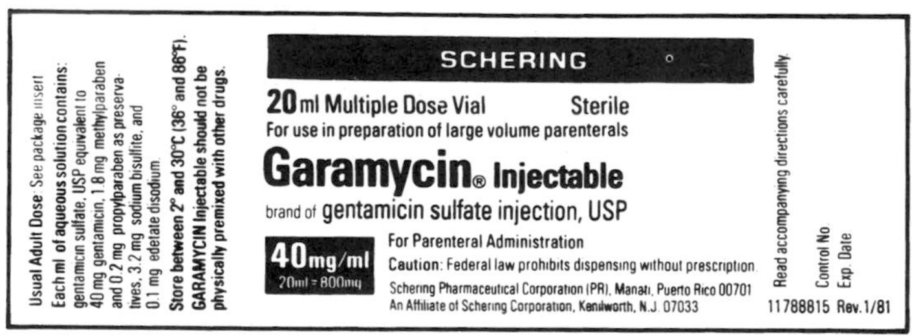

57. Mr. Ali receives Thorazine 0.2 mL IM q4 h for severe hiccups. How many milligrams does Mr. Ali receive in each dose? ______ .

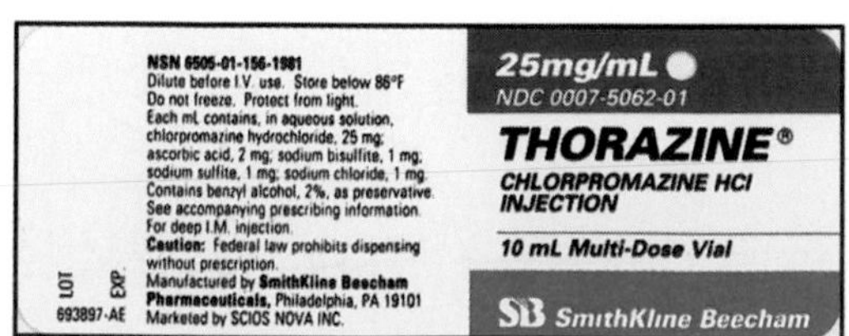

58. Your patient with sinusitis receives ampicillin 500 mg IV q12 h. You have ampicillin 100 mg per mL. How many milliliters will you prepare? ______ .

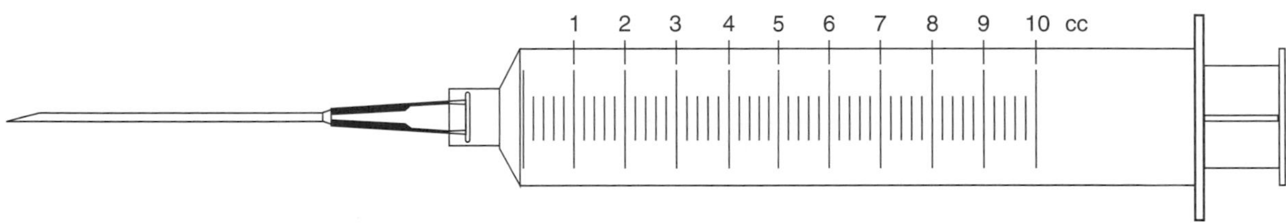

59. Ordered meperidine 50 mg IM q4 h prn. How many milliliters will the nurse administer? ______ .

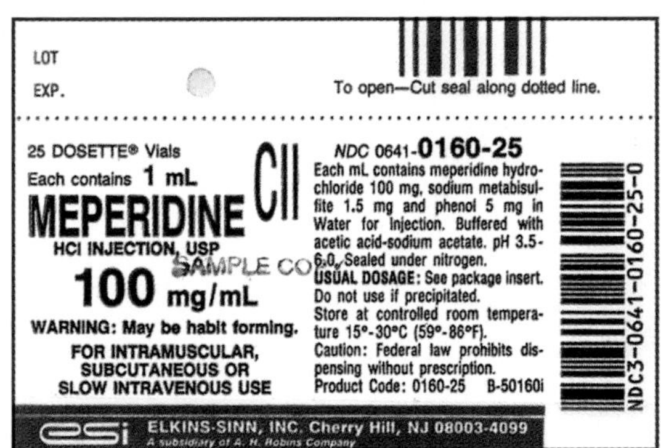

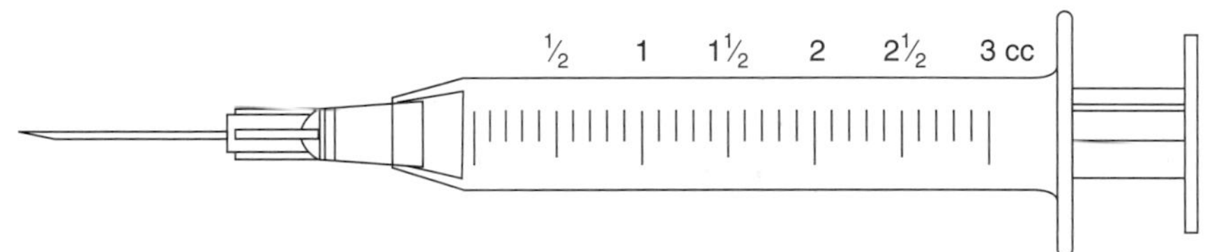

60. The physician orders Ativan 0.5 mg IM stat for your patient with severe anxiety. The drug is supplied in a 1-mL vial containing 2 mg per mL. How many milliliters will you administer? ______ .

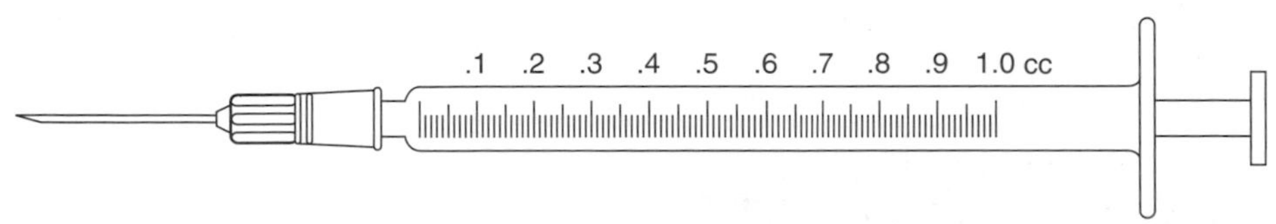

61. Aminophylline 0.2 g IV tid. Aminophylline is supplied in a 10-mL ampule containing 0.25 g per 10 mL. How many milliliters will the nurse prepare? ______ .

62. Codeine 15 mg IM q4 h. Codeine is available in a vial containing gr ss per mL. How many milliliters will the nurse administer? ______ .

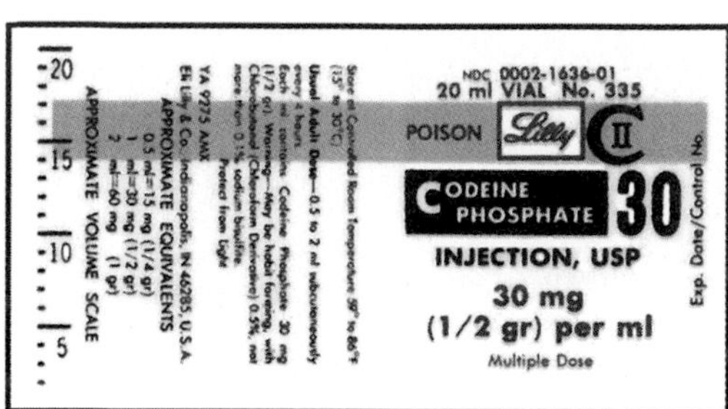

63. Mr. Ciele, who has undergone partial craniotomy, receives Dilantin 100 mg IV q8 h. You have available Dilantin 50 mg per mL. How many milliliters will you prepare? ______ .

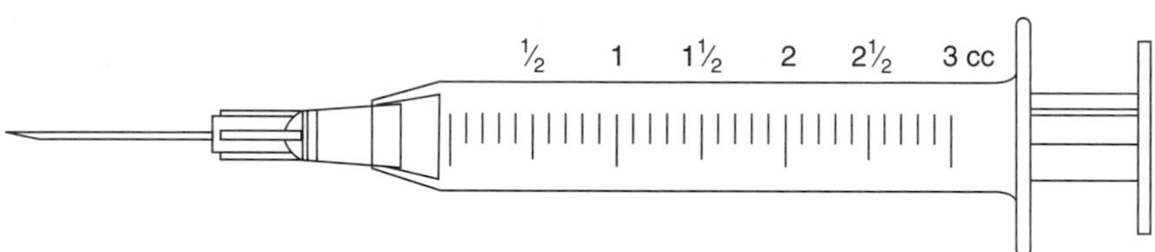

64. The physician orders digoxin 0.25 mg IV qd for your patient with atrial flutter. Digoxin is supplied in a 2-mL ampule containing 0.5 mg. How many milliliters will you prepare? ______ .

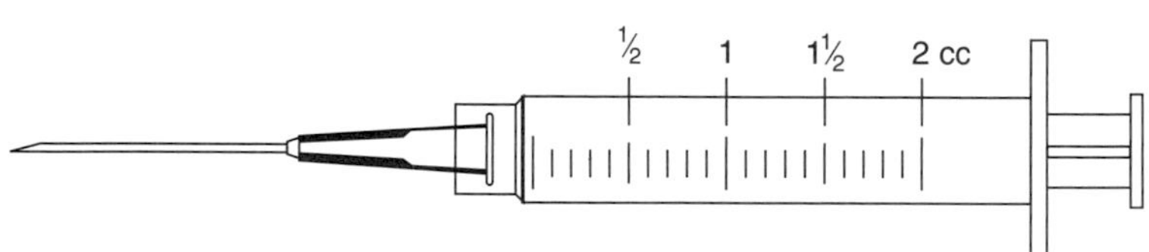

65. Mrs. Peterson needs meperidine 35 mg IM q3 h for severe pain after a total hip replacement. How many milliliters will the nurse administer? ______ .

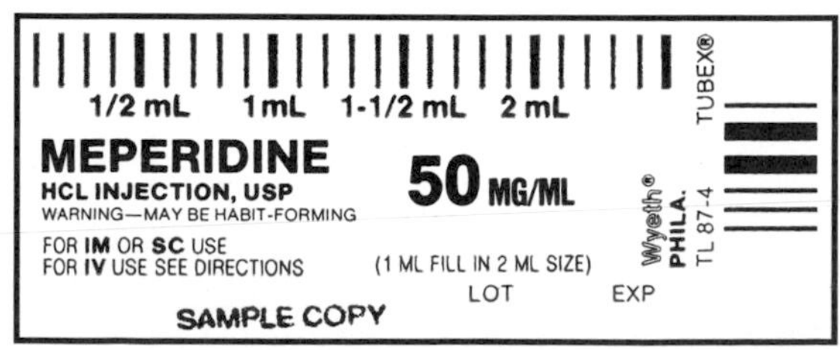

66. Ordered D_5W 250 mL plus calcium gluconate 5 mEq at 2 mL IV per h. Calcium gluconate is supplied in a 10-mL ampule containing 4.8 mEq. How many milliliters of calcium gluconate will be added to the 250 mL of D_5W? ______ .

67. Mr. Thompson, admitted with erythrasma, receives Cleocin 50 mg IV q8 h. How many milliliters will the nurse prepare? ______ .

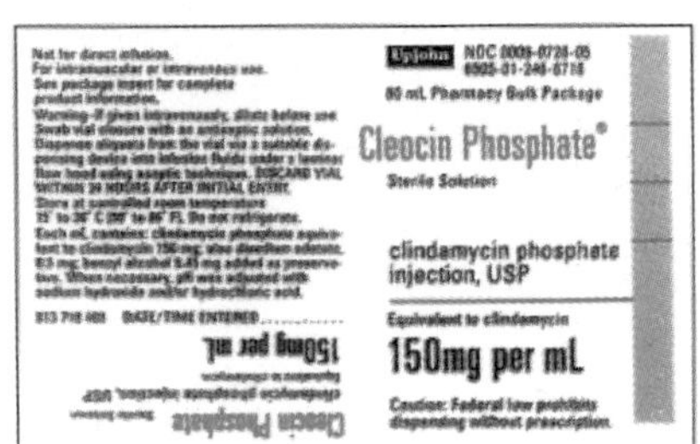

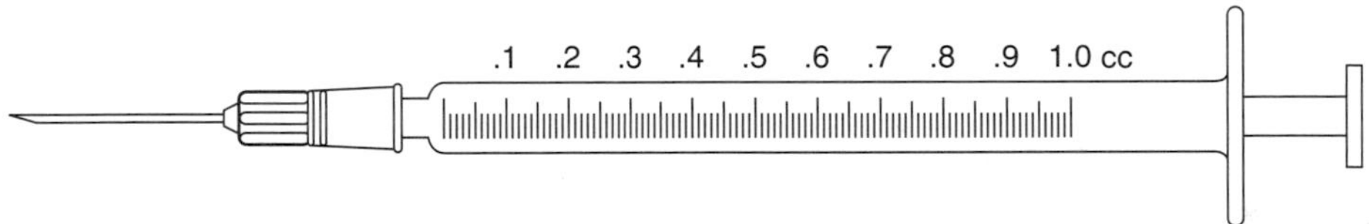

68. Atropine 0.2 mg IM at 7:30 AM. How many milliliters will the nurse administer? ______ .

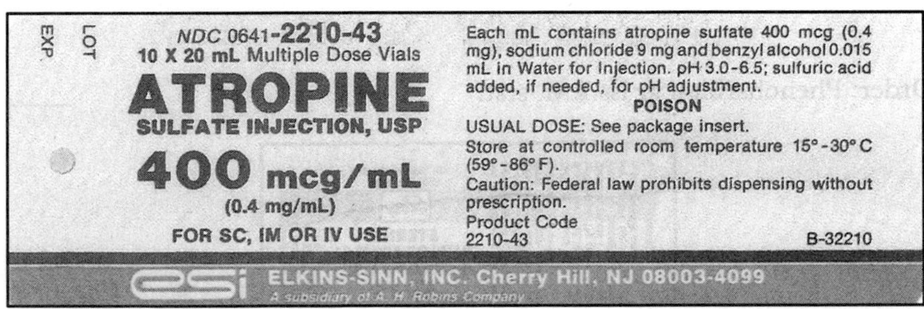

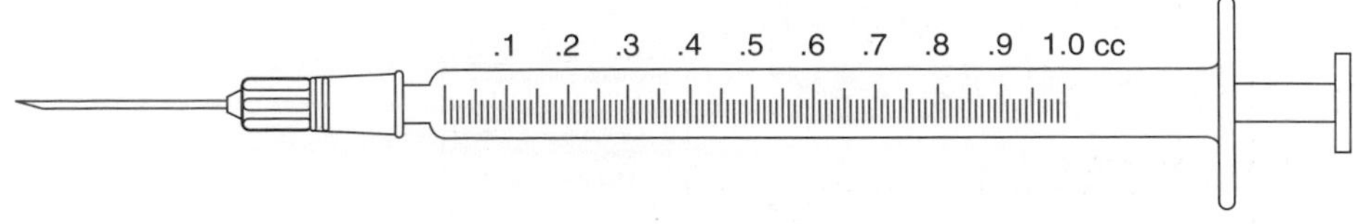

69. Mr. Riley receives tobramycin 55 mg IV q8 h for sepsis. How many milliliters will the nurse prepare? ______ .

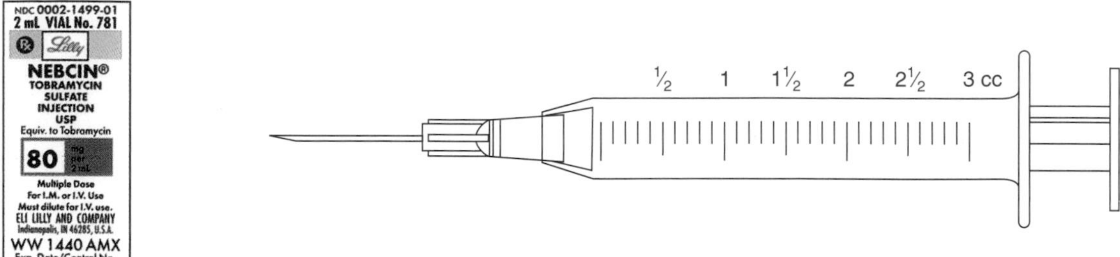

70. Phenobarbital 22 mg IM is ordered as an anticonvulsant. Phenobarbital is supplied in 1-mL ampules containing 65 mg. How many milliliters will the nurse administer? ______ .

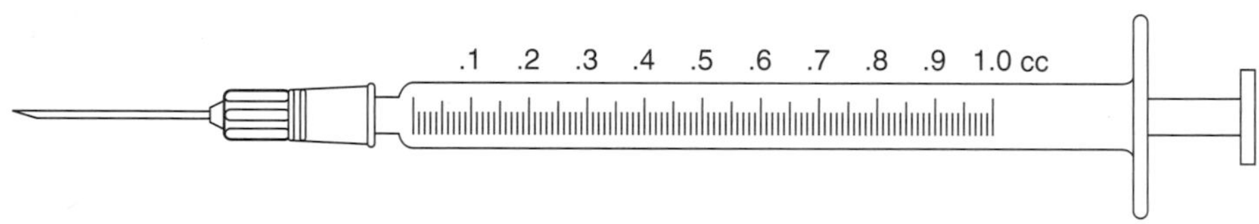

71. Your patient needs morphine gr 1/6 SQ stat for myocardial infarction. How many milliliters will you administer? ______ .

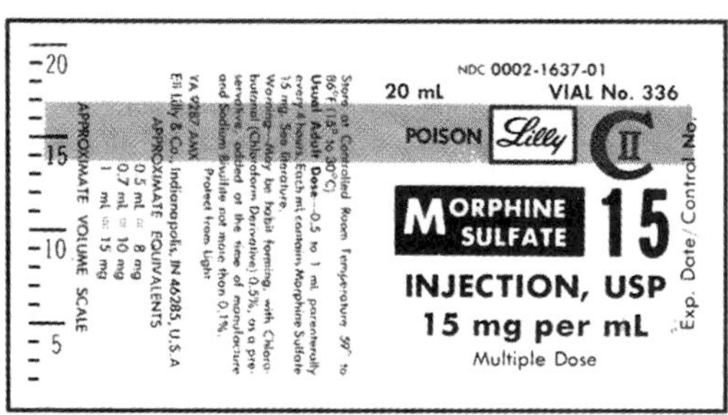

72. Ordered vitamin B_{12} 1 mg IM q Monday. How many milliliters will the nurse administer? _______ .

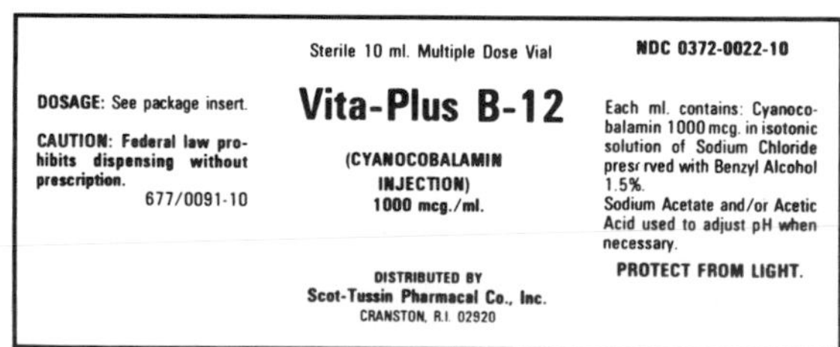

73. Ordered Monocid 800 mg IM qd. How many milliliters will the nurse administer? ______ .

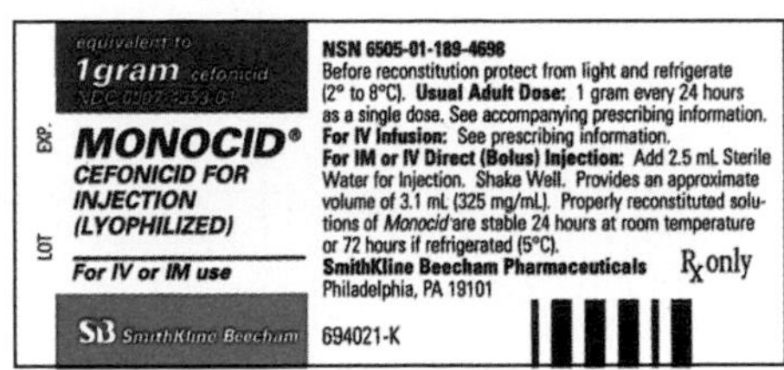

74. Mr. Paley receives Phenergan 12.5 mg IM at 9:30 AM for relief of nausea after a colonoscopy. Phenergan is supplied in an ampule containing 25 mg per mL. How many milliliters will the nurse administer? ______ .

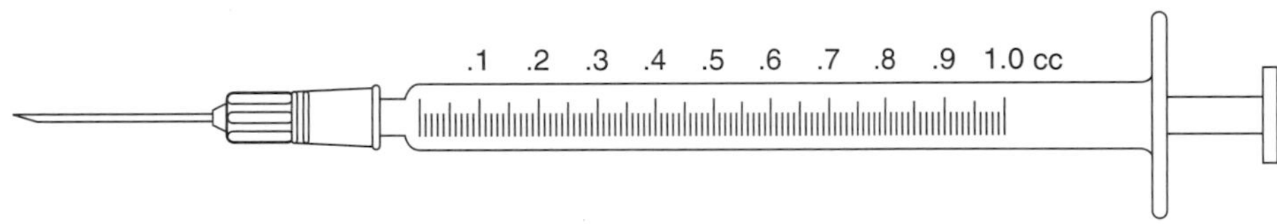

75. Your patient receives Robinul 0.28 mg IM at 6:00 AM. How many milliliters will you administer? ______ .

5 mL Multiple Dose Vial NDC 0031-7890-93
Robinul® Injectable
(Glycopyrrolate Injection, USP)
0.2 mg/mL
Water for Injection, USP q.s./Benzyl Alcohol, NF (preservative) 0.9%.
NOT FOR USE IN NEWBORNS
pH adjusted, when necessary, with hydrochloric acid and/or sodium hydroxide.

CAUTION: Federal law prohibits dispensing without prescription.
For I.M. or I.V. administration.
For dosage and other directions for use, consult accompanying product literature.
Store at Controlled Room Temperature, Between 15°C and 30°C (59°F and 86°F).
MANUFACTURED FOR PHARMACEUTICAL DIVISION
A.H. ROBINS COMPANY, RICHMOND, VA. 23220
by ELKINS-SINN, INC., CHERRY HILL, N.J. 08003
a subsidiary of A.H. Robins 10.87
LOT
EXP.

76. Mr. Eli receives Demerol 10 mg IM q6 h for pain after denervation from a gunshot wound. Demerol is available in an ampule containing 25 mg per mL. How many milliliters will the nurse administer? ______ .

77. Ordered D_5W 1000 mL plus NaCl 15 mEq at 30 mL IV per h. NaCl is supplied in a 40-mL vial containing 100 mEq. How many milliliters of NaCl will be added to the 1000 mL of D_5W? ______ .

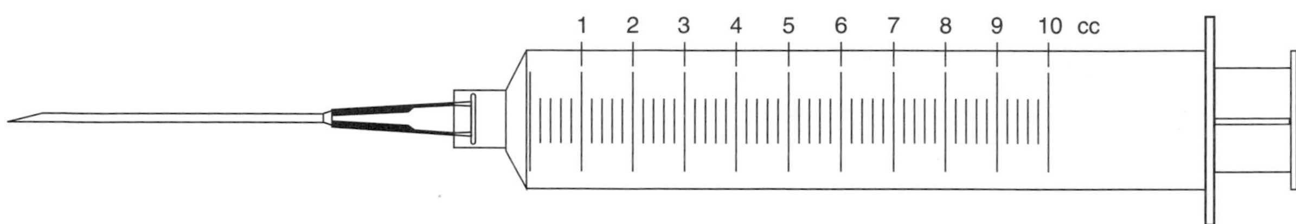

78. Mr. Neal receives Kefzol 250 mg IV q6 h for 12 doses after an ethmoidectomy. The drug is available in a vial containing 125 mg per mL. How many milliliters will the nurse prepare? ______ .

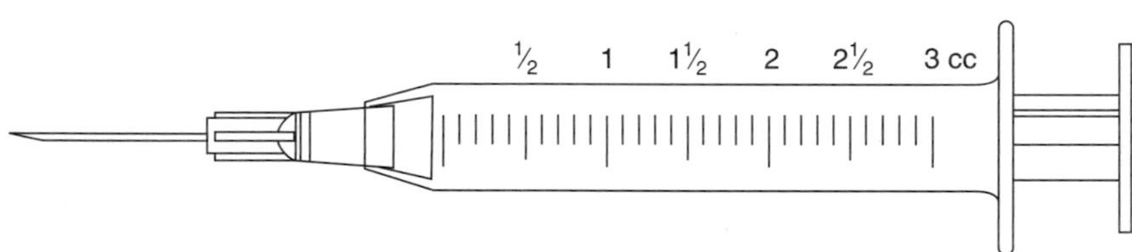

79. Your patient receives the antibiotic Cleocin 300 mg IV q6 h for treatment of diphtheria. Cleocin is available in a 4-mL ampule containing 600 mg. How many milliliters will you prepare? ______ .

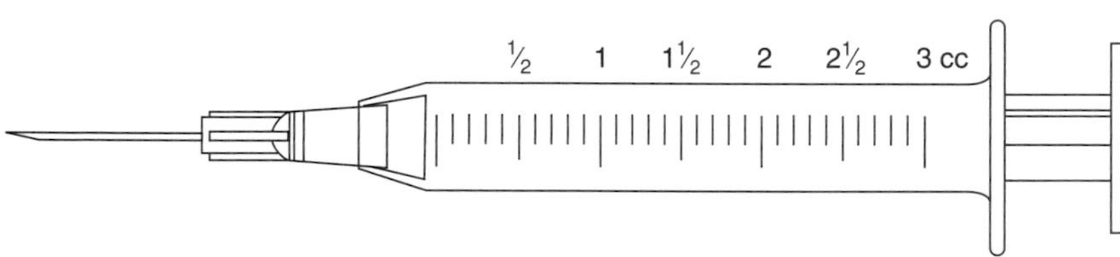

80. Ordered lidocaine 75 mg IV stat. Lidocaine is available in a 5-mL vial containing 100 mg per 5 mL. How many milliliters will the nurse prepare? ______ .

81. Ordered Ticar 0.8 g IV q6 h. How many milliliters will the nurse prepare? ______ .

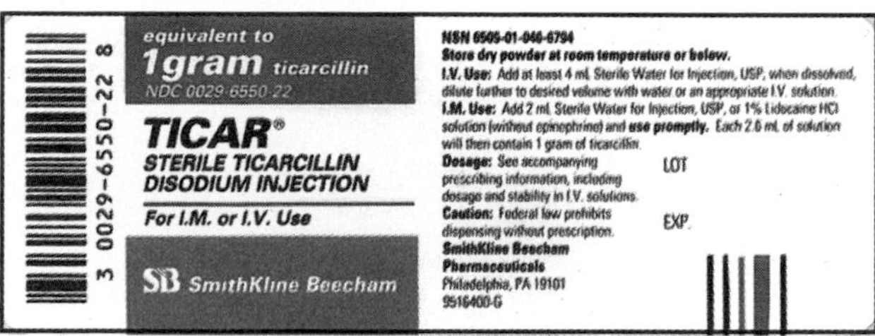

82. Ordered Solu-Medrol 100 mg IV stat. How many milliliters will the nurse prepare? ______ .

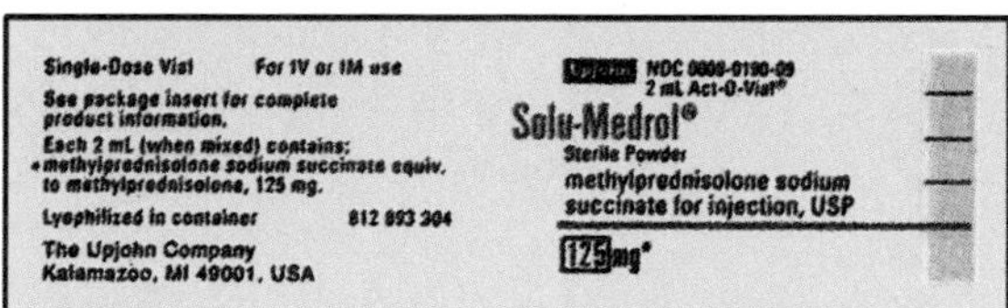

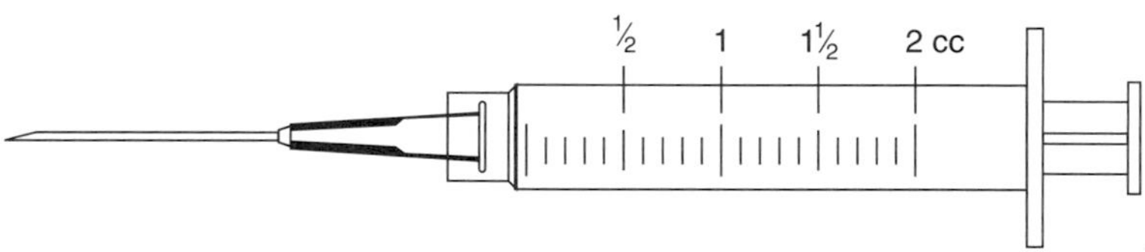

83. Your preop patient has Demerol 25 mg IM ordered on call to the operating room. Demerol is available in an ampule containing 50 mg per mL. How many milliliters will you administer? ______ .

84. Ordered Scopolamine gr 1/150 at 7 AM. How many milliliters will the nurse administer? _______ .

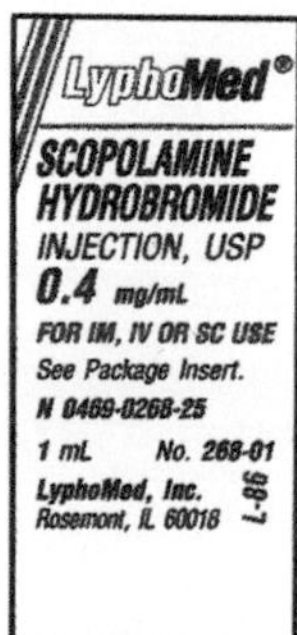

85. Your patient requires Phenergan 0.2 mL IM stat for relief of nausea and vomiting. Phenergan is supplied in an ampule containing 25 mg per mL. How many milligrams will the patient receive? _______ .

86. Ordered Dilaudid gr 1/60 IM q4 h prn. How many milliliters will the nurse administer? _______ .

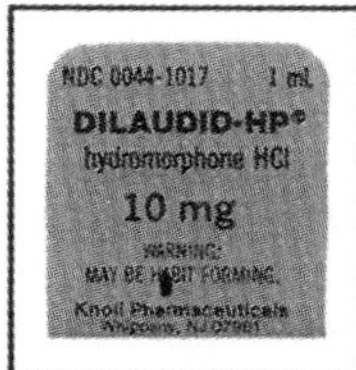

87. Your patient requires Vistaril 50 mg IM q4 h prn for severe agitation. How many milliliters will you administer? ______ .

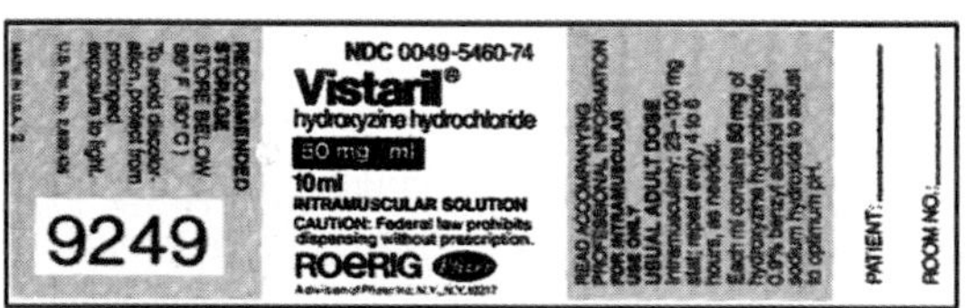

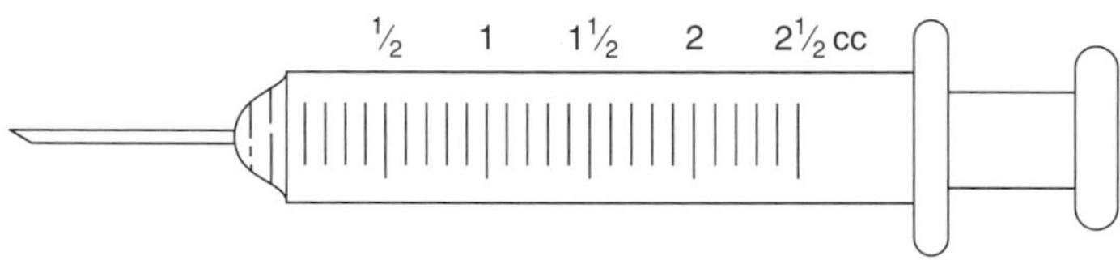

88. D_5W 500 mL plus KCl 10 mEq at 42 mL IV per h. How many milliliters of KCl will be added to the 500 mL of D_5W? _______ .

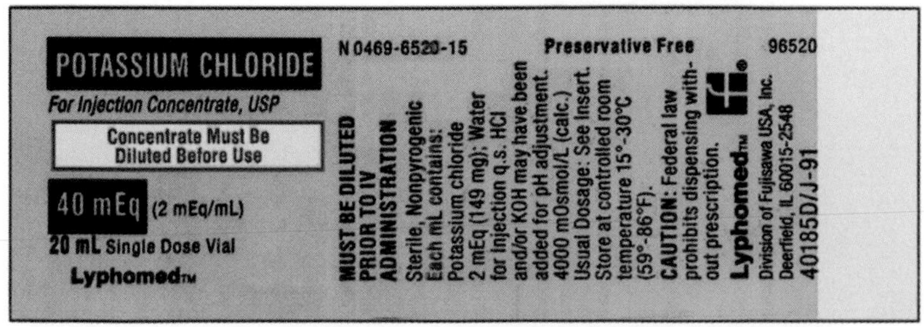

89. Atropine gr 1⁄120 IM stat. How many milliliters will the nurse administer? ______ .

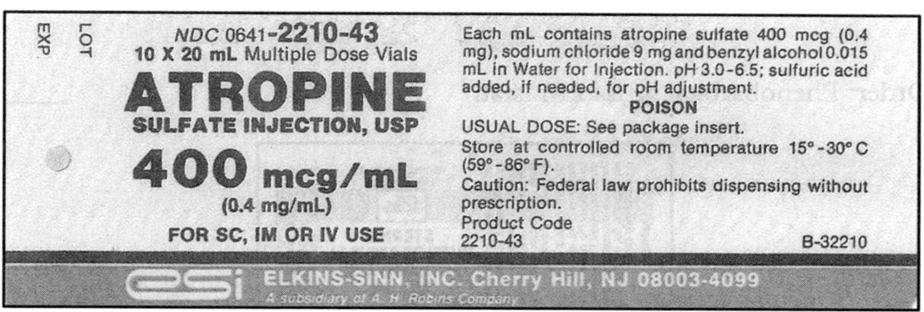

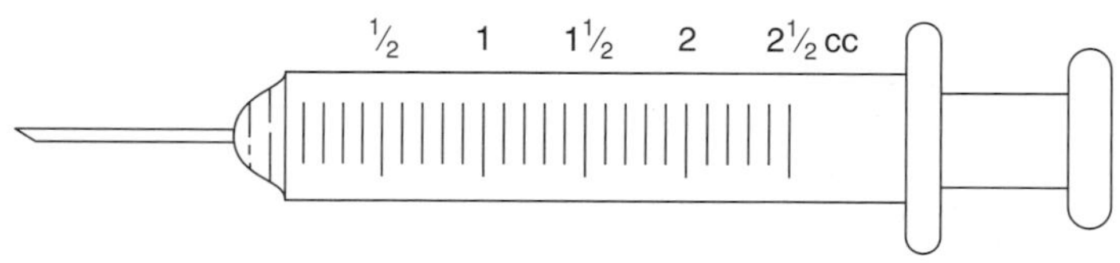

90. Your patient has Thorazine 15 mg IM q6 h ordered for severe agitation. How many milliliters will you administer? ______ .

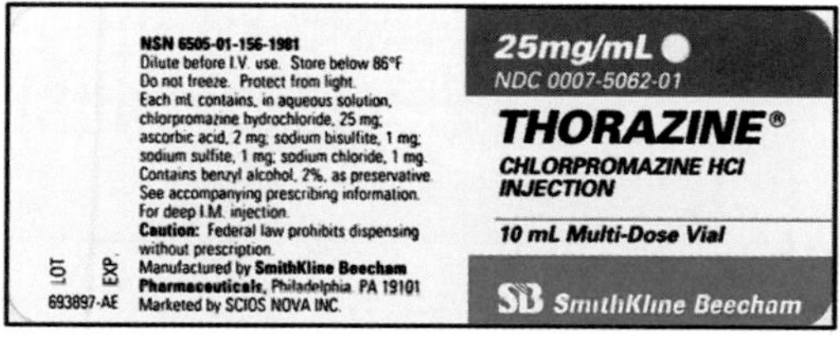

91. Ordered Vancocin 500 mg IVSS q12 h. Vancocin 250 mg per 5 mL is available after reconstitution. How many milliliters will the nurse prepare? ______ .

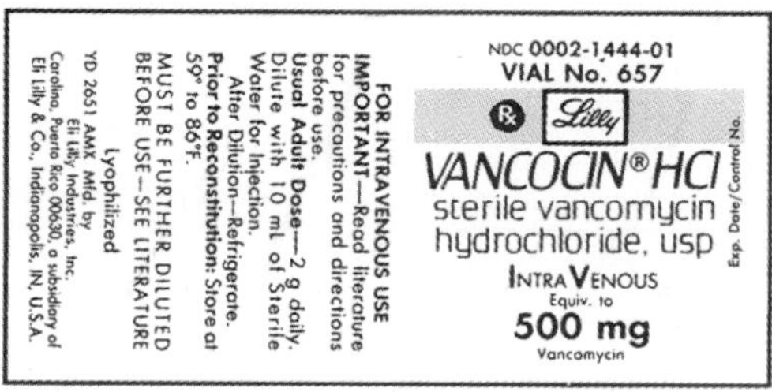

92. Mr. Ray receives tobramycin 90 mg IVPB q8 h for his abdominal wound infection. You have tobramycin 80 mg per 2 mL. How many milliliters will you prepare? ______ .

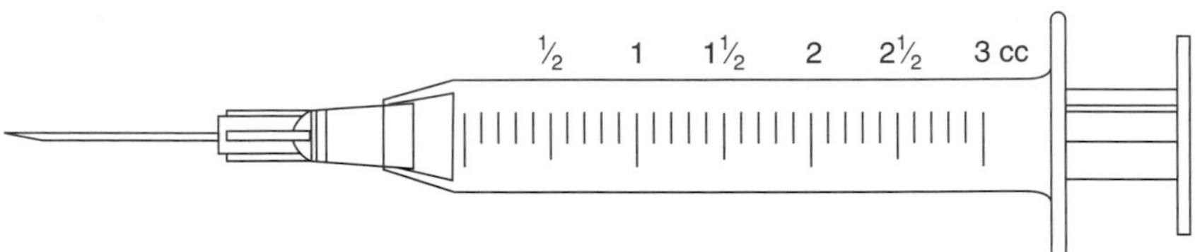

93. Your patient with delerium tremens receives diazepam 2 mg IM q6 h. How many milliliters will you administer? ______ .

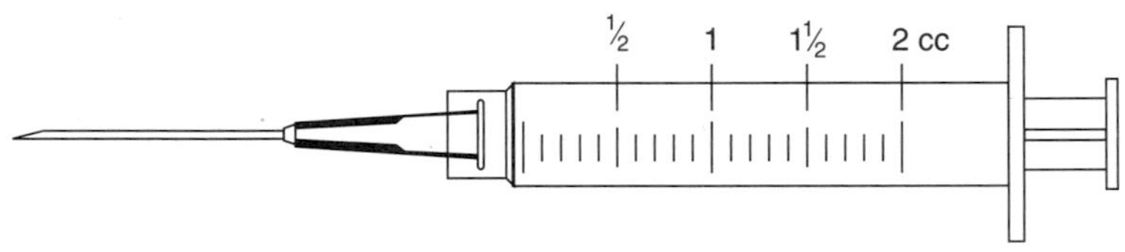

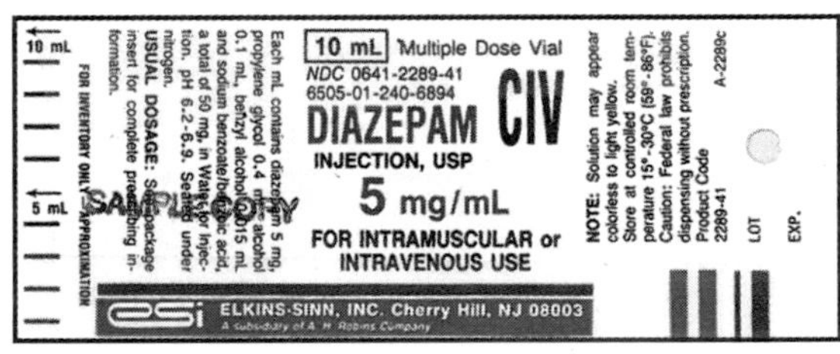

94. The physician orders Flagyl 500 mg IV q6 h to treat Ms. King's yeast infection. After reconstitution you have Flagyl 100 mg per mL. How many milliliters will you prepare? _______ .

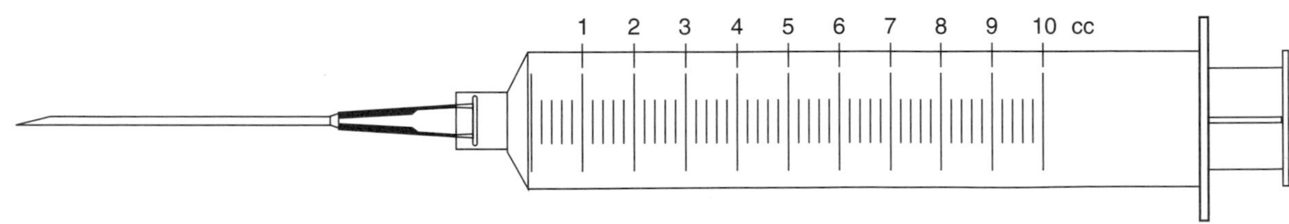

95. Ordered streptomycin 0.64 g IM qd. After reconstitution you have streptomycin 400 mg per mL. How many milliliters will you administer? ______ .

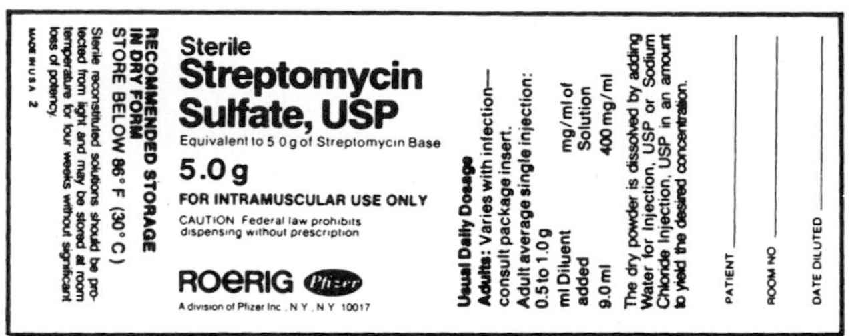

96. Your patient receives nafcillin 500 mg IM q6 h for treatment of a *Staphylococcus aureus* infection. You have nafcillin 250 mg per mL. How many milliliters will you administer? ______ .

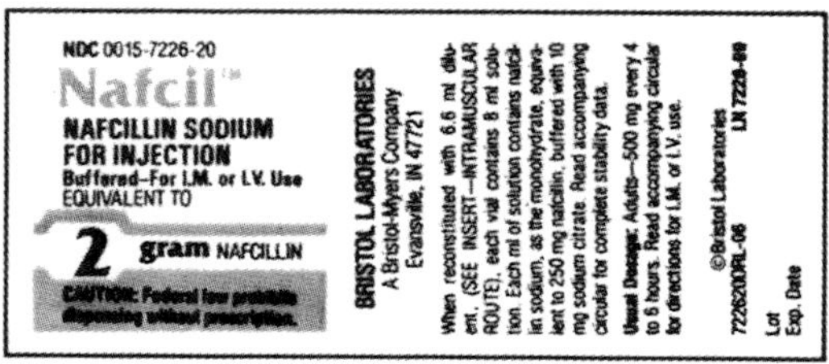

97. Ordered Isuprel 0.2 mg stat IM. The drug is available in 5-mL ampules containing 1 mg of Isuprel. How many milliliters will the nurse administer? ______ .

98. The physician orders Imferon 100 mg IM qod for your patient with pernicious anemia. The drug is supplied in ampules containing 25 mg per 0.5 mL. How many milliliters will you administer? ______ .

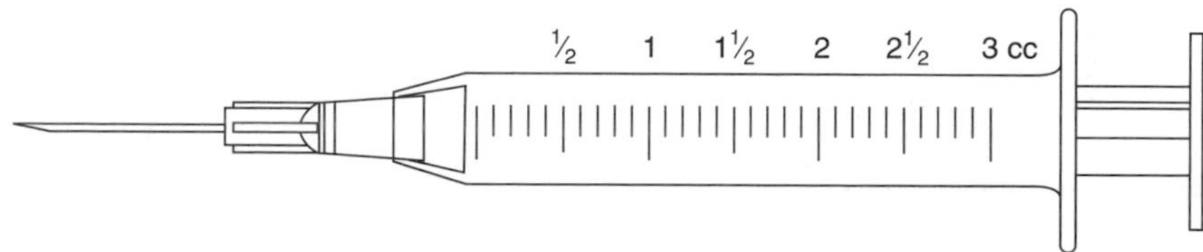

99. Your patient with arthritis receives Solganal 10 mg IM. Solganal is supplied 50 mg per mL. How many milliliters will you administer? ______ .

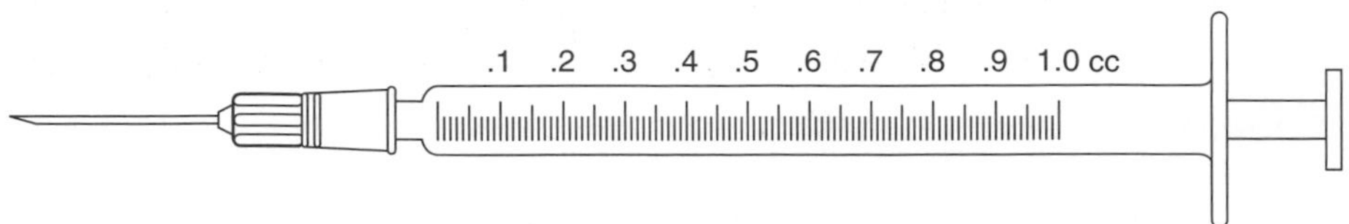

100. Ordered Aramine 4 mg IM stat. How many milliliters will the nurse administer? ______ .

Protect from light. Store container in carton until contents have been used.
USUAL ADULT DOSAGE: See accompanying circular.
CAUTION: Federal (USA) law prohibits dispensing without prescription.
10 ml | No. 3222X 7217609
MSD NDC 0006-3222-10
10 ml INJECTION
ARAMINE®
(METARAMINOL BITARTRATE, MSD)
1% Metaraminol Equivalent
10 mg per ml
MERCK SHARP & DOHME
DIVISION OF MERCK & CO., INC.
WEST POINT, PA 19486, USA
MULTIPLE DOSE VIAL
Lot
Exp.

Answers on pp. 467-475.

Name ______________________________

Date ______________________________

ACCEPTABLE SCORE 18

YOUR SCORE ______

POSTTEST 1

Directions: The medication order is listed at the beginning of each problem. Calculate the parenteral dosages. Show your work. Shade the syringe when provided to indicate the correct dosage.

1. The physician orders Vistaril 25 mg IM tid q4-6 h prn to enhance the effects of pain medication for your patient with a thyroidectomy. How many milliliters will you administer? ______ .

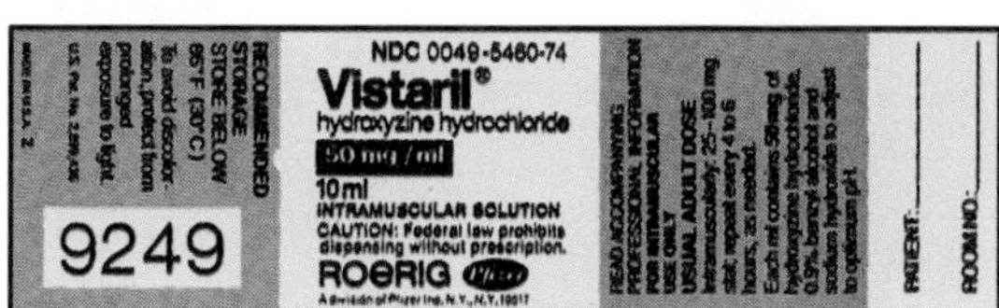

2. Your patient with a septoplasty complains of nausea and has Phenergan 5.5 mg IM qid ordered. Phenergan 25 mg per mL is available. How many milliliters will you administer? ______ .

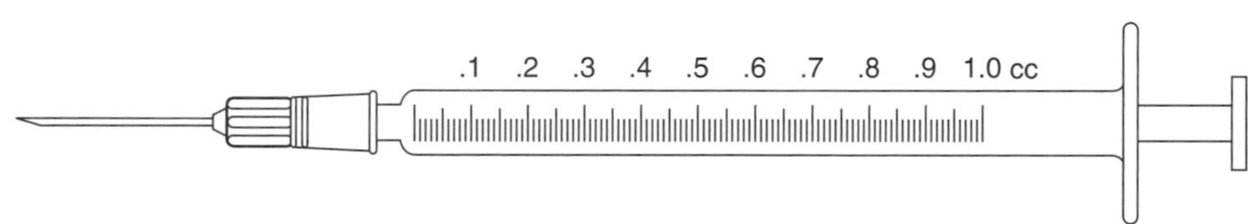

3. Your patient who has undergone tympano-mastoidectomy complains of pain and has codeine 30 mg IM q2 h prn ordered. Codeine is supplied in a 1-mL ampule containing gr ¼. How many milliliters will you administer? ______ .

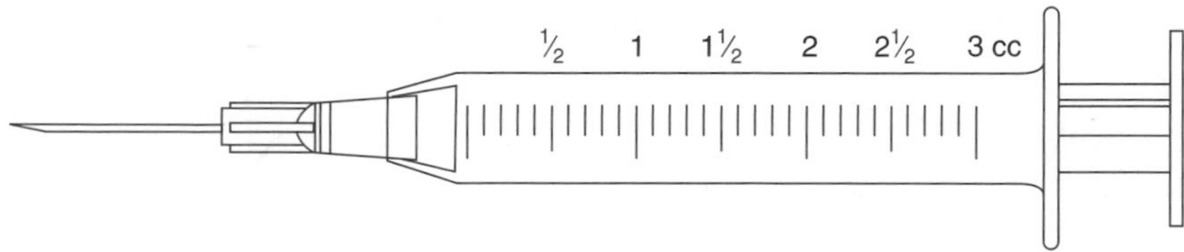

4. The physician orders Keflin 500 mg IM q6 h for your patient with a *Klebsiella* infection. Keflin 1 g per 10 mL is available. How many milliliters will you administer? ______ .

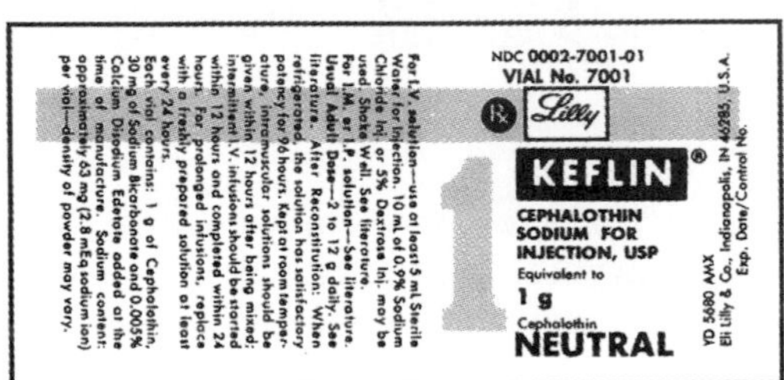

5. Your patient, who has undergone medullary carcinoma excision, has hydrocortisone 50 mg IM bid ordered. You have hydrocortisone 100 mg per 2 mL available. How many milliliters will you administer? ______ .

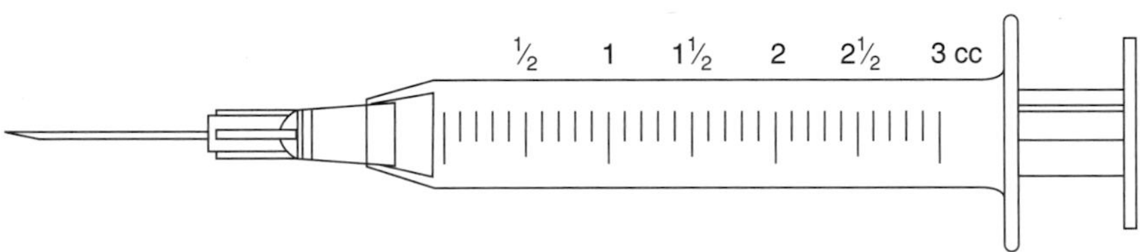

6. Ordered Dilaudid 0.5 mg IM q4 h prn. How many milliliters will the nurse administer? ______ .

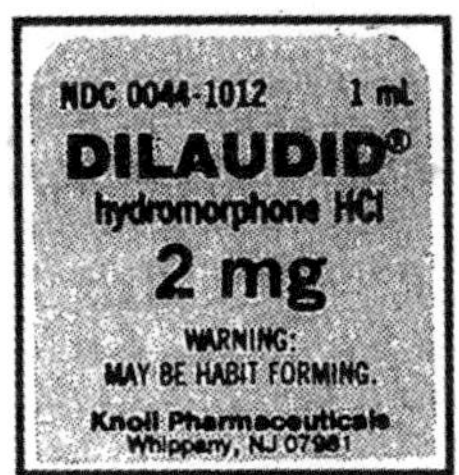

7. Your patient with epilepsy has phenobarbital gr iv IM bid ordered. Phenobarbital is supplied in a 1-mL ampule containing 120 mg per mL. How many milliliters will you administer? ______ .

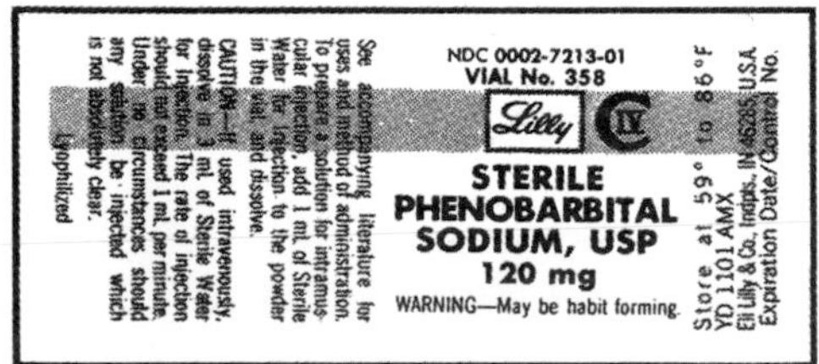

8. The physician orders scopolamine gr 1⁄300 IM at 6 AM before surgery. How many milliliters will the nurse administer? ______ .

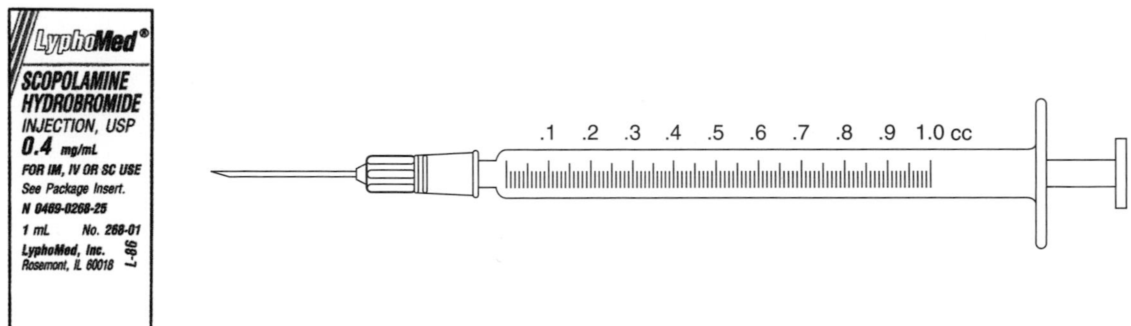

9. Ordered Thorazine 100 mg IM stat. Thorazine is supplied in a 10-mL vial containing 25 mg per mL. How many milliliters will the nurse administer? ______ .

10. Your severely agitated patient has diazepam 2 mg IM q6 h prn ordered. How many milliliters will you administer? ______ .

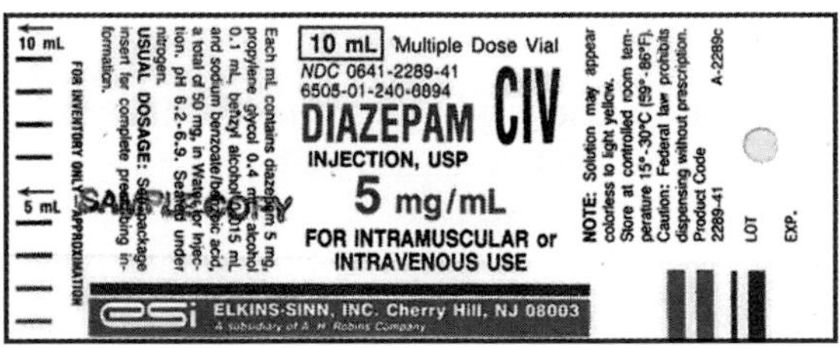

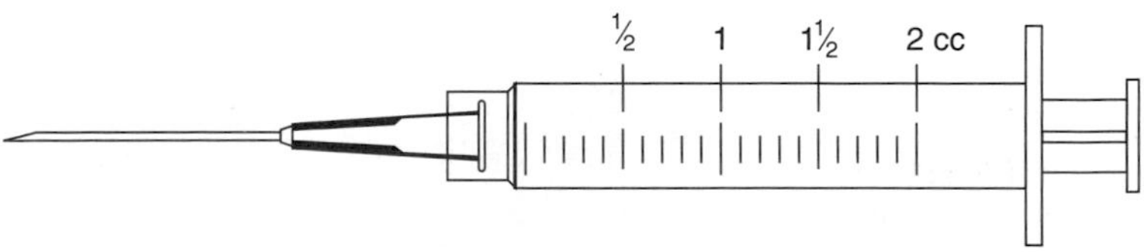

11. Atropine 0.7 mg IM stat is ordered for your patient before surgery. You have atropine gr $\frac{1}{120}$ per mL. How many milliliters will you administer? ______ .

12. Your patient with a medication reaction complains of pruritis and has Benadryl 25 mg IM prn ordered. You have Benadryl 50 mg per mL available. How many milliliters will you administer? ______ .

13. Ordered Depo-Medrol 50 mg IM bid. How many milliliters will the nurse administer? ______ .

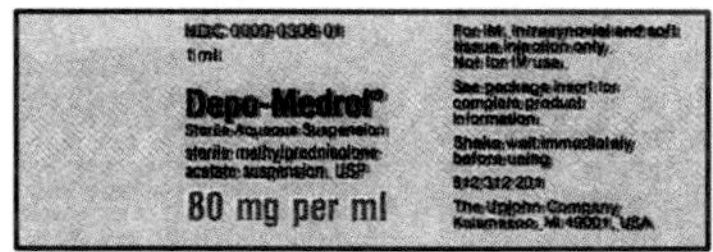

14. The physician orders ampicillin 500 mg IM q4 h for a patient who has undergone lumbar laminectomy. How many milliliters will the nurse administer? ______ .

NDC 0015-7403-20
NSN 6505-00-946-4700
EQUIVALENT TO
500 mg AMPICILLIN
STERILE AMPICILLIN SODIUM, USP
For IM or IV Use
CAUTION: Federal law prohibits dispensing without prescription.

For IM use, add 1.8 mL diluent (read accompanying circular). Resulting solution contains 250 mg ampicillin per mL.
Use solution within 1 hour.
This vial contains ampicillin sodium equivalent to 500 mg ampicillin.
Usual Dosage: Adults—250 to 500 mg IM q. 6h.
READ ACCOMPANYING CIRCULAR for detailed indications, IM or IV dosage and precautions.
APOTHECON®
A Bristol-Myers Squibb Company
Princeton, NJ 08540 USA 740320DRL-2

Cont:
Exp. Date:

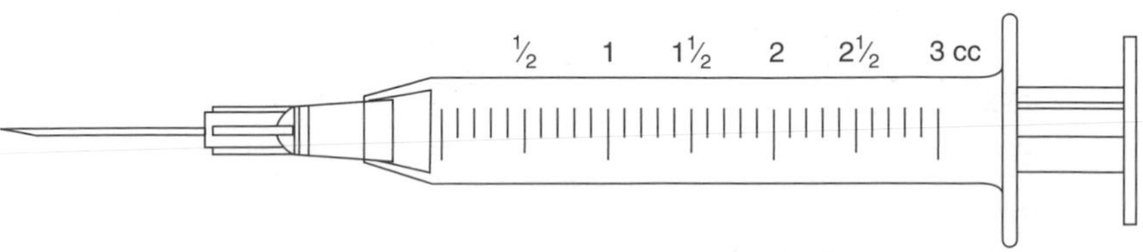

15. Ordered Ancef 300 mg IM q8 h. You have Ancef 1 g/50 mL vial available. How many milliliters will you administer? ______ .

16. Ordered morphine 6 mg IM q3 h prn. How many milliliters will the nurse administer? ______ .

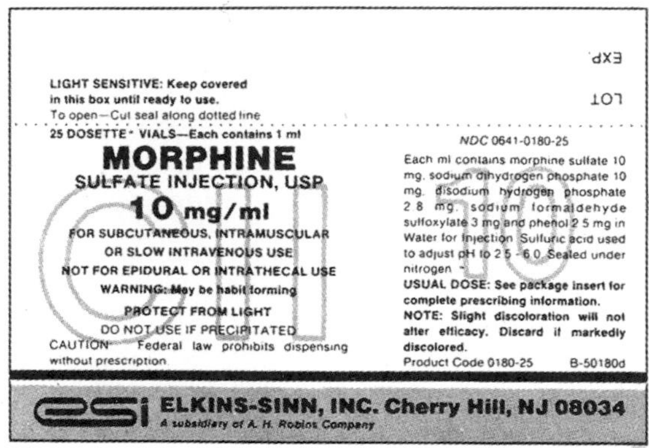

17. Ordered dexamethasone 6 mg IM stat. You have dexamethasone 10 mg/mL. How many milliliters will you administer? ______ .

18. Your patient with congestive heart failure has furosemide 10 mg IM q6 h ordered. How many milliliters will you administer? ______ .

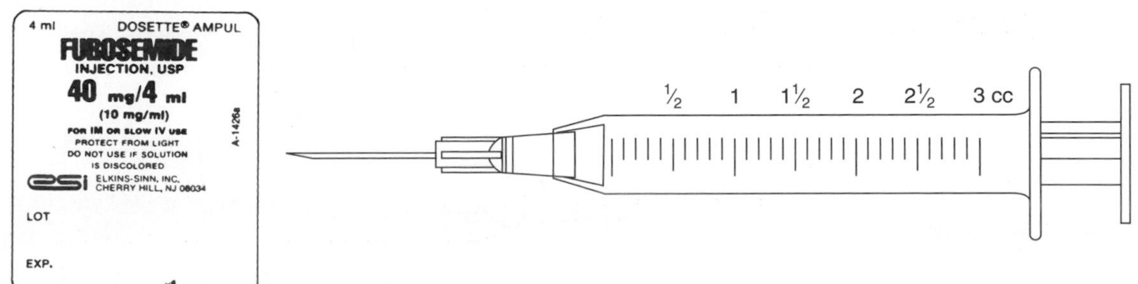

19. The physician orders Lanoxin 0.3 mg IM now. How many milliliters will the nurse administer? ______ .

LANOXIN® 2mL
(digoxin) Injection
500 µg (0.5 mg) in 2 mL
(250 µg [0.25 mg] per mL)
Store at 15° to 25°C (59° to 77°F).
PROTECT FROM LIGHT.
Glaxo Wellcome Inc.
Research Triangle Park, NC 27709
Rev. 1/96
542308
LOT
EXP

20. Ordered D_5W 500 mL plus KCl 5 mEq at 40 mL IV per h. KCl is supplied in a 10-mL ampule containing 20 mEq per mL. How many milliliters of KCl will be added to the 500 mL of D_5W? ______ .

Answers on pp. 485-489.

Name ______________________________

Date ______________________________

ACCEPTABLE SCORE 18

YOUR SCORE ______

POSTTEST 2

Directions: The medication order is listed at the beginning of each problem. Calculate the parenteral dosages. Show your work. Shade the syringe when provided to indicate the correct dosage.

1. Your patient who was involved in a motor vehicle accident complains of pain and has Dilaudid 2 mg IM q3 h prn ordered. How many milliliters will you administer? ______ .

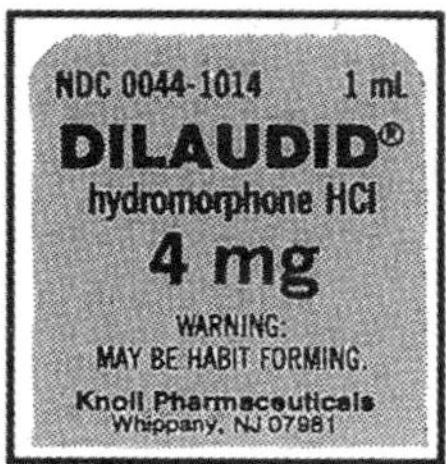

2. Your preop patient complains of anxiety and has Ativan 2 mg IM q6 h ordered. Ativan is supplied 4 mg per mL. How many milliliters will you administer? ______ .

3. Ordered erythromycin 0.4 g IV today. The drug is supplied in vials containing 500 mg per 10 mL. How many milliliters will the nurse prepare? ______ .

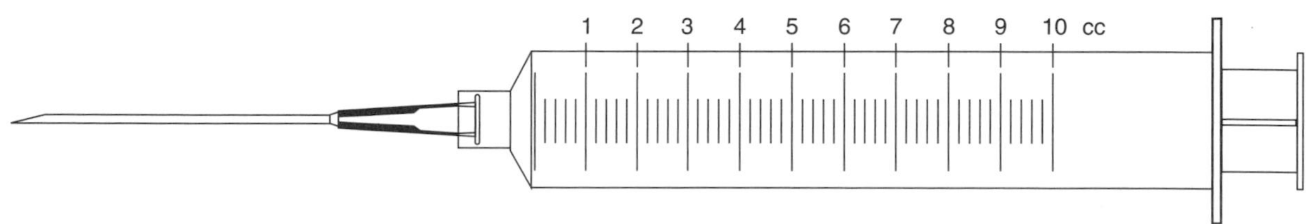

4. The physician orders Seconal 75 mg IM hs prn for your patient with a septoplasty. How many milliliters will you administer? ______ .

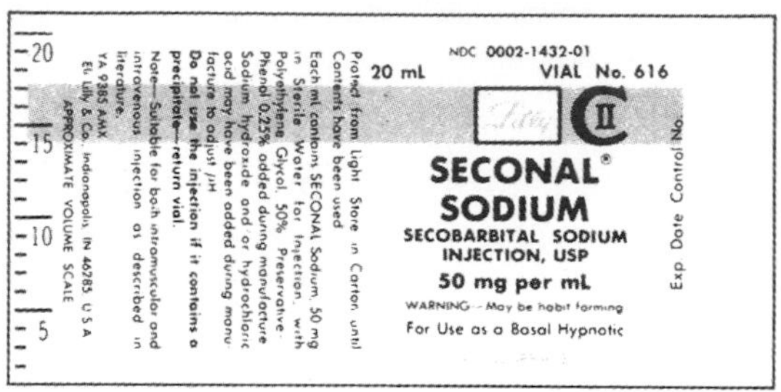

5. Your patient who has had a lumpectomy has codeine 60 mg IM q3 h ordered. How many milliliters will you administer? ______ .

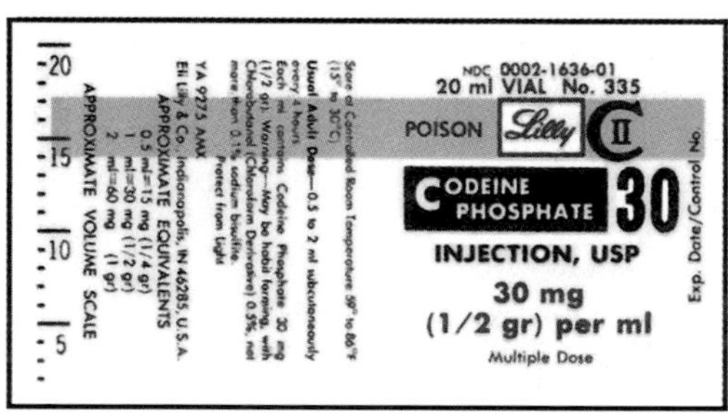

6. Ordered Demerol 15 mg IM q4 h prn. Demerol is available in an ampule containing 25 mg per 0.5 mL. How many milliliters will the nurse administer? ______ .

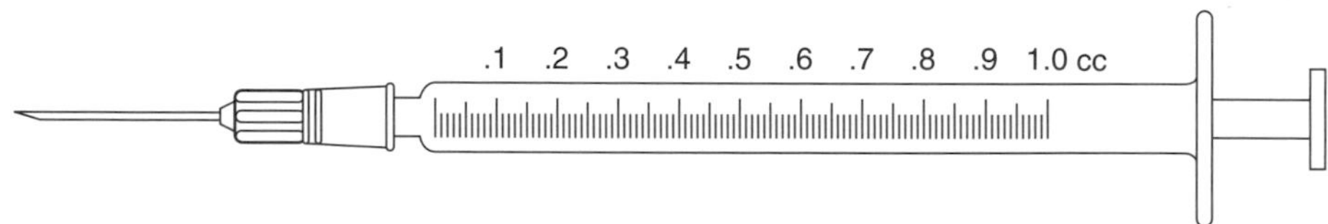

7. Ordered atropine gr $\frac{1}{200}$ IM at 6 AM. How many milliliters will the nurse administer? ______ .

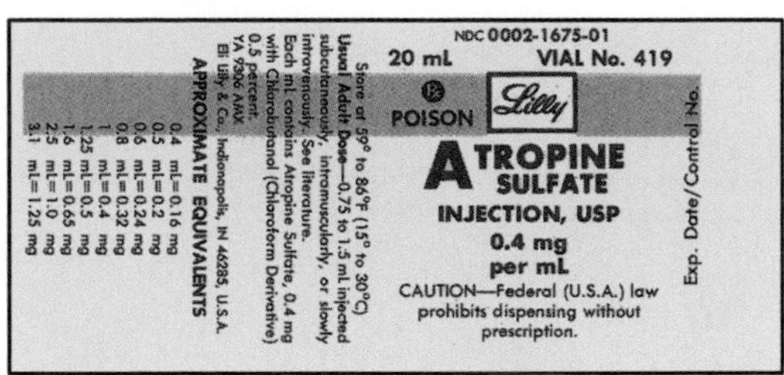

8. The physician orders Benadryl 25 mg IV now for your patient with a mild medication reaction. Benadryl 10 mg per mL is available. How many milliliters will you prepare? ______ .

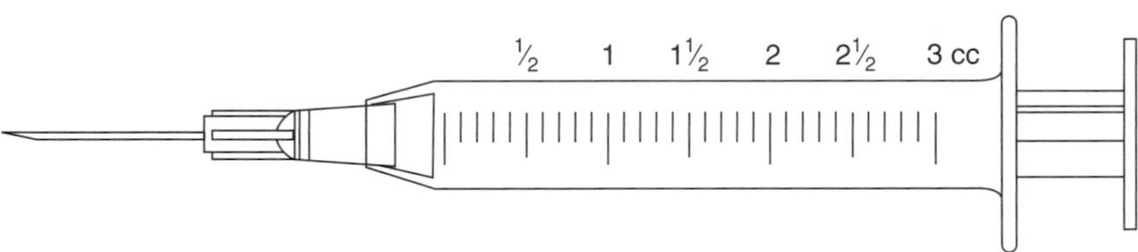

9. Your patient who has had an ethmoidectomy receives tobramycin sulfate 55 mg IV q8 h. Tobramycin 40 mg per mL is available. How many milliliters will you prepare? ______ .

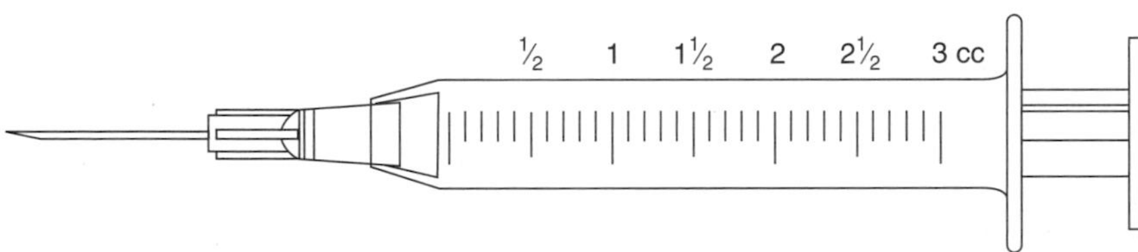

10. The physician orders Thorazine 30 mg IM prn for your patient with obsessive-compulsive disorder. Thorazine is supplied in 10-mL vial containing 25 mg per mL. How many milliliters will you administer? ______ .

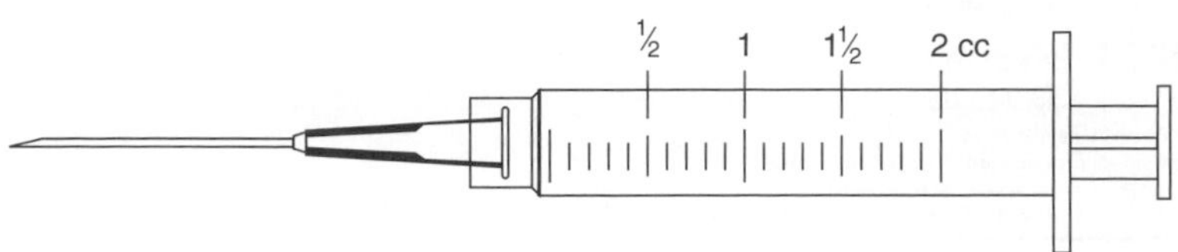

11. Your patient who has undergone parathyroidectomy receives ampicillin 200 mg IV q6 h. Ampicillin 100 mg per mL is available. How many milliliters will you prepare? ______ .

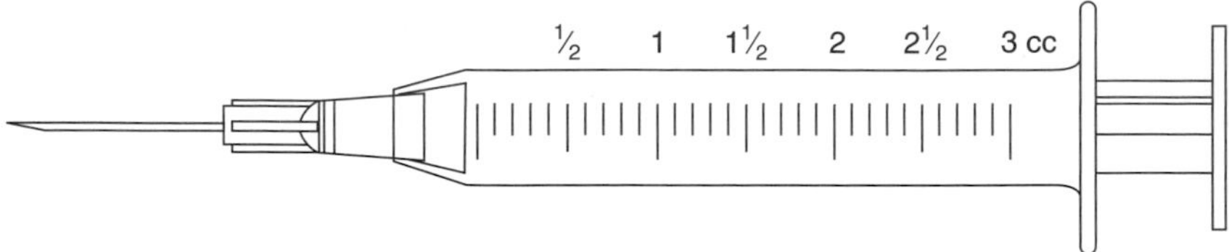

12. Ordered scopolamine gr 1/150 IM at 7 AM. Scopolamine gr 1/200 per mL is available. How many milliliters will the nurse administer? ______ .

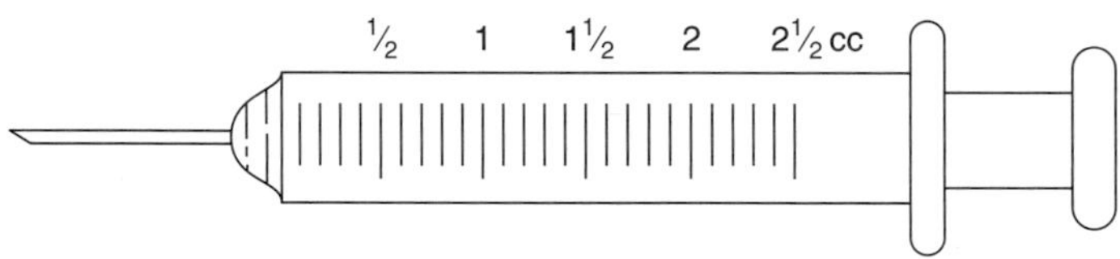

13. The physician orders piperacillin 2 g IV q8 h for your patient with sepsis. Piperacillin 1 g per 2.5 mL is available. How many milliliters will you prepare? ______ .

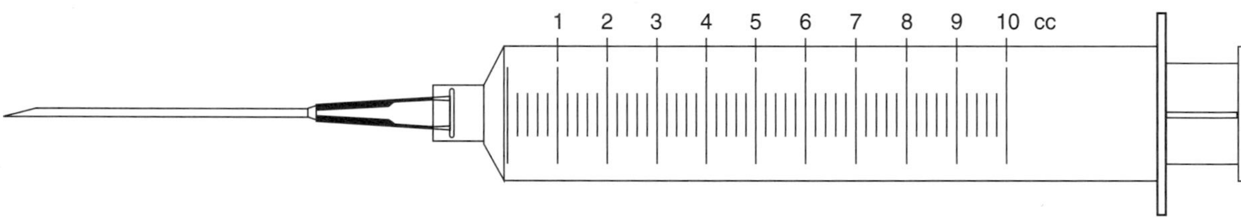

14. Ordered gentamicin 26 mg IV q8 h. How many milliliters will the nurse prepare? ______ .

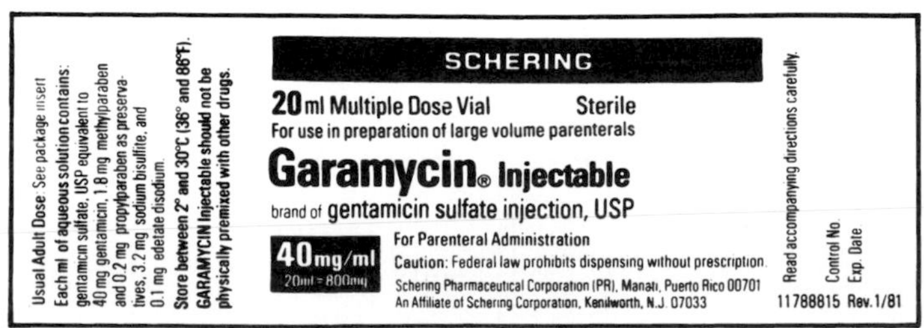

15. Ordered Lovenox 85 mg SQ q12 h qd. The drug is available 60 mg/0.6 mL. How many milliliters will the nurse administer? ______ .

16. Your patient, who has undergone tricuspid valve repair, has Lanoxin 80 mcg IM bid ordered. How many milliliters will you administer? ______

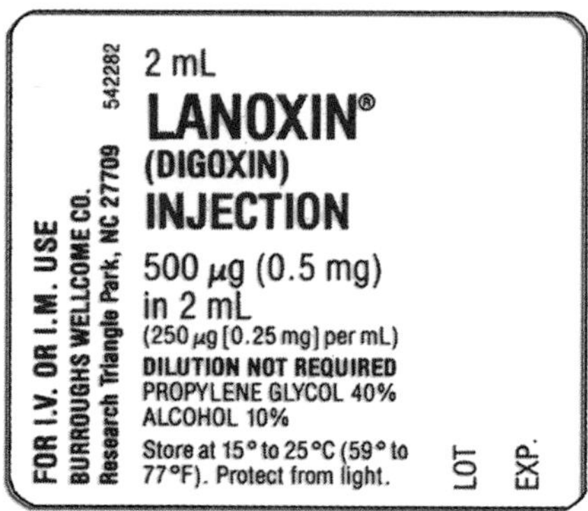

17. Ordered morphine 4 mg SQ q4 h prn. Morphine is supplied in a 1-mL ampule containing gr ⅛. How many milliliters will the nurse administer? ______

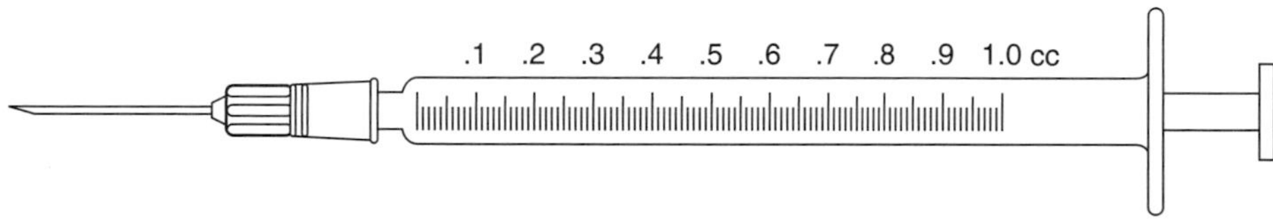

18. Your patient with a history of seizures has Dilantin 100 mg IV q8 h ordered. Dilantin 50 mg per 2 mL is available. How many milliliters will you prepare? ______

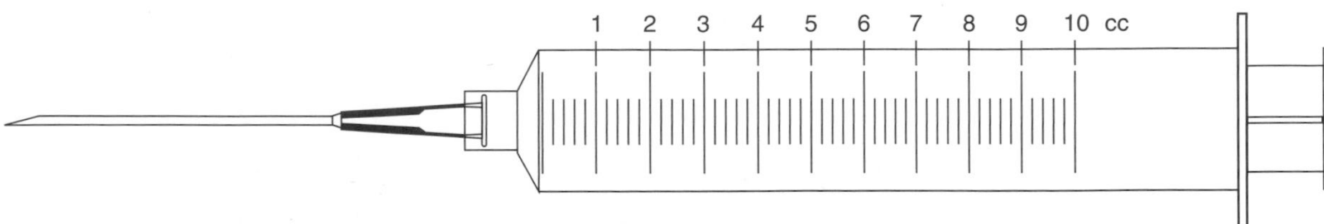

19. The physician orders phenobarbital 0.2 g IM q4 h for your patient with epilepsy. Phenobarbital is supplied in a 1-mL ampule containing 120 mg. How many milliliters will you administer? ______

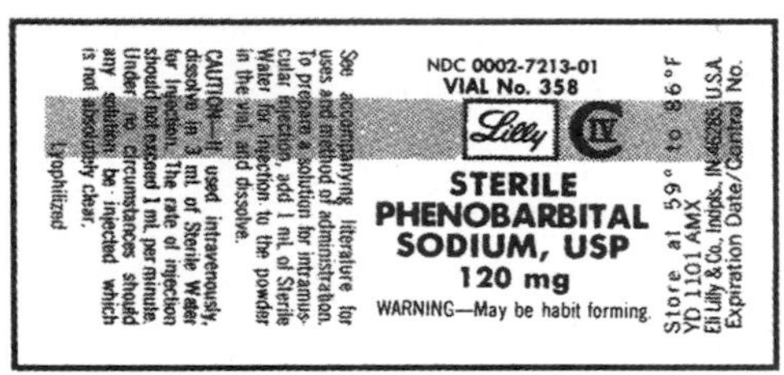

20. Ordered D_5W 500 mL plus calcium chloride ($CaCl_2$) 10 mEq at 10 mL per h IV. $CaCl_2$ is supplied in a 10-mL ampule containing 13.6 mEq. How many milliliters of $CaCl_2$ will be added to the 500 mL of D_5W? _______ .

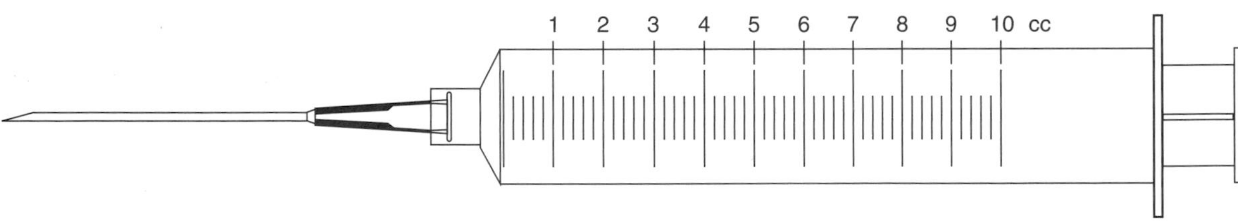

Answers on pp. 489-493.

CHAPTER

14

Dosages Measured in Units

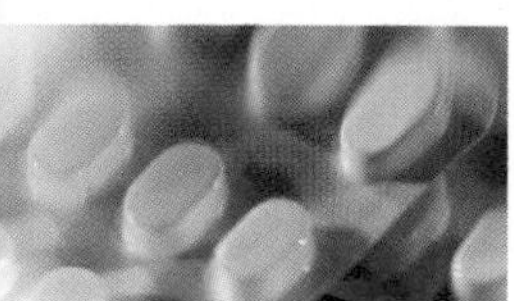

LEARNING OBJECTIVES

On completion of the materials provided in this chapter, you will be able to perform computations accurately by mastering the following mathematical concepts:

1. Using a proportion to solve problems involving drugs measured in unit dosages
2. Calculating drug dosage problems that first require reconstitution of a powdered drug into a liquid form
3. Drawing a line through an illustration of an insulin syringe to indicate the dosage of units desired

A unit (U) is the amount of a drug needed to produce a given result. Various drugs are measured in units; the examples used in this chapter are among the more common drugs used in hospitals and health care centers daily.

Drugs used in this chapter include the following:

Penicillin—An antibiotic that reduces organisms within the body that cause infection.

Heparin—An anticoagulant that inhibits clotting of the blood.

Insulin—A hormone secreted by the pancreas that lowers blood sugar.

Penicillin can be administered orally or parenterally, but heparin and insulin must be given subcutaneously or intravenously.

Before administering penicillin, the nurse must confer with the patient regarding previous allergies to the drug. After administration of the drug, the nurse must still observe the patient for signs of an allergic reaction.

Because heparin prolongs the time blood takes to clot, the dosage must be accurate. A larger dose may cause hemorrhage, and an insufficient dose may not have the desired result. After the administration of the drug, the nurse should observe the patient for signs of hemorrhage.

Insulin is used in the treatment of diabetes mellitus. Accuracy is important in the preparation of insulin. A higher dosage than needed may cause insulin shock. An insufficient amount of insulin may result in diabetic coma. Both conditions are extremely serious, and the nurse must be able to recognize the symptoms of each condition so that immediate treatment may be initiated to stabilize the patient. In many institutions, both insulin and heparin dosages are checked for accuracy by another nurse before the drug is administered to the patient.

A U-100 insulin syringe and U-100 insulin are necessary to ensure an accurate insulin dosage. U-100 insulin means that 100 U of insulin is contained in 1 mL of liquid. U-100 insulin is a universal insulin preparation that all persons requiring insulin can use. Another type of U-100 syringe is the U-100 Lo-Dose syringe, which measures 50 U; however, for accuracy, no more than 40 U should be measured in the U-100 Lo-Dose syringe. Because the doses are minute, the U-100 syringe provides the most accurate measurement of insulin dosages. The 30-unit, U-100 syringe is used for insulin doses that equal less than 30 units.

IMPORTANT NOTE: Only insulin is measured and given in the syringes that are marked in units. Heparin, penicillin, and other medication measured in units can only be measured and given in syringes marked in milliliters.

Powder Reconstitution

A drug in powdered form is necessary when a medication is unstable as a liquid form for a long period. This powdered drug must be reconstituted—dissolved with a sterile diluent—before administration. The diluents commonly used include sterile water, sterile normal saline solution, and 5% dextrose solution.

Before reconstituting the medication, several principles must be followed.

1. Carefully read the information and directions on the vial or package insert for reconstitution of the medication.
2. If no directions are available with the medication, consult the Physicians Desk Reference (PDR), hospital drug formulary, pharmacology text, or hospital pharmacy.
3. Identify the type and amount of diluent as well as the route of administration.
4. Note the drug strength or concentration after reconstitution and circle or place on the label, if not already written when you use a multidose vial.
5. Note the length of time for which the medication is good once reconstituted as well as the directions for storage.
6. Be aware that the total reconstitution amount may be greater than the amount of diluent.
7. After reconstitution, place your initials, date of preparation, time of preparation, date of expiration, and time of expiration on the label when you reconstitute a multidose vial.

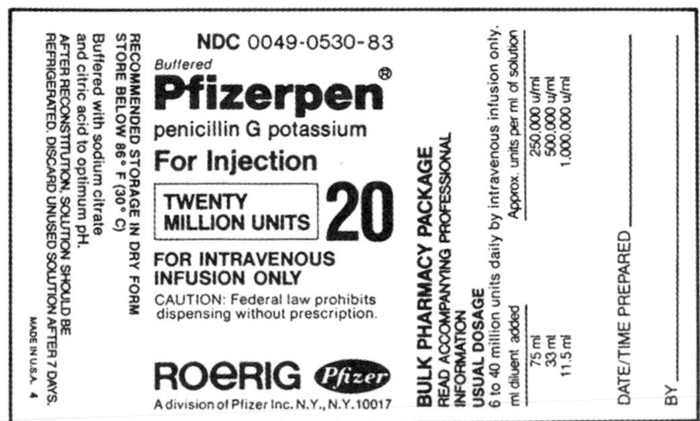

Example:

a. What is the route of administration? IV
b. What type of diluent can be used? Check insert
c. How much diluent must be added? 75 mL
d. What is the medication concentration? 250,000 U/mL
e. How long will the medication maintain its potency at room temperature? 7 days
f. The physician orders 2,000,000 U IV q4h. How many milliliters will you give? Shade the syringe. 8 mL

a. 250,000 U : 1 mL ::
b. 250,000 U : 1 mL :: _____ U : _____ mL
c. 250,000 U : 1 mL :: 2,000,000 U : x mL
d. $250{,}000x = 2{,}000{,}000$

$$x = \frac{2{,}000{,}000}{250{,}000}$$

$x = 8$

e. $x = 8$ mL

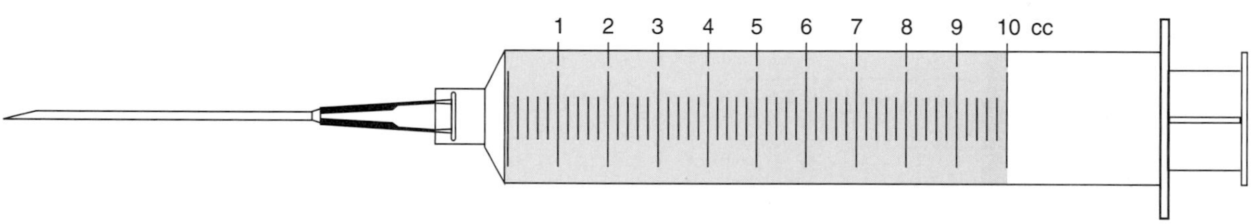

Dosages Measured in Units Involving Oral Medications

Example: Ordered mycostatin 400,000 U po qid. The drug is supplied 100,000 U per mL after reconstitution. How many milliliters will the nurse administer? _______ .

a. On the left side of the proportion, place what you know or have available. In this example, each mL contains 100,000 U. So the left side of the proportion would be

100,000 U : 1 mL ::

b. The right side of the proportion is determined by the physician's order and the abbreviations on the left side of the proportion. Only *two* different abbreviations may be used in a single proportion. The abbreviations must be in the same position on the right side as on the left side.

100,000 U : 1 mL :: 400,000 U : _______ mL

We need to find the number of milliliters to be administered, so we use the symbol x to represent the unknown.

100,000 U : 1 mL :: 400,000 U : x mL

c. Rewrite the proportion without using the abbreviations.

100,000 : 1 :: 400,000 : x

d. Solve for x.

$$100{,}000 : 1 :: 400{,}000 : x$$

$$100{,}000x = 400{,}000$$

$$x = \frac{400{,}000}{100{,}000}$$

$$x = 4$$

e. Label your answer as determined by the abbreviation placed next to x in the original proportion.

$$x = 4 \text{ mL}$$

4 mL would be measured to administer 400,000 U of mycostatin.

Dosages Measured in Units Involving Parenteral Medications

Example: Ordered heparin 12,000 U SQ q8 h. How many milliliters will the nurse administer? ______ .

a. 10,000 U : 1 mL ::
b. 10,000 U : 1 mL :: ______ U : ______ mL

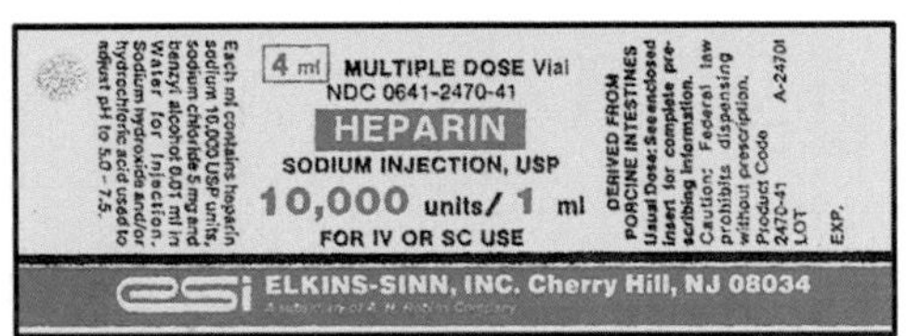

10,000 U : 1 mL :: 12,000 U : x mL

c. $10{,}000 : 1 :: 12{,}000 : x$

d. $10{,}000x = 1 \times 12{,}000$

$$10{,}000x = 12{,}000$$

$$x = \frac{12{,}000}{10{,}000}$$

$$x = 1.2$$

e. $x = 1.2$ mL

Therefore 1.2 mL of heparin would be the amount of each individual dose of heparin given q8 h.

Insulin Given with a Lo-Dose Insulin Syringe

Example: Ordered Humulin L Lente U100 insulin 36 U SQ in AM. A U-100 Lo-Dose syringe is available. Draw a vertical line through the syringe to indicate the correct dosage.

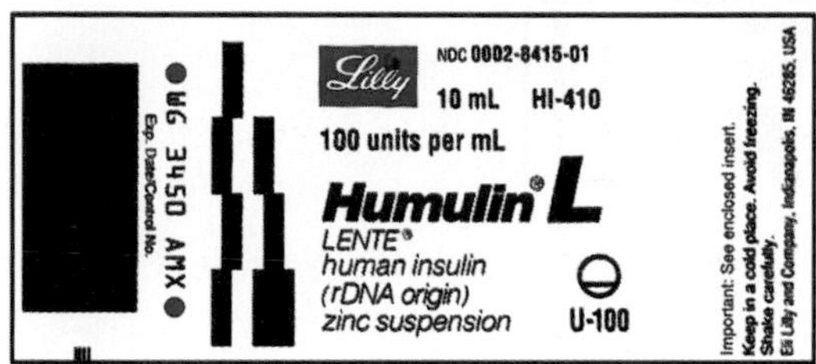

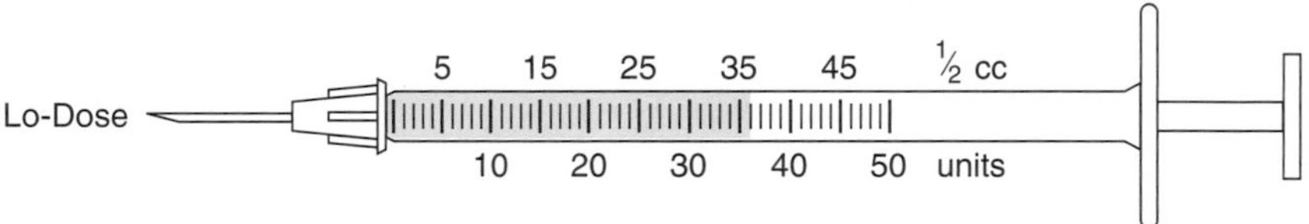

With a Lo-Dose insulin syringe, 36 U of U-100 insulin would be measured as indicated.

Mixed Insulin Administration

The physician may prescribe two types of insulin to be administered at the same time. These insulins will be drawn up in the same syringe to avoid injecting the patient twice.

Several guidelines apply to this type of administration.

1. Air equal to the amount of insulin being withdrawn should be injected into each vial. Do *not* touch the solution with the tip of the needle.
2. Using the same syringe, draw up the desired amount of insulin from the regular insulin bottle first.
3. Remove the syringe from the regular insulin bottle. Check the syringe for any air bubbles and remove them.
4. Using the same syringe, draw up the amount of cloudy insulin to the desired dosage.
5. Some hospitals require that you check your insulin with another nurse before administration. Consult your hospital policy and procedures.

Example 1: The physician orders administration of Humulin R Regular U100 10 U plus Humulin NPHU100 20 U SQ.

The total amount of insulin is 30 U (10 U + 20 U = 30 U).

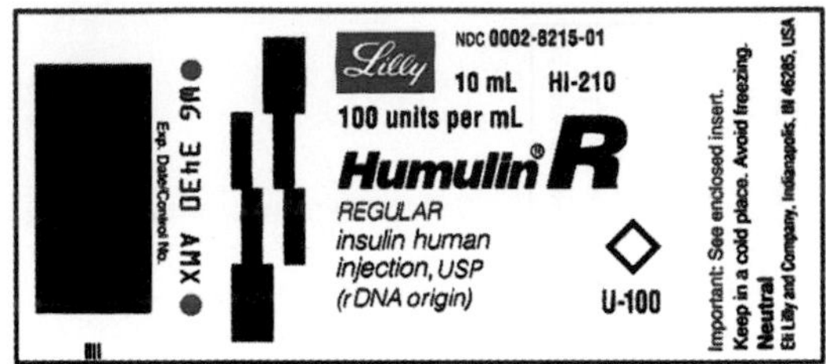

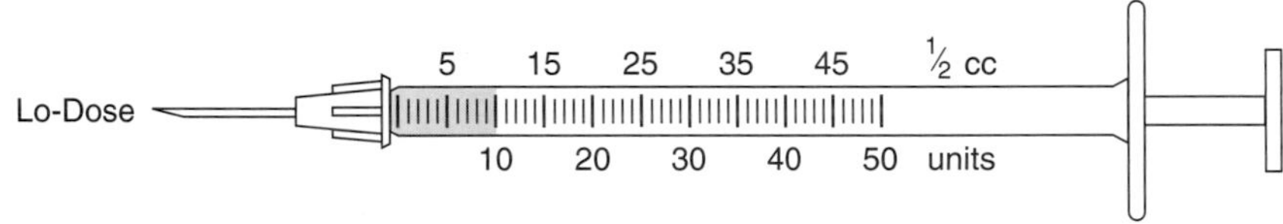

10 U of regular insulin

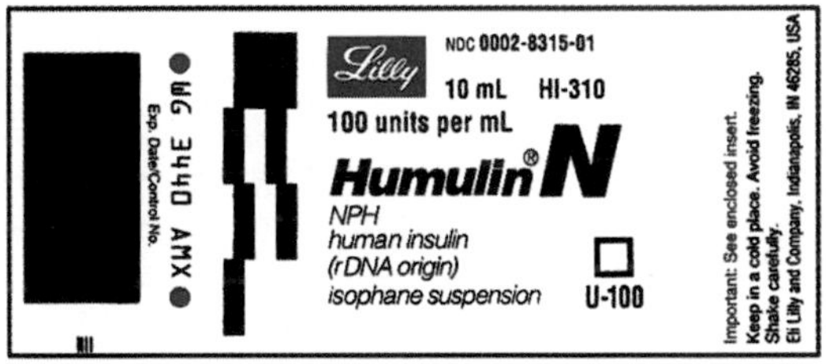

10 U of regular insulin + 20 U of NPH insulin = 30 U of insulin

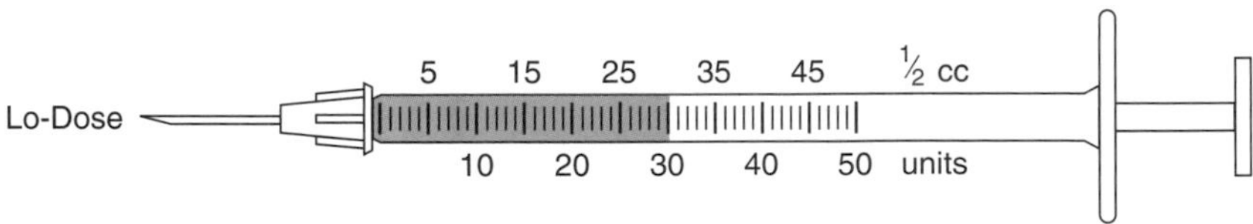

Example 2: Ordered Humulin L Lente U100 46 U SQ qAM. Regular Humulin R U100 20 U. A U-100 insulin syringe is available. Draw a vertical line through the syringe to indicate the amount of Lente Humulin insulin to be given, and a second line to indicate the total dosage.

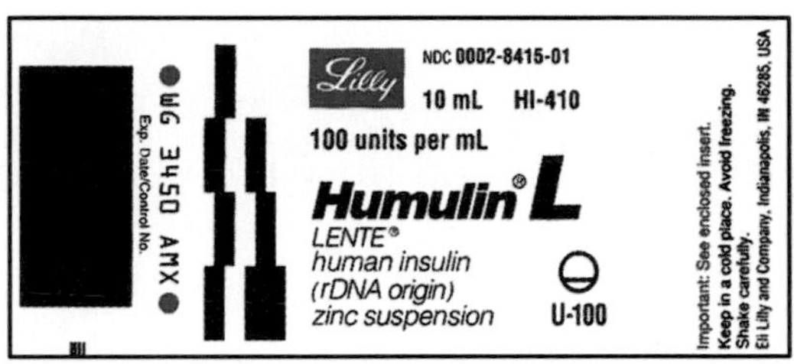

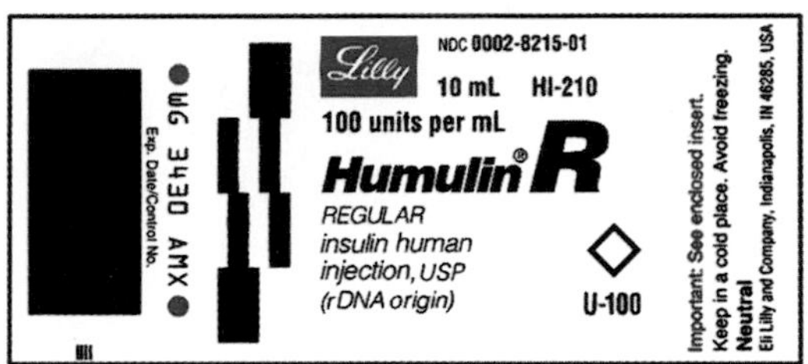

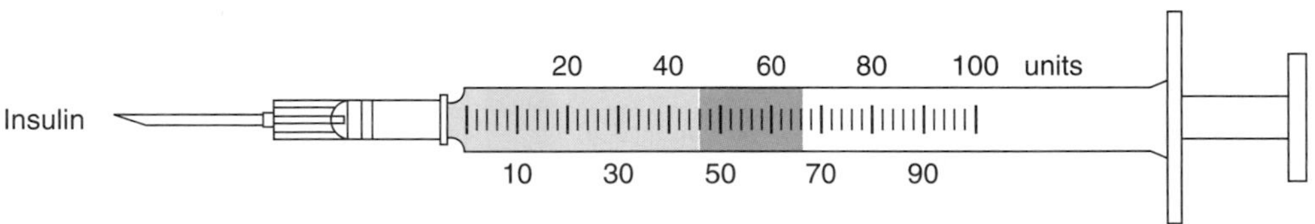

The Humulin Lente insulin dosage is indicated at 46 U. Add 20 U of Humulin regular insulin for a total dosage of 66 U of insulin.

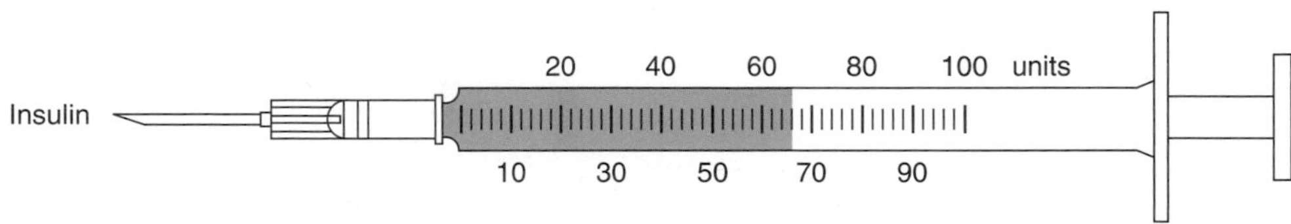

Complete the following work sheet, which provides for extensive practice in the calculation of dosages measured in units. Check your answers. If you have difficulties, go back and review the necessary material. When you feel ready to evaluate your learning, take the first posttest. Check your answers. An acceptable score as indicated on the posttest signifies that you have successfully completed this chapter. An unacceptable score signifies a need for further study before taking the second posttest.

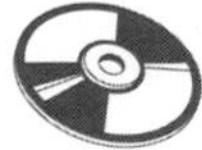

Refer to Calculating Dosages on the CD for additional help and practice problems.

WORK SHEET

Directions: The medication order is listed at the beginning of each problem. Calculate the dosages. Show your work. Mark the syringe when provided to indicate the correct dosage.

1. Your patient with pneumonia receives penicillin V 200,000 U po qid. You have penicillin V oral solution 400,000 U per 5 mL available. Draw a vertical line through the syringe to indicate the number of milliliters to be given.

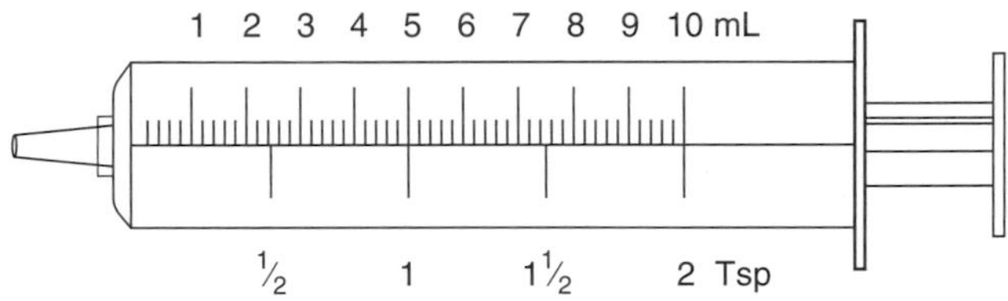

2. The physician orders heparin 7500 U SQ q12 h for your postoperative patient. You have heparin 5000 U per mL available. How many milliliters will you administer? ______ .

3. Ordered NPH U100 insulin 20 U SQ qAM. Draw a vertical line through the syringe to indicate the amount of NPH insulin to be given.

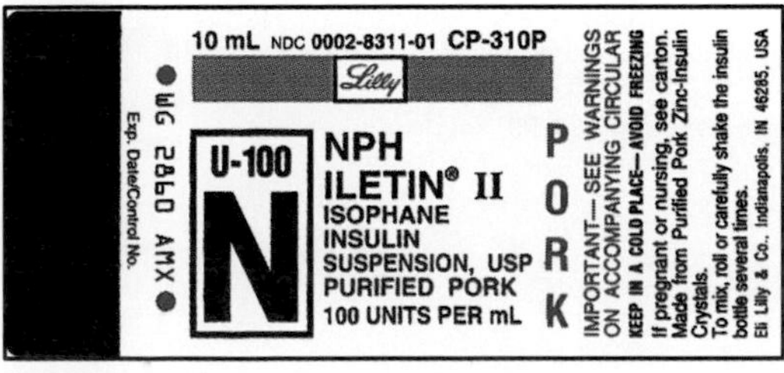

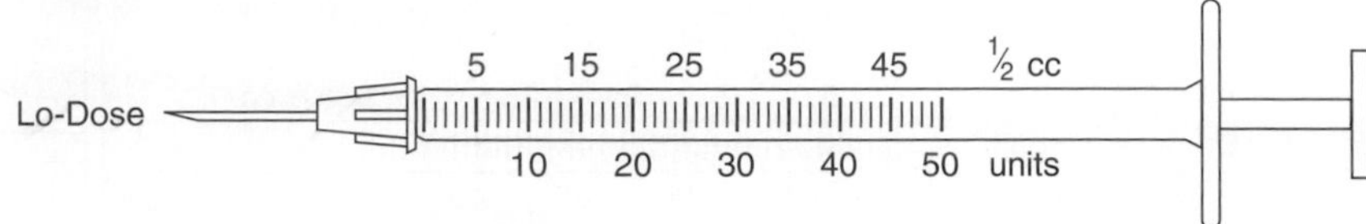

4. A patient with a temporal bone infection receives penicillin G 500,000 U IM q6 h. How much diluent should be added? _______ . What is the medication concentration? _______ . How many milliliters will you administer? _______ . What would you circle on the label to indicate concentration? _______ .

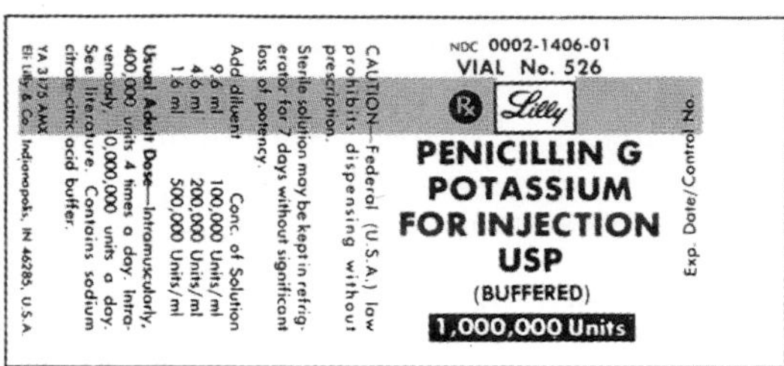

5. The physician orders heparin 2500 U SQ q12 h for your patient with a jejunostomy. You have heparin 5000 U per mL available. How many milliliters will you administer? _______ . Draw a vertical line through the syringe to indicate the dosage.

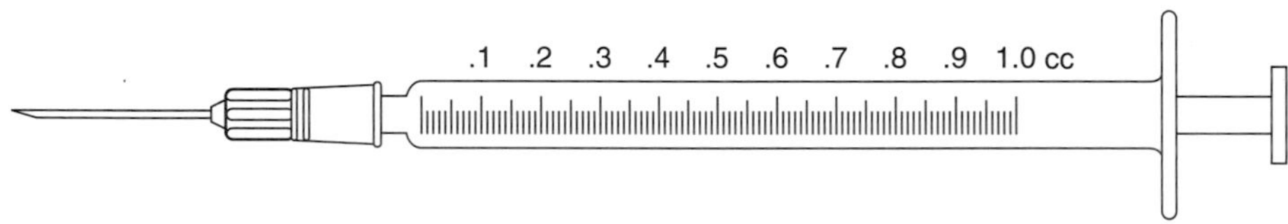

6. Ordered regular humulin insulin 2 U SQ qPM. Draw a vertical line through the syringe to indicate the dosage.

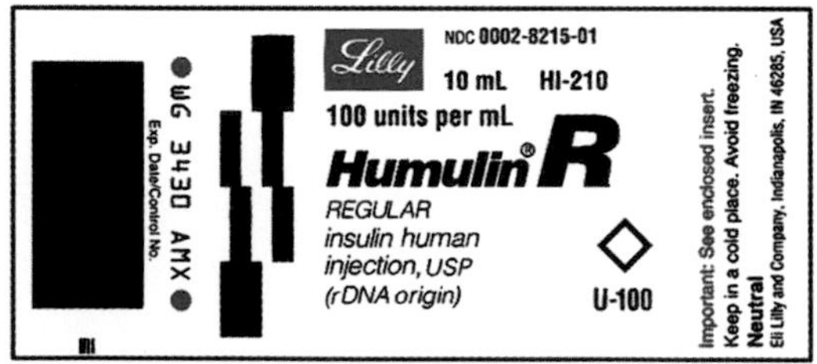

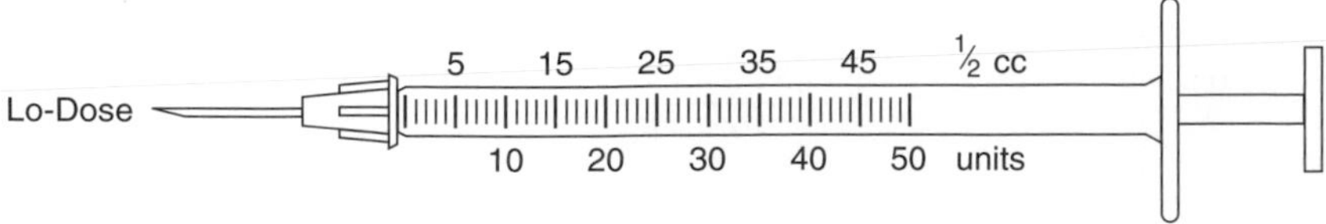

7. Your patient with a gastric pull-up receives heparin 5000 U SQ q8 h. How many milliliters will you administer? _______ .

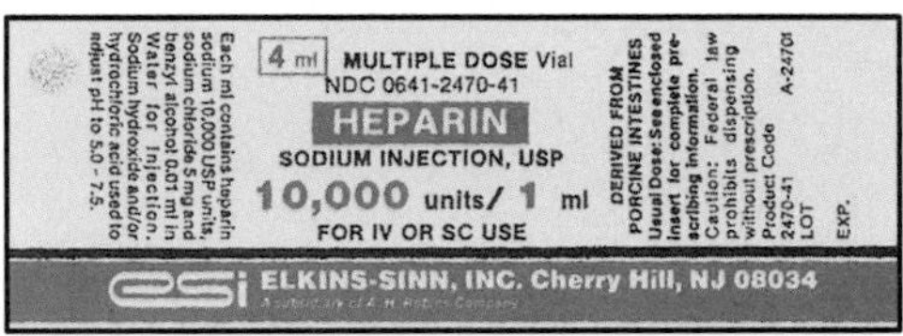

8. Ordered V-Cillin K suspension 400,000 U po q6 h. V-Cillin K suspension is supplied 200,000 U per 5 mL. How many milliliters will the nurse administer? _______ .

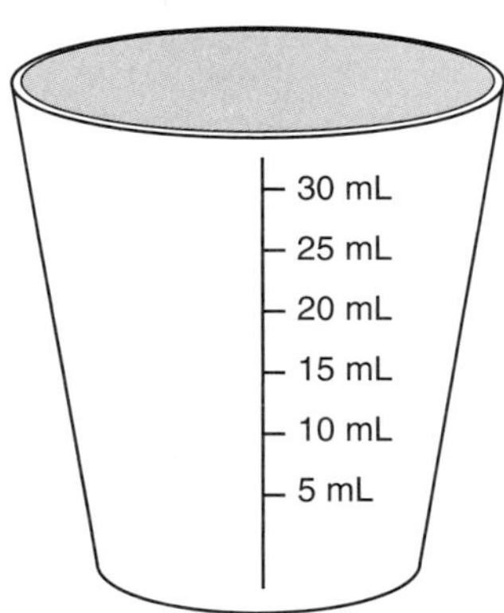

9. Ordered Lente insulin 14 U, regular insulin 6 U SQ qAM. Lente insulin U-100, regular insulin U-100, and a U-100 Lo-Dose syringe are supplied. Draw a vertical line through the syringe to indicate the amount of Lente insulin to be given and a second line to indicate the total dosage.

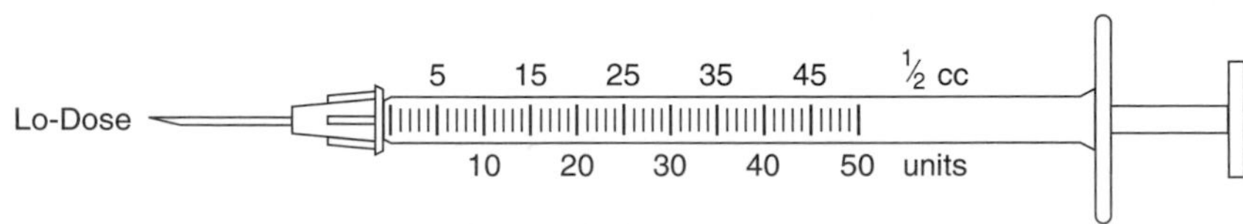

10. Your patient with an appendectomy has penicillin V 300,000 U po qid ordered. You have penicillin V oral solution 400,000 U per 5 mL available. How many milliliters will you administer? _______ . Draw a vertical line through the syringe to indicate the dosage.

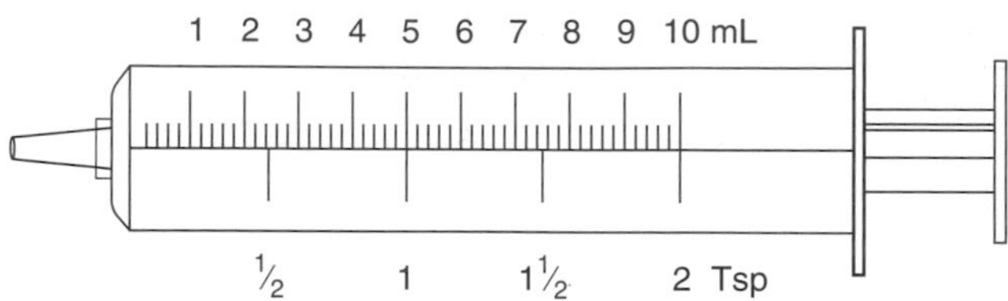

11. The physician orders heparin 6000 U SQ qd for your patient with a corneal transplant. How many milliliters will you administer? _______ .

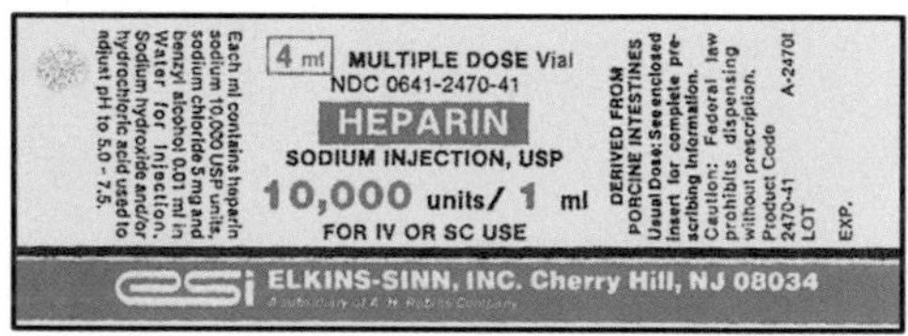

12. Ordered regular insulin 18 U SQ qAM. Draw a vertical line through the syringe to indicate the dosage.

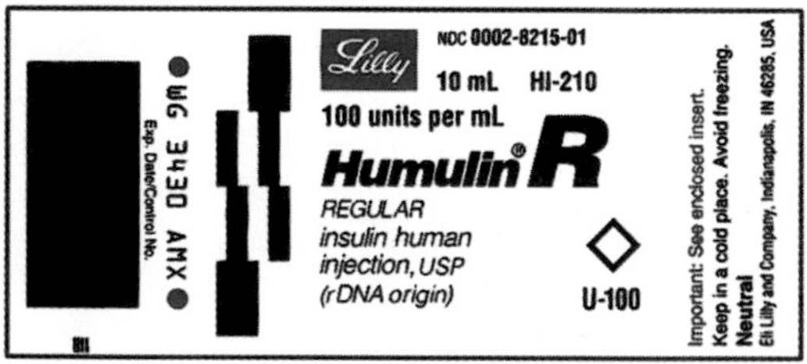

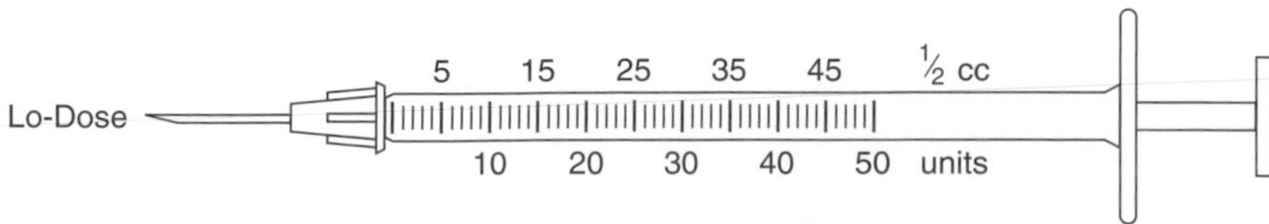

13. Ordered NPH insulin 32 U SQ tomorrow at 7:45 AM. You have NPH insulin U-100 and a U-100 Lo-Dose syringe. Draw a vertical line through the syringe to indicate the dosage.

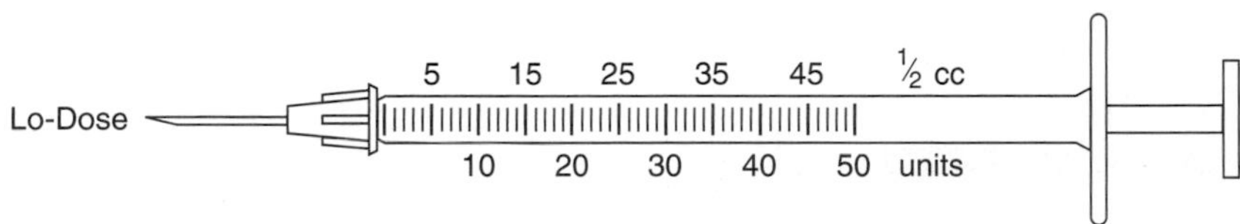

14. Your patient with a thoracotomy receives penicillin G 600,000 U IM bid. How much diluent should be added? _______ . What is the medication concentration? _______ . How many milliliters will you administer? _______ .

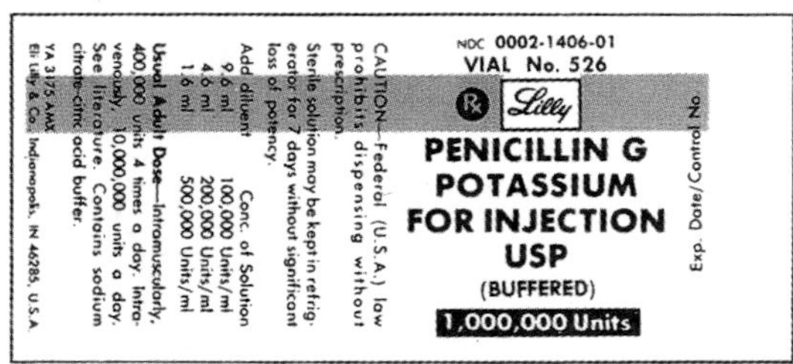

15. The physician orders heparin 10,000 U SQ q12 h for your patient with a below-the-knee amputation. You have heparin 5000 U per mL available. How many milliliters will you administer? _______ . Draw a vertical line through the syringe to indicate the dosage.

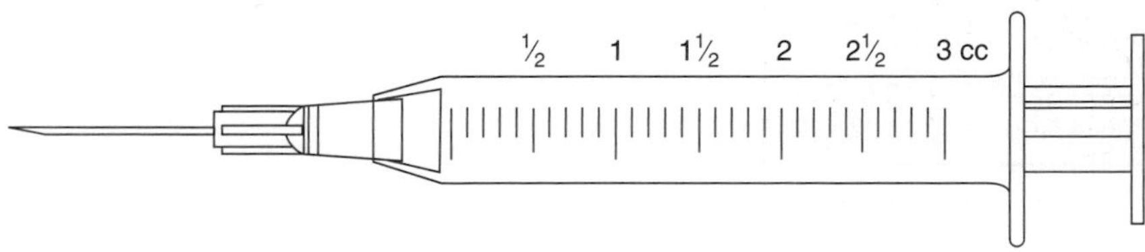

16. Your patient who has undergone a Nissen procedure receives heparin 5000 U SQ q12 h. How many milliliters will you administer? _______ .

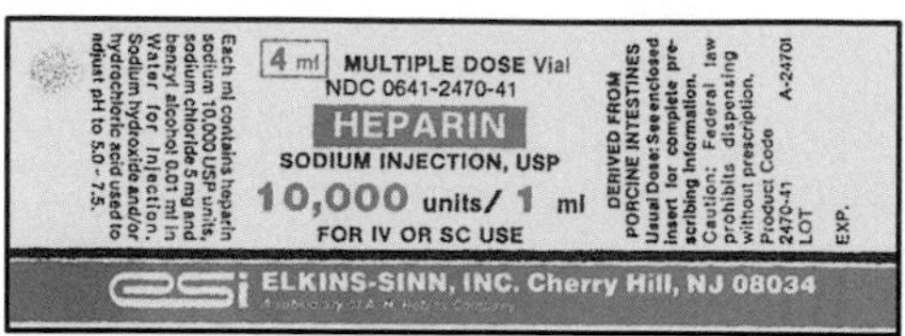

17. Your patient with a stapedectomy receives penicillin V 300,000 U po qid. The drug is supplied in oral solution 200,000 U per 5 mL. How many milliliters will you administer? _______ .

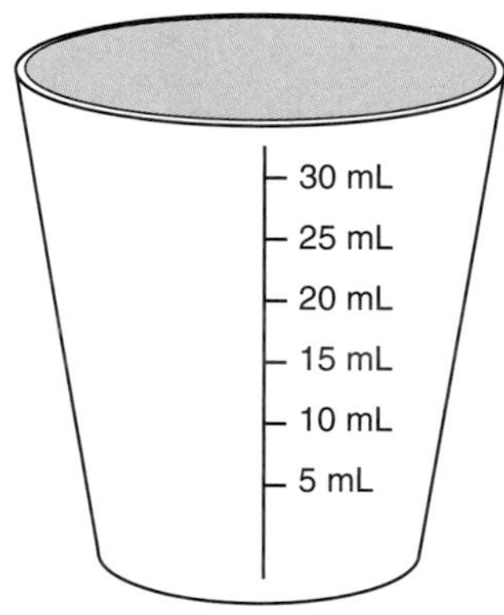

18. Your patient with insulin-dependent diabetes receives NPH Insulin 24 U SQ qAM. Draw a vertical line through the syringe to indicate the dosage.

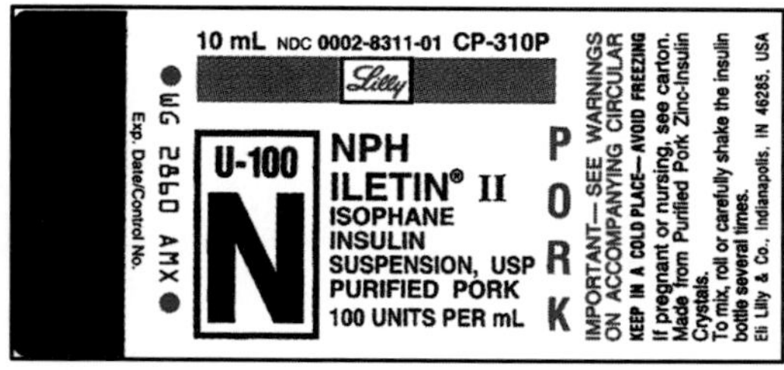

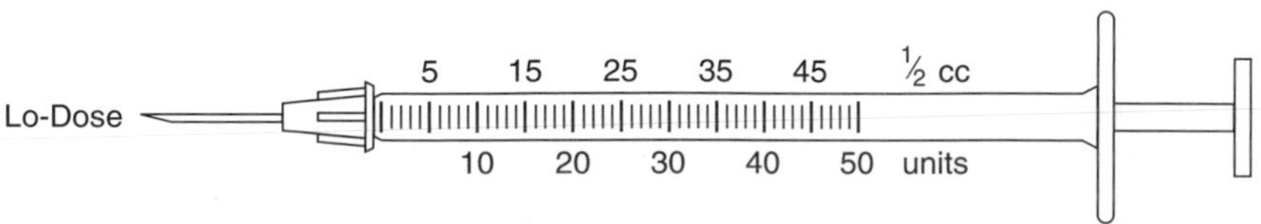

19. Your patient with a lumbar laminectomy receives heparin 0.5 mL SQ. How many units will you administer? ______ . Draw a vertical line through the syringe to indicate the dosage.

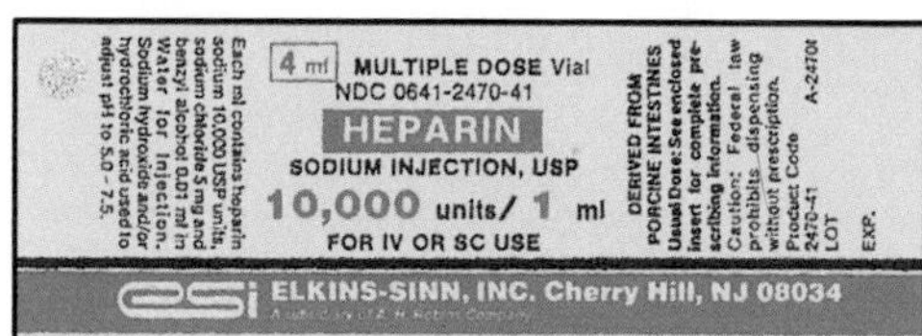

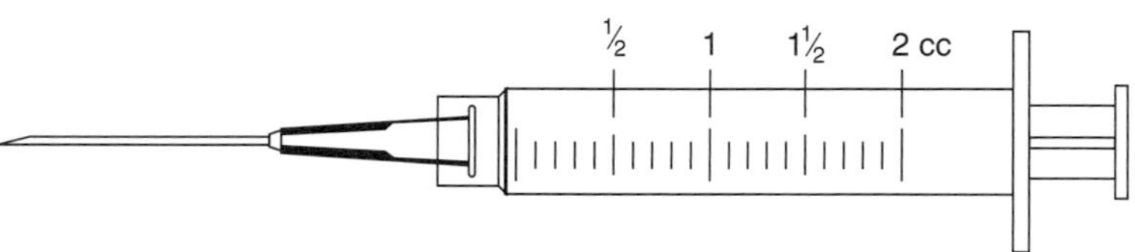

20. Your patient with a gastric pull-up receives penicillin G 200,000 U IM q6 h. You have penicillin G 250,000 U per mL available. How many milliliters will you administer? ______ . Draw a vertical line through the syringe to indicate the dosage.

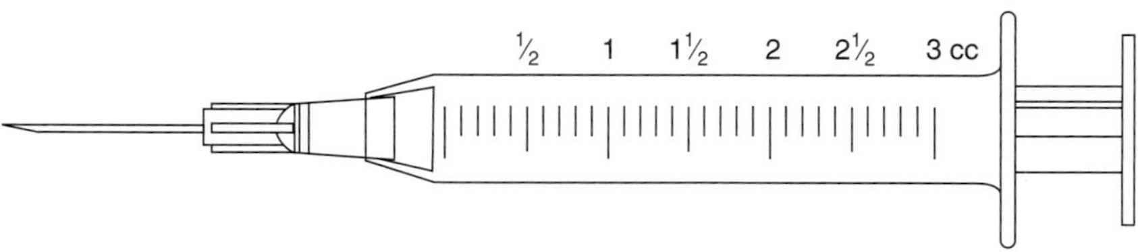

Answers on pp. 493-497.

CHAPTER 14 **Dosages Measured in Units**

Name ______________________

Date ______________________

ACCEPTABLE SCORE 13

YOUR SCORE ______

POSTTEST 1

Directions: The medication order is listed at the beginning of each problem. Calculate the dosages. Show your work. Mark the syringe when provided to indicate the correct dosage.

1. The physician orders penicillin V 500,000 U po qid for your patient with a hysterectomy. Penicillin V pediatric suspension 400,000 U per 5 mL is supplied. How many milliliters will you administer? _______ . Draw a vertical line through the syringe to indicate the dosage.

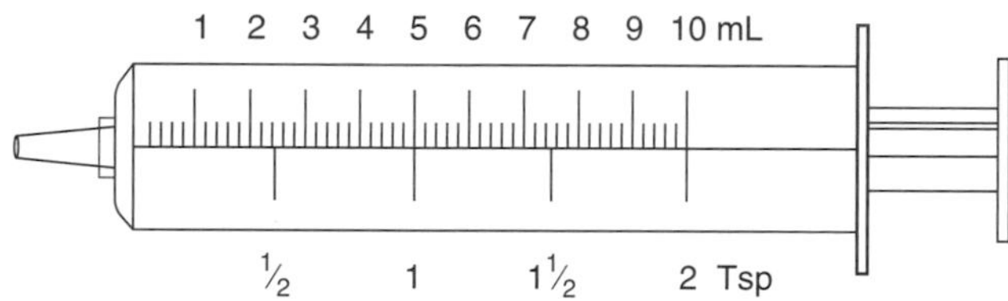

2. Ordered Lente insulin 40 U SQ qAM. Draw a vertical line through the syringe to indicate the dosage.

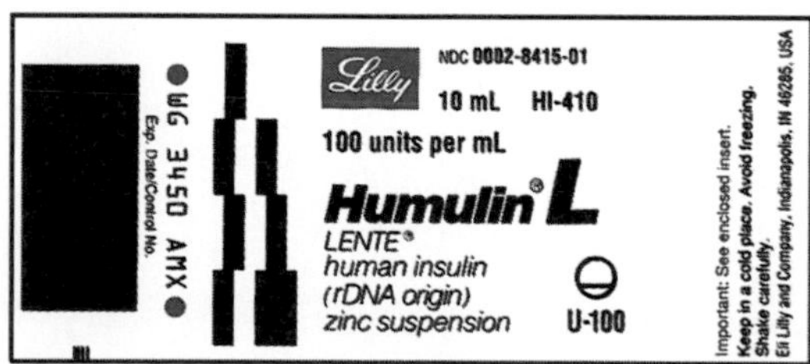

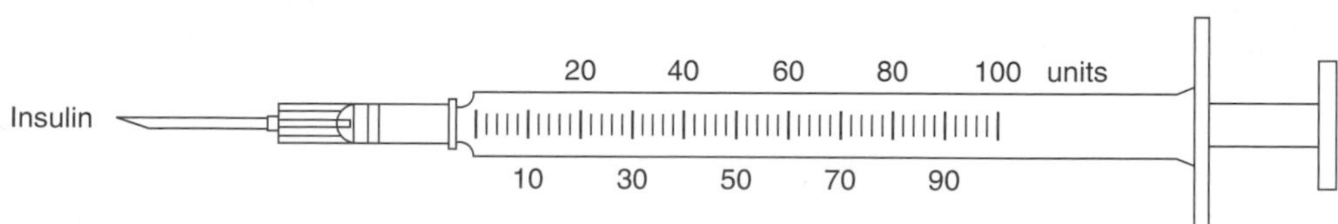

3. Your patient with a lumbar laminectomy receives heparin 7500 U SQ qid. You have heparin 5000 U per mL available. How many milliliters will you administer? _______ .

4. Ordered Humulin regular insulin 6 U SQ. Draw a vertical line through the syringe to indicate the dosage.

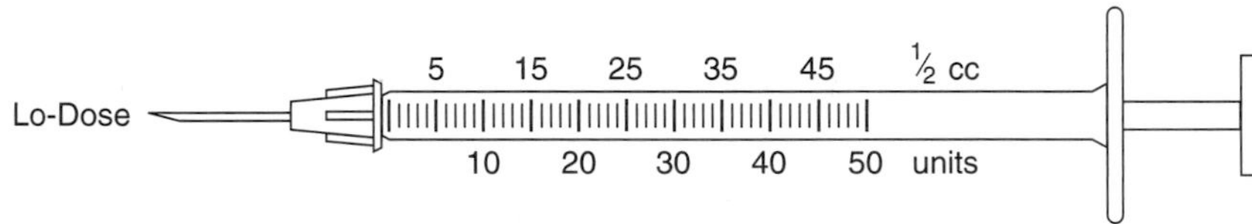

5. The physician orders penicillin G potassium 3,000,000 U IM q6 h for your patient with an ethmoidectomy. What is the best amount of diluent to add? _______ . What is the medication concentration? _______ . How many milliliters will you administer? _______ .

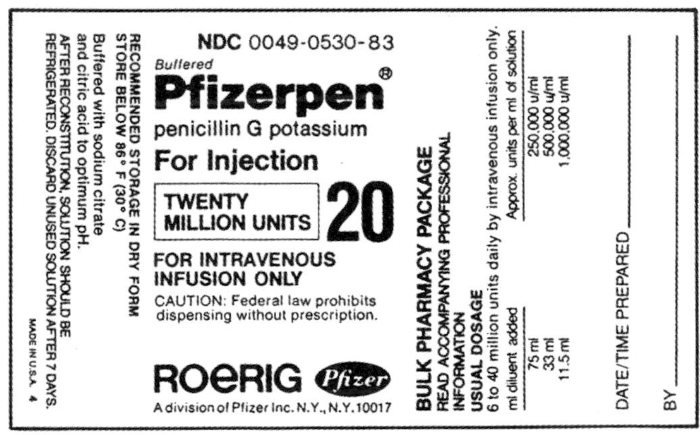

6. Your patient with insulin-dependent diabetes has NPH insulin 60 U SQ qAM. You have NPH insulin U-100 and a U-100 syringe. Draw a vertical line through the syringe to indicate the dosage.

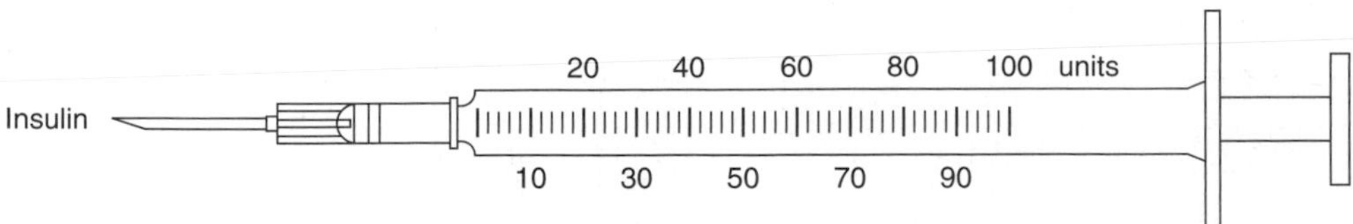

7. Ordered heparin 20,000 U SQ today. How many milliliters will the nurse administer? _______ .

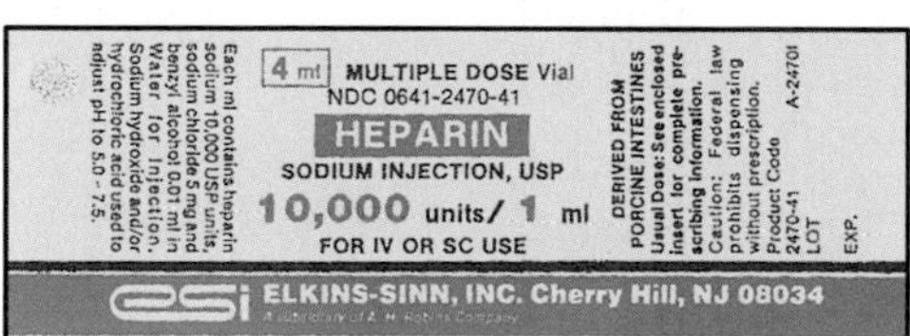

8. Ordered Lente insulin 38 U, regular insulin 18 U SQ qAM. Lente U-100, regular insulin U-100, and a U-100 syringe are supplied. Draw a vertical line through the syringe to indicate the amount of regular insulin to be given and a second line to indicate the total dosage.

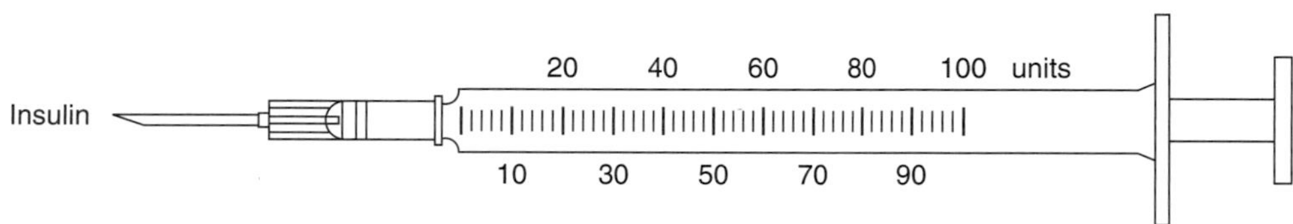

9. The physician orders penicillin V 300,000 U po qid for your patient with chronic otitis. The drug is supplied in oral solution 200,000 U per 5 mL. How many milliliters will you administer? _______ .

10. Ordered Pfizerpen 1.2 million U IM in a single dose today. How much diluent should be added? _______ . What is the medication concentration? _______ . How many milliliters will the nurse administer? _______ .

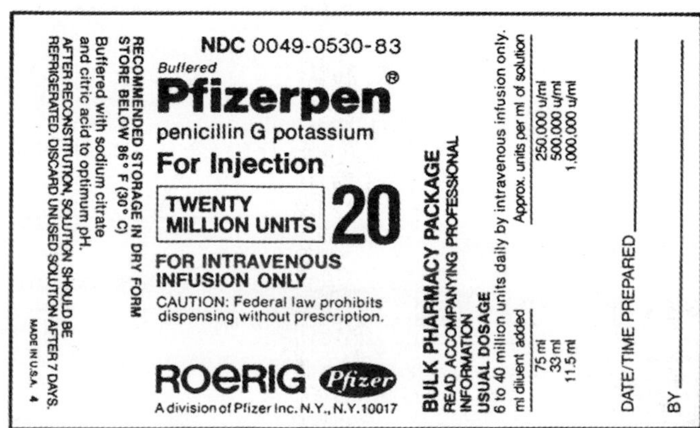

11. Your patient with a sacral decubitus receives penicillin V 200,000 U po qid. You have penicillin V oral solution 400,000 U per 5 mL. How many milliliters will you administer? _______ .

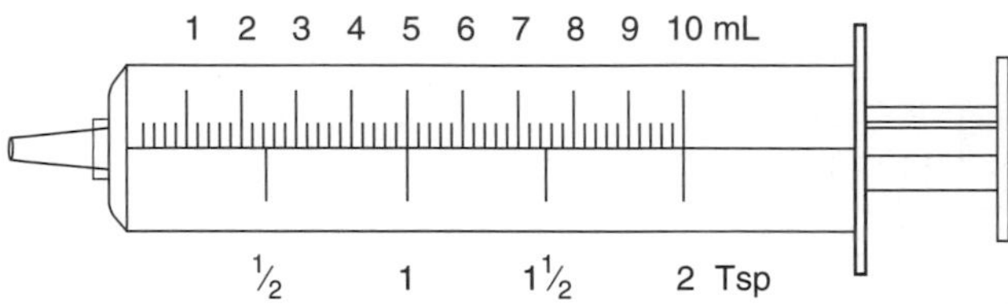

12. Your patient with a lumbar laminectomy receives heparin 7500 U SQ q12 h. Heparin 5000 U per mL is available. How many milliliters will you administer? _______ .

13. Your patient with meningitis receives penicillin G 500,000 U IM q6 h. How many milliliters will you administer? _______ .

14. Mrs. Daisy receives nystatin oral suspension 600,000 U po qid. How many milliliters will the nurse administer? _______ .

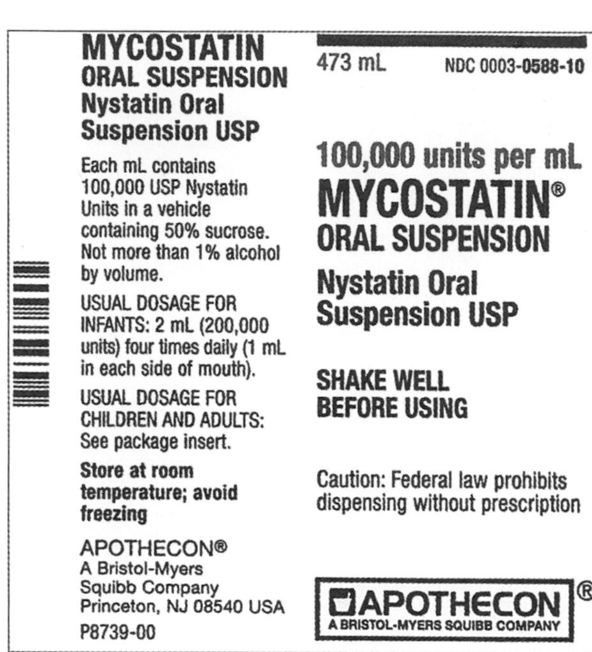

15. Your patient with a lumbar discectomy requires heparin 5000 U SQ q8 h. How many milliliters will you administer? _______ .

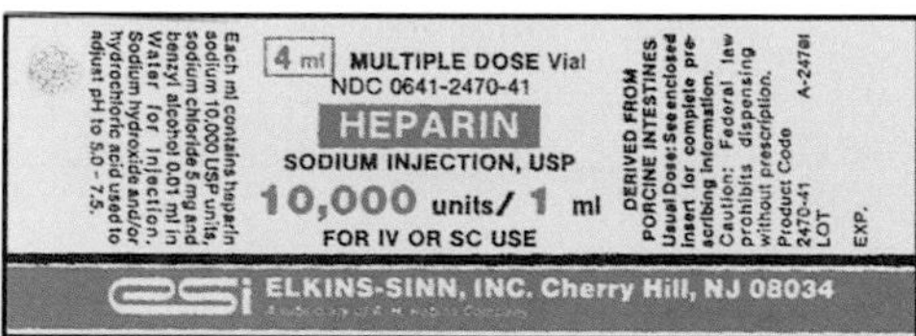

Answers on pp. 498-500.

Name ______________________

Date ______________________

ACCEPTABLE SCORE 13

YOUR SCORE ______

POSTTEST 2

Directions: The medication order is listed at the beginning of each problem. Calculate the dosages. Show your work. Mark the syringe when provided to indicate the correct dosage.

1. Ordered regular insulin 10 U SQ tomorrow AM. Regular insulin U-100 and a U-100 Lo-Dose syringe are supplied. Draw a vertical line through the syringe to indicate the dosage.

Lo-Dose

5 15 25 35 45 ½ cc

10 20 30 40 50 units

2. Ordered heparin 1000 U per L to be added to IV fluids. How many milliliters will you add to 1 L? ______ .

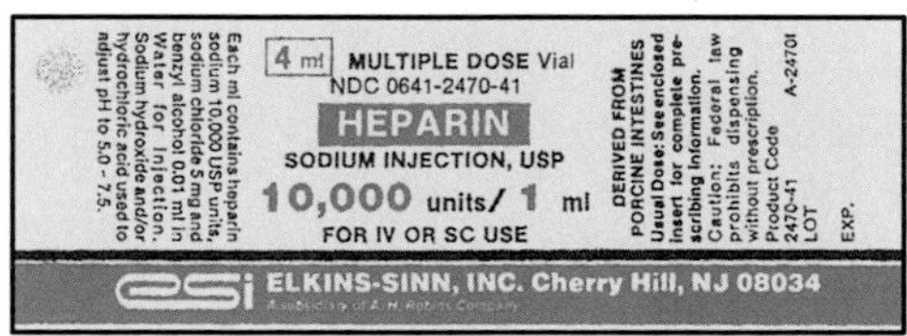

3. Your patient with a septoplasty receives V-Cillin K 500,000 U po q6 h. You have 200,000 U per 5 mL available. How many milliliters will you administer? ______ .

4. Ordered NPH insulin 28 U SQ at 7:45 AM. Draw a vertical line through the syringe to indicate the dosage of NPH insulin to be given.

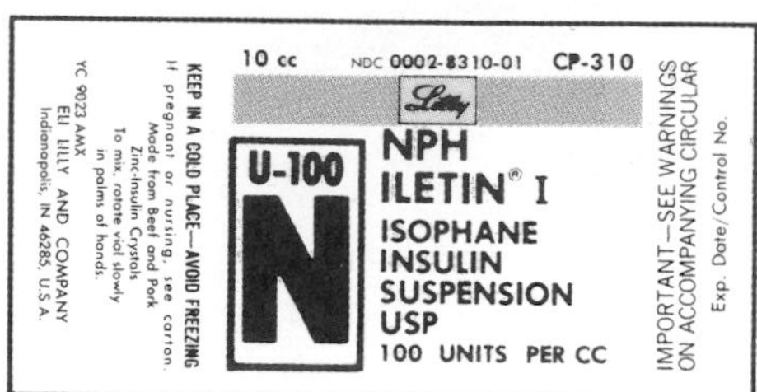

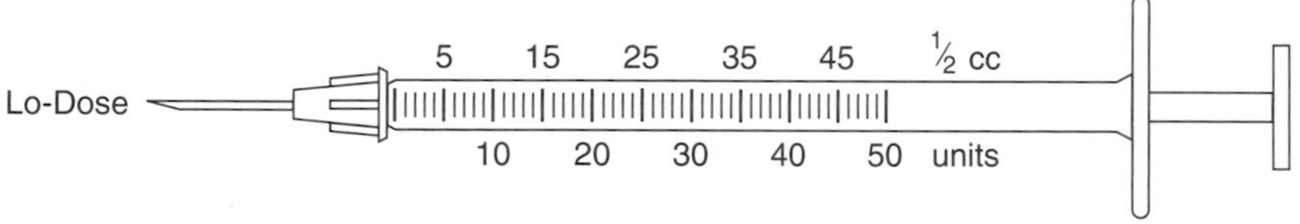

5. The physician orders heparin 1500 U SQ today for your patient with a total hip replacement. How many milliliters will you administer? _______ .

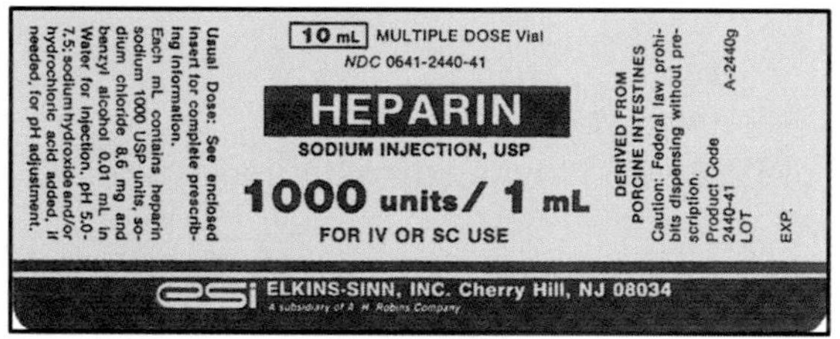

6. The physician orders penicillin G potassium 1.2 million U IV q4 h for your patient after dental extraction. You have a vial containing 1,000,000 U per mL. How many milliliters will you prepare? _______ .

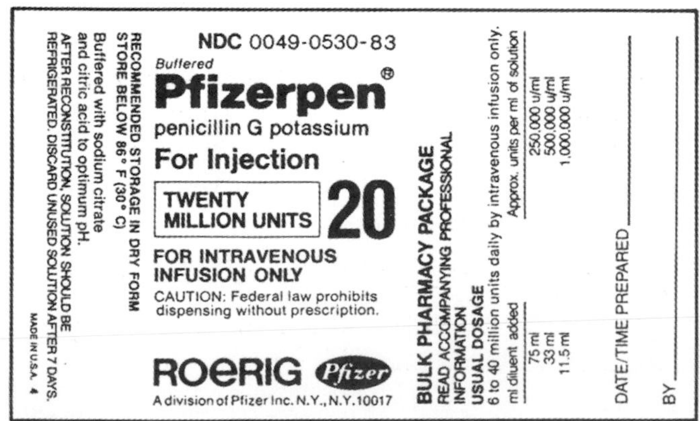

7. Ordered Lente insulin 54 U SQ qAM. You have Lente insulin U-100 and a U-100 syringe. Draw a vertical line through the syringe to indicate the amount of Lente insulin to be given.

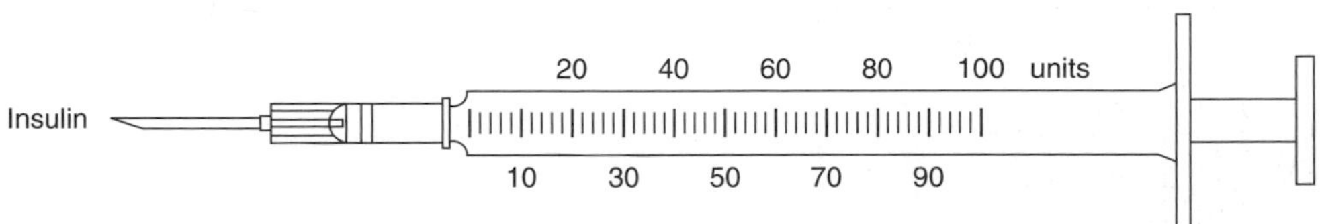

8. Ordered NPH insulin 16 U, regular insulin 8 U SQ qAM. You have NPH insulin U-100, regular insulin U-100, and a U-100 Lo-Dose syringe. Draw a vertical line through the syringe to indicate the amount of regular insulin to be given and a second line to indicate the total dosage.

Lo-Dose
5 15 25 35 45 ½ cc
10 20 30 40 50 units

9. Your patient with chronic sinusitis receives penicillin V 300,000 U po qid. You have penicillin V oral solution 400,000 U per 5 mL. How many milliliters will you administer? ______ .

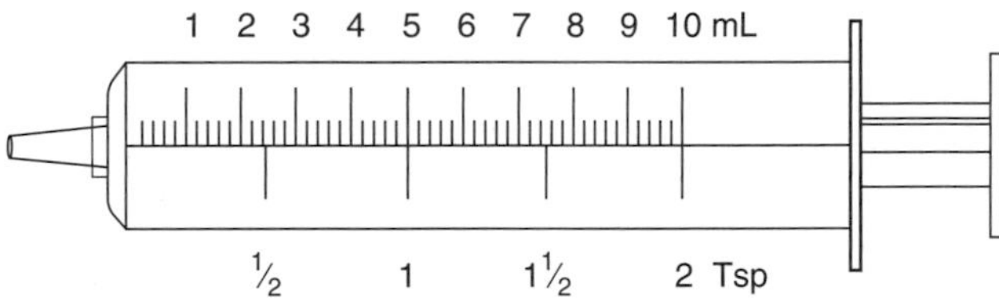

10. Your patient with a jejunostomy requires heparin 6000 U SQ qd. You have heparin 5000 U per mL available. How many milliliters will you administer? ______ . Draw a vertical line through the syringe to indicate the dosage.

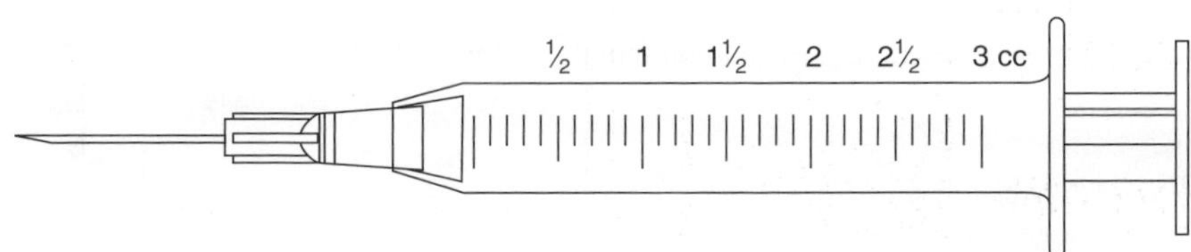

11. Your patient with osteomyelitis receives penicillin G 600,000 U IM bid. How much diluent should be added? _______ . What is the medication concentration? _______ . How many milliliters will you administer? _______ .

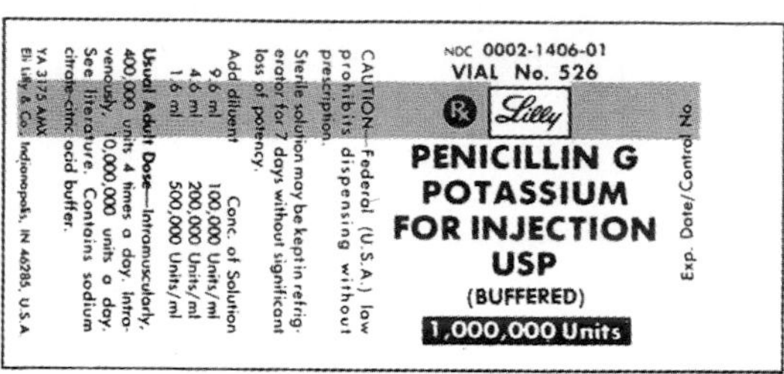

12. Your patient who has had a total hip replacement requires heparin 10,000 U SQ q12 h. You have heparin 5000 U per mL available. How many milliliters will you administer? _______ .

13. Your patient with insulin-dependent diabetes receives Lente insulin 25 U SQ qAM. Draw a vertical line through the syringe to indicate the amount of Lente insulin to be given.

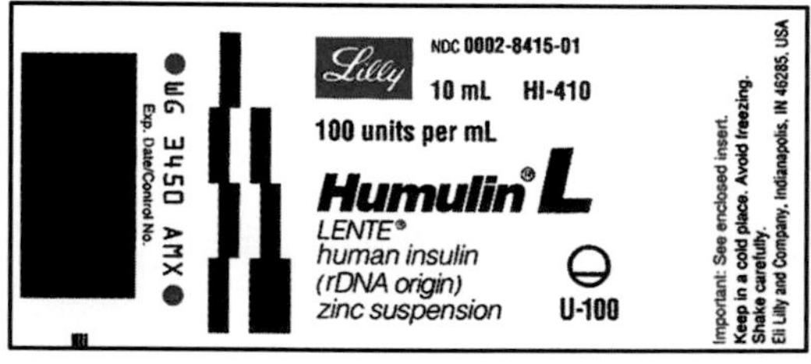

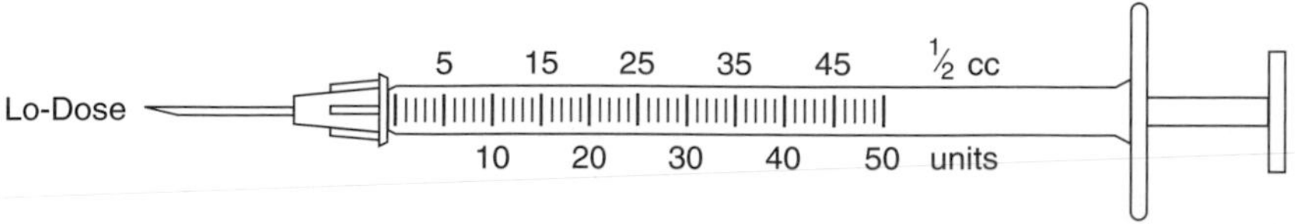

14. Your patient who has had a gastrectomy requires heparin 7500 U SQ qid. You have heparin 5000 U per mL. How many milliliters will you administer? _______ .

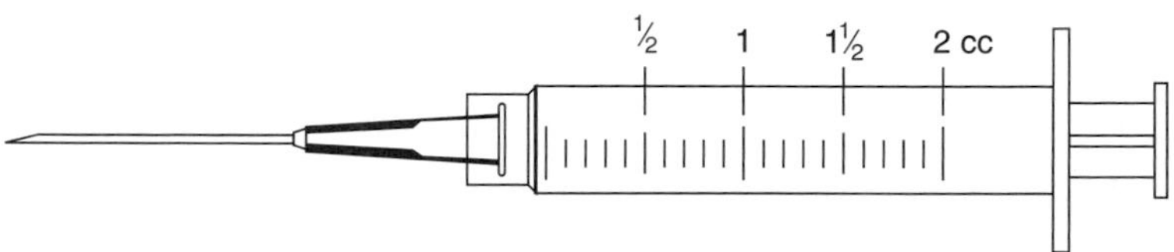

15. Your patient with a cholecystectomy receives heparin 20,000 U SQ today. How many milliliters will you administer? _______ .

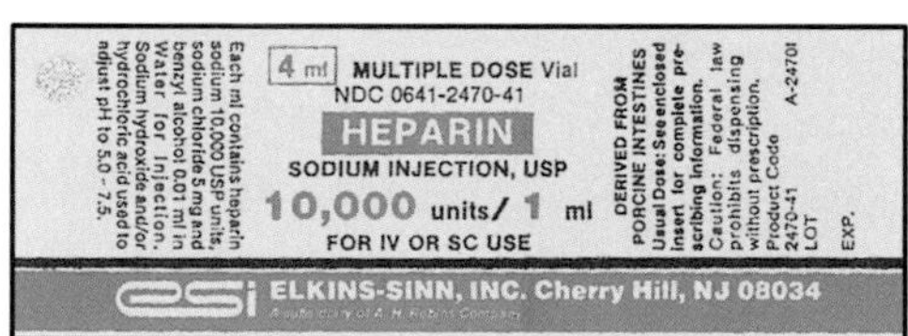

Answers on pp. 500-502.

CHAPTER

15

Intravenous Flow Rates*

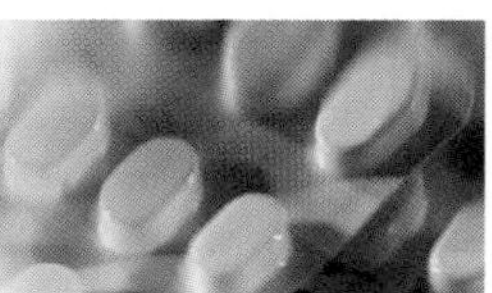

LEARNING OBJECTIVES

On completion of the materials provided in this chapter, you will be able to perform computations accurately by mastering the following mathematical concepts:

1 Calculating milliliters per hour (mL/h) when given the total volume and time over which an IV solution or intravenous piggyback is to be infused

2 Calculating drops per minute (gtt/min) when given the total volume and time over which an IV solution or intravenous piggyback is to be infused

It is sometimes necessary to deliver fluids and medications to a patient intravenously. Intravenous (IV) solutions and medications are placed directly into a vein. Infusions are injections of moderate to large quantities of fluids and nutrients into the patient's venous system. An IV medication or infusion may be prepared and administered by a physician, nurse, or technician as regulated by state law and the policies of the particular health care agency. Medications and electrolyte milliequivalents are commonly ordered as additives to IV fluids. Medications may also be diluted and given in conjunction with IV solutions.

IV fluids are administered via an intravenous infusion set. This set includes the sealed bottle or bag containing the fluids, a drip chamber connected to the bottle or bag by a small tube or spike, and tubing that leads from the drip chamber down to and connecting with the needle or catheter at the site of insertion into the patient (Figure 15-1). The flow rate is adjusted to the desired drops per minute by a clamp placed around the tubing. The nurse must be knowledgeable about the equipment being used and, in particular, about the flow rate or drops per milliliter that a particular set of tubing will deliver.

*Linda Fluharty, MSN, RN, contributed to this chapter.

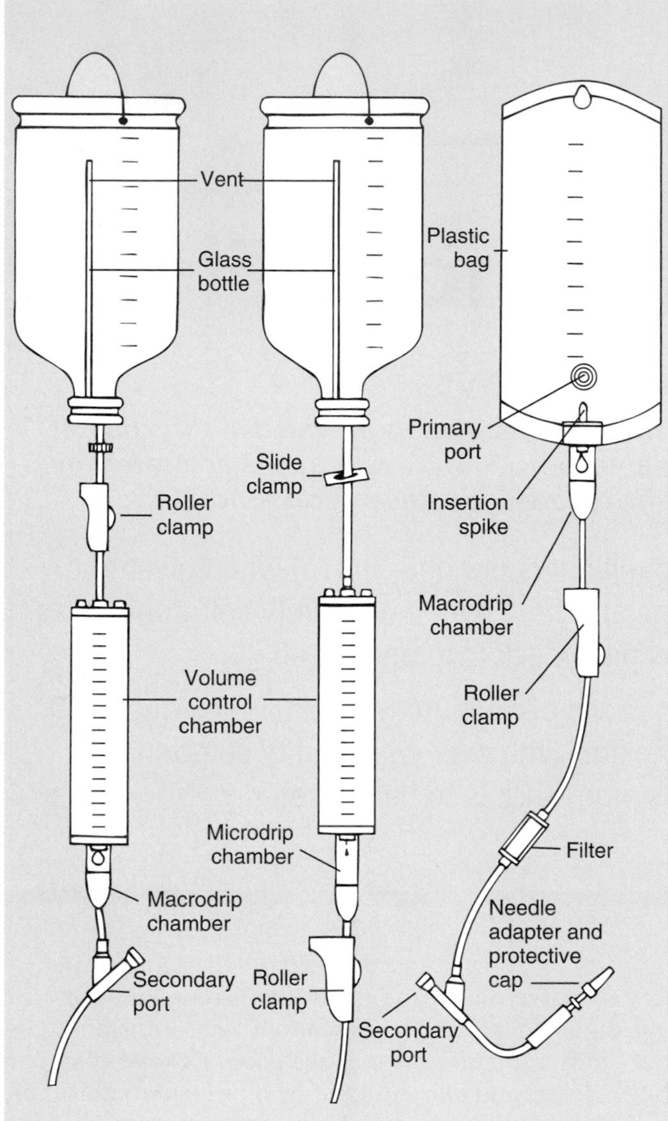

FIGURE 15-1 Intravenous infusion sets. (From Clayton BD, Stock YN: *Basic pharmacology for nurses,* ed 12, St Louis, 2001, Mosby.)

Infusion sets come in a variety of sizes. The larger the diameter of the tubing where it enters the drip chamber, the bigger the drop will be. The drop factor of an infusion set is the number of drops contained in 1 mL (1 cc). This equivalent may vary with different manufacturers. The most common drop factors are 10, 15, 20, and 60. Sets that deliver 10, 15, or 20 drops per milliliter are called *macrodrip sets.* A set that delivers 60 drops per milliliter is called *a microdrip set.* Macrodrip sets are larger than microdrip sets.

If large volumes of fluid must be administered (125 mL/h or more), a macrodrip set is required. Microdrip sets are unable to deliver large volumes per hour because their drop size is so small. When an IV solution is to run at a rate of 50 mL/h or less, a microdrip set should be used. Some hospitals may even require a microdrip set for rates of 60 to 80 mL/h, for accuracy of flow rate and to help maintain the patency of the line. The number of drops per milliliter for the IV administration set is written on the outside of the box. This information is essential for solving problems related to the regulation of IV flow rates (Figure 15-2).

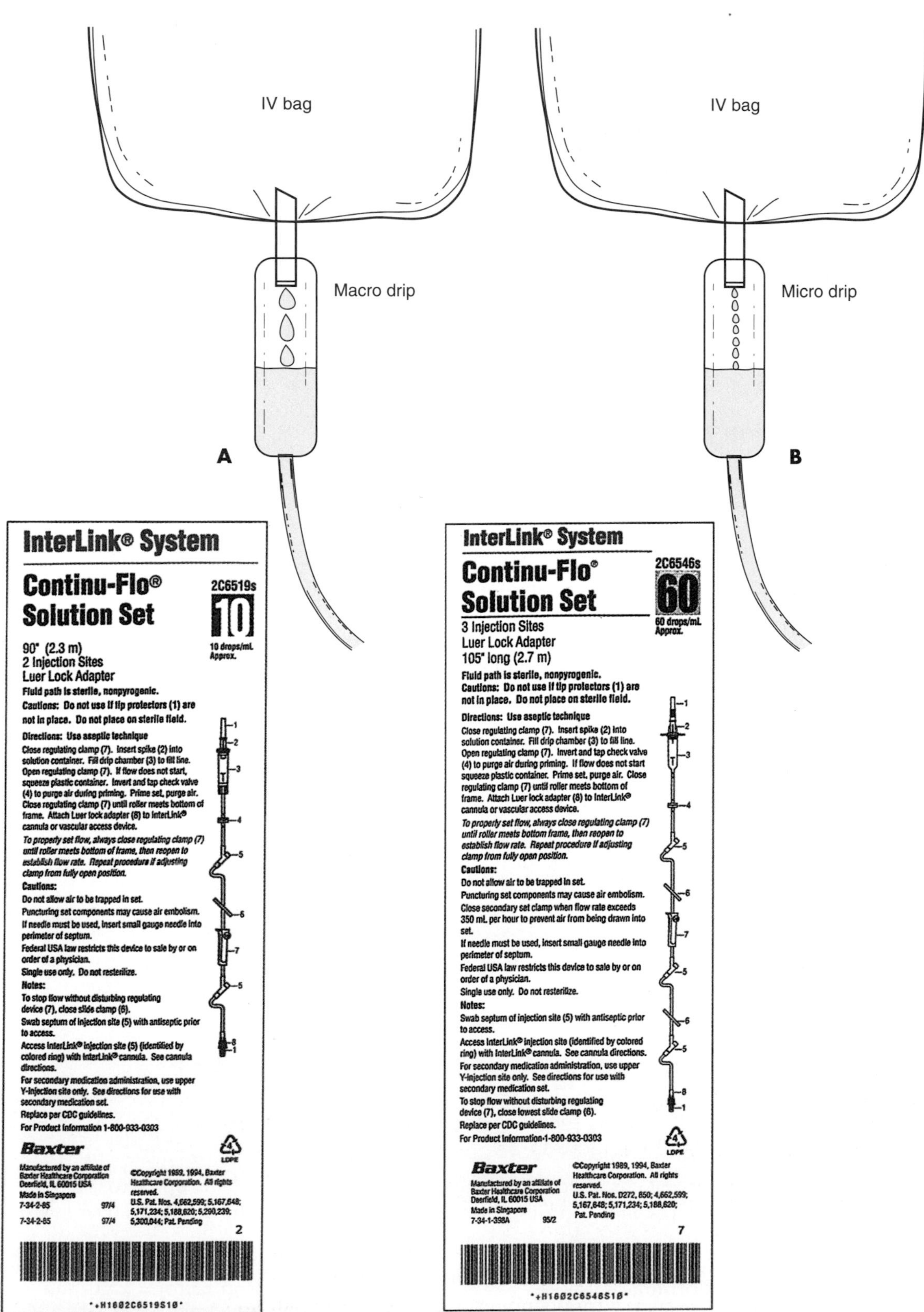

FIGURE 15-2 Administration sets. **A,** Set delivers 10 gtt per mL. **B,** Set delivers 60 gtt per mL. (From Morris DG: *Calculate with confidence,* ed 3, St Louis, 2002, Mosby.)

The physician is responsible for writing the order for the type and amount of IV or hyperalimentation fluids. The number of hours or rate of infusion is also ordered by the physician. It is usually the nurse's responsibility to regulate and maintain the infusion flow rate. It is the nurse's goal to ensure that the IV flow is regular. If the rate is irregular, too much or too little fluid may be infused. This may lead to complications such as fluid overload, dehydration, or medication overdose. Sometimes the rate of flow must be adjusted because of interruptions caused by needle placement, condition of the vein, or infiltration.

The nurse must be able to determine the number of drops per minute (gtt/min) the patient must receive for the infusion to be completed within the specified time.

When the volume, time or length of the infusion, and the constant drip factor are known, a simple formula may be used.

$$\frac{\text{V (Volume}}{\text{T (Time)}} \times \text{C (Constant drip factor)} = \text{R (gtt/min)}$$

IV Administration of Fluids by Gravity

Example 1: Hespan 500 mL is ordered to be infused over 3 hours. The drop factor is 15 gtt/min. How many gtt/min should be given to infuse the total amount of Hespan over 3 hours? _______ .

$$\text{The formula: } \frac{\text{Total volume to be infused}}{\text{Total amount of time in minutes}} \times \text{Drop factor} = x \text{ gtt/min}$$

Step 1: Convert total hours to minutes

$1 \text{ h} : 60 \text{ min} :: 3 \text{ h} : x \text{ min}$

$x = 180$ Therefore 3 hours equals 180 minutes.

Step 2: Calculate gtt/min

(This calculation depends on the drop factor of the tubing being used. Remember, this information is found on the package. For the problems in this work text, the drop factor is indicated. The drop factor for this problem is 15.)

$$\text{(Formula setup)} \quad \frac{500 \text{ mL}}{180 \text{ min}} \times \frac{15 \text{ gtt/mL}}{} = x \text{ gtt/min}$$

$$\text{(Cancel)} \quad \frac{500 \not{\text{mL}}}{\underset{12}{\not{180}} \text{ min}} \times \frac{\overset{1}{\not{15}} \text{gtt/}\not{\text{mL}}}{} = x \text{ gtt/min}$$

$$\text{(Calculate)} \quad \frac{500}{12 \text{ min}} \times \frac{1 \text{ gtt}}{} = \frac{500}{12} = 41.6 \text{ or } 42 \text{ gtt/min}$$

Therefore the nurse will regulate the IV to drip at 42 drops per minute, and the 500 mL of Hespan will be infused over 3 h (Figure 15-3).

Example 2: 1000 mL of D_5W is ordered to be infused over 5 hours. The drop factor is 10 gtt/mL. How many gtt/min should be given to infuse the 1000 mL over 5 hours? _______ .

$$\text{The formula: } \frac{\text{Total volume to be infused}}{\text{Total amount of time in minutes}} \times \text{drop factor} = x \text{ gtt/min}$$

$$\frac{V}{T} \times C = R$$

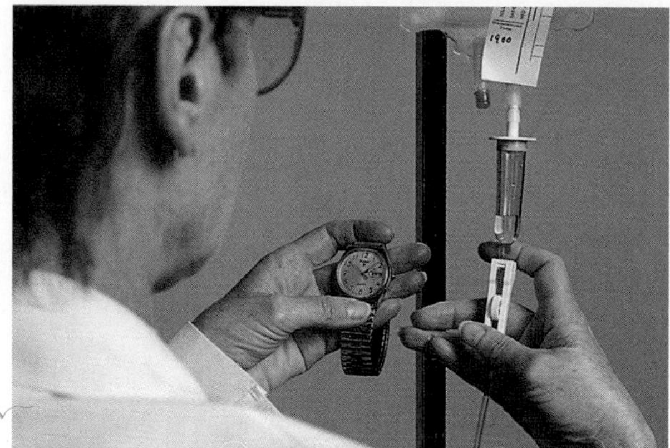

FIGURE 15-3 Count drops per minute by watching the drip chamber for 1 minute and adjusting the roller clamp as needed to deliver the desired number of drops per minute. (From Potter PA, Perry AG: *Fundamentals of nursing,* ed 5, St Louis, 2001, Mosby.)

Step 1: Convert the total hours to minutes

1 h : 60 min :: 5 h : x min
x = 300 Therefore 5 hours equals 300 minutes

Step 2: Calculate gtt/min

(Formula setup) $$\frac{1000 \text{ mL}}{300 \text{ min}} \times \frac{10 \text{ gtt/mL}}{} = x \text{ gtt/min}$$

(Cancel) $$\frac{1000 \not{\text{mL}}}{\underset{30}{\cancel{300}} \text{ min}} \times \frac{\overset{1}{\cancel{10}} \text{ gtt/}\not{\text{mL}}}{} = x \text{ gtt/min}$$

(Calculate) $$\frac{1000}{30 \text{ min}} \times \frac{1 \text{ gtt}}{} = \frac{1000}{30} = 33.3 \text{ or } 33 \text{ gtt/min}$$

The nurse will regulate the IV to drip at a rate of 33 gtt/min, and the 1000 mL of D_5W will be infused over 5 hours.

Infusion of IV Piggybacks by Gravity

Sometimes the physician will order medications to be administered in a small amount of IV fluid. This medication will need to be infused in addition to the regular IV fluids; it is called an *IV piggyback* (IVPB) (Figure 15-4). The medication for the IVPB may be received premixed by the pharmacy or may need to be prepared by the nurse. The time frame for the IVPB infusion is usually 60 minutes or less.

If the physician does not include an infusion time or rate, it is the responsibility of the nurse to follow the manufacturer's guidelines. The hospital pharmacy and drug books such as the *Hospital Formulary* and *A Handbook for Intravenous Medication* published by Mosby are known resources for fluid rates. The nurse should always refer to any standing fluid limits and rates before IVPB administration.

When the volume, time of infusion, and tubing drip factor are known, the same formula that was used for *IV Administration of Fluids by Gravity* is used to calculate the flow rate for the IVPB.

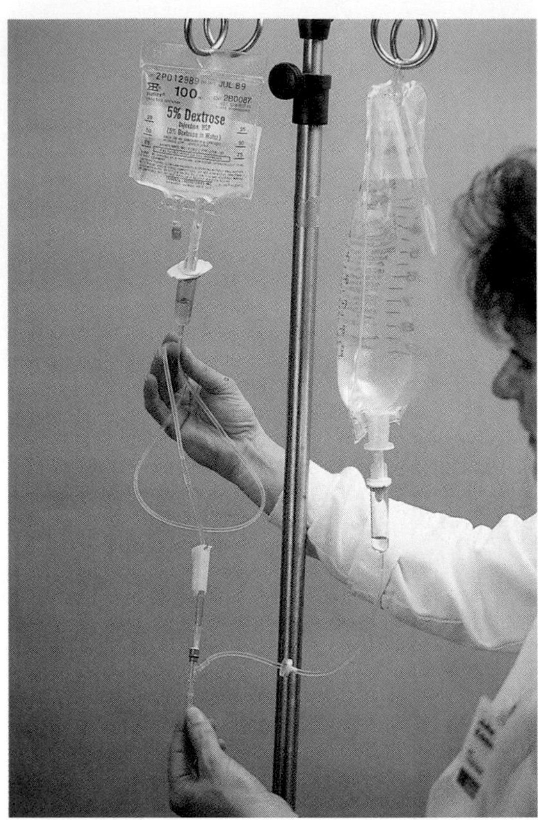

FIGURE 15-4 Tandem/intravenous piggyback (IVPB) administration setup. (From Potter PA, Perry AG: *Fundamentals of nursing,* ed 5, St Louis, 2001, Mosby.)

Example 1: The physician orders cefuroxime 1.0 g in 50 mL of normal saline solution (NS) to be infused over 30 minutes. The tubing drop factor is 60 gtt/mL. How many gtts/min should be given to infuse the total amount of cefuroxime over 30 minutes?_______ .

The formula: $\dfrac{\text{Total volume to be infused}}{\text{Total amount of time in minutes}} \times \text{Drop factor} = x \text{ gtt/min}$

Step 1: Calculate gtt/min

(Formula setup) $\dfrac{50 \text{ mL}}{30 \text{ min}} \times \dfrac{60 \text{ gtt/mL}}{} = x \text{ gtt/min}$

(Cancel) $\dfrac{50 \not{\text{mL}}}{\underset{1}{\not{30}} \text{ min}} \times \dfrac{\overset{2}{\not{60}} \text{ gtt/}\not{\text{mL}}}{} = x \text{ gtt/min}$

(Calculate) $\dfrac{50}{1} \times 2 = 100 \text{ gtt/min}$

Therefore the nurse will regulate the IVPB to drip at 100 gtt/min, and the cefuroxime will be infused over 30 minutes.

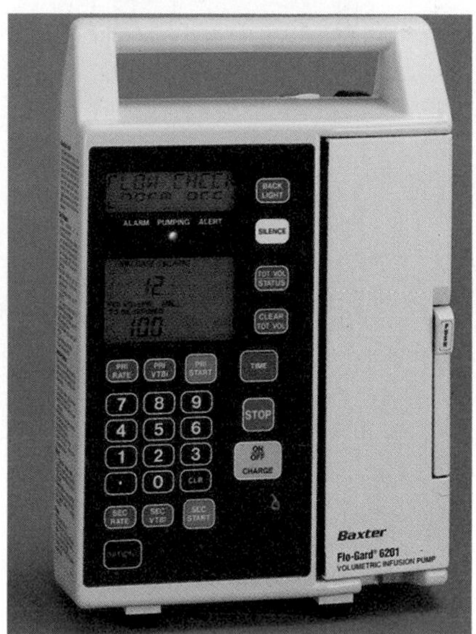

FIGURE 15-5 Single infusion pump. (From Morris DG: *Calculate with confidence,* ed 3, St Louis, 2002, Mosby. Courtesy Baxter Healthcare Corporation, Deerfield, Illinois.)

Example 2: The physician orders gentamicin 80 mg in 100 mL D_5W to be infused over 1 hour. The tubing drop factor is 60 gtt/mL. How many gtt/min should be given to infuse the gentamicin over 1 hour? ______ .

Step 1: Convert the total hours to minutes

1 h :: 60 min

Step 2: Calculate the gtt/min

(Formula setup) $$\frac{100\text{ mL}}{60\text{ min}} \times \frac{60\text{ gtt/mL}}{} = x\text{ gtt/min}$$

(Cancel) $$\frac{100\ \cancel{\text{mL}}}{\underset{1}{\cancel{60}}\text{ min}} \times \frac{\overset{1}{\cancel{60}}\text{ gtt/}\cancel{\text{mL}}}{} = x\text{ gtt/min}$$

(Calculate) $$\frac{100}{1\text{ min}} \times \frac{1\text{ gtt}}{} = 100\text{ gtt/min}$$

Therefore the nurse will regulate the IVPB to drip at 100 gtt/min, and the gentamicin will be infused over 1 hour.

Note: If the infusion time is 60 minutes and a microdrip set (drop factor of 60 gtt/mL) is used, the drops per minute will be the same as the number of milliliters per hour.

IV flow rates are often controlled by an electronic device or pump. The IV pumps are programmed to deliver a set amount of fluid per hour. Safety for the patient is an advantage of electronic IV pumps. The pumps are used for patients in regular medical-surgical units, critical care areas, pediatrics, the operating room, and ambulatory care settings.

Many electronic pumps are on the market today. These vary from simple one-channel models to those that are four multichannel pumps. Many of the newer models will actually calculate flow rates and automatically start infusions at a later time. Convenience, safety, accuracy, and time-saving options are driving forces in the innovations currently available.

Some examples of equipment are pictured in Figures 15-5, 15-6, and 15-7; in Figure 15-6, the Medley™ Medication Safety System and the Medley™ pump module (attached to the programming module) are shown. In Figure 15-7, the Medley™ Medication Safety System is being used on a patient in a critical care setting. Each company offers special tubing for use with its pumps.

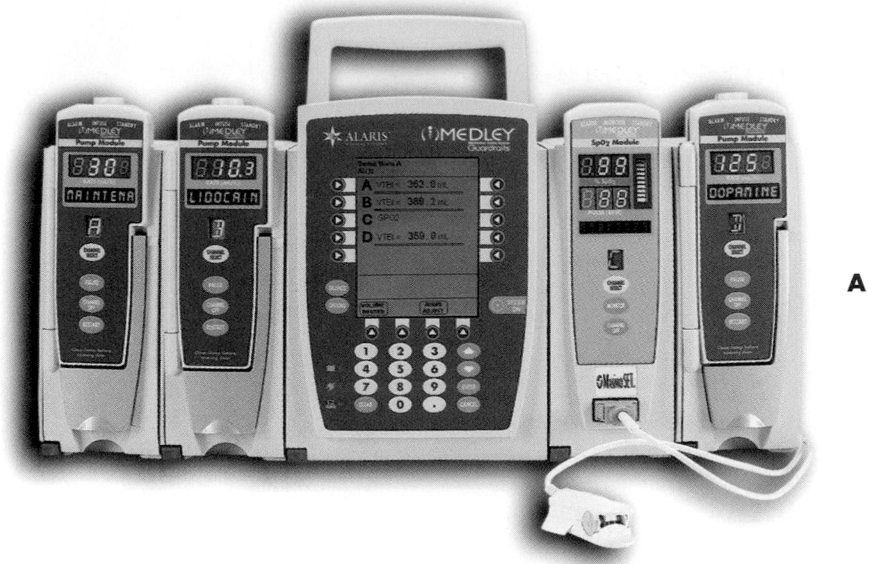

A

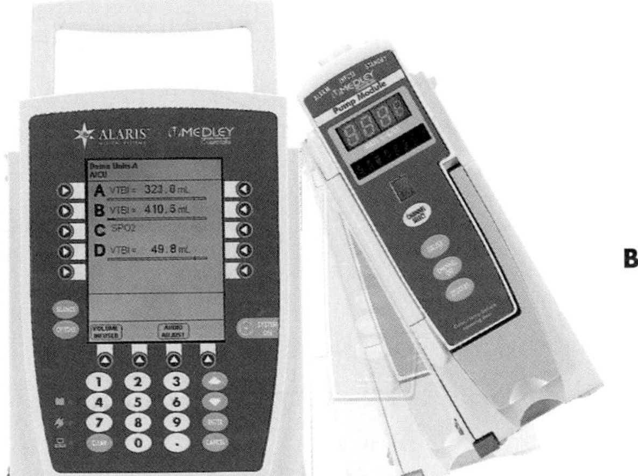

B

FIGURE 15-6 **A,** Medley™ Medication Safety System. **B,** Example of the Medley™ pump module attached to the Medley™ programming module. (Courtesy ALARIS Medical Systems, Inc., San Diego, California.)

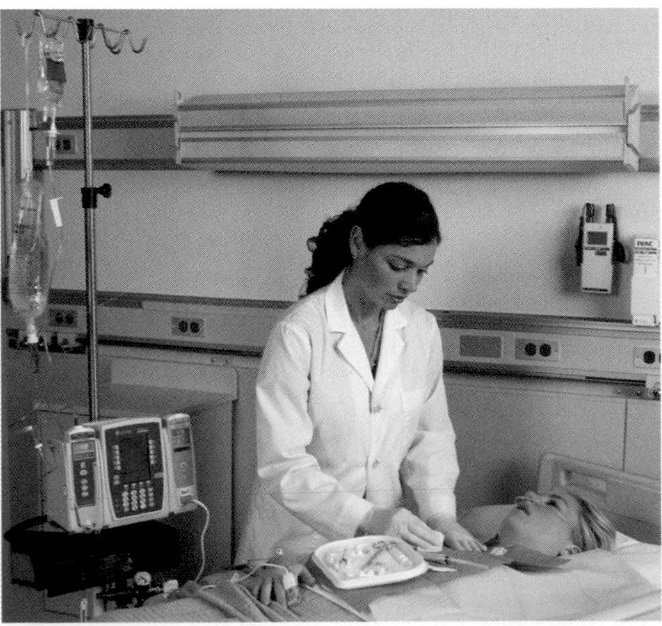

FIGURE 15-7 Medley™ Medication Safety System being used on a patient in a critical care setting. (Courtesy ALARIS Medical Systems, Inc., San Diego, California.)

Infusion of IV Fluids with an IV Pump

In many facilities, IV fluids are infused by using an IV pump. IV pumps are programmed to infuse IV fluids by milliliters per hour (mL/h).

$$\text{The formula: } \frac{\text{Total volume in milliliters}}{\text{Total time in hours}} = x \text{ mL/h}$$

Example 1: Infuse 250 mL of 0.9% NS over 2 hours. How many mL/h should the IV pump be programmed for to infuse 250 mL over 2 hours? ______ .

$$\text{The formula: } \frac{\text{Total volume in milliliters}}{\text{Time in hours}} = x \text{ mL/h}$$

Step 1: Calculate mL/h

$$\text{(Formula setup)} \quad \frac{250 \text{ mL}}{2 \text{ h}} = 125 \text{ mL/h}$$

Therefore the nurse will program the IV pump for 125 mL/h, and the 250 mL of NS will be infused over 2 hours.

Example 2: Infuse 1000 mL of lactated Ringer's solution (LR) over 12 hours. How many mL/h should the IV pump be programmed for? ______.

Step 1: Calculate mL/h

$$\text{(Formula setup)} \quad \frac{1000 \text{ mL}}{12 \text{ h}} = 83.3 \text{ or } 83 \text{ mL/h}$$

Therefore the nurse will program the IV pump for 83 mL/h, and the 1000 mL of LR will be infused over 12 hours.

Infusion of IV Medications with an IV Pump

In some situations the health care professional will be required to infuse medications using an IV pump. Whether the medication is an electrolyte replacement, an antiinfective agent, or another type of medication to be infused by IVPB, the health care professional needs to calculate the rate, in milliliters per hour, for which the IV pump should be programmed.

Example 1: Dilute potassium 40 mEq in 250 mL of D_5W and administer IV now. The facility's policy states to infuse potassium at a rate of 10 mEq per hour. How many mL/h should the IV pump be programmed for to infuse the potassium at a rate of 10 mEq per hour? ______ .

Using the ratio-proportion method:

Calculate mL/h

(Formula setup) $40 \text{ mEq} : 250 \text{ mL} :: 10 \text{ mEq} : x \text{ mL}$

(Calculate) $40x = 2500$

$$x = \frac{2500}{40}$$

$$x = 62.5 \text{ or } 63 \text{ mL}$$

Therefore the nurse will program the IV pump for 63 mL/h, and the potassium will be infused at 10 mEq/h as stated in the facility's policy. (Note: Follow your facility's policy when you calculate the rate for any electrolyte replacement.)

Using the $\frac{D}{A} \times Q = x$ mL/h method:

Calculate mL/h

(Formula setup) $\frac{10 \text{ mEq}}{40 \text{ mEq}} \times 250 \text{ mL} = x \text{ mL}$

(Cancel) $\frac{\overset{1}{\cancel{10}} \cancel{\text{mEq}}}{\underset{4}{\cancel{40}} \cancel{\text{mEq}}} \times 250 \text{ mL} = x \text{ mL}$

(Calculate) $\frac{1}{4} \times 250 \text{ mL} = \frac{250}{4} = 62.5$ or 63 mL/h

Example 2: Administer 1 g of vancomycin over 60 minutes. The vancomycin is dissolved in 100 mL of D_5W. How many mL/h should the IV pump be programmed for? _______ .

The formula: $\frac{\text{Total volume in milliliters}}{\text{Total time in hours}} = x$ mL/h

Step 1: Convert minutes to hours

60 min : 1 h

Step 2: Calculate mL/h

(Formula setup) $\frac{100 \text{ mL}}{1 \text{ h}} = 100$ mL/h

The nurse will program the IV pump for 100 mL/h, and the 100 mL of vancomycin will be infused over 1 hour (60 minutes).

Example 3: The physician orders Kefzol 1 g dissolved in 50 mL of D_5W to be infused over 30 minutes. The IVPB may be given by using an IV pump. How many mL/h should the IV pump be programmed for to infuse the Kefzol over 30 minutes? _______ .

Step 1: Convert minutes to hours

1 h : 60 min :: x h : 30 min

$60x = 30$

$x = \frac{30}{60} = 0.5$ h

Step 2: Calculate mL/h

(Formula setup) $\frac{50 \text{ mL}}{0.5 \text{ h}} = 100$ mL/h

IV or Heparin (Saline) Locks

IV or heparin locks are commonly used in a variety of health care settings. A heparin lock is an IV catheter that is inserted into a peripheral vein. It may be used for medications or fluids, usually on an intermittent basis. The use of a heparin lock prevents the patient from having to endure numerous venipunctures. Also, when fluid is not being infused, the patient enjoys greater mobility and freedom of movement. Each institution will have its own policy concerning the use and care of heparin locks. The locks may be flushed with 2 to 3 cc of normal saline solution alone or also with heparin flush solution of 10 units of heparin per 1 cc. This practice is called *heparinization,* and it prevents clotting of the heparin lock (Figure 15-8).

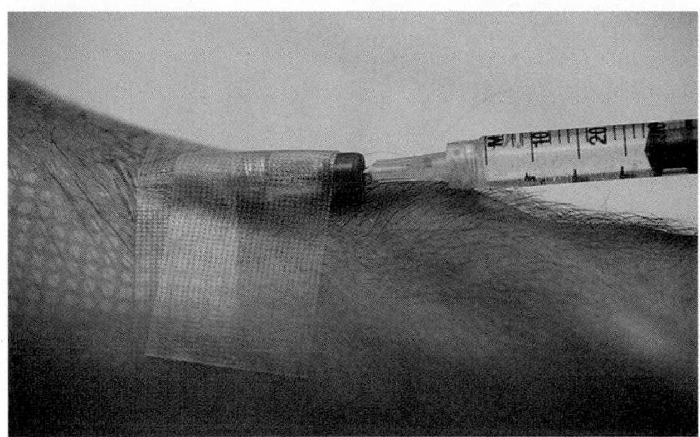

FIGURE 15-8 An IV or heparin/saline lock. (From Potter PA, Perry AG: *Fundamentals of nursing,* ed 5, St Louis, 2001, Mosby.)

Central Venous Catheters

Occasionally, a patient will need a central venous catheter. Central venous catheters are indwelling, semipermanent central lines that are inserted into the right atrium of the heart via the cephalic, subclavian, or jugular vein (Figure 15-9).

This type of catheter may be required for clients who need frequent venipuncture, long-term IV infusions, hyperalimentation, chemotherapy, intermittent blood transfusions, or antibiotics. These catheters may be referred to as *triple lumen catheters* or *Hickman lines*.

Central venous catheter management involves flushing the catheter with 2.5 cc of heparin (10 U/cc) when the catheter access is routinely capped or clamped after blood draws. Please consult your institution's procedure or policy guidelines about central venous line flushes. If continuous fluids are ordered, these fluids must be regulated via an infusion pump. All central venous catheter management must be done under the supervision of a registered nurse.

The central venous catheter site must be assessed regularly. The catheter site should always remain sterile under an occlusive dressing that is changed according to the institution's procedure regarding central venous catheters.

Patient-Controlled Analgesia

Patient-controlled analgesia (PCA) or a PCA pump involves patients giving themselves an IV narcotic. This IV narcotic is given at intervals via an infusion pump (Figure 15-10). Only a registered nurse can be accountable for dispensing analgesia to be given in this manner. In addition, only a registered nurse may administer a PCA loading dose.

Several considerations are crucial in the administration of PCA. IV narcotics may cause depressed respirations, hypotension, sedation, dizziness, and nausea or vomiting in the patient. The patient must not be allergic to the narcotic, must be able to understand and comply with instructions, and must have a desire to use the PCA. The materials needed for infusion include a PCA pump, PCA tubing, a PCA pump key, a narcotic injector vial, and maintenance IV fluids through which the intravenous narcotic will be infused.

Example 1: The physician orders morphine sulfate 1 mg every 10 minutes to a maximum of 30 mg in 4 hours. Morphine concentration is 1 mg/mL per 30-cc injector vial. What is the pump setting?

1 mL per 10 min, 4-hour limit is 30 mL

Example 2: The physician orders Demerol 10 mg every 10 minutes to a maximum of 300 mg in 4 hours. Demerol concentration is 10 mg/mL per 30-cc injector vial. What is the pump setting?

1 mL per 10 min, 4-hour limit is 30 mL

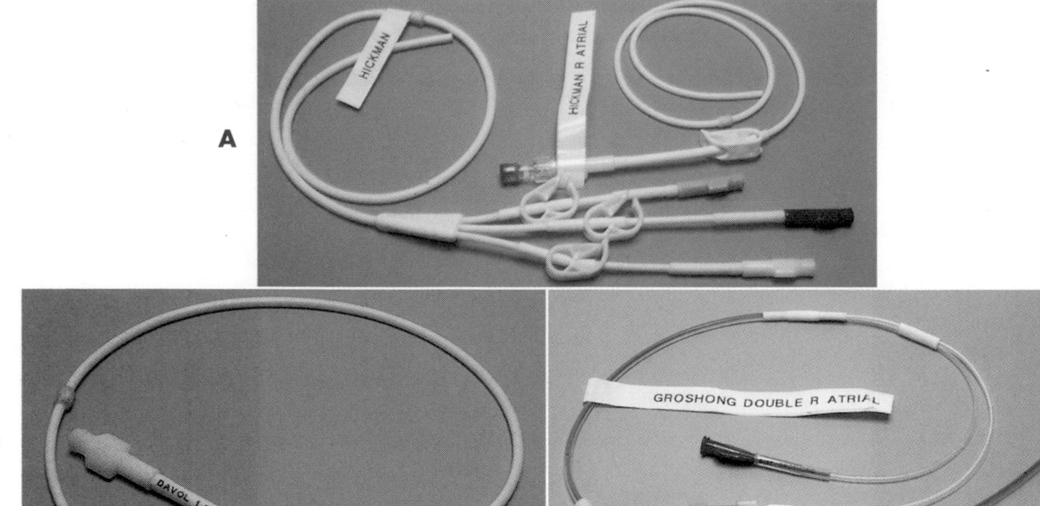

FIGURE 15-9 **A,** Hickman catheter. **B,** Brovia catheter. **C,** Groshong catheter. (From Clayton BD, Stock YN: *Basic pharmacology for nurses,* ed 12, St Louis, 2001, Mosby. Courtesy of Chuck Dresner.)

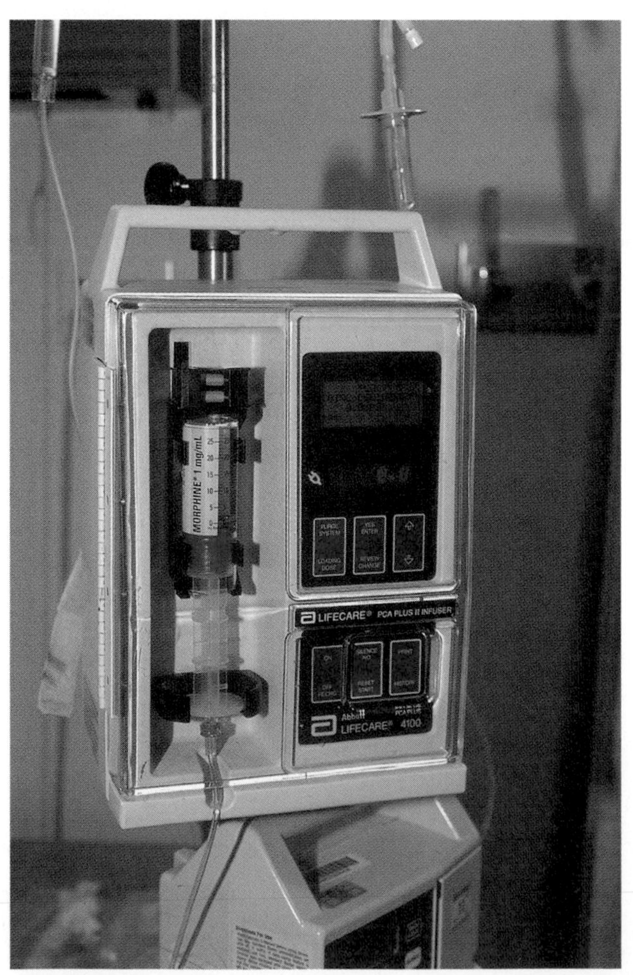

FIGURE 15-10 Patient-controlled analgesia (PCA) infusion pump. (From Potter PA, Perry AG: *Fundamentals of nursing,* ed 5, St Louis, 2001, Mosby.)

Complete the following work sheet, which provides for practice in the calculation of IV solutions and IVPB by either the IV pump or gravity. Check your answers. If you have difficulties, go back and review the necessary material. When you feel ready to evaluate your learning, take the first posttest. Check your answers. An acceptable score, indicated on the posttest, signifies that you have successfully completed the chapter. An unacceptable score signifies a need for further study before taking the second posttest.

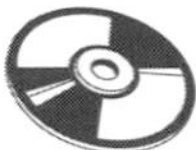

Refer to Calculating Dosages on the CD for additional help and practice problems.

WORK SHEET

Directions: The IV fluid or medication order is listed in each problem. Calculate the IV flow rates using the appropriate formula. Show your work.

1. The physician orders 500 mL of dextran to be infused over 24 hours. How many mL/h should the IV pump be programmed for? _______ .

2. A patient with genital herpes has an order for acyclovir 400 mg IVPB every 8 hours. The acyclovir is dissolved in 100 mL 0.9% NS and is to be infused over 1 hour. How many mL/h should the IV pump be programmed for? _______ .

3. Amikacin 80 mg is ordered IVPB q12 h. The amikacin is dissolved in 100 mL D_5W and is to be infused over 30 minutes. With a tubing drop factor of 15 gtt/mL, how many gtt/min should be given? _______ .

4. 3000 mL of total parenteral nutrition (TPN) is ordered to be infused from 7:00 PM to 7:00 AM. How many mL/h should the IV pump be programmed for? _______ .

5. A patient with peptic ulcer disease has Pepcid 20 mg in 100 mL D_5W ordered q12 h. The Pepcid is to be infused over 30 minutes. With a tubing drop factor of 10 gtt/mL, how many gtt/min should be given? _______ .

6. A malnourished patient has an order for 500 mL of Intralipid 10% to be infused over 6 hours. How many mL/h should the IV pump be programmed for? ______.

7. An order is received to infuse penicillin G 4,000,000 U in 100 mL of D_5W every 12 hours. The tubing drop factor is 10 gtt/mL. The penicillin should be infused over 60 minutes. How many gtt/min should be given? ______.

8. A patient with hypokalemia has an order for potassium 60 mEq in 250 mL of D_5W. The facility's policy states to infuse the potassium at 20 mEq/h. How many mL/h should the IV pump be programmed for? ______.

9. A postoperative patient has Kefzol 1 g ordered q8 h. The Kefzol is dissolved in 50 mL of D_5W and is to be infused over 30 minutes. The tubing drop factor is 60 gtt/mL. How many gtt/min should be given? ______.

10. A postoperative patient has an order for 1000 mL of D_5LR over 10 hours. How many mL/h should the IV pump be programmed for? ______.

11. A patient with sepsis has an order for Kefzol 1 g in 50 mL of D_5W IVPB over 15 minutes. The drip factor is 60 gtt/mL. How many gtt/min should be given? _______ .

12. A patient with a methicillin-resistant *Staphylococcus aureus* infection has Cipro 400 mg in 200 mL D_5W ordered. The pharmacy recommends that the Cipro be infused at a rate of 200 mg/h with an IV pump. How many mL/h should the IV pump be programmed for? _______ .

13. A patient with anuria has an order for 1000 mL of 0.9% NS to be infused over 1 hour. The tubing drop factor is 10 gtt/mL. How many gtt/min should be given? _______ .

14. A postoperative patient has an order for 1000 mL of D_5W 0.45 NS with 20 mEq of potassium to be infused over 8 hours. How many mL/h should the IV pump be programmed for? _______ .

15. After a total hip replacement, a patient has an order for Toradol 60 mg IVPB q6 h over 15 minutes. The Toradol is diluted in 25 mL of D_5W. The tubing drop factor is 15 gtt/mL. How many gtt/min should be given? _______ .

16. A terminal patient has an order for Dilaudid at 0.5 mg/h by continuous drip. Given a bag with a concentration of 20 mg Dilaudid in 100 mL of D_5W, how many mL/h should the IV pump be programmed for? _______ .

17. A patient with peptic ulcer disease has an order for Pepcid 20 mg IVPB q12 h over 15 minutes. The Pepcid is diluted in 25 mL of D_5W. The tubing drop factor is 20 gtt/mL. How many gtt/min should be given? _______ .

18. A patient with alcoholism has an order for magnesium sulfate 2 g in 100 mL of D_5W. The pharmacy recommends that the magnesium be infused at a rate of 1 g/h with an IV pump. How many mL/h should the IV pump be programmed for? _______ .

19. A patient with aplastic anemia has an order for 1 unit of packed red blood cells (250 mL) to be infused. The facility's policy states to infuse the blood over 4 hours. The tubing drop factor is 20 gtt/mL. How many gtt/min should be given? _______ .

20. A patient with oliguria has an order for 500 mL of 0.9% NS IV over 4 hours. The drop factor is 10 gtt/mL. How many gtt/min should be given? _______ .

21. A patient with hypokalemia has an order for 40 mEq of potassium to be infused IV now. The potassium is diluted in 200 mL of D_5W. The facility's policy states to infuse IV potassium at a rate of 10 mEq per hour. How many mL/h should the IV pump be programmed for? ______ .

22. A patient with Crohn's disease has an order for TPN from 10:00 PM to 8:00 AM. The total volume of the TPN bag is 1350 mL. How many mL/h should the IV pump be programmed for? ______ .

23. A patient with hypomagnesemia has an order for magnesium sulfate 2 g in 50 mL D_5W IV. The pharmacist recommends that the magnesium be infused at 1 g/h. How many mL/h should the IV pump be programmed for? ______ .

Answers on pp. 503-504.

Name ____________________

Date ____________________

ACCEPTABLE SCORE 13

YOUR SCORE ______

POSTTEST 1

Directions: The IV fluid order is listed in the problem. Calculate the appropriate infusion rate for each problem.

1. A patient with hypotension has an order for 500 mL of Plasmanate to be infused over 2 hours. How many mL/h should the IV pump be programmed for? ______ .

2. An order is received to infuse amphotericin B 240 mg in 500 mL D_5W over 4 hours. How many mL/h should the IV pump be programmed for? ______ .

3. An NPO patient has an order for 0.9% NS at 120 mL/h. The drop factor is 12 gtt/mL. How many gtt/min should be given? ______ .

4. A postpartum patient is to receive 1500 mL of LR over the next 8 hours. How many mL/h should the IV pump be programmed for? ______ .

5. A patient with a burn injury is to receive 500 mL of blood plasma over 4 hours. The tubing drop factor is 15 gtt/mL. How many gtt/min should be given? ______ .

6. A patient is admitted with pernicious anemia. The physician orders a unit of packed red blood cells (250 mL) to be infused over 3 hours. The tubing drop factor is 12 gtt/mL. How many gtt/min should be given? ______ .

7. A patient has an order for 500 mL of LR over 6 hours. The tubing drop factor is 15 gtt/mL. How many gtt/min should be given? ______ .

8. A patient with hypomagnesemia has an order for infusion of magnesium sulfate 4 g diluted in 250 mL D_5W. Policy states that the magnesium be infused at a rate of 2 g/h. How many mL/h should the IV pump be programmed for? ______ .

9. Mr. Simpson has an order for NS to be infused at 150 mL/h after a transesophageal echocardiogram. The tubing drop factor is 60 gtt/mL. How many gtt/min should be given? ______ .

10. A patient has an order for 2500 mL of TPN to be infused over 24 hours. How many mL/h should the IV pump be programmed for? ______ .

11. A patient with hypokalemia and hypophosphatemia has an order for potassium phosphate 30 mMos in 200 mL of 0.9% NS IV. The facility's policy states to infuse the potassium phosphate at 10 mMos per hour. How many mL/h should the IV pump be programmed for? ______ .

12. A postoperative patient has an order for ceftazidime 1 g in 25 mL of D_5W over 15 minutes. The tubing drop factor is 60 gtt/mL. How many gtt/min should be given? _______ .

13. A patient with metastatic cancer has an order for morphine sulfate 15 mg/h IV. Given a bag with a concentration of 100 mg of morphine sulfate in 200 mL of D_5W, how many mL/h should the IV pump be programmed for? _______ .

14. A patient with a methicillin-resistant *S. aureus* infection has an order for vancomycin 1.5 g in 200 mL of D_5W IVPB every 12 hours. The physician orders the vancomycin to be infused over 4 hours. How many mL/h should the IV pump be programmed for? _______ .

15. A patient with sepsis has an order for Timentin 3.1 g in 100 mL of D_5W IVPB over 1 hour. The drop factor is 60 gtt/mL. How many gtt/min should be given? _______ .

Answers on pp. 505-506.

Name ______________________________

Date ______________________________

ACCEPTABLE SCORE 13

YOUR SCORE _____

POSTTEST 2

Directions: The IV fluid order is listed in each problem. Calculate the appropriate infusion rate for each problem.

1. A patient with poor wound healing has ascorbic acid 300 mg in 200 mL of 0.9% NS ordered to be infused over 6 hours. How many mL/h should the IV pump be programmed for? _______ .

2. A patient with osteomyelitis has cefoxitin 2 gm q8 h IVPB ordered. The cefoxitin is dissolved in 50 mL of D_5W and is to be infused over 30 minutes. The tubing drop factor is 10 gtt/mL. How many gtt/min should be given? _______ .

3. A patient with iron-deficiency anemia has an order for iron dextran 100 mg in 200 mL of 0.9% NS over 6 hours. How many mL/h should the IV pump be programmed for? _______ .

4. A patient with hypotension has an order for 500 mL of 0.9% NS over 3 hours. The tubing drop factor is 10 gtt/mL. How many gtt/min should be given? _______ .

5. Your patient with a gastrointestinal (GI) bleed has an order for 1 unit of whole blood (500 mL) to be given over 3 hours. The tubing drop factor is 15 gtt/mL. How many gtt/min should be given? _______ .

6. An order for a patient with hypocalcemia states to infuse 1 g of calcium chloride 10% over 30 minutes. The calcium chloride is diluted in 50 mL of 0.9% NS. How many mL/h should the IV pump be programmed for? ______ .

7. A terminal patient has morphine sulfate ordered at 8 mg per hour. The medication concentration is morphine 100 mg diluted in 100 mL of D_5W. How many mL/h should the IV pump be programmed for? ______ .

8. A patient who has undergone hip replacement has an order for Toradol 30 mg q6 h. The Toradol is diluted in 50 mL of 0.9% NS and is to be infused over 15 minutes. The tubing drop factor is 60 gtt/mL. How many gtt/min should be given? ______ .

9. A patient with severe nausea and vomiting has a one-time order for Zofran 8 mg IVPB over 15 minutes. The Zofran is diluted in 50 mL of D_5W. The tubing drop factor is 15 gtt/mL. How many gtt/min should be given? ______ .

10. A postoperative patient has an order for 1000 mL of LR over 6 hours. How many mL/h should the IV pump be programmed for? ______ .

11. A postoperative patient experiences bradypnea after intrathecal administration of anesthesia. An order for Narcan 0.4 mg/h is written. Given a bag with a concentration of 8 mg in 100 mL of 0.9% NS, how many mL/h should the IV pump be programmed for? ______ .

12. A patient with a total gastrectomy has TPN ordered to be infused from 10:00 PM to 6:00 AM. The total volume of the TPN bag is 1200 mL. How many mL/h should the IV pump be programmed for? _______ .

13. A postoperative patient has an order for Kefzol 1 g in 25 mL of D_5W over 15 minutes. The medication will be infused with an IV pump. How many mL/h should the IV pump be programmed for? _______ .

14. A patient with oliguria has an order for 1000 mL of 0.9% NS over 3 hours. The tubing drop factor is 10 gtt/mL. How many gtt/min should be given? _______ .

15. An NPO patient has an order for 1000 mL of D_5W 0.45% NS with 30 mEq of potassium over 12 hours. How many mL/h should the IV pump be programmed for? _______ .

Answers on pp. 506-507.

CHAPTER 16

Critical Care IV Flow Rates*

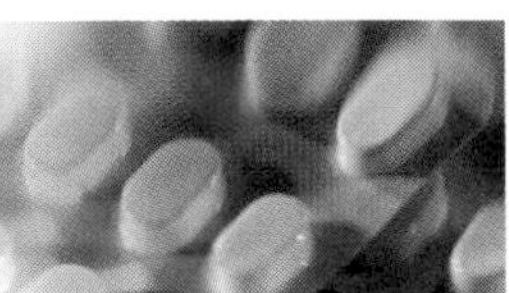

LEARNING OBJECTIVES

On completion of the materials provided in this chapter, you will be able to perform computations accurately by mastering the following mathematical concepts:

1. Calculating the IV flow rate of medications in units per hour (U/h) or international units per hour (IU/h)
2. Calculating the IV flow rate of medications in micrograms per kilogram per minute (mcg/kg/min)
3. Calculating the IV flow rate of medications in micrograms per minute (mcg/min)
4. Calculating the IV flow rate of medications in milligrams per minute (mg/min)

Critically ill patients in a hospital often receive special medications that are very potent and therefore need to be monitored closely. Some of these medications may be ordered as a set amount of the drug measured in units to be infused over a given period, for example, regular insulin or heparin. Other drugs used in the critical care setting may be ordered to be infused by amount of drug per kilogram of body weight per minute. These are called titrations. They are based on the manufacturer's provided recommended dosage and the patient's body weight measured in kilograms. In most health care institutions, these situations will occur in the emergency department, an intensive care unit, or a step-down unit. It is extremely important to accurately monitor the flow of these medications; therefore most are delivered through an IV machine. Because of the nature of these drugs, route of administration, and state of the patient, it cannot be overemphasized how important the accuracy of the calculation of the drug dosage and IV flow rates is. It is truly a matter of life and death.

*Linda Fluharty, MSN, RN, contributed this chapter.

The following sections focus on medications that are ordered by units per hour (U/h), international units per hour (IU/h), micrograms per kilogram per minute (μg/kg/min), micrograms per minute (μg/min), and milligrams per minute (mg/min). All of the following medications *must* be delivered with an IV controller or pump for safe administration. Since infusion pumps are set by milliliters per hour (mL/h), the health care provider needs to be familiar with the steps to convert the ordered drug dosage to mL/h.

Facilities that administer medications with a hemodynamic effect usually have IV controllers that allow the health care professional to program medication rates with a decimal. Therefore answers should be rounded to the nearest tenth decimal place.

IV Administration of Medications by Units/Hour or International Units/Hour

Example 1: 200 U of regular insulin has been added to 500 mL of 0.9% NS. The order states to infuse the regular insulin IV at 10 U/h. The nurse needs to calculate how many mL/h the IV pump should be programmed for.

Using the Ratio-Proportion Method

(Formula setup) 200 U : 500 mL :: 10 U : x mL

$$200x = 5000$$

$$x = \frac{5000}{200}$$

$$x = \frac{25}{1}$$

$$x = 25 \text{ mL}$$

Therefore the nurse will program the IV pump for 25 mL/h to infuse the insulin at 10 U/h.

Using the $\frac{D}{A} \times Q$ Method

(Formula setup) $\frac{10 \text{ U}}{200 \text{ U}} \times 500 \text{ mL} = x \text{ mL}$

(Cancel) $\frac{10 \text{ U}}{\overset{2}{\cancel{200}} \text{ U}} \times \overset{5}{\cancel{500}} \text{ mL} = x \text{ mL}$

(Calculate) $\frac{50}{2} = 25 \text{ mL}$

Example 2: 20,000 U of heparin has been added to 500 mL of D_5W. The order is to infuse the heparin drip at 2000 U/h. The health care provider needs to calculate how many mL/h to program the IV pump for.

Using the Ratio-Proportion Method

(Formula setup) 20,000 U : 500 mL :: 2000 U : x mL

$$20{,}000x = 1{,}000{,}000$$

$$x = \frac{1{,}000{,}000}{20{,}000}$$

$$x = \frac{100}{2}$$

$$x = 50 \text{ mL}$$

Therefore the nurse will program the IV pump for 50 mL/h to deliver the heparin at 2000 U/h.

Using the $\frac{D \times Q}{H}$ Method

(Formula setup) $\frac{2000 \text{ U}}{40{,}000 \text{ U}} \times 1000 \text{ mL} = x \text{ mL}$

(Cancel) $\frac{2000 \cancel{\text{U}}}{\underset{40}{\cancel{40{,}000}} \cancel{\text{U}}} \times \overset{1}{\cancel{1000}} \text{ mL} = x \text{ mL}$

(Calculate) $\frac{2000 \text{ mL}}{40} = 50 \text{ mL}$

IV Administration of Medications by Microgram/Kilogram/Minute

Example: 800 mg of dopamine is added to 250 mL of 0.9% NS. The order is to begin the infusion at 3 mcg/kg/min. The patient's weight is 70 kg. The nurse needs to calculate how many mL/h the IV pump should be set for.

The formula for calculating the mL/h is:

$$\frac{\text{Ordered µg/kg/min} \times \text{Patient's weight in kg} \times 60 \text{ min/1 h*}}{\text{Medication concentration (No. of mcg/1 mL)}}$$

*60 min/1 h is a constant fraction in the formula and represents the equivalency of 60 min = 1 h.

When this formula is used, the result will always be expressed in mL/h because the pair of values in mcg cancel each other, as do the pair of values in kg and the pair of values in minutes.

Step 1: Before the medication concentration can be determined, the total mg in the IV bag must be converted to mcg.

$$1 \text{ mg} : 1000 \text{ mcg} :: 800 \text{ mg} : x \text{ mcg}$$

$$x = 800{,}000 \text{ mcg}$$

Step 2: Determine the concentration (No. of mcg/1 mL) by dividing the total mcg in the IV bag by the total amount of fluid in the IV bag.

$$\frac{800{,}000 \text{ mcg}}{250 \text{ mL}} = \frac{3200 \text{ mcg}}{1 \text{ mL}} = 3200 \text{ mcg/mL}$$

Step 3: Calculate mL/h

(Formula setup) $\frac{3 \text{ mcg/kg/min} \times 70 \text{ kg} \times 60 \text{ min/h}}{3200 \text{ mcg/mL}} = x \text{ mL/h}$

(Cancel) $\frac{3 \cancel{\text{mcg/kg/min}} \times 70 \cancel{\text{kg}} \times 60 \cancel{\text{min}}\text{/h}}{3200 \cancel{\text{mcg}}\text{/mL}} = x \text{ mL/h}$

(Calculate) $\frac{3 \times 70 \times 60}{3200} = \frac{12{,}600}{3200} = 3.93 = 3.9 \text{ mL/h}$

IV Administration of Medications by Microgram/Minute

Example: 50 mg of nitroglycerin has been added to 500 mL 0.9% NS. The order is to infuse the nitroglycerin at 5 mcg/min. The nurse needs to calculate how many mL/h the IV pump needs to be set for.

$$\text{The formula: } \frac{\text{Ordered mcg/min} \times 60 \text{ min/1 h}}{\text{Medication concentration (No. of mcg/mL)}}$$

When this formula is used, the answer will always be expressed in mL/h because the pair of values in mg will cancel each other, as will the pair of values in minutes.

Step 1: Convert total mg in the IV bag to mcg.

$$1 \text{ mg} : 1000 \text{ mcg} :: 50 \text{ mg} : x \text{ mcg}$$

$$x = 50{,}000 \text{ mcg}$$

Step 2: Calculate the concentration (No. of mcg/1 mL) by dividing the total mcg by the total amount of fluid in the IV bag.

$$\frac{50{,}000 \text{ mcg}}{500 \text{ mL}} = 100 \text{ mcg/mL}$$

Step 3: Calculate the mL/h.

$$\text{(Formula setup)} \quad \frac{5 \text{ mcg/min} \times 60 \text{ min/h}}{100 \text{ mcg/mL}} = x \text{ mL/h}$$

$$\text{(Cancel)} \quad \frac{\overset{1}{\cancel{5}} \,\cancel{\text{mcg}}/\cancel{\text{min}} \times 60 \,\cancel{\text{min}}/\text{h}}{\underset{20}{\cancel{100}} \,\cancel{\text{mcg}}/\text{mL}} = x \text{ mL/h}$$

$$\text{(Calculate)} \quad \frac{1 \times 60}{20} = \frac{60}{20} = 3 \text{ mL/h}$$

IV Administration of Medications by Milligram/Minute

Example: Lidocaine 1 g has been added to 500 mL of D_5W. The order states to infuse the lidocaine at 2 mg/min. The nurse needs to calculate how many mL/h the IV pump should be set for.

$$\text{The formula: } \frac{\text{Desired mg/min} \times 60 \text{ min/1 h}}{\text{Medication concentration (No. mg/mL)}}$$

When this formula is used, the answer will always be expressed in mL/h because the pair of values in mg will cancel each other, as will the pair of values in minutes.

Step 1: Convert total g in the IV bag to mg.

$$1 \text{ g} = 1000 \text{ mg}$$

Step 2: Calculate mL/h.

(Formula setup) $$\frac{2 \text{ mg/min} \times 60 \text{ min/h}}{2 \text{ mg/mL}} = x \text{ mL/h}$$

(Simplify) $$\frac{\overset{1}{\cancel{2}} \text{ mg/min} \times 60 \text{ min/h}}{\underset{1}{\cancel{2}} \text{ mg/mL}} = x \text{ mL/h}$$

(Calculate) $$\frac{1 \times 60}{1} = 60 \text{ mL/h}$$

Complete the following work sheet, which provides for practice in the calculation of critical care IV flow rates. Check your answers. If you have difficulties, go back and review the necessary material. An acceptable score as indicated on the posttest signifies that you have successfully completed the chapter. An unacceptable score signifies a need for further study before taking the second posttest.

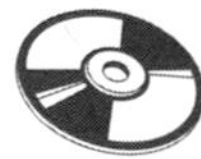

Refer to Calculating Dosages on the CD for additional help and practice problems.

CHAPTER 16 **Critical Care IV Flow Rates**

WORK SHEET

Directions: The IV fluid order is listed in each problem. Calculate the IV flow rates using the appropriate formula required for the problem.

1. You have a patient who has undergone aortic valve repair and has orders for heparin at 1000 U/h. The concentration is heparin 25,000 U in 250 mL 0.9% NS. How many mL/h should the IV pump be programmed for? ______ .

2. You have an order for your patient with diabetes to receive regular insulin IV at 12 U/h. The concentration is insulin 100 U in 250 mL of 0.9% NS. How many mL/h should the IV pump be programmed for? ______ .

3. The insulin order for the patient in problem 2 is reduced to 8 U/h. How many mL/h should the IV pump be programmed for? ______ .

4. A patient who has undergone mitral valve repair has heparin ordered at 1000 U/h. The concentration is heparin 10,000 U in 500 mL of D_5W. How many mL/h should the IV pump be programmed for? ______ .

5. The physician orders dobutamine at 12 μg/kg/min for a patient weighing 75 kg. The concentration is dobutamine 1 g in 250 mL of D_5W. How many mL/h should the IV pump be programmed for? _______ .

6. Mr. Baxter is having chest pain and has an order for nitroglycerin at 10 μg/min. The concentration is nitroglycerin 100 mg in 500 mL of D_5W. How many mL/h should the IV pump be programmed for? _______ .

7. The physician orders dopamine at 5 μg/kg/min. The concentration is dopamine 2 g in 250 mL of 0.9% NS. The patient's weight is 80 kg. How many mL/h should the IV pump be programmed for? _______ .

8. A patient with a brachial thrombus has streptokinase ordered at 100,000 IU/h. The concentration is 250,000 IU of streptokinase in 45 mL of 0.9% NS. How many mL/h should the IV pump be programmed for? _______ .

9. The physician has ordered amiodarone at 0.5 mg/min. The concentration is amiodarone 900 mg in 500 mL of D_5W. How many mL/h should the IV pump be programmed for? ______ .

10. Your patient with malignant hypertension is ordered to have nitroprusside at 3 μg/kg/min. The concentration is nitroprusside 50 mg in 250 mL of D_5W. The patient's weight is 70 kg. How many mL/h should the IV pump be programmed for? ______ .

11. A patient with heart failure has dobutamine ordered at 10 μg/kg/min. The patient weighs 100 kg. The concentration is dobutamine 2 g in 500 mL of D_5W. How many mL/h should the IV pump be programmed for? ______ .

12. A patient has propofol ordered at 30 μg/kg/min. The propofol concentration is 15 mg/mL. The patient's weight is 75 kg. How many mL/h should the IV pump be programmed for? ______ .

13. A patient with a ventricular dysrhythmia has procainamide ordered at 4 mg/min. The concentration is procainamide 2 g/250 mL of D_5W. How many mL/h should the IV pump be programmed for? ______ .

14. A patient who has been resuscitated has Levophed ordered at 10 µg/min. The concentration is Levophed 2 mg in 250 mL of 0.9% NS. How many mL/h should the IV pump be programmed for? ______ .

15. A patient with a dysrhythmia has an order for amiodarone 0.75 mg/min. The concentration is amiodarone 900 mg in 500 mL D_5W. How many mL/h should the IV pump be programmed for? ______ .

16. A patient with hypotension has Vasopressor ordered at 15 µg/min. The concentration is Vasopressor 4 mg in 250 mL D_5W. How many mL/h should the IV pump be programmed for? ______ .

17. A patient has lidocaine ordered at 2 mg/min. The concentration is lidocaine 2 g in 250 mL of D_5W. How many mL/h should the IV pump be programmed for? _______ .

18. A patient with a deep vein thrombosis has an order for a heparin infusion at 750 U/h. The heparin bag has a concentration of 25,000 U per 500 mL of D_5W. How many mL/h should the IV pump be programmed for? _______ .

19. A patient with diabetic ketoacidosis has an order for insulin at 10 U/h. The insulin comes in a concentration of 100 U in 100 mL of 0.9% of NS. How many mL/h should the IV pump be programmed for? _______ .

20. The physician orders dopamine at 10 µg/kg/min. The concentration is dopamine 2 g in 250 mL of 0.9% NS. The patient's weight is 90 kg. How many mL/h should the IV pump be programmed for? _______ .

Answers on pp. 507-509.

Name ______________________________

Date ______________________________

ACCEPTABLE SCORE 9

YOUR SCORE ______

POSTTEST 1

Directions: The IV fluid order is listed in each problem. Calculate the appropriate mL/h rate for each problem.

1. Your patient with diabetes has an order for regular insulin IV at 9 U/h. The concentration is insulin 500 U in 500 mL of 0.9% NS. How many mL/h should the IV pump be programmed for? ______ .

2. A patient with a deep vein thrombosis has an order for heparin at 800 U/h. The concentration is heparin 50,000 U in 500 mL of D_5W. How many mL/h should the IV pump be programmed for? ______ .

3. Your patient with hypertension has orders for Nipride at 5 μg/kg/min. The concentration is Nipride 100 mg in 250 mL D_5W. The patient weighs 62 kg. How many mL/h should the IV pump be programmed for? ______ .

4. Your patient with pulmonary edema has dobutamine ordered at 5 μg/kg/min. The concentration is dobutamine 1 g in 250 mL of 0.9% NS. The patient's weight is 50 kg. How many mL/h should the IV pump be programmed for? ______ .

5. A patient with an acute myocardial infarction has IV nitroglycerin ordered at 20 μg/min. The concentration is nitroglycerin 50 mg in 250 mL of D_5W. How many mL/h should the IV pump be programmed for? _______ .

6. A patient with a ventricular dysrhythmia has lidocaine ordered at 3 mg/min. The concentration is lidocaine 2 g in 500 mL of D_5W. How many mL/h should the IV pump be programmed for? _______ .

7. A patient has been resuscitated and now has Levophed ordered at 5 μg/min. The concentration is Levophed 1 mg in 250 mL of 0.9% of NS. How many mL/h should the IV pump be programmed for? _______ .

8. An intubated patient has propofol ordered at 25 μg/kg/min. The concentration of propofol is 10 mg/mL. The patient's weight is 50 kg. How many mL/h should the IV pump be programmed for? _______ .

9. A patient with a thrombosis is to receive heparin at 1050 U/h. The concentration is heparin 25,000 U in 250 D_5W. How many mL/h should the IV pump be programmed for? ______ .

10. A patient with atrial fibrillation has amiodarone ordered at 0.5 mg/min. The concentration is amiodarone 900 mg in 250 mL of D_5W. How many mL/h should the IV pump be programmed for? ______ .

Answers on pp. 509-510.

CHAPTER 16 Critical Care IV Flow Rates

Name ______________________

Date ______________________

ACCEPTABLE SCORE 9

YOUR SCORE ______

POSTTEST 2

Directions: The IV fluid order is listed in each problem. Calculate the mL/h needed in each problem to deliver the correct dose.

1. A patient with hypotension has dopamine ordered at 3 µg/kg/min. The patient weighs 85 kg. The concentration is dopamine 2 g in 500 mL of D_5W. How many mL/h should the IV pump be programmed for? ______ .

2. A patient with a pulmonary embolus has an order for streptokinase to be infused at 100,000 IU/h. The concentration is streptokinase 750,000 IU in 200 mL of 0.9% NS. How many mL/h should the IV pump be programmed for? ______ .

3. A patient with tachycardia has an order for Brevibloc to be started at 50 µg/kg/min. The concentration is Brevibloc 5 g in 500 mL of D_5W. The patient weighs 80 kg. How many mL/h should the IV pump be programmed for? ______ .

4. A patient with a ventricular dysrhythmia has an order for amiodarone at 0.5 mg/min. The concentration is amiodarone 900 mg in 250 mL of D_5W. How many mL/h should the IV pump be programmed for? ______ .

5. A patient has an order for Vasopressor at 10 μg/min. The concentration is Vasopressor 4 mg in 500 mL of D_5W. How many mL/h should the IV pump be programmed for? ______ .

6. A patient has an order for procainamide at 4 mg/min. The concentration is procainamide 2 g in 500 mL of D_5W. How many mL/h should the IV pump be programmed for? ______ .

7. A patient has an order for dobutamine at 7 μg/kg/min. The concentration is dobutamine 1 g in 200 mL of 0.9% NS. The patient's weight is 55 kg. How many mL/h should the IV pump be programmed for? ______ .

8. A patient in shock has an order for Isuprel to be infused at 2 μg/min. The concentration is Isuprel 1 mg in 500 mL of D_5W. How many mL/h should the IV pump be programmed for? ______ .

9. Your patient has a blood clot in his arm, and the physician has ordered heparin to be infused at 1500 U/h. The concentration is heparin 20,000 U in 200 mL of D_5W. How many mL/h should the IV pump be programmed for? ______ .

10. A patient with diabetic ketoacidosis has an order for regular insulin to be infused at 8 U/h. The concentration is insulin 50 U in 100 mL of 0.9% NS. How many mL/h should the IV pump be programmed for? ______ .

Answers on pp. 510-511.

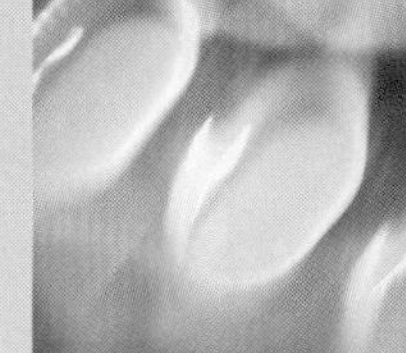

CHAPTER 17

Pediatric Dosages

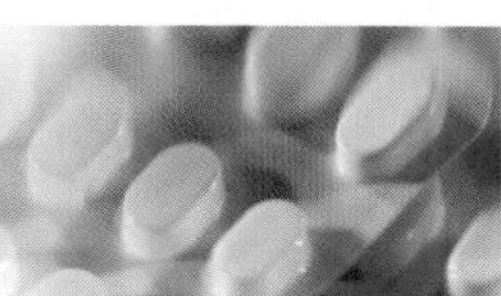

LEARNING OBJECTIVES

On completion of the materials provided in this chapter, you will be able to perform computations accurately by mastering the following mathematical concepts:

1. Converting the weight of a child from pounds to kilograms
2. Using a formula based on body weight to determine the correct dosage of a medication to be administered to a child
3. Calculating body surface area (BSA) using the West nomogram
4. Estimating body surface area using a formula
5. Calculating pediatric dosages using a formula based on body surface area expressed as square meters (m^2)
6. Calculating the rate of infusion in both gtt/min and mL/h for pediatric dosages
7. Calculating the appropriate concentration of IV medications for pediatric patients

Because of their age, weight, height, and physical condition, children are more sensitive to medications than adults. Therefore careful attention must be paid to the preparation and administration of medications to children. The right amount of the right medication must be given to the right child at the right time, in the right way.

Although the physician prescribes the medication, the nurse who administers it is responsible for errors in the calculation of the dosage and in the preparation and administration of the drug. The medication order must be accurate; a dosage that is too high may be unsafe, and a dosage that is too low may not have the desired therapeutic effect.

Pediatric Dosages Calculated by Milligram/Kilogram/Hour

Pediatric dosages are most commonly calculated by the mg/kg/h method. This is the amount of drug in relation to the child's weight in kilograms, usually for a 24-hour period. Package inserts and reference books such as the current year's *Mosby's Nursing Drug Reference* show the safe amount of the drug that should be given in milligrams per kilogram per hour (mg/kg/h). Normally the amount of medication given to children is less than that given to adults. The amount of medication to be given in 24 hours is calculated and then divided into an equal number of doses. The number of doses is determined by the recommended frequency of administration.

Example: Amoxicillin 125 mg po tid for a child weighing 34.32 lb is prescribed. You have amoxicillin suspension 125 mg/5 mL. The recommended daily oral dose for a child is 20 to 40 mg/kg/day in divided doses q8 h. a. Child's weight is ______ kg. b. What is the safe recommended dosage or range for this child? ______ . c. Is the order safe? ______ . d. If yes, how many millimeters will you administer? ______ .

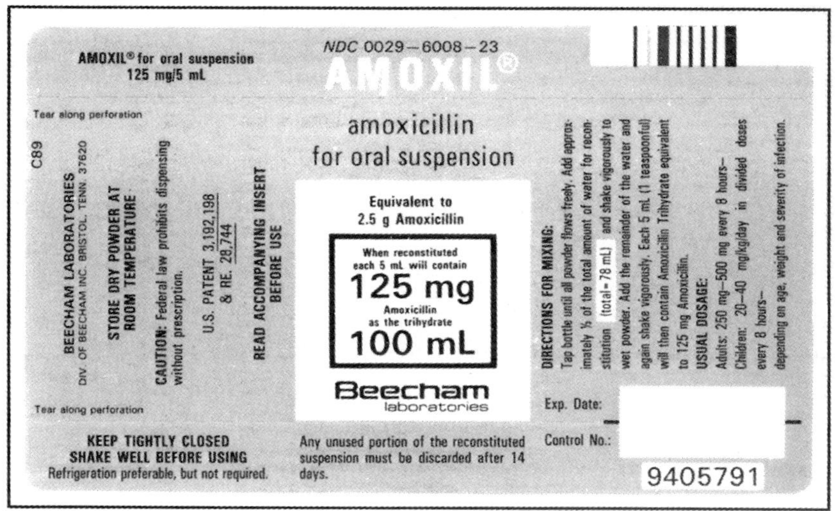

a. Change the child's weight to kg (see Chapter 8). Remember, there are 2.2 lb in each kilogram.

$$2.2 \text{ lb} : 1 \text{ kg} :: 34.32 \text{ lb} : x \text{ kg}$$

$$2.2 : 1 :: 34.32 : x$$

$$2.2x = 34.32$$

$$x = \frac{34.32}{2.2}$$

$$x = 15.6 \text{ kg}$$

b. Write a proportion(s) using the recommended dosage and child's weight as your known values to determine the safe recommended dosage or range for this child.

$$20 \text{ mg} : 1 \text{ kg} :: x \text{ mg} : 15.6 \text{ kg}$$

$$20 : 1 :: x : 15.6$$

$$x = 312 \text{ mg}$$

$$40 \text{ mg} : 1 \text{ kg} :: x \text{ mg} : 15.6 \text{ kg}$$

$$40 : 1 :: x : 15.6$$

$$x = 624 \text{ mg}$$

The safe recommended range for this child, who weighs 15.6 kg, is 312 to 624 mg in a 24-hour period.

c. Determine the total amount of medication ordered per 24-hour period.

$$125 \text{ mg} : 1 \text{ dose} :: x \text{ mg} : 3 \text{ doses}$$

$$125 : 1 :: x : 3$$

$$x = 375 \text{ mg/24-hour period}$$

The order is safe because it falls within the recommended 24-hour range of 312 to 624 mg for this medication and this child.

d. Calculate the actual dosage amount to be given by the use of a proportion (see Chapter 10).

$$125 \text{ mg} : 5 \text{ mL} :: 125 \text{ mg} : x \text{ mL}$$

$$125 : 5 :: 125 : x$$

$$125x = 625$$

$$x = 5 \text{ mL}$$

Therefore 5 mL is the amount of each individual dose given three times a day (tid).

Body Surface Area Calculations

Body surface area (BSA) is determined by using a child's height and weight along with the West nomogram. If the child has a normal height and weight for his or her age, the BSA may be ascertained by the weight alone. For example, in Figure 17-1 showing the West nomogram, you can see that a child who weighs 70 pounds has a BSA of 1.10 m^2.

When using the West nomogram, take a few minutes to assess the markings of each column. Note that the markings are not at the same intervals throughout each column.

If the child is not of normal height and weight for his or her age, an extended use of the nomogram is required. The far right column is for weight measured in pounds and kilograms. The far left column is for height measured in centimeters and inches. Place a ruler on the nomogram and draw a line connecting the height and weight points. Where the line crosses the surface area (SA) column, the SA in square meters (m^2) will be indicated.

Practice Problems. Using the West nomogram, state the BSA in square meters for each child of normal height and weight listed below:

1. Child weighs 22 lb BSA = _______
2. Child weighs 4 lb BSA = _______
3. Child weighs 75 lb BSA = _______
4. Child weighs 10 lb BSA = _______
5. Child weighs 32 lb BSA = _______

Answers

1. 0.46 m^2
2. 0.15 m^2
3. 1.15 m^2
4. 0.27 m^2
5. 0.62 m^2

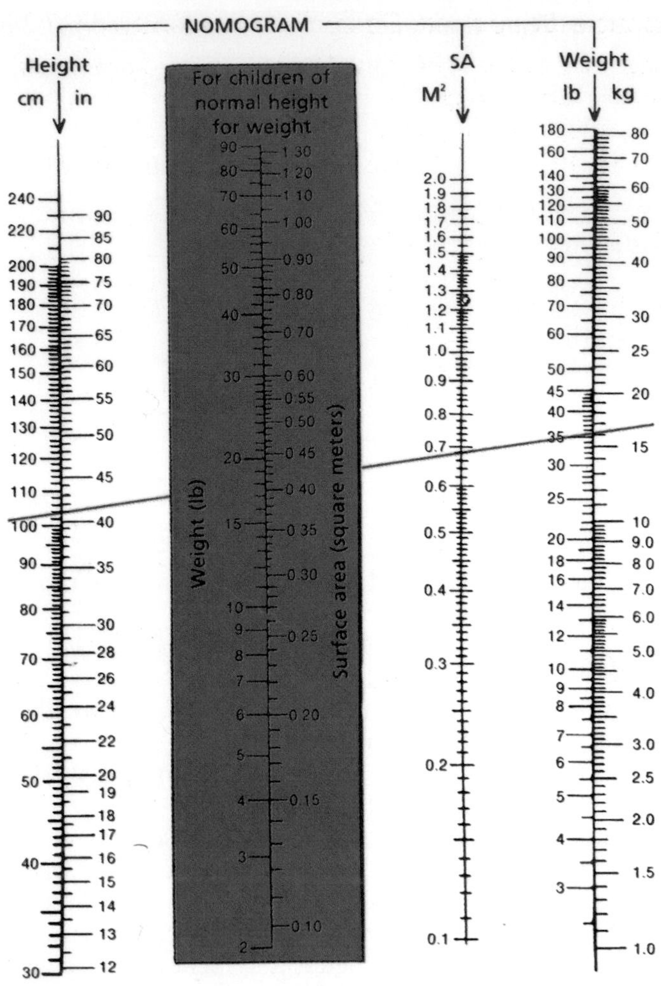

FIGURE 17-1 West nomogram for estimation of body surface areas in children. A straight line is drawn between height and weight. The point where the line crosses the surface area column is the estimated body surface area. (From Behrman RE, Kliegman RM, Jenson HB, eds: *Nelson textbook of pediatrics,* ed 16, Philadelphia, 2000, Saunders; modified from data of E Boyd, by CD West.)

Practice Problems. Using the West nomogram, calculate the BSA for each child with the following heights and weights:

1. Child weighs 6 kg, height is 110 cm BSA = ________
2. Child weighs 5 lb, height is 19 in BSA = ________
3. Child weighs 25 kg, height is 70 cm BSA = ________
4. Child weighs 30 lb, height is 90 cm BSA = ________
5. Child weighs 160 lb, height is 200 cm BSA = ________

Answers

1. 0.41 m^2
2. 0.18 m^2
3. 0.74 m^2
4. 0.58 m^2
5. 2.0 m^2

Calculation of Dosage Based on Body Surface Area

The calculation of dosage may be based on BSA. The BSA method provides a means of converting an adult dosage to a safe pediatric dosage. There are three steps to the calculation with this method.

1. Determine the child's weight in kilograms.
2. Calculate the BSA in square meters (m^2). The formula for this calculation is as follows:

$$\frac{4\text{ W (Child's weight in kilograms)} + 7}{\text{W (Child's weight in kilograms)} + 90} = \text{BSA in square meters}$$

3. Calculate the pediatric dosage using the following formula. The formula is based on the premise that an adult who weighs 140 pounds has a BSA of 1.7 m^2.

$$\frac{\text{BSA in m}^2}{1.7} \times \text{Adult dose} = \text{Child's dose}$$

Example: Child weighs 24 lb and the adult dose is 100 mg.

1. First, convert the child's weight to kilograms.

$$2.2\text{ lb} : 1\text{ kg} :: 24\text{ lb} : x\text{ kg}$$

$$2.2 : 1 :: 24 : x$$

$$2.2x = 24$$

$$x = \frac{24}{2.2}$$

$$x = 10.9$$

$$x = 10.9\text{ kg}$$

The child weighs approximately 10.9 kg.

2. Next, calculate the child's BSA in m^2.

$$\frac{4(10.9) + 7}{10.9 + 90} = \frac{43.6 + 7}{10.9 + 90} = \frac{50.6}{100.9} = 0.5$$

Child's BSA = 0.5 m^2

3. Finally, calculate the appropriate dosage for this child.

$$\frac{0.5}{1.7} \times 100 = 29.4\text{ mg}$$

Practice Problems. Calculate the following children's dosages.

1. Child weighs 40 lb, adult dose = 300 mg child's dose = ________
2. Child weighs 65 lb, adult dose = 30 mL child's dose = ________
3. Child weighs 20 lb, adult dose = 50 mg child's dose = ________
4. Child weighs 90 lb, adult dose = 10 mL child's dose = ________
5. Child weighs 14 lb, adult dose = 2 g child's dose = ________

Answers

1. 132 mg
2. 18.5 mL
3. 13 mg
4. 7.65 mL
5. 0.4 g

Calculation of Pediatric IV Solutions

Pediatric patients require smaller volumes of IV fluids and medications. An IV pump, a buretrol (soluset), or both may be used for the pediatric patient. Each facility will have guidelines for preparing and administering IV solutions and medications to the pediatric patient. Also, for a pediatric patient, IV tubing with a drop factor of 60 gtt/mL is usually recommended.

The concentration of the IV medication is also an important factor in medication administration. Administering a medication with a higher concentration than recommended is avoided because of the vein irritation that can result.

Example 1: Infuse 100 mL of 0.9% NS over 5 h to a 6-month-old child. How many milliliters per hour (mL/h) should the IV pump be programmed for? ______ .

The formula: $\frac{\text{Total volume to be infused}}{\text{Total amount of time in hours}} = x \text{ mL/h}$

(Formula setup) $\frac{100 \text{ mL}}{5 \text{ h}} = 20 \text{ mL/h}$

Example 2: Infuse 150 mL of D5LR over 3 hours to a 3-year-old child. How many mL/h should the IV pump be programmed for? ______ .

(Formula setup) $\frac{150 \text{ mL}}{3 \text{ h}} = 50 \text{ mL/h}$

If an IV pump is not used, IV fluids may be given by gravity. In this case, the formula is:

$$\frac{\text{Total volume to be given}}{\text{Total time in minutes}} \times \text{Tubing drop factor} = x \text{ gtt/min}$$

Example 3: Infuse 200 mL lactated Ringer's solution (LR) over 4 hours to an 8-year-old child. The tubing drop factor is 60 gtt/mL. How many drops per minute (gtt/min) of lactated Ringer's solution should be infused? ______ .

(Formula setup) $\frac{200 \cancel{\text{mL}}}{\underset{4}{\cancel{240}} \text{ min}} \times \overset{1}{\cancel{60}} \text{ gtt/}\cancel{\text{mL}} = x \text{ gtt/min}$

$$\frac{200}{4} \times \frac{1 \text{ gtt}}{} = 50 \text{ gtt/min}$$

Example 4: Infuse 500 mL of D_5W over 8 hours to a 14-year-old child. The tubing drop factor is 60 gtt/mL. How many gtt/min of D_5W should be infused? ______ .

Step 1: Convert hours to minutes
1 h : 60 min :: 8 h : x min

x = 480 min

Step 2: Calculate gtt/min

(Formula setup) $\dfrac{500 \cancel{mL}}{\overset{}{\cancel{480}}_{8} \text{ min}} \times \overset{1}{\cancel{60}} \text{ gtt}/\cancel{mL} = x \text{ gtt/min}$

$\dfrac{500}{8 \text{ min}} \times 1 \text{ gtt} = 62.5 \text{ or } 63 \text{ gtt/min}$

IV Administration of Medications to Pediatric Patients

The formulas to calculate the administration rate of IV medications to pediatric patients are not different from those used for adults. The difference in administration of medications to a pediatric patient lies in the volume of solution used. Pediatric patients require a smaller volume of IV solutions; therefore care must be taken to give the medication at the recommended infusion concentration. Using a concentration that is higher than recommended may result in vein irritation and phlebitis. Unit policies and IV drug books provide the guidelines needed for appropriate concentration of IV medications for the pediatric patient.

If the medication is to be infused with an IV pump, the formula would be:

$$\frac{\text{Total volume to be infused (in mL)}}{\text{Total amount of time for infusion (in h)}} = x \text{ mL/h}$$

If the medication is to be infused with a buretrol (soluset) by gravity (Figure 17-2), then the formula would be:

$$\frac{\text{Total volume to be infused (in mL)}}{\text{Total amount of time for infusion (in min)}} \times \text{drop factor} = x \text{ gtt/min}$$

Example 1: An 18-month-old child has Ancef 450 mg q 4 h IVPB over 15 minutes ordered. The child weighs 19 kg. The maximum recommended infusion concentration is 50 mg/mL. The vial of medication has a concentration of Ancef 250 mg/mL. How many milliliters of medication will provide 450 mg? ______. How many milliliters of IV solution needs to be added to the medication to equal the recommended final concentration? ______. How many mL/h should the IV pump be programmed for? ______.

Step 1: Calculate volume of medication to withdraw from the vial

(Formula setup) $250 \text{ mg} : 1 \text{ mL} :: 450 \text{ mg} : x \text{ mL}$

$250x = 450$

$x = \dfrac{450}{250}$

$x = 1.8 \text{ mL}$

Therefore the nurse would withdraw 1.8 mL from the vial to administer 450 mg of Ancef.

Step 2: Calculate the volume of IV solution to provide the recommended final concentration.

The formula: $\text{Ordered dose} \times \dfrac{1 \text{ mL}}{\text{Recommended concentration}} = x \text{ mL}$

(Formula setup) $450 \text{ mg} \times \dfrac{1 \text{ mL}}{50 \text{ mg}} = 9 \text{ mL}$

Therefore to the 1.8 mL of Ancef, the nurse must add enough IV solution to give a **TOTAL** of 9 mL.

$$9 \text{ mL} - 1.8 \text{ mL} = 7.2 \text{ mL}$$

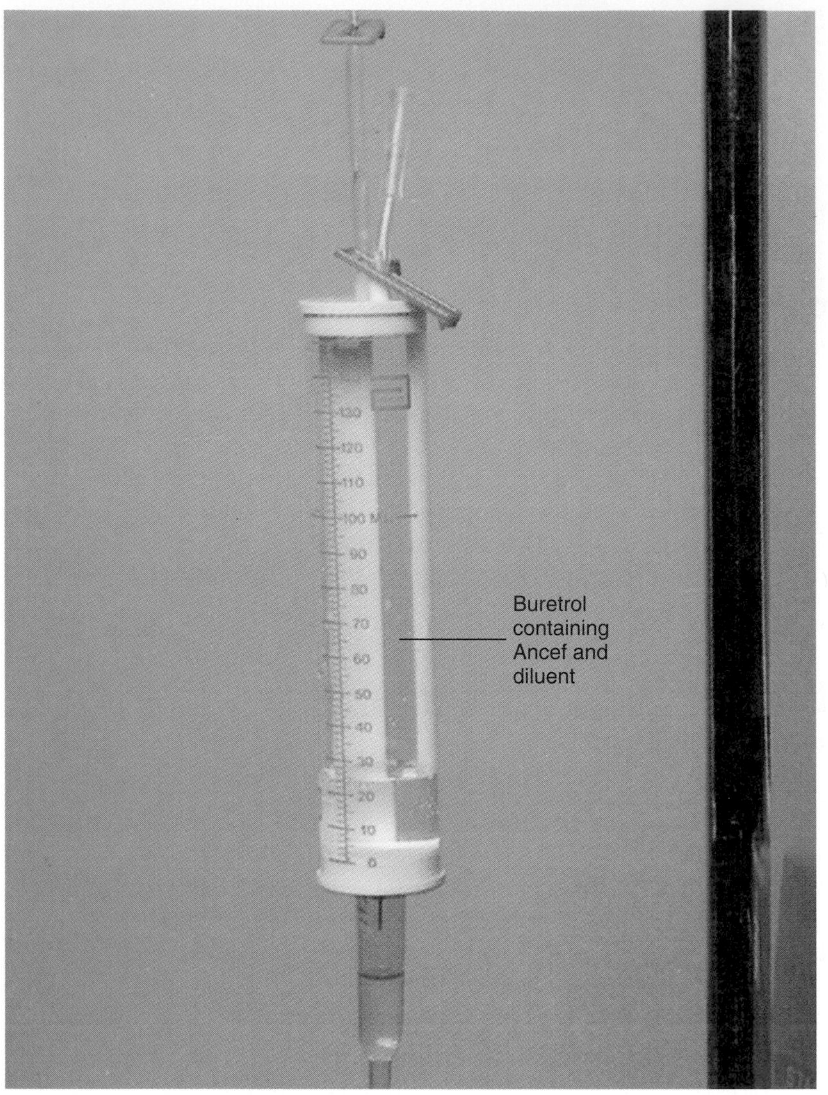

1. Add 1.8 mL of Ancef to an empty buretrol.
2. Add 7.2 mL of compatible IV fluid diluent to make a total volume of 9 mL.

$$\begin{array}{r} 1.8 \text{ mL} \\ + \ \underline{7.2 \text{ mL}} \\ 9.0 \text{ mL} \end{array}$$

Final concentration: 50 mg/mL

FIGURE 17-2 Dilution of Ancef in a volume control device, also known as a buretrol or soluset. (From Elkin MK, Perry AG, Potter PA: *Nursing interventions and clinical skills,* ed 2, St Louis, 2000, Mosby.)

Therefore the nurse will add an additional 7.2 mL of IV solution to the 1.8 mL of Ancef to give a total of 9 mL.

Step 3: Calculate the milliliters per hour to program the IV pump.

(Formula setup) $\frac{9 \text{ mL}}{0.25 \text{ h}} = 36 \text{ mL/h}$

Therefore the nurse would program the IV pump for 36 mL/h to infuse the Ancef over 15 minutes.

Example 2: A child weighing 30 kg has an order for nafcillin 850 mg IVPB q6h over 10 minutes. The nafcillin vial gives a concentration of 250 mg/mL. The recommended infusion concentration of nafcillin is 100 mg/mL. How many milliliters of medication will provide 850 mg of nafcillin? ______ . How many milliliters of IV solution needs to be added to the medication to equal the recommended final concentration? ______ . How many gtt/min should the IVPB be programmed for? ______ .

Step 1: Calculate the volume of medication to withdraw from the vial

(Formula setup) $250 \text{ mg} : 1 \text{ mL} :: 850 \text{ mg} : x \text{ mL}$

$$250x = 850$$

$$x = \frac{850}{250}$$

$$x = 3.4 \text{ mL}$$

Therefore the nurse will withdraw 3.4 mL from the vial to administer 850 mg of nafcillin.

Step 2: Calculate the volume of IV solution to provide the recommended final concentration

(Formula setup) $850 \cancel{\text{mg}} \times \frac{1 \text{ mL}}{100 \cancel{\text{mg}}} = 8.5 \text{ mL}$

Therefore to the 3.4 mL of nafcillin, the nurse must add IV solution to give a **TOTAL** of 8.5 mL.

$$8.5 \text{ mL} - 3.4 \text{ mL} = 5.1 \text{ mL}$$

Therefore the nurse will add an additional 5.1 mL of IV solution to the 3.4 mL of nafcillin to give a total of 8.5 mL.

Step 3: Calculate gtt/min (a buretrol or soluset has a drop factor of 60 gtt/mL)

(Formula setup) $\frac{8.5 \cancel{\text{mL}}}{10 \text{ min}} \times 60 \text{ gtt/}\cancel{\text{mL}} = x \text{ gtt/min}$

$$\frac{510}{10} = x \text{ gtt/min}$$

$$x = 51 \text{ gtt/min}$$

Complete the following work sheet, which provides for extensive practice in the calculation of pediatric dosages. Check your answers. If you have difficulties, go back and review the necessary material. When you feel ready to evaluate your learning, take the first posttest. Check your answers. An acceptable score as indicated on the posttest signifies that you have successfully completed this chapter. An unacceptable score signifies a need for further study before taking the second posttest.

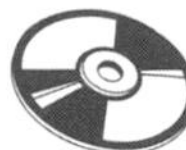

Refer to Introducing Drug Measures: Measuring Dosages on the CD for additional help and practice problems.

WORK SHEET

Directions: The medication order is listed at the beginning of each problem. Calculate the child's weight in kilograms, determine the safe recommended dosage or range, determine the safety of the order, and calculate the drug dosage. Show your work.

1. Ordered Keflex 250 mg PO qid for a child weighing 50 lb. You have Keflex 250-mg capsules. The recommended daily PO dosage for a child is 25 to 50 mg/kg/day in divided doses q6 h. a. Child's weight is _______ kg. b. What is the safe recommended dosage or range for this child? _______ . c. Is the order safe? _______ . d. If yes, how many capsules will you administer? _______ .

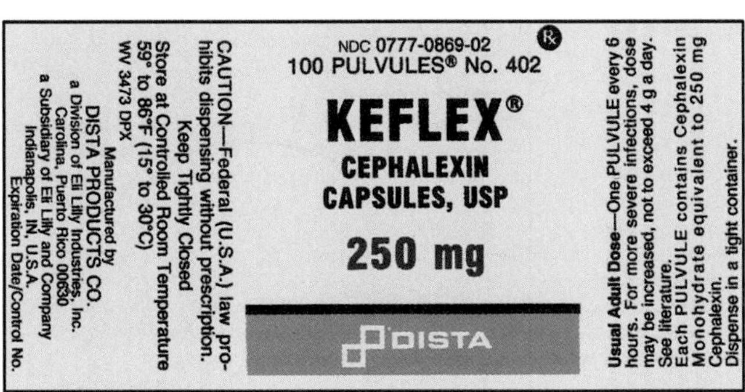

2. Ordered Lanoxin 12.5 mg PO qd for an infant weighing 6 lb 8 oz. You have Lanoxin 0.05 mg/mL. The recommended daily dosage for an infant is 0.035 to 0.06 mg/kg/day in divided doses q8 h. a. Child's weight is _______ kg. b. What is the safe recommended dosage or range for this child? _______ . c. Is the order safe? _______ . d. If yes, how many milliliters will you administer? _______ .

60 mL NDC 0173-0264-27
LANOXIN®
(DIGOXIN)
ELIXIR
PEDIATRIC
Each mL contains
50 µg (0.05 mg)
PLEASANTLY FLAVORED
GlaxoWellcome
Glaxo Wellcome Inc.
Research Triangle Park, NC 27709
Made in U.S.A. Rev. 2/96 542404
Alcohol 10%, Methylparaben 0.1% (added as a preservative)
For indications, dosage, precautions, etc., see accompanying package insert.
Store at 15° to 25°C (59° to 77°F) and protect from light.
CAUTION: Federal law prohibits dispensing without prescription.
LOT
EXP

3. Ordered Benadryl 25 mg IV q6 h for a child weighing 50 lb. You have Benadryl 10 mg/mL. The recommended daily dosage for a child weighing more than 12 kg is 5 mg/kg/day in four divided doses. a. Child's weight is _______ kg. b. What is the safe recommended dosage or range for this child? _______ . c. Is the order safe? _______ . d. If yes, how many milliliters will you prepare? _______ .

4. Ordered Thorazine 10 mg IV q6 h for a child weighing 44 lb. You have Thorazine 25 mg/mL. The recommended daily dosage is 0.55 mg/kg/day q6 to 8 h. a. Child's weight is _______ kg. b. What is the safe recommended dosage or range for this child? _______ . c. Is the order safe? _______ . d. If yes, how many milliliters will you prepare? _______ .

5. Ordered thioguanine 60 mg PO today for a child weighing 78 lb. You have thioguanine 40-mg tablets. The recommended PO dosage is 2 mg/kg/day. a. Child's weight is _______ kg. b. What is the safe recommended dosage or range for this child? _______ . c. Is the order safe? _______ . d. If yes, how many tablets will you administer? _______ .

6. Ordered initial dose of Furadantin 10 mg PO qd for a child weighing 30.31 lb. You have Furadantin 5 mg/mL. The recommended PO dosage is 2 mg/kg/day. a. Child's weight is _______ kg. b. What is the safe recommended dosage or range for this child? _______ . c. Is the order safe? _______ . d. If yes, how many milliliters will you administer? _______ .

7. Ordered theophylline 16 mg PO q6 h for a child weighing 28 lb. You have theophylline elixir 11.25 mg/mL. The recommended PO dosage should not exceed 12 mg/kg/24 h. a. Child's weight is _______ kg. b. What is the safe recommended dosage or range for this child? _______ . c. Is the order safe? _______ . d. If yes, how many milliliters will you administer? _______ .

8. Ordered Dilantin 75 mg PO q12 h for a child weighing 66 lb. You have Dilantin chewable 50-mg tablets. The recommended PO dosage for a child is 5 to 7 mg/kg/day in divided doses q12 h. a. Child's weight is _______ kg. b. What is the safe recommended dosage or range for this child? _______ . c. Is the order safe? _______ . d. If yes, how many tablets will you administer? _______ .

9. Ordered Kantrex 250 mg IV q12 h for a child weighing 78 lb. You have Kantrex 75 mg/2 mL. The recommended daily IV dosage for a child is 15 mg/kg/day in divided doses q8 to 12 h. a. Child's weight is _______ kg. b. What is the safe recommended dosage or range for this child? _______ . c. Is the order safe? _______ . d. If yes, how many milliliters will you prepare? _______ .

NDC 0015-3512-20
6505-00-926-9202
Kantrex®
KANAMYCIN SULFATE
PEDIATRIC INJECTION
FOR I.M. OR I.V. USE
EQUIVALENT TO
75 mg KANAMYCIN
per 2 ml
BRISTOL LABORATORIES
Div of Bristol-Myers Company
Syracuse, NY 13221-4755
0.099% sodium bisulfite added as an antioxidant, buffered with 0.33% sodium citrate. • Adjusted to pH 4.5 with H_2SO_4. • Kantrex Pediatric Injection should not be physically mixed with other antibacterial agents.
READ ACCOMPANYING CIRCULAR
CAUTION: Federal law prohibits dispensing without prescription.
©Bristol Laboratories
351220DRL-13
MAXIMUM DOSE: 15 MG/KG/DAY
Lot
Exp. Date

10. Ordered Amoxil 375 mg PO q8 h for a child weighing 42 lb. You have Amoxil 125 mg/5 mL. The recommended daily PO dosage for a child is 20 to 50 mg/kg/day in divided doses q8 h. a. Child's weight is _______ kg. b. What is the safe recommended dosage or range for this child? _______ . c. Is the order safe? _______ . d. If yes, how many milliliters will you administer? _______ .

11. Ordered Compazine 2.5 mg PO tid for a child weighing 63 lb. You have Compazine 5 mg/5 mL. The recommended PO dosage for a child is 2.5 mg tid or 5 mg bid. a. Child's weight is _______ kg. b. What is the safe recommended dosage or range for this child? _______ . c. Is the order safe? _______ . d. If yes, how many milliliters will you administer? _______ .

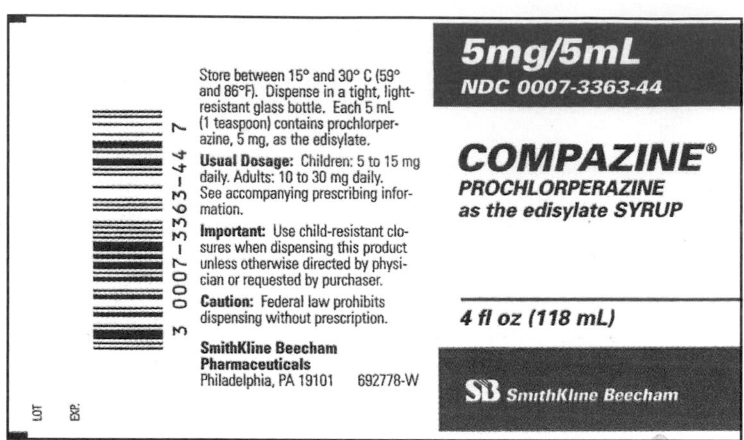

12. Ordered Tegretol 150 mg PO tid for a child weighing 58 lb. You have Tegretol 100 mg/5 mL. The recommended daily PO dosage for a child is 10 to 20 mg/kg/day in divided doses bid or tid. a. Child's weight is _______ kg. b. What is the safe recommended dosage or range for this child? _______ . c. Is the order safe? _______ . d. If yes, how many milliliters will you administer? _______ .

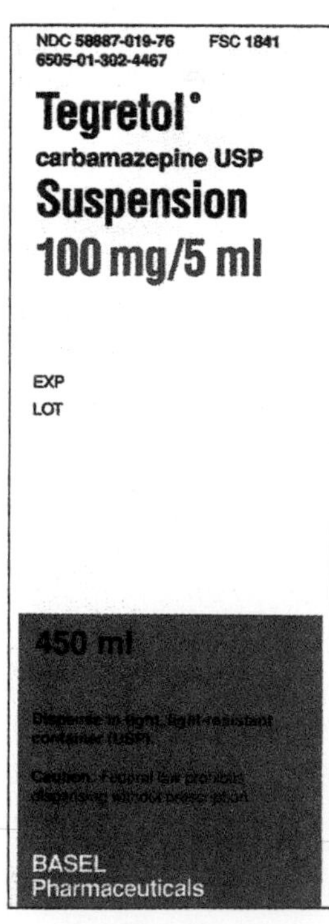

13. Ordered Dilaudid 1.5 mg PO q6 h for a child weighing 36 lb. You have Dilaudid oral solution 5 mg/mL. The recommended daily PO dosage for a child is 0.03 to 0.08 mg/kg in divided doses q4 to 6 h (maximum of 5 mg/dose). a. Child's weight is _______ kg. b. What is the safe recommended dosage or range for this child? _______ . c. Is the order safe? _______ . d. If yes, how many milliliters will you administer? _______ .

14. Ordered Naprosyn 150 mg PO bid for a child weighing 66 lb. You have Naprosyn 125 mg/5 mL. The recommended daily PO dosage for a child is 10 mg/kg/day in two divided doses. a. Child's weight is _______ kg. b. What is the safe recommended dosage or range for this child? _______ . c. Is the order safe? _______ . d. If yes, how many milliliters will you administer? _______ .

15. Ordered Kefzol 350 mg IV q8 h for a child weighing 81 lb. You have Kefzol 125 mg/mL. The recommended daily IV dosage for a child is 25 to 50 mg/kg/day in divided doses q6 to 8 h. a. Child's weight is _______ kg. b. What is the safe recommended dosage or range for this child? _______ . c. Is the order safe? _______ . d. If yes, how many milliliters will you prepare? _______ .

NDC 0002-1496-01
VIAL No. 766
℞ Lilly
KEFZOL®
STERILE CEFAZOLIN SODIUM, USP
Equiv. to
250 mg
Cefazolin

CAUTION—Federal (U.S.A.) law prohibits dispensing without prescription.
For I.M. or I.V. Use
Dosage—See Literature
To prepare solution add 2 mL Sterile Water for Injection or 0.9% Sodium Chloride Injection. Provides an approximate volume of 2 mL (125 mg per mL.)
SHAKE WELL Protect from light
Prior to Reconstitution: Store at Controlled Room Temperature 59° to 86°F (15° to 30°C)
After reconstitution—Store in a refrigerator. For Storage Time - See Accompanying Literature. If kept at room temperature, use within 24 hours.
Lyophilized
WV 6980 AMX
Eli Lilly & Co., Indianapolis, IN 46285, U.S.A.
Exp. Date/Control No.

16. Ordered Diuril 100 mg PO bid for a child weighing 16 lb 8 oz. You have Diuril 250 mg/5 mL. The recommended daily PO dosage for a child is 10 to 20 mg/kg/day in divided doses bid. a. Child's weight is _______ kg. b. What is the safe recommended dosage or range for this child? _______ . c. Is the order safe? _______ . d. If yes, how many milliliters will you administer? _______ .

17. Ordered Nebcin 16 mg IV q6 h for a child weighing 13 lb. You have Nebcin 20 mg/2 mL. The recommended daily IV dosage for a child is 6 to 7.5 mg/kg/day in divided doses q6 to 8 h. a. Child's weight is _______ kg. b. What is the safe recommended dosage or range for this child? _______ . c. Is the order safe? _______ . d. If yes, how many milliliters will you prepare? _______ .

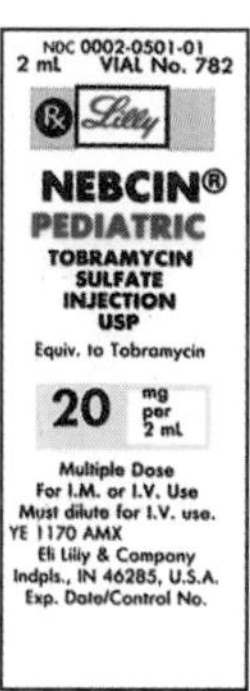

18. Ordered prednisone 8 mg PO q12 h for a child weighing 19 lb. You have prednisone syrup 5 mg/5 mL. The recommended daily PO dosage for a child is 0.05 to 2 mg/kg/day in divided doses q6 to 12 h. a. Child's weight is _______ kg. b. What is the safe recommended dosage or range for this child? _______ . c. Is the order safe? _______ . d. If yes, how many milliliters will you administer? _______ .

19. Ordered erythromycin 75 mg PO q6 h for a child weighing 22 lb. You have erythromycin 125 mg/5 mL. The recommended daily PO dosage for a child is 30 to 50 mg/kg/day in divided doses q6 h. a. Child's weight is _______ kg. b. What is the safe recommended dosage or range for this child? _______ . c. Is the order safe? _______ . d. If yes, how many milliliters will you administer? _______ .

20. Ordered Ancef 400 mg IV q8 h for a child weighing 32 lb. You have Ancef 330 mg/mL. The recommended daily IV dosage for a child is 100 mg/kg/day in divided doses q6 to 8 h. a. Child's weight is ______ kg. b. What is the safe recommended dosage or range for this child? ______ . c. Is the order safe? ______ . d. If yes, how many milliliters will you prepare? ______ .

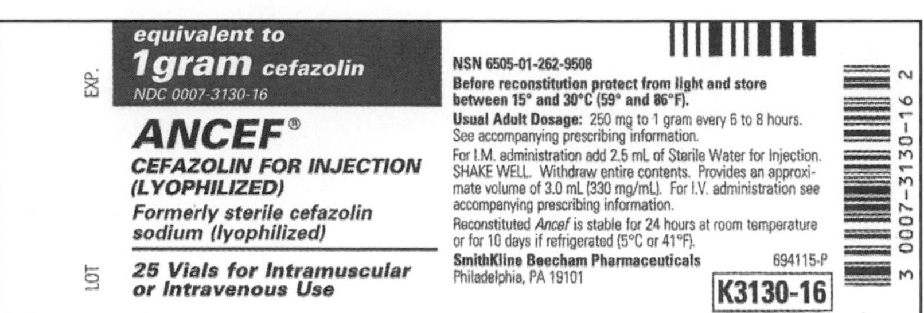

21. Infuse 250 mL of D_5W over 3 hours to an 11-year-old child. How many mL/h should the IV pump be programmed for? ______ .

22. A 25-kg child has an order for gentamicin 40 mg IVPB bid over 20 minutes. The concentration of the vial states 10 mg/mL. The recommended infusion concentration is 2 mg/mL. Step 1: How many milliliters of medication will provide 40 mg of gentamicin? ______ . Step 2: How many milliliters of IV solution needs to be added to the medication to equal the recommended final concentration? ______ . Step 3: How many gtt/min of gentamicin should be infused? ______ .

Answers on pp. 511-514.

Name ______________________________

Date ______________________________

ACCEPTABLE SCORE 17

YOUR SCORE ______

POSTTEST 1

Directions: The medication order is listed at the beginning of each problem. Calculate the child's weight in kilograms, determine the safe recommended dosage or range, determine the safety of the order, and calculate the drug dosage. Show your work.

1. Ordered phenobarbital 60 mg PO q12 h for a child weighing 55 lb. Elixir of phenobarbital 20 mg/5 mL is available. The recommended daily dosage for a child is 4 to 6 mg/kg/day in divided doses q12 h. a. Child's weight is _______ kg. b. What is the safe recommended dosage or range for this child? _______ . c. Is the order safe? _______ . d. If yes, how many milliliters will the nurse administer? _______ .

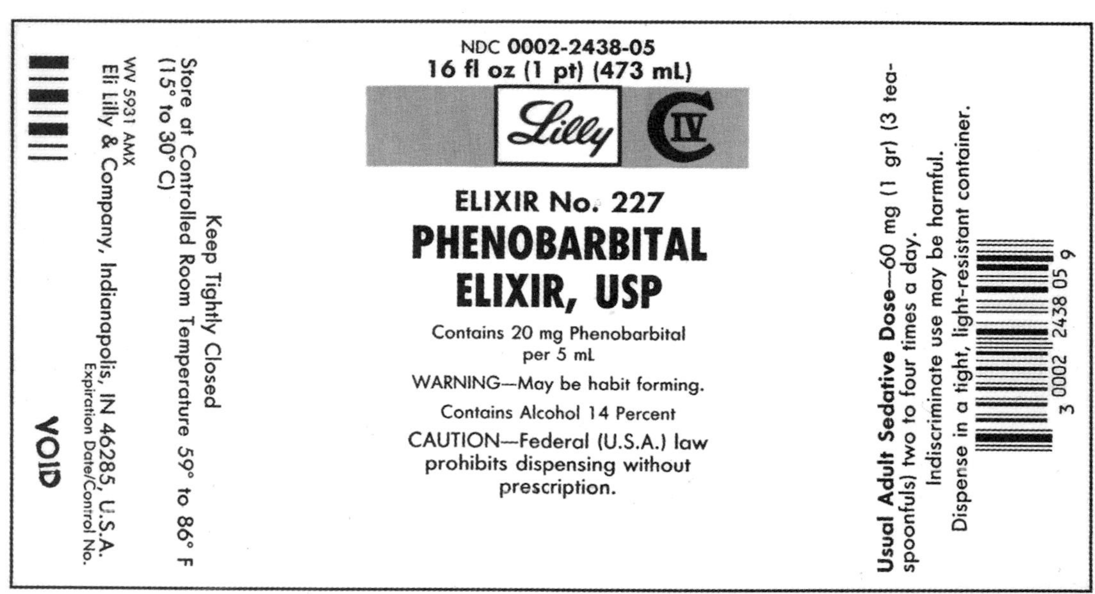

2. Ordered Lincocin 500 mg PO q6 h for a child weighing 44 lb. Lincocin is supplied in 250-mg capsules. The recommended daily PO dosage for a child is 30 to 60 mg/kg/day in divided doses q6 h. a. Child's weight is _______ kg. b. What is the safe recommended dosage or range for this child? _______ . c. Is the order safe? _______ . d. If yes, how many capsules will the nurse administer? _______ .

3. Ordered procaine penicillin G 150,000 U IM q12 h for a child weighing 6 lb 12 oz. You have procaine penicillin G 300,000 U/mL. The recommended daily IM dosage for a child is 50,000 U/kg IM. a. Child's weight is _______ kg. b. What is the safe recommended dosage or range for this child? _______ . c. Is the order safe? _______ . d. If yes, how many milliliters will you administer? _______ .

4. Ordered Keflex 250 mg PO tid for a child weighing 44 lb. Keflex is supplied in an oral suspension at 125 mg/5 mL. The recommended daily PO dosage for a child is 20 to 40 mg/kg/day in divided doses q8 h. a. Child's weight is ______ kg. b. What is the safe recommended dosage or range for this child? ______ . c. Is the order safe? ______ . d. If yes, how many milliliters will the nurse administer? ______ .

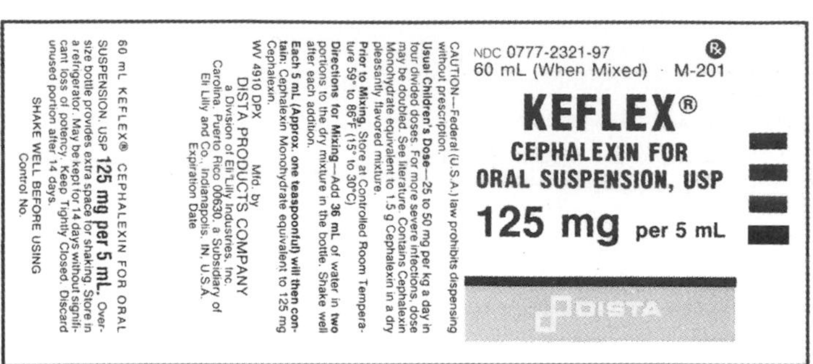

5. Ordered morphine 4 mg IM stat for a child weighing 78 lb. You have morphine sulfate 15 mg/mL. The recommended IM dosage for a child is 0.1 to 0.2 mg/kg/day. a. Child's weight is ______ kg. b. What is the safe recommended dosage or range for this child? ______ . c. Is the order safe? ______ . d. If yes, how many milliliters will you administer? ______ .

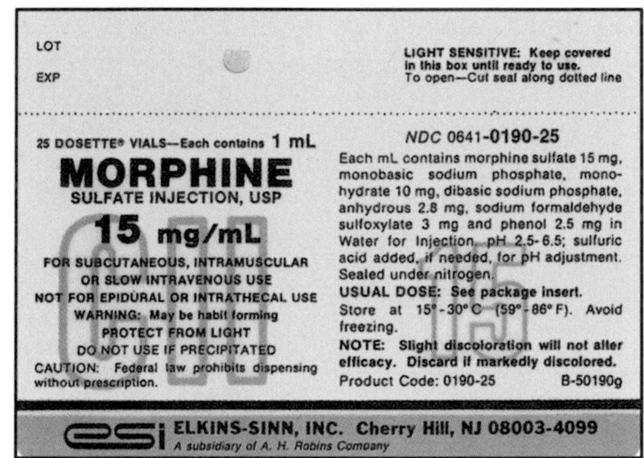

6. Ordered Biaxin 300 mg PO bid for a child weighing 92 lb. You have Biaxin 125 mg/5 mL. The recommended daily PO dosage for a child is 15 mg/kg/day in divided doses q12 h. a. Child's weight is _______ kg. b. What is the safe recommended dosage or range for this child? _______ . c. Is the order safe? _______ d. If yes, how many milliliters will you administer? _______ .

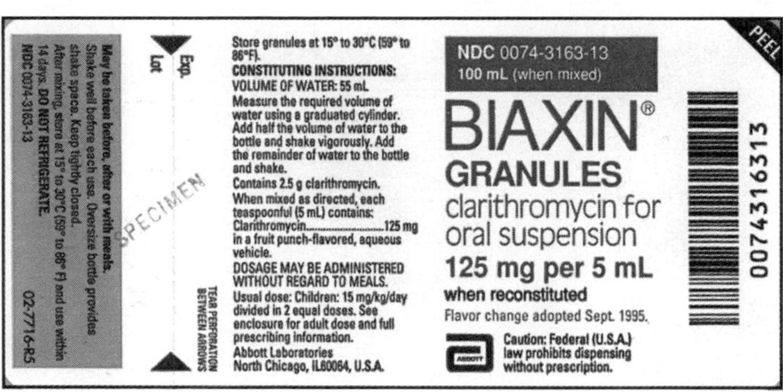

7. Ordered Zithromax 180 mg PO qd for a child weighing 35 lb. You have Zithromax 200 mg/5 mL. The recommended daily PO dosage for a child is 12 mg/kg/day for 5 days. a. Child's weight is _______ kg. b. What is the safe recommended dosage or range for this child? _______ . c. Is the order safe? _______ d. If yes, how many milliliters will you administer? _______ .

8. Ordered Lufyllin 25 mg PO q6 h for a child weighing 52 lb. You have Lufyllin 100 mg/15 mL. The recommended daily PO dosage for a child is 4 to 7 mg/kg/day in divided doses q6 h. a. Child's weight is _______ kg. b. What is the safe recommended dosage or range for this child? _______ . c. Is the order safe? _______ d. If yes, how many milliliters will you administer? _______ .

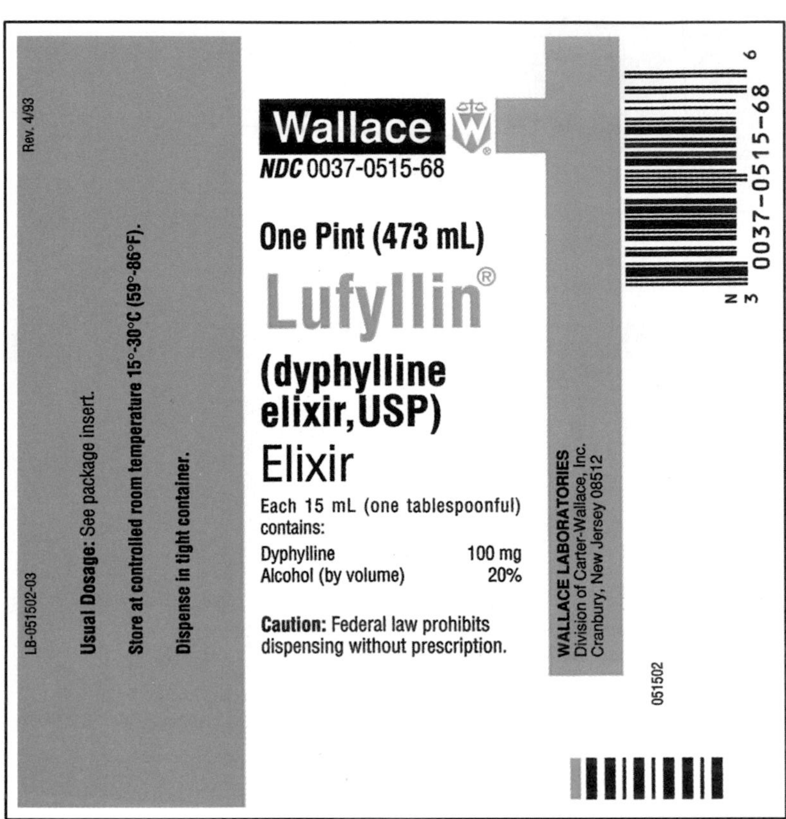

9. Ordered Dolophine 0.5 mg SQ q6 h for a child weighing 6 lb 4 oz. You have Dolophine 10 mg/mL. The recommended daily dosage for a child is 0.05 to 0.1 mg/kg/day in divided doses q6-12 h. a. Child's weight is _______ kg. b. What is the safe recommended dosage or range for this child? _______ . c. Is the order safe? _______ d. If yes, how many milliliters will you administer? _______ .

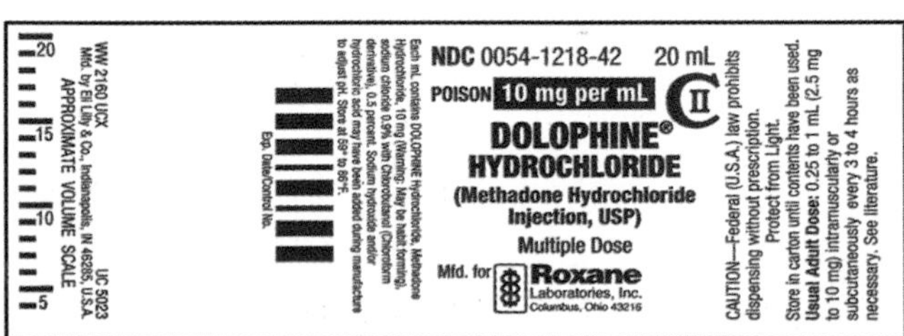

10. Ordered Ceclor 525 mg PO q12 h for a child weighing 66 lb. You have Ceclor 375 mg/ 5 mL. The recommended daily PO dosage for a child is 15 mg/kg/day q12 h. a. Child's weight is _______ kg. b. What is the safe recommended dosage or range for this child? _______ . c. Is the order safe? _______ . d. If yes, how many milliliters will you administer? _______ .

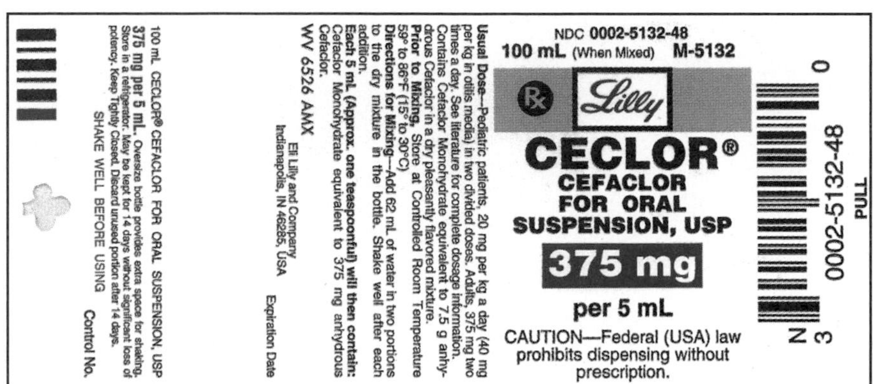

11. A 10-month-old infant has an order for 100 mL 0.9% NS to be infused over 6 hours. How many mL/h should the IV pump be programmed for? _______ .

12. A 15-kg infant has an order for ampicillin 400 mg IVPB over 30 minutes. The ampicillin vial gives a concentration of 250 mg/mL. The recommended infusion concentration is 50 mg/mL. Step 1: How many milliliters of medication will provide 400 mg of ampicillin? _______ . Step 2: How many milliliters of IV solution need to be added to the medication to equal the recommended final concentration? _______ . Step 3: How many gtt/min of ampicillin should be infused? _______ .

Answers on pp. 515-516.

Name ______________________

Date ______________________

ACCEPTABLE SCORE 17

YOUR SCORE ______

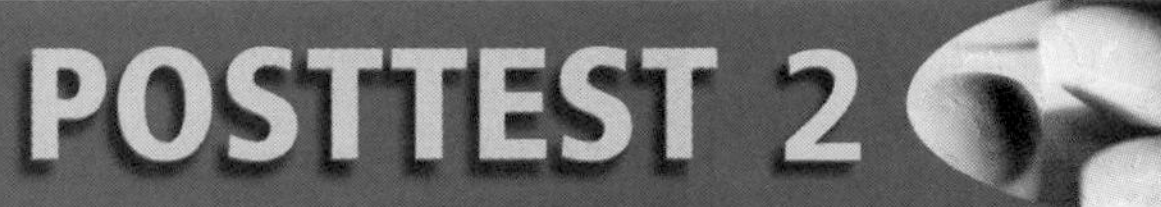

Directions: The medication order is listed at the beginning of each problem. Calculate the child's weight in kilograms, determine the safe recommended dosage or range, determine the safety of the order, and calculate the drug dosage. Show your work.

1. Ordered Cleocin 225 mg IV q6 h for a child weighing 58 lb. You have Cleocin 150 mg/mL. The recommended daily dosage for a child is 15 to 40 mg/kg/day in divided doses q6-8 h. a. Child's weight is ______ kg. b. What is the safe recommended dosage or range for this child? ______ . c. Is the order safe? ______ . d. If yes, how many milliliters will you prepare? ______ .

2. Ordered Dilantin 50 mg PO q12 h for a child weighing 70 lb. You have Dilantin 125 mg/5 mL. The recommended daily PO dosage for a child is 5 to 7 mg/kg/day in divided doses q12 h. a. Child's weight is ______ kg. b. What is the safe recommended dosage or range for this child? ______ . c. Is the order safe? ______ . d. If yes, how many milliliters will you administer? ______ .

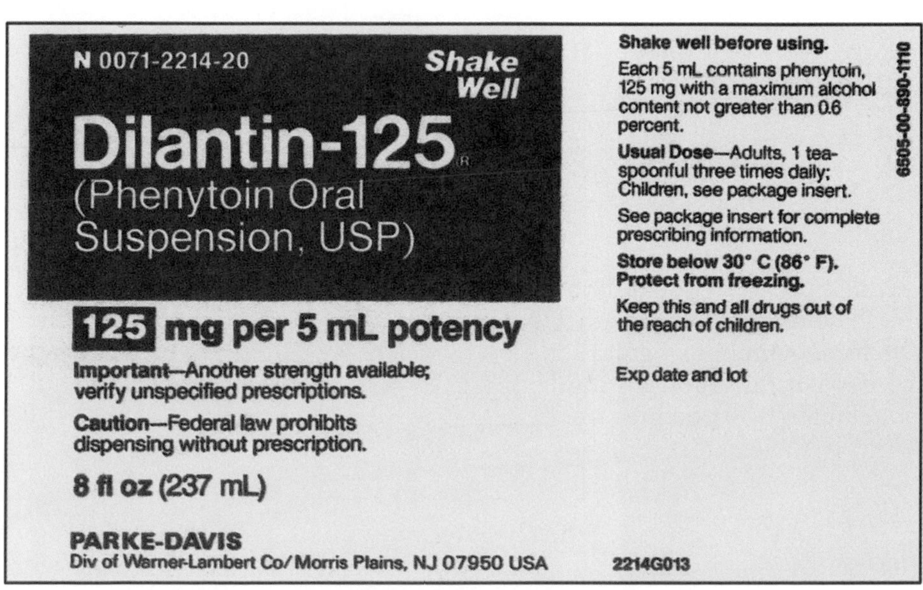

3. Ordered Amoxil 250 mg PO q8 h for a child weighing 58 lb. You have Amoxil 125 mg/ 5 mL. The recommended daily PO dosage for the child is 20 to 40 mg/kg/day in divided doses q8 h. a. Child's weight is _______ kg. b. What is the safe recommended dosage or range for this child? _______ . c. Is the order safe? _______ . d. If yes, how many milliliters will you administer? _______ .

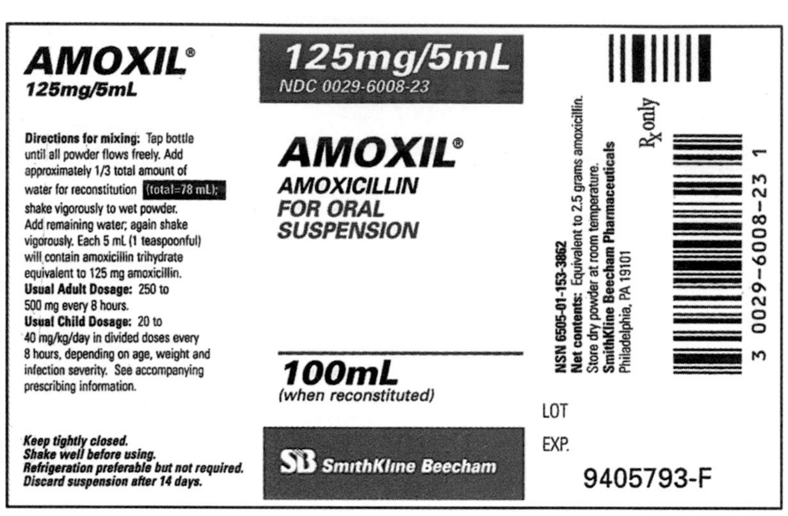

4. Ordered Keflex 500 mg PO q6 h for a child weighing 99 lb. You have Keflex 250-mg capsules available. The recommended daily PO dosage for a child is 25 to 50 mg/kg/day in four equal doses q6 h. a. Child's weight is _______ kg. b. What is the safe recommended dosage or range for this child? _______ . c. Is the order safe? _______ . d. If yes, how many capsules will you administer? _______ .

5. Ordered Cloxacillin 500 mg PO q6 h for a child weighing 66 lb. You have cloxacillin 125 mg/mL available. The recommended daily PO dosage for a child is 50 to 100 mg/kg in divided doses q6 h (maximum of 4 g/day). a. Child's weight is _______ kg. b. What is the safe recommended dosage or range for this child? _______ . c. Is the order safe? _______ . d. If yes, how many milliliters will you prepare? _______ .

6. Ordered Lorabid 250 mg PO q12 h for a child weighing 39 lb. You have Lorabid 200 mg/5 mL. The recommended daily PO dosage for a child is 15 to 30 mg/kg/day in divided doses q12 h. a. Child's weight is _______ kg. b. What is the safe recommended dosage or range for this child? _______ . c. Is the order safe? _______ . d. If yes, how many milliliters will you administer? _______ .

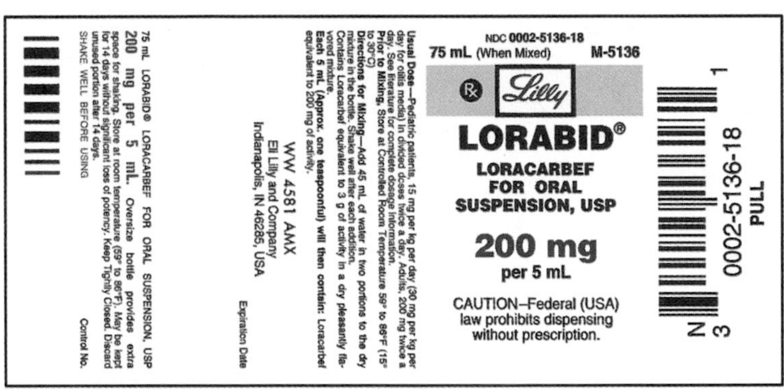

7. Ordered Amoxil 0.4 mg PO q8 h for a child weighing 42 lb. You have Amoxil 250 mg/5 mL. The recommended daily PO dose for a child is 20-50 mg/kg/day in divided doses q8 h. a. Child's weight is _______ kg. b. What is the safe recommended dosage or range for this child? _______ . c. Is the order safe? _______ . d. If yes, how many milliliters will you administer? _______ .

AMOXIL®
250mg/5mL

Directions for mixing: Tap bottle until all powder flows freely. Add approximately 1/3 total amount of water for reconstitution (total=59 mL); shake vigorously to wet powder. Add remaining water; again shake vigorously. Each 5 mL (1 teaspoonful) will contain amoxicillin trihydrate equivalent to 250 mg amoxicillin.
Usual Adult Dosage: 250 to 500 mg every 8 hours.
Usual Child Dosage: 20 to 40 mg/kg/day in divided doses every 8 hours, depending on age, weight and infection severity. See accompanying prescribing information.

Keep tightly closed.
Shake well before using.
Refrigeration preferable but not required.
Discard suspension after 14 days.

250mg/5mL
NDC 0029-6009-21

AMOXIL®
AMOXICILLIN
FOR ORAL
SUSPENSION

80mL (when reconstituted)

SB SmithKline Beecham

NSN 6505-01-153-3442
Net contents: Equivalent to 4.0 grams amoxicillin.
Store dry powder at room temperature.
Caution: Federal law prohibits dispensing without prescription.
SmithKline Beecham Pharmaceuticals
Philadelphia, PA 19101

LOT
EXP.

3 0029-6009-21 4

9405783-E

8. Ordered Vancocin 300 mg PO q6 h for a child weighing 70 lb. You have Vancocin 250 mg/5 mL. The recommended daily PO dosage for a child is 40 mg/kg/day in divided doses q6 h. a. Child's weight is _______ kg. b. What is the safe recommended dosage or range for this child? _______ . c. Is the order safe? _______ . d. If yes, how many milliliters will you administer? _______ .

9. Ordered morphine 0.9 mg IV q4 h for a child weighing 53 lb. You have 0.5 mg/mL. The recommended daily IV dosage for a child is 0.1 to 0.2 mg/kg/day in divided doses q4 h. a. Child's weight is _______ kg. b. What is the safe recommended dosage or range for this child? _______ . c. Is the order safe? _______ . d. If yes, how many milliliters will you prepare? _______ .

10. Ordered Epivir 9 mg PO q12 h for a child weighing 10 lb 4 oz. You have Lamivudine 10 mg/mL. The recommended daily PO dosage for a child is 4 mg/kg/day in divided doses q12 h. a. Child's weight is _______ kg. b. What is the safe recommended dosage or range for this child? _______ . c. Is the order safe? _______ . d. If yes, how many milliliters will you administer? _______ .

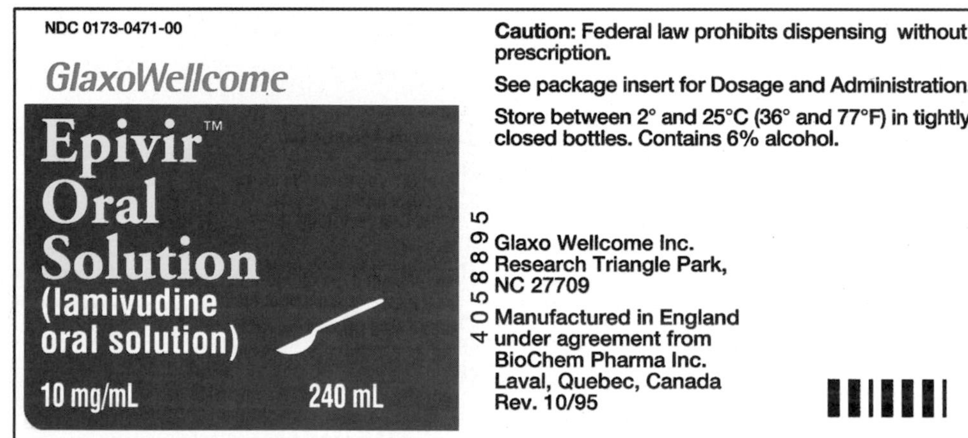

11. Infuse 200 mL LR over 6 hours to a 2-year-old child. How many mL/h should the IV pump be programmed for? _______ .

12. A 60-kg child has an order for vancomycin 500 mg IVPB bid over 1 hour. The vial concentration is 50 mg/mL. The recommended infusion concentration is 5 mg/mL. Step 1: How many milliliters of medication will provide 500 mg of vancomycin? _______ . Step 2: How many milliliters of IV solution need to be added to the medication to equal the recommended final concentration? _______ . Step 3: How many gtt/min of vancomycin should be infused? _______ .

Answers on pp. 517-518.

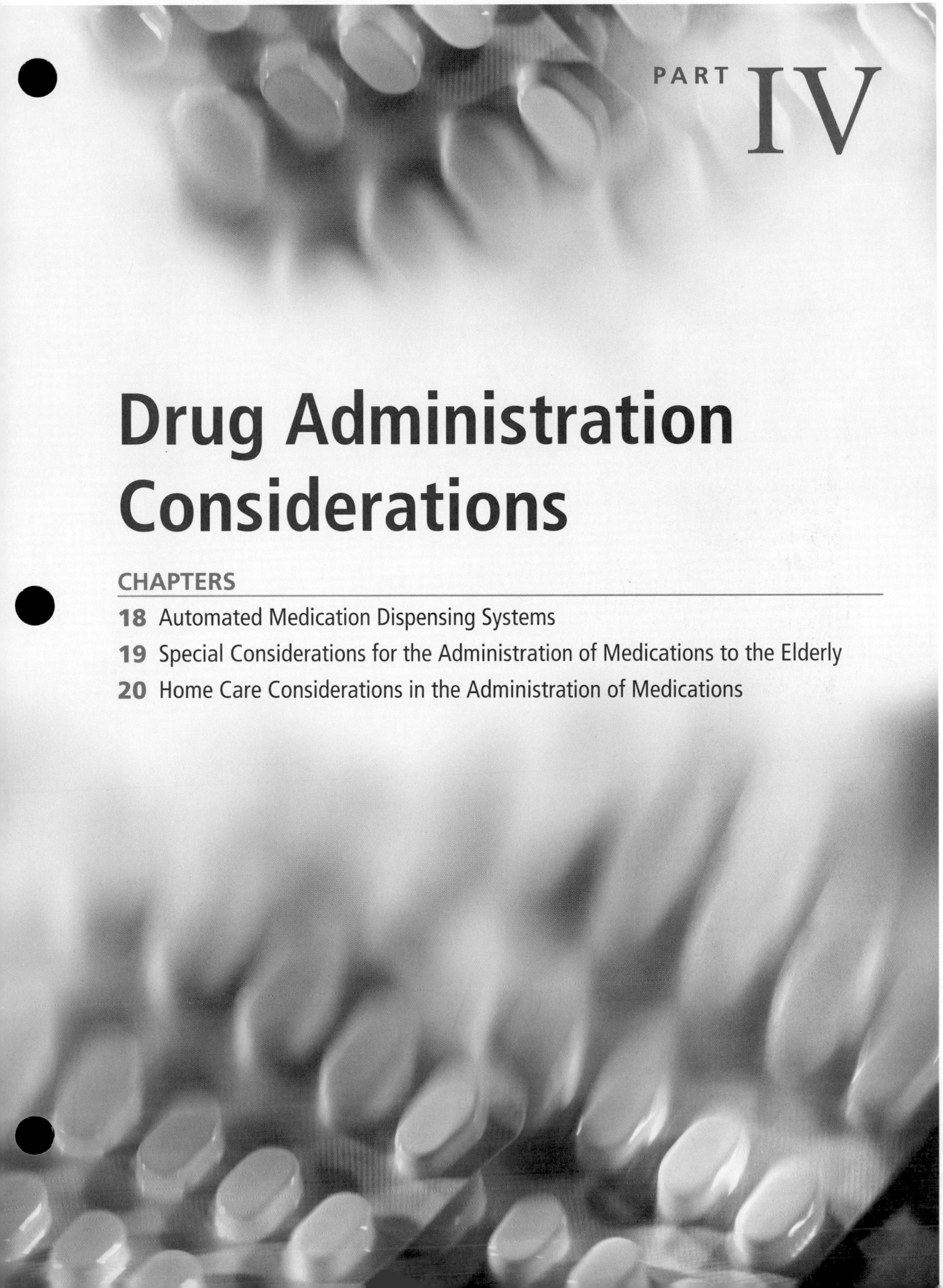

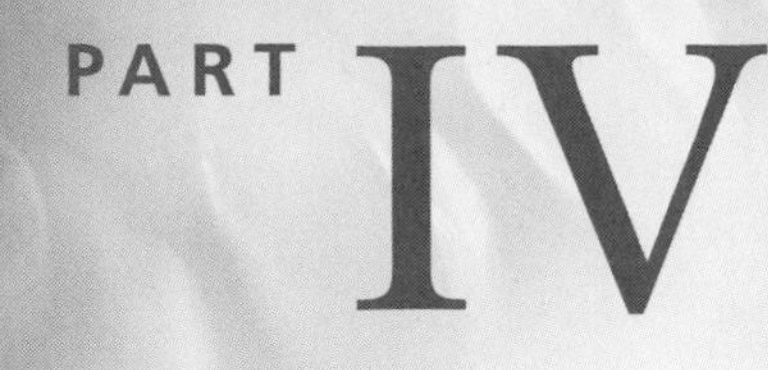

Drug Administration Considerations

CHAPTERS

CHAPTER 18

Automated Medication Dispensing Systems

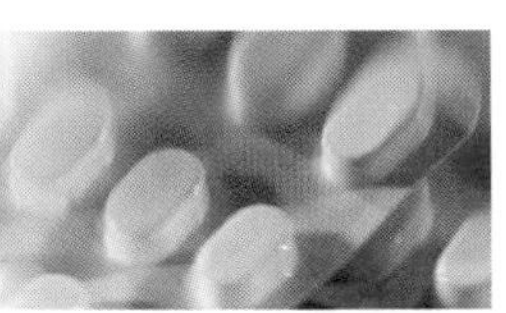

LEARNING OBJECTIVES

On completion of the materials provided in this chapter, you will be able to:

1. Recognize an automated medication dispensing system
2. Identify the advantages of using an automated medication dispensing system

Health care delivery systems continue to strive to improve the accuracy and efficiency of the delivery of medications to patients. In recent years, more and more hospitals and other care center areas have moved to the use of automated medication dispensing systems.

Each patient care unit is provided with a special cabinet that houses the medications that will be dispensed from that unit. The medications in the machine are usually listed by both their trade and generic names. This feature helps to expedite location of the medications by the nurse. These cabinets are connected to the central pharmacy for order verifications and accuracy, as well as for automation of usage reports that are provided for many facets of the medication process. Depending on the vendor chosen by the institution, a variety of medications may be housed in the cabinet, ranging from only controlled substances to inclusion of first doses, as-needed (prn) doses, and regularly scheduled medications. Having a wide range of medications within the patient care area allows a quick response to changes in a patient's condition. For example, a new medication order does not require a special trip to the central pharmacy to obtain the needed medication, allowing the new drug regimen to be initiated quickly. With a computerized system, the patient has the added benefit of more time being available to the nurse for all aspects of patient care, and the pharmacist has more time to confer with physicians and resource nurses and to analyze drug studies and usage.

An automatic drug dispensing system also leads to a reduction in medication errors. This is especially true as vendors market new options that allow only the designated drawer housing the medication that is being given at that time to open. The automated medication dispensing system also enhances patient satisfaction. This is especially evident in postsurgical patients or patients with cancer who require the administration of pain medications in a timely manner. Pain medications are usually controlled substances that require the nurse to first locate and obtain the narcotic keys from a peer, then open the narcotic supply, find and remove the right medication, relock the supply area, sign out the controlled substance, and then take the medication to the patient for administration. With an automated system, the nurse is able to access the medication from the cabinet. The machine then allows the nurse to confirm the accuracy of the controlled substance count immediately. The medication may then be given quickly to the patient with the least amount of time and effort expended (Figure 18-1). All of these systems are password-

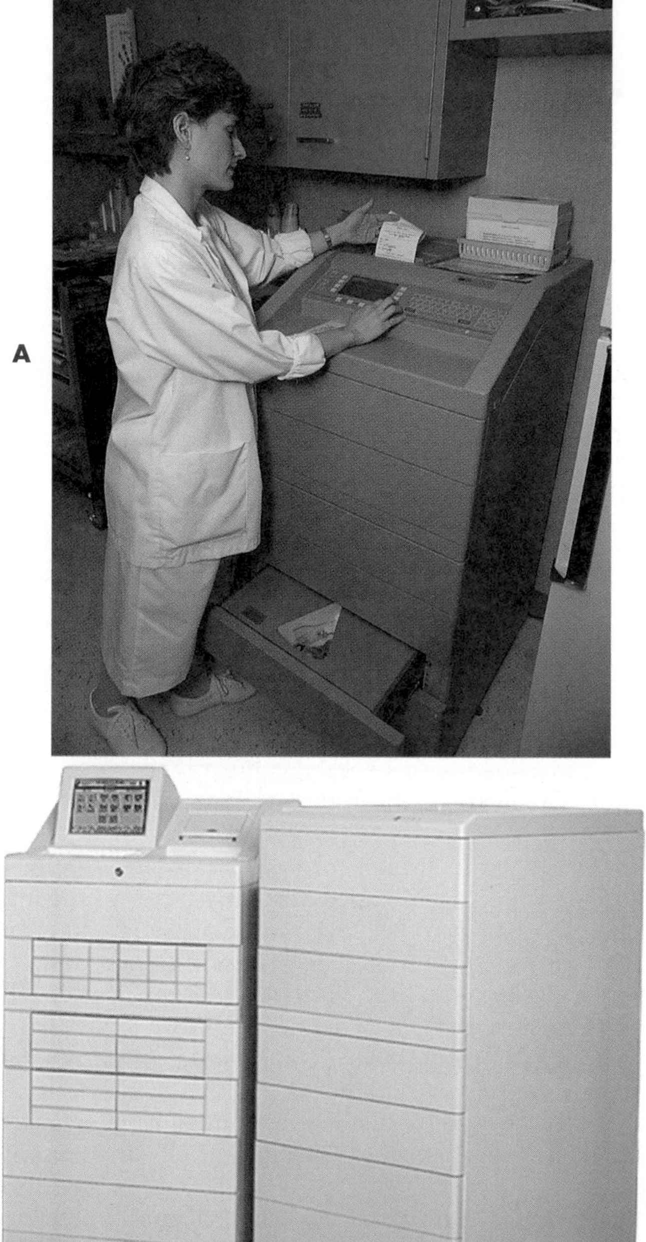

FIGURE 18-1 **A,** Nurse using computer-controlled dispensing system. **B,** Medstation® automated drug dispensing system. (**A,** from Potter PA, Perry AG: *Fundamentals of nursing,* ed 5, St Louis, 2001, Mosby. **B,** Courtesy Pyxis Corporation.)

secured. Continuous documentation is occurring while the cabinet is in use. The nurse can review records, but at the same time the cabinet records how long the nurse has been "logged in." This is important for quality control and evaluation of nursing actions in relationship to patient care.

Another advantage of an automated medication dispensing system is reduction in the time that is required for end-of-shift narcotic counts. This count is performed by two nurses, usually one from the ending shift and one from the starting shift. It is also standard practice that until the narcotic count is completed and correct, all staff that are ending their shift may not leave. This results in staff dissatisfaction and unnecessary overtime costs that can be better spent on actual patient care. This scenario is prevented because automated systems require the confirmation of the count of controlled substance medications after each withdrawal.

These medication dispensing systems are also beneficial for patients who are transferred from one unit to another. The medications are already housed in the cabinet if it is one that has been expanded to include most patient medications (Figure 18-2). This allows the patient to continue to progress without delays caused by medications being unavailable.

Some of the systems currently on the market interface with the health care system's program for charting of medications. With some dispensing systems, charting is done at the cabinet in the unit, whereas other manufacturers are designing programs to document the administration of medication at the bedside. With the automatic documentation of the administration of the patient's medications, the nurse is not required to return to the paper medication administration record and manually chart that the medicine has been given.

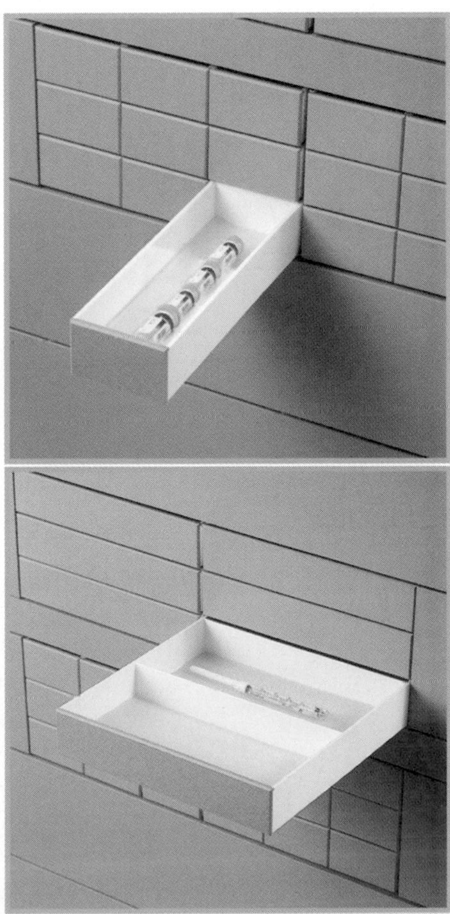

FIGURE 18-2 Pyxis MiniDrawers for medication storage. (Courtesy Pyxis Corporation.)

There are some disadvantages to the automated dispensing systems. Because some of the drawers have open compartments, it is possible for the wrong medication to be placed in the drawer. This makes the three medicine checks the nurse performs when he or she prepares a patient's medicines to be absolutely paramount. Technology is *not* perfect, and mistakes can and do occur in the delivery of medication. The pharmacy, as the cabinet is being restocked, or another nurse may have mishandled the medications while searching the drawers for the medication that is currently needed. If the machine houses all of the patient medications, lines may form when several nurses need to obtain patient medications at the same time. The nurse needs to be well organized and plan ahead for access to the cabinet.

As health care facilities continue to monitor costs and at the same time strive to improve patient and staff satisfaction, the use of automated medication dispensing systems will become more widespread. This is a new area in which nursing students will need to become knowledgeable and competent because the accurate and efficient delivery of medications is one of the most important tasks of patient care that the nurse is required to perform.

CHAPTER 19

Special Considerations for the Administration of Medications to the Elderly

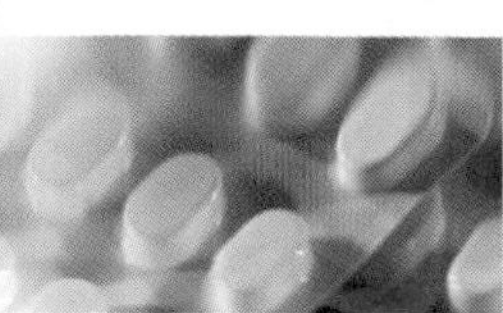

LEARNING OBJECTIVES

On completion of the materials provided in this chapter, you will be able to:

1. Understand the implications of the physiological changes of aging on medication administration to the elderly
2. Understand the special problems and issues related to medication administration for the elderly

People are now living longer than at any period in history, and we are continuing to increase our knowledge of how to protect our health and prevent illness. By practicing good health habits, such as proper diet, an exercise program, and a positive attitude, people are enjoying better health. As research continues, cures and maintenance regimens for major health problems are being found. Life expectancy continues to increase. "Old-old" persons over the age of 85 are the most rapidly increasing portion of the population in the United States. This group is also using more of the nation's health care resources.

Aging is a normal process, beginning at infancy and continuing throughout the life cycle. Aging is not the cause of specific diseases, but certain chronic illnesses are more prevalent in the elderly and may lead to additional health problems. Chronic illnesses usually require an increase in drug use to control the symptoms or progression of the condition.

Changes Experienced by the Elderly

Biological and physiological changes that affect all body systems occur and conflict with the action of some medications. Medication problems are more likely to occur in the older age group. These problems can be drug interactions, adverse reactions, drug and food interactions, or medication errors. Reflexes slow, and there is an inability to adapt quickly to changes in temperature. A decrease in the sense of touch may be a safety issue. There is a decrease in saliva, which may slow the absorption of buccal medications. Some elderly persons may have difficulty in swallowing, especially large tablets. An advantage of aging is a diminished sense of taste: elderly people may have no difficulty with some of the bitter-tasting medications.

Biological and physiological changes also affect the metabolism and excretion of drugs. Chronic conditions, such as hypertension, diabetes, heart conditions, and arthritis, interfere with homeostasis and may cause medications to be less effective. Absorption is affected by age-related changes in the motility of the gastrointestinal tract. A decrease in motility may cause an increase in drug actions. Many elderly persons resort to the regular use of laxatives. Laxatives increase the motility of the gastrointestinal tract and therefore allow less time for the prescribed medication to be absorbed.

Changes in cardiac output may also decrease the flow of blood to the liver and kidneys. Another major change with aging is the decrease in renal function. This may lead to medications being removed from the body more slowly and perhaps less completely.

A decrease in body weight of many elderly persons is reason to reassess the dosages of medications ordered. The actual weight of the patient should be used to validate the correct dosage of each drug. Many drug reference manuals now list the appropriate dosages for geriatric as well as pediatric and adult patients. At times it may be difficult to select a proper site for an injection. This is because of a decrease in muscle mass. However, an advantage to aging may be a decrease in the perception of pain from injections because of a decrease in some sensory perceptions.

These changes, in concert with a person's genetic programming, add to the severity of health problems in the elderly. It is difficult for a person who has had an active life to deal with these changes. The nurse must be understanding in order to assist an elderly person to adapt to a limited lifestyle.

Physical illness often affects the mental state of a person, which adds to anxiety and further deterioration. Occasionally, an elderly person feels unable to make the most basic decisions. The nurse, in collaboration with other members of the health care team, can assist the patient, the family, and the person(s) responsible for giving care to understand the process of change or aging. Alzheimer's disease negatively affects a person's ability to safely assume responsibility for taking his or her own medications, especially as the stages advance. It is important for family members and caregivers to be aware of this.

Problems of the Elderly

Some older persons are in the habit of visiting an internist for an annual physical examination. Because the elderly have more aches and pains than other age groups, they may also visit a physician in family practice to deal with minor problems. If these aches and pains do not resolve, they may visit a third physician. If each physician writes a prescription(s), the patient may be prescribed several medications that duplicate actions or cause drug interaction or overdosage.

The patient should be encouraged to visit only one physician unless referred to a specialist. Should the patient visit another physician, he or she should prepare a list of all medications taken routinely or as needed and give it to the new physician. The physician can then prescribe medication and instruct the patient to delete duplicate medications or those that cause drug interactions.

Older patients should be encouraged to have all of their prescriptions filled at the same pharmacy. This allows the pharmacist to have a complete listing of the medications they have been prescribed. The pharmacist is then able to monitor for adverse interactions of the patient's medicines.

Inadequate income is a major problem for many older people. To lower medical costs, they may take less than the prescribed amount of a prescription drug so that it will last longer. They may also stop taking the medication if they perceive it to be ineffective. They may go to the drug store and buy nonprescription drugs. Such drugs will save a physician's fee and are less expensive than prescription drugs, but they may be ineffective. However, the patient may perceive them to be a cure.

Another method used to lower costs of drugs is to take medication prescribed for a family member or friend. Misuse of drugs is widespread among the elderly and may cause various problems, such as fluid imbalance, nutritional disturbances, and psychological or neurological problems.

As older persons become forgetful, they may not take their medications or may not take them at the prescribed time. Often family members find medications on the floor, and they do not know whether the medication was taken.

When it becomes unsafe for an elderly person to stay at home alone, a day-care center can relieve the pressure on family members who are employed. People enjoy being with others of their age to discuss memories and similar experiences. They can join in crafts and activities as they wish. There are opportunities to discuss thoughts and concerns with personnel at the center. Then the medication regimen can be continued during the day, and meals can be served and activities planned. Activities at the center stimulate the elderly and give them something interesting to discuss at home in the evening.

More elderly persons are electing to live in their own homes rather than in a retirement home or a nursing home. Sometimes they share their home with someone near their age. If an elderly person or couple cannot care for themselves, they may choose to share their home with an individual or a couple who will not only be homemakers but also give care as needed. Apart from providing a home for the one(s) giving care, monetary compensation may be provided.

Medical Alert System

A medical alert system is a valuable tool for a homebound person living alone or for times when the caregiver must be away for a few minutes. It is also used in retirement homes. In an emergency a button is pushed on the monitoring system or on a chain worn by the patient. The system alerts medical personnel to the emergency situation. Such a system gives a feeling of security to homebound persons and their families.

Medications for the Elderly in the Home

When purchasing medications from a pharmacy, elderly persons should request that childproof containers *not* be used. Containers that are available to prepare medications for a day or a week at a time should be purchased and used (Figure 19-1). Such containers have a special compartment for each hour the medications are to be given. The time can be written on the lid of the individual compartment and easily removed if the time changes. These containers are especially helpful if someone outside the home assists the patient in preparing medications.

An appointment book with the day and date, a spiral notebook, or a writing tablet with the day and date added can be used as an efficient and safe way to plan medications taken in the home. The medications and the times they are to be taken each day are listed. The entry is crossed off after the medication has been taken (Box 19-1).

The used medication sheet is discarded, and a new one is completed each day.

The Visiting Nurse

At times when the patient, the family, or the person giving care believes that an assessment of the patient's health status is needed, a request can be made to the physician for assistance from a visiting nurse. The visiting nurse provides skilled care and consultation in the home under the supervision of the patient's physician.

The nurse assesses the patient's condition, gives nursing care as needed, and assists the family and the person giving care to better understand the patient. The nurse should review the patient's medication regimen with the person giving care. If some time has elapsed since the medication was ordered, the nurse should review the medication orders with the physician. The service provided by the visiting nurse will help the patient and family feel secure that the patient is receiving optimum health care in the home.

A

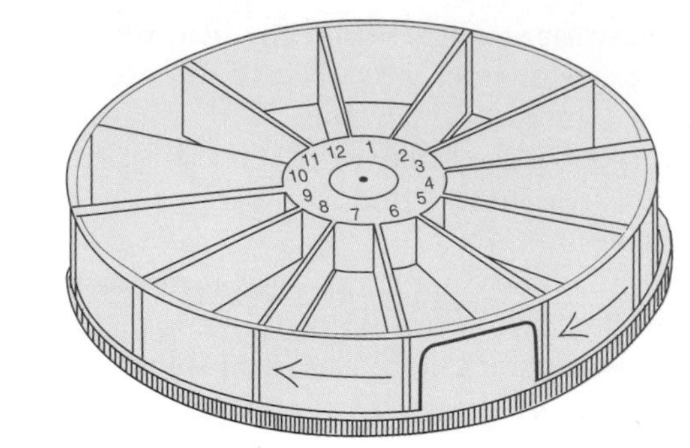

B

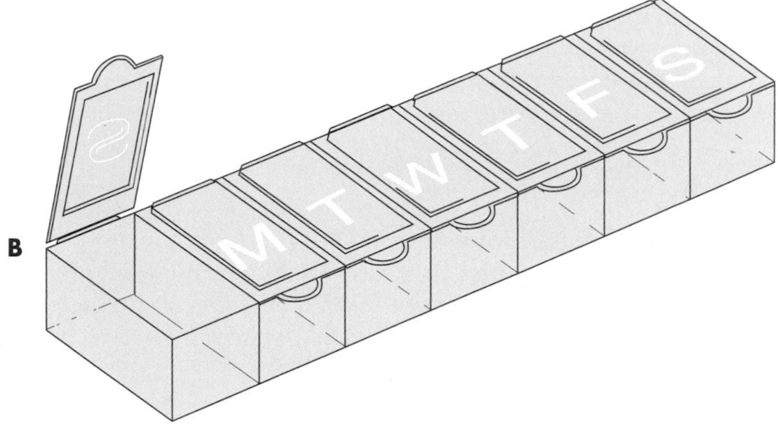

FIGURE 19-1 Examples of containers that hold medications for a day **(A)** or a week **(B)** at a time.

BOX 19-1 ■ MEDICATION SHEET EXAMPLE

Thursday, March 25
Motrin 300 mg after each meal
~~8:00~~ AM 1:00 PM 6:00 PM
Naprosyn 250 mg two times a day
~~8:00~~ AM 4:00 PM
Persantin 25 mg two times a day
10:00 AM 6:00 PM
Lanoxin 40 mg daily
10:00 AM
Mylanta 2 tablespoons after meals

Medication Errors with the Elderly

The elderly at home are more prone to medication errors than those in health care facilities. The most common error is that of omission. This may be because of the cost of medication or the person's forgetfulness. An incorrect dosage, wrong time, or lack of understanding of directions may be the cause of other medication errors.

The decrease in gross and fine motor skills may affect how well the packaging of medications can be handled. For example, arthritis may make it difficult for a patient with insulin-dependent diabetes to draw up and self-administer the correct dose of insulin.

It is important for the nurse to make sure that elderly patients understand the directions for taking their medications safely. Many elderly persons are hearing impaired to some degree. The nurse should ask the patient to verbally repeat the instructions. Older people, beginning with middle age, often are also visually impaired. It is necessary to make certain they can read the labels of their drugs, and any written directions should be printed in a large, easy-to-read format.

Medication errors with the elderly can be reduced if time is taken to explain the reason for the medication, its importance, and how it works. This is especially important if timing is critical in maintaining a therapeutic blood level of the medication. Some elderly patients fear becoming addicted to their medication because they do not understand its purpose.

A careful and complete drug history should be obtained from all patients, but especially older ones. This history should include over-the-counter drugs. Many people think that over-the-counter drugs are completely safe. However, they may be unaware of the negative interactions that may occur if these products are taken with other medicines that have been prescribed by their physician.

Alcohol is one of the most abused drugs in the elderly population. The combination of alcohol and certain medicines may be a problem for the chronic drinker and the occasional drinker. The nurse's assessment should include the patient's use of alcohol. This information should be validated with other family members.

Medications for the Elderly in the Hospital

Professional nurses will plan nursing care for older patients in the hospital. As our older population continues to increase, nurses will be employed not only in hospitals and nursing homes but also in day-care centers and retirement communities. The nurse will work with the patient and the family, as well as other health care practitioners, including the physician, dietitian, pharmacist, occupational therapist, social worker, and clinical nurse specialist or nurse practitioner.

Although the physician orders the medications and the pharmacist prepares them, the nurse is responsible for administering the medication to the patient. It is important that the right amount of the right medicine be given to the right patient at the right time in the right way. The patient must also be observed for reactions. The physician must be notified if drug reactions occur. The nurse must record the date, time, medication, dosage, and route of administration. It is important to follow the six rights of medication administration with the elderly as well as with all other patients (Box 19-2).

Before administering the medication to the patient, the nurse should tell the patient the name of the drug and why it was prescribed. The nurse must also be sure that the medication was taken. Sometimes an older patient may hold the medication in the mouth and then remove it after the nurse leaves the bedside. The patient may save the medication in case he or she needs it later. This could cause an overdose.

The nurse should observe the patient after administering the medication for any unusual symptoms and record these observations on the patient's chart. The patient's physician must be notified if serious symptoms occur.

BOX 19-2 ■ SIX RIGHTS OF MEDICATION ADMINISTRATION

1. Drug
2. Dose
3. Patient
4. Route
5. Time
6. Documentation

Administration of medications is one of the most important responsibilities of the nurse. However, without good skin care, oral hygiene, body alignment and exercise, and a well-balanced diet, the patient will not maintain the potential for health and a satisfying life. Care of the whole person is essential for health and well-being.

Remember, the elderly should be viewed as experienced and mature adults, no matter what the functional state of the body. The older adult is using the Internet more and more for health education information. Older adults are capable of learning, but their learning is most successful when there is no time constraint. Allow for plenty of time for their learning to take place and relate the new material to something familiar, if possible. For these reasons discharge planning needs to be done *before the day of discharge.* When teaching the elderly, use visual material, simple language, and large print and involve their support persons. The elderly should be encouraged to administer their own medications in the hospital if possible. This allows the nurse to answer questions and assess the level of learning that has occurred.

CHAPTER

20

Home Care Considerations in the Administration of Medications

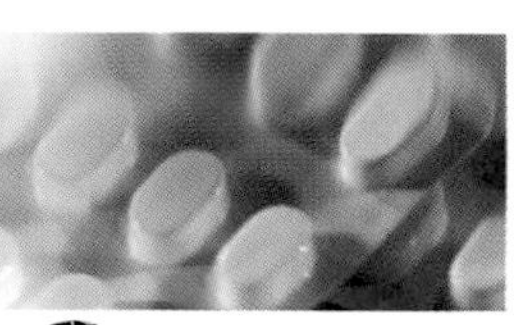

LEARNING OBJECTIVES

On completion of the materials provided in this chapter, you will be able to:

1. Understand the unique issues of nursing practice in a home care setting
2. Understand the administration of intravenous therapy in a home care setting

HOME HEALTH NURSING

Home health nursing is one of the fastest growing sectors in the health care industry. Quality nursing care is being delivered to patients in their homes to promote cost-effective health care. These services may be provided on a scheduled or intermittent basis. Home health care is often more conducive to restoring or maintaining a patient's quality of life. Patient satisfaction may also be increased by being at home rather than separated from family in an acute-care setting.

Nurses working in the field of home care enjoy an increase in autonomy of practice. They must have a medical-surgical background (usually 1 year of clinical experience) and be able to demonstrate expert critical thinking skills. These skills include assessment, communication, judgment, and problem solving. Home care nurses need to be self-directed. Their patients are more likely to need specialized care because of the shortened length of stays in hospitals, resulting in an increase in the technology used in the home. These nurses need to be independent and innovative in their practice. The technical skills required of them are often the same as for nurses working in intensive care units. Many states require home care agencies to have nurses available 24 hours a day.

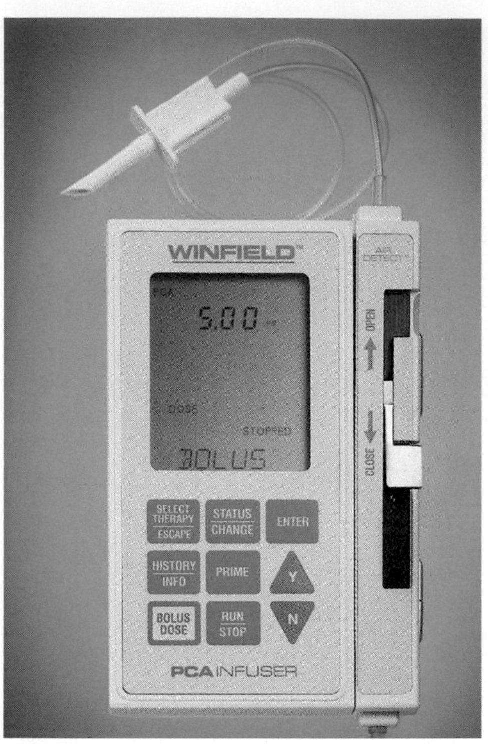

FIGURE 20-1 Ambulatory infusion pump with patient-controlled analgesia (PCA). (From Elkin MK, Perry AG, Potter PA: *Nursing interventions & clinical skills,* ed 2, St Louis, 2000, Mosby.)

BOX 20-1 ■ SIX RIGHTS OF MEDICATION ADMINISTRATION

1. Drug
2. Dose
3. Patient
4. Route
5. Time
6. Documentation

Home care nursing may involve dressing changes, tracheostomy and/or ventilator care, patient/family teaching, bathing, rehabilitation services, and hospice care. However, the home infusion market is the area of greatest growth in home care. This involves the administration and management of medications in the home. Administration of intravenous medications at home costs substantially less than it would in a hospital. The design of portable infusion pumps has improved the safety, accuracy, and ease of home infusion therapy (Figures 20-1 and 20-2).

The principles of medication administration are the same in the home setting as in a hospital. The physician writes the order for the medication. Medication calculations are done in exactly the same way as discussed earlier in this book. The guiding principles include the six rights of medication administration (Box 20-1). The nurse must follow the rights as discussed in Chapter 9, "Interpretation of the Physician's Orders."

The sixth right of *documentation* is also required in home administration of medications. This is not only for a legal record; it also plays a significant role in cost reimbursement and

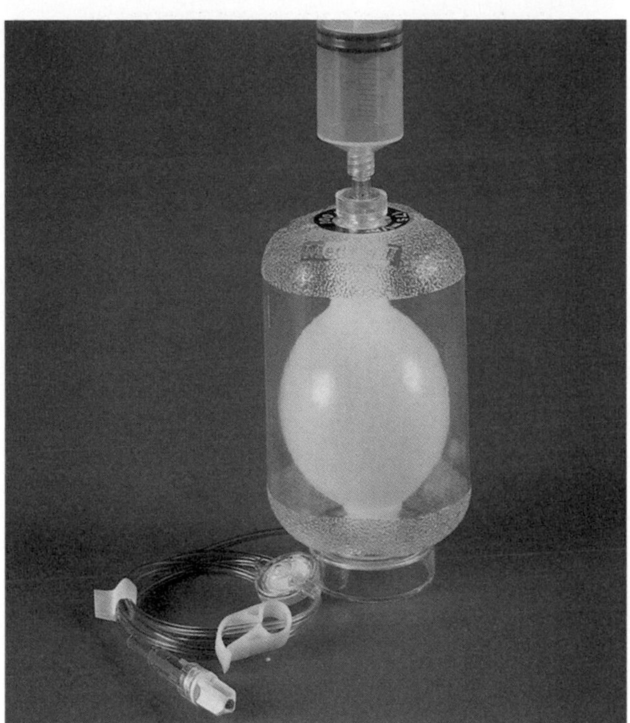

FIGURE 20-2 MedFlo® Postoperative Pain Management System ambulatory infusion device. (Courtesy Smith & Nephew Endoscopy, Andover, Maryland.)

payments. The nurse needs to be very knowledgeable about home health care policies. This information is then used to provide the clinical documentation that results in the greatest amount of reimbursement for the patient.

IV THERAPY IN THE HOME

Central Venous Catheter

A central venous catheter (CVC) is often used in home care. The CVC may be used for antibiotic therapy, fluid replacement, chemotherapy, hyperalimentation, narcotic pain control, and delivery of blood components. These devices prevent repeated venipunctures in the treatment of patients with cancer, malnutrition, and long-term antibiotic needs. Central lines may also be used for drawing blood from a patient without another needlestick.

Depending on the brand name, the CVC may be called a *Hickman, Broviac,* or *Groshong.* The line is placed by a physician using sterile technique, after local or general anesthesia has been induced. The line is threaded into a subclavian, jugular, or superior vena cava. The catheter is sutured on the outside of the body to secure placement. Before the line is used for administration of fluids or medications, a radiograph is obtained to confirm appropriate placement. A subclavian catheter is for short-term use of less than 60 days. Tunneled catheters, such as a Hickman, are for long-term use of 1 to 2 years (Figure 20-3).

Peripherally Inserted Central Catheter

A current trend in home care is to favor the use of a peripherally inserted central catheter (PICC) line. The line is inserted peripherally by a physician or specially certified nurse at the bedside, using strict aseptic technique (Figure 20-4). This catheter is used for 1 to 8 weeks of therapy. Placement should be confirmed by radiography.

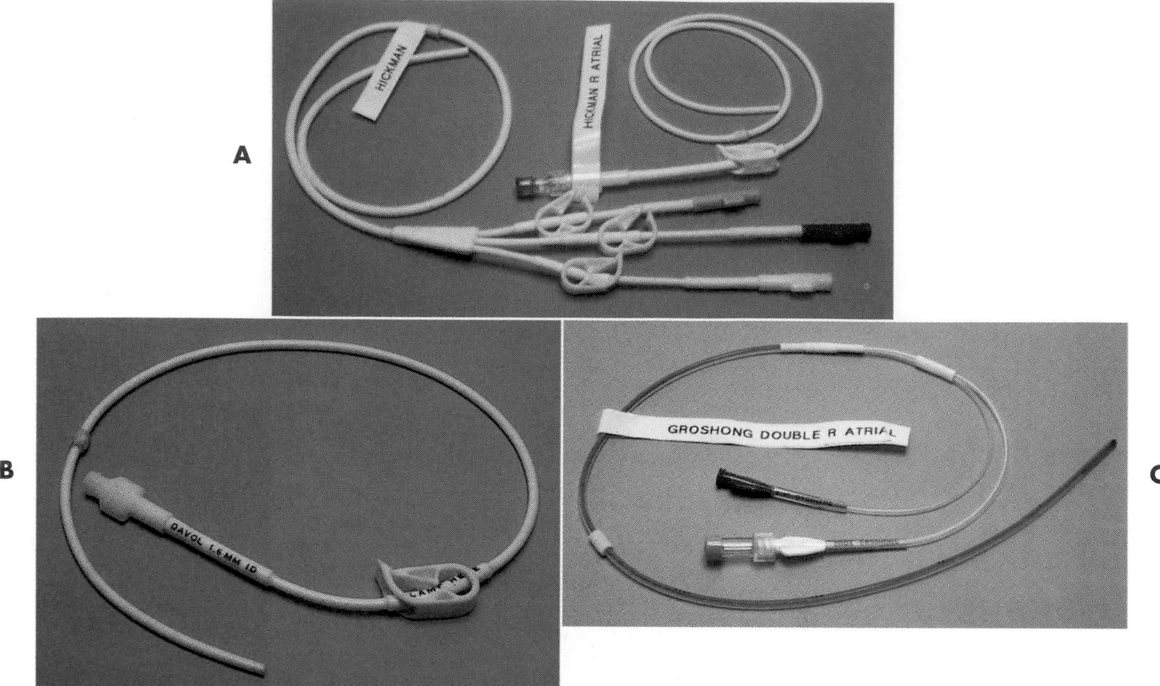

FIGURE 20-3 **A,** Hickman catheter. **B,** Brovia catheter. **C,** Groshong catheter. (From Clayton BD, Stock YN: *Basic pharmacology for nurses,* ed 12, St Louis, 2001, Mosby. Courtesy of Chuck Dresner.)

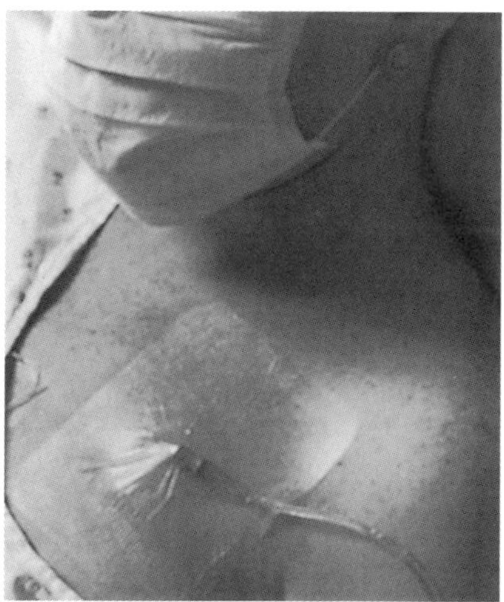

FIGURE 20-4 Continuous infusion with a peripherally inserted central catheter (PICC). (From Perry A, Potter P: *Clinical nursing skills and techniques,* ed 4, St Louis, 1998, Mosby.)

Implantable Venous Access Devices, or Ports

An implantable or subcutaneous port is placed in the subcutaneous layer beneath the skin of the patient. The port is seen as a raised area of 0.2 inch beneath the skin (Figures 20-5 and 20-6). The dome of the port is made of a self-sealing silicone septum. This access device may be used for long-term therapy of 1 to 2 years.

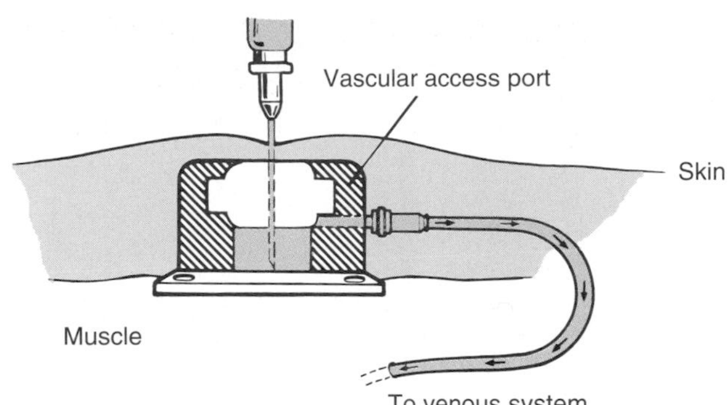

FIGURE 20-5 Example of an implantable vascular access device. (From Potter PA, Perry AG: *Fundamentals of nursing,* ed 5, St Louis, 2001, Mosby.)

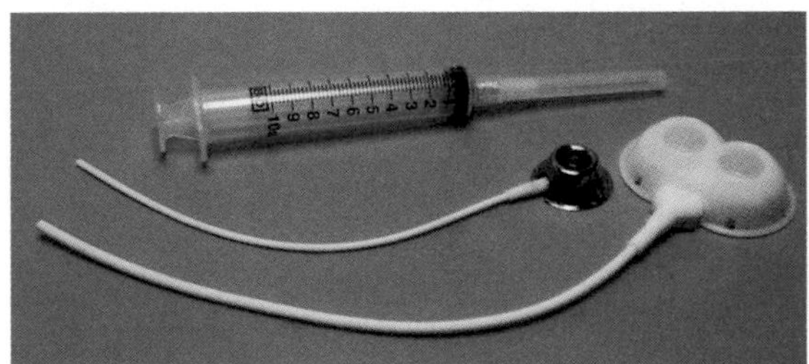

FIGURE 20-6 Silicone venous catheters with infusion ports. (From Clayton BD, Stock YN: *Basic pharmacology for nurses,* ed 12, St Louis, 2001, Mosby.)

Landmark Midline Venous Access Device

The midline catheter follows the same principle of other peripherally inserted central catheters with one exception. This catheter is inserted into the antecubital area and is advanced into the upper veins of the arm. It does not advance into the chest area. Therefore placement does not require a confirmation by radiography.

The Landmark catheter is constructed of a material called *Aquavane.* This catheter is introduced by an over-the-needle method. After placement, the Aquavane material absorbs fluid from the blood and softens. At the same time, the gauge expands and provides an increased flow rate. This catheter should also be placed by using strict aseptic technique.

Implications for Home Care Nursing

With home IV therapy, it is important that the nurse treating the patient be aware of the care and precautions required for an IV line. Routine dressing changes and assessment of the insertion site and area are mandatory. Assessment for infiltration and signs and symptoms of infection are necessary also. Education of the patient and the family is vital for the successful use of home IV therapies. Routine line care must be followed accurately to prevent clotting and infection. The patient also needs to be assessed for systemic complications such as circulatory overload and an air embolus. The routine care will be delineated by the physician and per agency policies.

For home infusion therapy to be successful, the patient and family need to be informed and educated. The areas to include are medication information, how to administer and manage the IV fluids, what complications may occur and how to handle them, principles of infection control, operation of equipment, and clear guidelines as to when to notify the physician. With physicians, nurses, patients, and families working together, true continuity of care may be attained in the home.

Name ______________________________

Date ______________________________

ACCEPTABLE SCORE 68

YOUR SCORE ______

COMPREHENSIVE POSTTEST

Directions: This test contains 39 questions with a total of 75 points (pts) possible. Each of the five separate case sections includes a variety of patient diagnoses. Test items focus on medication dosages, medication calculations, and medication transcription. Use the forms provided and mark syringes where indicated.

CASE 1 *(20 pts)*

Mr. Jones is transferred to your floor from the ICU. You receive Mr. Jones and look over his orders. It is 1700 on 2/3/07. Refer to the physician's order sheet and medication profile sheet for the following questions. Show your work where applicable.

1. Mr. Jones complains of pain to his incision. Percocet tablets are ordered on the physician's order sheet. Percocet is supplied in single tablets issued from the pharmacy. Give ______ .

(1 pt)

2. What regularly scheduled medications would Mr. Jones receive at 0900 each day? Include the amount of medication. a. ______ . b. ______ . c. ______ . d. ______ .

(4 pts)

3. How much IV fluid will Mr. Jones receive every 8 hours? ______ mL.

(1 pt)

PHYSICIAN'S ORDERS	
1. ADDRESSOGRAPH BEFORE PLACING IN PATIENT'S CHART 	Mr. Jones
2. INITIAL AND DETACH COPY EACH TIME PHYSICIAN WRITES ORDERS	
3. TRANSMIT COPY TO PHARMACY	
4. ORDERS MUST BE DATED AND TIMED	

DATE	ORDERS	TRANS BY
	Diagnosis: S/P Coronary Art. Bypass Graff Weight: 184.5# Height: 5'11"	
	Sensitivities/Drug Allergies: NKDA	
2/3/07	1. Transfer to step-down unit from ICU	
	2. VS q.4 h. × 24 hours then q.shift	
	3. Up in chair 3×day, asst. to walk in hall 2×day	
	4. I+O q.shift	
	5. Daily WT.	
	6. TED Hose	
	7. Incentive Spirometer q.1 h. while awake	
	8. Diet: 3 gm Na^+, low cholesterol	
	9. Percocet $\dot{\dot{\overline{i}}}\dot{\dot{i}}$ tabs p.o. q.4 h. p.r.n. pain	
	10. Tylenol GrX p.o. q.4 h. p.r.n. pain or Temp. >38.°	
	11. MOM 30cc p.o. q.day p.r.n. constipation	
	12. Mylanta 30cc p.o. q.4 h. p.r.n. indigestion	
	13. Restoril 15mg p.o. q.h.s. p.r.n. insomnia	
	14. $O_2$3L per nasal cannula	
	15. IVF: D_5 $^1/_2$ NS @ $50^{cc}/_{hr}$, maximum 1200 cc IVF/day	
	16. Digoxin 0.25mg p.o. q.day	
	17. E.C. ASA Gr. V p.o. q.day	
	18. Cimetidine 300mg p.o. t.i.d.	
	19. Lasix 20mg I.V. q.8 h.	
	20. Slow-K 10meq p.o. b.i.d.	
	21. Labs A_7, CBC, CXR q. a.m.	
	M. Doctor, M.D.	

Do Not Write Orders If No Copies Remain; Begin New Form **Copies Remaining**

MEDICAL RECORDS COPY				**PHYSICIAN'S ORDERS**				**T-5**
B-CLIN. NOTES	E-LAB	G-X-RAY	K-DIAGNOSTIC	M-SURGERY	Q-THERAPY	T-ORDERS	W-NURSING	Y-MISC.

4. Transcribe each as-needed (prn) medication from the physician's orders. Include date, medication, dose, route, interval, and time schedule.

(5 pts)

1												
	dose	route	interval									
2												
	dose	route	interval									
3												
	dose	route	interval									
4												
	dose	route	interval									
5												
	dose	route	interval									

5. Transcribe each regularly scheduled medication from the physician's order sheet. Include date, medication, dose, route, interval, and time schedule.

(5 pts)

1												
	dose	route	interval									
2												
	dose	route	interval									
3												
	dose	route	interval									
4												
	dose	route	interval									
5												
	dose	route	interval									

6. Mr. Jones complains of insomnia at 2300. What prn medication is available for him? _______ . How many pills will you administer? _______ .

(1 pt)

7. It is time to give Mr. Jones his Lasix. You have a premixed intravenous piggyback (IVPB) of Lasix 20 mg in 50 cc of normal saline solution (NS). Infusion time is 30 minutes. Drop factor is 60 gtt/mL. You will administer how many gtt/min? ______ .

(1 pt)

8. Mr. Jones complains of constipation. What is the medication you will give? ______ . How much will you administer? ______ .

(1 pt)

9. What regularly scheduled medications would Mr. Jones receive at 0800 each day? Include the amount of medication. Give ______ .

(1 pt)

CASE 2 *(12 pts)*

Mrs. Smith is received by you from the recovery room. You review her orders. It is 1700 on 2/3/07. Refer to the physician's order sheet for the following questions. Show your work where applicable.

1. What regularly scheduled medication(s) would Mrs. Smith receive at 0900 each day? Include the amount of medication. Give _______ .

   (2 pts)

2. Mrs. Smith complains of nausea. You have Phenergan 25 mg per 2 mL available. How many milliliters will you administer? _______ .

   (1 pt)

3. How much intravenous (IV) fluid will Mrs. Smith receive per shift? per day? _______ mL/shift. _______ mL/day.

   (2 pts)

PHYSICIAN'S ORDERS	Mrs. Smith
1. ADDRESSOGRAPH BEFORE PLACING IN PATIENT'S CHART 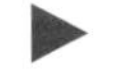	
2. INITIAL AND DETACH COPY EACH TIME PHYSICIAN WRITES ORDERS	
3. TRANSMIT COPY TO PHARMACY	
4. ORDERS MUST BE DATED AND TIMED	☐ Inpatient ☐ Outpatient

DATE	TIME	ORDERS	TRANS BY
2/3/07	1650	Diagnosis: S/P Thyroidectomy Weight: 146.0# Height: 5'10"	
		Sensitivities/Drug Allergies: PCN	
		STATUS: ASSIGN TO OBSERVATION ☐ ; ADMIT AS INPATIENT ☐	
	1.	Transfer to ward from recovery room.	
	2.	VS q.1 hour ×2 hours, then q.4 hours	
	3.	HOB ↑45 degrees	
	4.	Up in chair 3× day	
	5.	I+O q. shift	
	6.	Incentive Spirometer q.1 hour while awake	
	7.	Diet: Full liquid.	
	8.	Demerol 25mg I.M. q.4 hours p.r.n. pain	
	9.	Phenergan 12.5mg. I.M. q.4-6 hours p.r.n. nausea	
	10.	Tylenol Gr. X p.o. q.4 hours p.r.n. pain or Temp >38°C	
	11.	Restoril 15mg p.o. q.h.s. p.r.n. insomnia	
	12.	O_2 4L per nasal cannula	
	13.	IVF: NS @ $75^{cc}/_{hr}$	
	14.	Synthroid 0.15mg. p.o. q.day	
	15.	Tagamet 300mg. p.o. q.day	
	16.	Labs: Ca^+ q. 8 hours × 3 days	
		A_7, CBC q. a.m.	
	17.	JP drains × 2 to bulb suction, record output q. shift	
		M. Doctor, M.D.	

Do Not Write Orders If No Copies Remain; Begin New Form **Copies Remaining**

MEDICAL RECORDS COPY				**PHYSICIAN'S ORDERS**				**T-5**
B-CLIN. NOTES	E-LAB	G-X-RAY	K-DIAGNOSTIC	M-SURGERY	Q-THERAPY	T-ORDERS	W-NURSING	Y-MISC.

4. Mrs. Smith complains of insomnia at 2200. Restoril is supplied in 30-mg tablets. Give _______ tablet(s).

(1 pt)

5. What prn medications are available for complaints of pain? a. _______ . b. _______ .

(2 pts)

6. Your patient complains of pain shortly after she is received on the ward from the recovery room. Demerol is available 100 mg in 2 mL for injection. You will administer how many milliliters? _______ .

(1 pt)

7. Your patient has a fever of 38.1° C. You have Tylenol 325-mg tablets available. You will administer how many tablets? _______ .

(1 pt)

8. Transcribe all regularly scheduled medications from the physician's orders.

(2 pts)

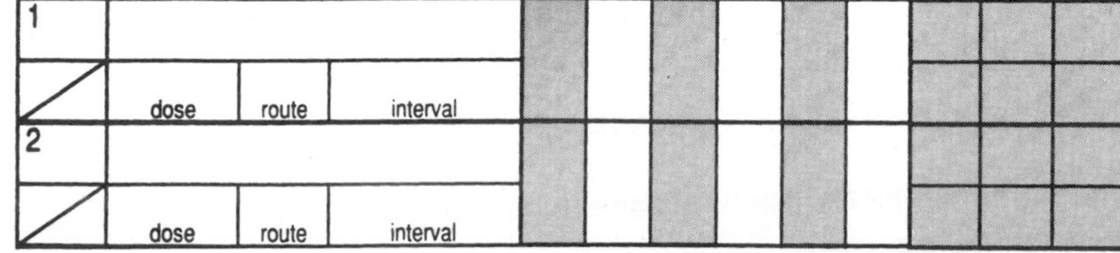

CASE 3

(11 pts)

Mrs. Hutsen is received by you after vaginal delivery childbirth without complications. Refer to the physician's order sheet for the following questions. Show your work where applicable.

PHYSICIAN'S ORDERS

1. ADDRESSOGRAPH BEFORE PLACING IN PATIENT'S CHART ▶
2. INITIAL AND DETACH COPY EACH TIME PHYSICIAN WRITES ORDERS
3. TRANSMIT COPY TO PHARMACY
4. ORDERS MUST BE DATED AND TIMED

Mrs. Hutsen

☐ Inpatient ☐ Outpatient

DATE	TIME	ORDERS	TRANS BY
4/27/07	0815	Diagnosis: S/P Childbirth Weight: 146.0# Height: 5'8"	
		Sensitivities/Drug Allergies: PCN	
		STATUS: ASSIGN TO OBSERVATION ☐; ADMIT AS INPATIENT ☐	
		Diet: Regular	
		Activity: Up ad lib $\bar{c}$ assistance as needed	
		Vital signs: Routine	
		Breast care: per protocol manual breast pump if desired.	
		Incentive spirometer ×10 breaths q.1 h. while awake	
		May shower as desired	
		If pt. unable to void within 6-8 h. or fundus boggy, bladder	
		distended, or uterus displaced, may I+O cath.	
		Notify M.D. if unable to void 6 h. after catheterization.	
		Call H.O. for Temp >38.5° C, u/o <240 cc/shift.	
		DSLR @ 50cc/hr, may D/C I.V. when tolerating p.o. well.	
		FESO4 0.3gm p.o. b.i.d.	
		Ibuprofen 600mg p.o. q.6 h. p.r.n. pain	
		Tucks to peri-area p.r.n. at bedside.	
		Senokot $\dot{\overline{\text{i}}}$ p.o. q.d. p.r.n.	
		Seconal 100 mg I.M. q.h.s. p.r.n. insomnia	
		Tylenol 650mg p.o. q.4 h. p.r.n. pain	
		M. Doctor, M.D.	

Do Not Write Orders If No Copies Remain; Begin New Form **Copies Remaining**

MEDICAL RECORDS COPY				**PHYSICIAN'S ORDERS**				**T-5**
B-CLIN. NOTES	E-LAB	G-X-RAY	K-DIAGNOSTIC	M-SURGERY	Q-THERAPY	T-ORDERS	W-NURSING	Y-MISC.

1. What regularly scheduled medication would your patient receive each day? Include the amount. _______ .

(2 pts)

2. Your patient is tolerating oral intake well. Her IV fluid was stopped 2 hours before the evening shift (1500-2330) ended. How many cubic centimeters did the patient receive on the evening shift? _______ cc.

(1 pt)

3. Your patient complains of insomnia and requests Seconal. Seconal is supplied as 200 mg per mL in a vial. How many milliliters will you administer? _______ . Mark the syringe at the appropriate amount.

(2 pts)

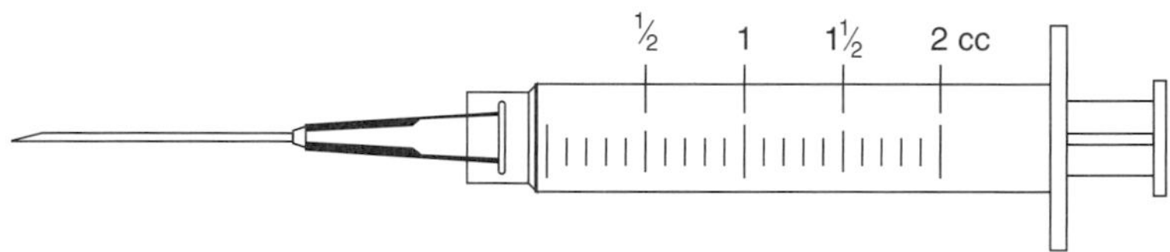

4. Your patient complains of pain and has Ibuprofen ordered. Ibuprofen is supplied as 1200-mg tablets. How many tablets will you administer? _______ .

(1 pt)

5. Transcribe all prn medications from the physician's orders.

(5 pts)

10			
	dose	route	interval
11			
	dose	route	interval
12			
	dose	route	interval
13			
	dose	route	interval
14			
	dose	route	interval

CASE 4 *(15 pts)*

J. Todd is received on your floor with a diagnosis of acute lymphocytic leukemia. Refer to the physician's order sheet for the following questions. Show your work where applicable.

PHYSICIAN'S ORDERS

1. ADDRESSOGRAPH BEFORE PLACING IN PATIENT'S CHART ▶
2. INITIAL AND DETACH COPY EACH TIME PHYSICIAN WRITES ORDERS
3. TRANSMIT COPY TO PHARMACY
4. ORDERS MUST BE DATED AND TIMED

Jason Todd

☐ Inpatient ☐ Outpatient

DATE	TIME	ORDERS	TRANS BY
10/13/07	0800	Diagnosis: Acute Lymphocytic Leukemia Weight: 28# Height: 3'0"	
		Sensitivities/Drug Allergies: Codeine	
		STATUS: ASSIGN TO OBSERVATION ☐; ADMIT AS INPATIENT ☐	
	1.	Diet: Regular	
	2.	Activity: ↑chair t.i.d., Ø rigorous play activity	
	3.	O_2–Biox to keep sats >93%	
	4.	Vital signs: q.4 h.	
	5.	I+O q. shift	
	6.	Daily WT.	
	7.	IVF: D5$^1/_2$ NS @ 25$^{cc}/_{hr.}$	
	8.	Allopurinol 50mg. p.o. t.i.d.	
	9.	Theophylline 16mg. p.o. q.6 h.	
	10.	Prednisone 2mg./kg/day	
	11.	Vincristine 5.0mg./m^2 in 50ml. of NaCl × ‡ now	
	12.	MVI ‡ q.day p.o.	
	13.	Compazine 0.07 mg./kg. I.M. q.day p.r.n. nausea	
	14.	Tylenol 120 mg. p.o. t.i.d. p.r.n. pain	
	15.	Call H.O. SBP >140<90, DBP >90<40, Temp. >38.5°C, SOB,	
		$^u/_o$ <200 ^{cc}/shift, any problems	
	16.	Labs: CBC c̄ diff., A_7, plts., CXR q.day	
		M. Doctor, M.D.	

Do Not Write Orders If No Copies Remain; Begin New Form Copies Remaining

MEDICAL RECORDS COPY			PHYSICIAN'S ORDERS					T-5
B-CLIN. NOTES	E-LAB	G-X-RAY	K-DIAGNOSTIC	M-SURGERY	Q-THERAPY	T-ORDERS	W-NURSING	Y-MISC.

1. Transcribe all regularly scheduled medications.

(4 pts)

1												
	dose	route	interval									
2												
	dose	route	interval									
3												
	dose	route	interval									
4												
	dose	route	interval									
5												
	dose	route	interval									

2. Transcribe all prn medications.

(2 pts)

7												
	dose	route	interval									
8												
	dose	route	interval									

3. Your patient requires theophylline 16 mg po q6 h. You have theophylline elixir 11.25 mg per mL available. Give _______ mL.

(1 pt)

4. Your patient requires the allopurinol dose now. You have allopurinol elixir 100 mg per 1 mL available. Give _______ mL.

(1 pt)

5. Your patient receives prednisone 2 mg/kg/day. You have 10 mg/mL available. Calculate the patient's weight in kilograms and the correct dose. _______ kg. Give _______ mL.

(2 pts)

6. Your patient requires a vincristine dosage now. The vincristine is supplied in 50 mL of NaCl to be infused over 60 minutes. Drop factor is 60 gtt/mL. _______ gtt/min.

(1 pt)

7. Your patient complains of nausea. You have Compazine 1 mg per mL available. Mark the syringe at the appropriate amount. How many milliliters will you administer? _______ . Mark the syringe at the appropriate amount.

(2 pts)

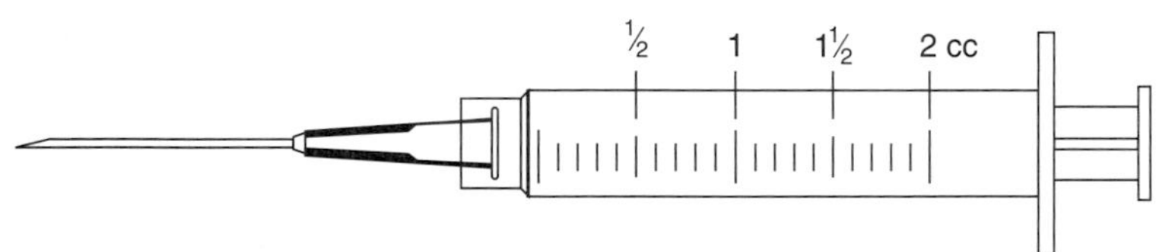

8. Your patient receives D_5 ½ NS at 25 cc/h. How much fluid will your patient receive during each 8 hour shift? _______ cc.

(1 pt)

9. Your patient complains of pain. You have Tylenol elixir 360 mg per 2 mL available. How many milliliters will you administer? _______ .

(1 pt)

CASE 5 *(18 pts)*

Mr. Miller is received on your floor from the recovery room. Refer to the physician's order sheet for the following questions. Show your work where applicable.

PHYSICIAN'S ORDERS

1. ADDRESSOGRAPH BEFORE PLACING IN PATIENT'S CHART 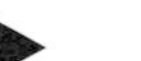
2. INITIAL AND DETACH COPY EACH TIME PHYSICIAN WRITES ORDERS
3. TRANSMIT COPY TO PHARMACY
4. ORDERS MUST BE DATED AND TIMED

Mr. Miller

☐ Inpatient ☐ Outpatient

DATE	TIME	ORDERS	TRANS BY
6/15/07	1600	Diagnosis: S/PⓇtotal hip replacement Weight: 197.0# Height: 6'2"	
		Sensitivities/Drug Allergies: NKDA	
		STATUS: ASSIGN TO OBSERVATION ☐ ; ADMIT AS INPATIENT ☐	
		Diet: NPO til fully awake, then clear liquids	
		Activity: Bedrest, log roll side-back-side q.2 h.	
		Vital signs: Every 4 hours	
		Overhead frame trapeze	
		Abductor pillow is necessary whenever pt. is supine.	
		Incentive spirometer q.1 h. while awake.	
		I+O q.8 h.	
		Hemovacs to own reservoirs, record output q.1 h. × 6 h., then q.6 h.	
		I+O catheterization q.shift p.r.n. inability to void.	
		Heparin 5,000 U. S.C. b.i.d.	
		Torecan 10mg. I.M. q.4 h. p.r.n. nausea	
		Mylanta 30cc p.o. p.r.n. indigestion	
		Restoril 15mg. p.o. q. h.s. p.r.n. insomnia	
		Tylenol c̄ codeine p.o. 1-2 tabs q.4 h. p.r.n. pain	
		Demerol PCA 10mg. I.V. q.10 minutes to maximum 250mg./4 h.	
		Dulcolax supp. ī p.r. q.shift p.r.n. constipation	
		Labs: CBC q.day × 3	
		Call Orders: Hemovac output $>500^{cc}$/shift,	
		U/o $<250^{cc}$/shift, Temp. >38.5°C, Hgb <10.0,	
		SBP >160<80, DBP >90<50.	
		IVF: D_5NS @ 50^{cc}/hr.	
		Cefuroxime 1gm. IVPB q.8 h.	
		M. Doctor, M.D.	

Do Not Write Orders If No Copies Remain; Begin New Form **Copies Remaining**

MEDICAL RECORDS COPY				**PHYSICIAN'S ORDERS**				**T-5**
B-CLIN. NOTES	E-LAB	G-X-RAY	K-DIAGNOSTIC	M-SURGERY	Q-THERAPY	T-ORDERS	W-NURSING	Y-MISC.

1. Transcribe the regularly scheduled medication below.

(2 pts)

1												
	dose	route	interval									
2												
	dose	route	interval									

2. Transcribe all prn medications ordered below.

(7 pts)

3												
	dose	route	interval									
4												
	dose	route	interval									
5												
	dose	route	interval									
6												
	dose	route	interval									
7												
	dose	route	interval									
8												
	dose	route	interval									
9												
	dose	route	interval									

3. Your patient requires 5000 U heparin SQ. You have a vial containing 10,000 U per mL. Give _______ mL. Mark the syringe at the appropriate amount.

(2 pts)

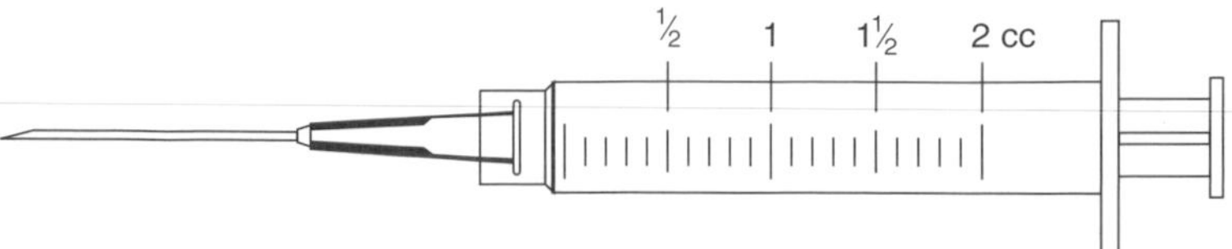

4. Your patient requires a Demerol patient-controlled analgesia (PCA) 10 mg every 10 minutes. You have a Demerol syringe with 300 mg/30 mL available. How many milliliters will the patient receive every 10 minutes? _______ mL/10 min.

(1 pt)

5. Your patient complains of nausea and requires Torecan as ordered. You have Torecan 20 mg per 2 mL available per vial. Give _______ mL.

(1 pt)

6. Your patient receives D_5 NS at 50 cc/h. How much IV fluid will your patient receive per 8-hour shift? per day? _______ /8-hour shift. _______ /day.

(2 pts)

7. Your patient receives cefuroxime 1 g in 100 cc NS IVPB 30 minutes q8 h. Drop factor is 60 gtt/mL. _______ mL/h. _______ mL/min. _______ gtt/min.

(3 pts)

Answers on pp. 519-521.

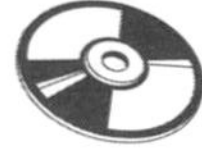

Refer to the Comprehensive Posttest on the CD for further testing of your knowledge base for calculations of all the various types of dosage problems.

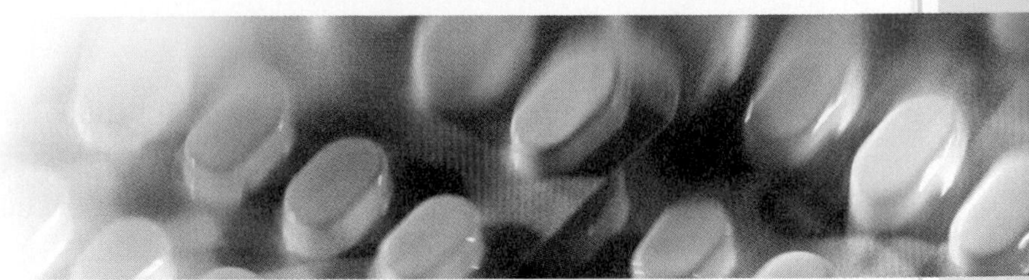

Glossary

Addends the numbers to be added

Ampule a sealed glass container; usually contains one dose of a drug

Buccal between teeth and cheek

Canceling dividing numerator and denominator by a common number

Capsule a small soluble container for enclosing a single dose of medicine

Complex Fraction a fraction whose numerator, denominator, or both contain fractions

Decimal Fraction a fraction consisting of a numerator that is expressed in numerals, a decimal point that designates the value of the denominator, and the denominator, which is understood to be 10 or some power of 10

Decimal Numbers include an integer, a decimal point, and a decimal fraction

Denominator the number of parts into which a whole has been divided

Difference the result of subtracting

Dividend the number being divided

Divisor the number by which another number is divided

Dosage the determination and regulation of the size, frequency, and number of doses

Dose the exact amount of medicine to be administered at one time

Drug a chemical substance used in therapy, diagnosis, and prevention of a disease or condition

Elixir a clear, sweet, hydroalcoholic liquid in which a drug is suspended

Equivalent equal

Extremes the first and fourth terms of a proportion

Fraction indicates the number of equal parts of a whole

Improper Fraction a fraction whose numerator is larger than or equal to the denominator

Infusion the therapeutic introduction of a fluid into a vein by the flow of gravity

Injection the therapeutic introduction of a fluid into a part of the body by force

Integer a whole number

Intramuscular within the muscle

Intravenous within the vein

Invert turn upside down

Lowest Common Denominator the smallest whole number that can be divided evenly by all denominators within the problem

Means the second and third terms of a proportion

Medicine any drug

Milliequivalent the number of grams of a solute contained in one milliliter of a normal solution

Minuend the number from which another number is subtracted

Mixed Number a combination of a whole number and a proper fraction

Multiplicand the number that is to be multiplied

Multiplier the number that another number is to be multiplied by

Numerator the number of parts of a divided whole

Oral Dosage a medication taken by mouth

Parenteral Dosage a dosage administered by routes that bypass the gastrointestinal tract and that is generally given by injection

Percent indicates the number of hundredths

Product the result of multiplying

Proper Fraction a fraction whose numerator is smaller than the denominator

Proportion two ratios that are of equal value and are connected by a double colon

Quotient the answer to a division problem

Ratio the relationship between two numbers that are connected by a colon

Reconstitution the return of a medication to its previous state by the addition of water or other designated liquid

Subcutaneous beneath the skin

Sublingual under the tongue

Subtrahend the number being subtracted

Sum the result of adding

Suspension a liquid in which a drug is distributed

Syrup a sweet, thick, aqueous liquid in which a drug is suspended

Tablet a drug compressed into a small disk

Topical on top of the skin or mucous membrane

Unit the amount of a drug needed to produce a given result

Vial a glass container with a rubber stopper; usually contains a number of doses of a drug

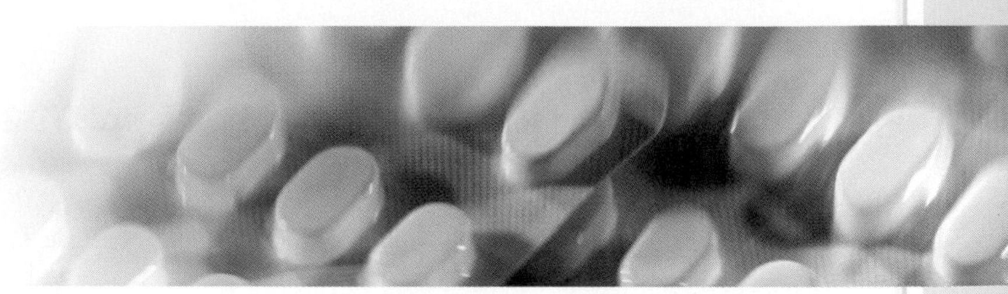

Answer Key

PART I REVIEW OF MATHEMATICS

Mathematics Review Pretest, pp. 3-6

1. $\frac{17}{24}$
2. $4\frac{2}{21}$
3. $4\frac{9}{40}$
4. 4.364
5. 34.659
6. $\frac{23}{30}$
7. $1\frac{5}{6}$
8. 1.053
9. 0.585
10. $1\frac{5}{7}$
11. 9
12. 1.827
13. 31.79484
14. $\frac{18}{25}$
15. $\frac{2}{15}$
16. $\frac{33}{80}$
17. 25.9924
18. 21.373
19. 6.4771
20. 0.003
21. 0.45
22. 0.0072
23. 0.058
24. 0.155
25. 0.8
26. 0.249
27. 2.99
28. 0.625
29. 0.68
30. $\frac{3}{8}$
31. $\frac{1}{20}$
32. 43.2%
33. $\frac{13}{20}$
34. 3 : 1000
35. 20%
36. 0.15
37. 292.5
38. 3 : 14
39. 9 : 16
40. 17 : 50
41. 400
42. 5
43. 24
44. $7\frac{1}{5}$ or 7.2
45. 20
46. 100
47. 500
48. 51
49. $2\frac{1}{2}$ or 2.5
50. 68

Chapter 1 Fractions—Pretest, pp. 7-8

1. $1\frac{10}{63}$
2. $10\frac{2}{3}$
3. $9\frac{3}{4}$
4. $5\frac{9}{16}$
5. $9\frac{1}{22}$
6. $7\frac{8}{9}$
7. $5\frac{23}{24}$
8. $\frac{3}{10}$
9. $\frac{7}{8}$
10. $2\frac{5}{8}$
11. $2\frac{17}{24}$
12. $1\frac{5}{6}$
13. $1\frac{4}{5}$
14. $1\frac{5}{6}$
15. $\frac{1}{15}$
16. 5
17. $7\frac{19}{63}$
18. $1\frac{1}{14}$
19. $\frac{1}{10,000}$
20. $4\frac{5}{18}$
21. $12\frac{1}{12}$
22. $2\frac{25}{28}$
23. $\frac{5}{16}$
24. $1\frac{1}{3}$
25. $33\frac{1}{3}$
26. $\frac{7}{8}$
27. $1\frac{1}{3}$
28. $\frac{5}{9}$
29. $1\frac{7}{10}$
30. 2

Chapter 1 Fractions—Work Sheet, pp. 21-24

Improper fractions to mixed numbers, p. 21

1. $1\frac{1}{3}$
2. 3
3. $3\frac{1}{5}$
4. $3\frac{1}{4}$
5. $1\frac{1}{2}$
6. $1\frac{1}{8}$
7. $1\frac{2}{3}$
8. $2\frac{1}{6}$
9. $3\frac{1}{2}$
10. $1\frac{3}{8}$
11. $3\frac{1}{2}$
12. $1\frac{3}{25}$

Mixed numbers to improper fractions, p. 21

1. $\frac{3}{2}$
2. $\frac{15}{4}$
3. $\frac{8}{3}$
4. $\frac{17}{6}$
5. $\frac{8}{5}$
6. $\frac{25}{7}$
7. $\frac{39}{8}$
8. $\frac{307}{100}$
9. $\frac{27}{10}$
10. $\frac{53}{8}$
11. $\frac{28}{25}$
12. $\frac{17}{4}$

Addition, p. 22

1. $1\frac{1}{2}$
2. $\frac{29}{35}$
3. $3\frac{19}{24}$
4. $3\frac{1}{4}$
5. $5\frac{13}{20}$
6. $3\frac{5}{39}$
7. $7\frac{5}{8}$
8. $6\frac{17}{22}$
9. $6\frac{4}{9}$
10. $6\frac{11}{30}$
11. 9
12. $8\frac{7}{30}$

Subtraction, pp. 22-23

1. $\frac{5}{21}$
2. $\frac{9}{16}$
3. $\frac{7}{48}$
4. $\frac{1}{2}$
5. $1\frac{1}{10}$
6. $1\frac{15}{16}$
7. $\frac{5}{8}$
8. $1\frac{1}{3}$
9. $2\frac{5}{8}$
10. $1\frac{5}{12}$
11. $1\frac{19}{24}$
12. $\frac{15}{16}$

Multiplication, p. 23

1. $\frac{4}{15}$
2. $\frac{7}{12}$
3. 4
4. $1\frac{1}{2}$
5. $8\frac{3}{4}$
6. $11\frac{7}{8}$
7. $12\frac{11}{16}$
8. $1\frac{25}{32}$
9. $\frac{1}{5}$
10. $\frac{3}{1000}$
11. $6\frac{5}{12}$
12. $3\frac{1}{9}$

Division, p. 24

1. $\frac{10}{21}$
2. $2\frac{1}{5}$
3. $1\frac{5}{9}$
4. $2\frac{1}{2}$
5. $1\frac{23}{26}$
6. $1\frac{7}{20}$
7. $1\frac{7}{11}$
8. $3\frac{47}{51}$
9. $3\frac{1}{2}$
10. $2\frac{5}{17}$
11. $2\frac{1}{16}$
12. $1\frac{1}{2}$

Chapter 1 Fractions—Posttest 1, pp. 25-26

1. $1\frac{1}{9}$
2. $\frac{17}{24}$
3. $5\frac{1}{12}$
4. $3\frac{2}{21}$
5. $\frac{39}{50}$
6. $8\frac{3}{20}$
7. $7\frac{7}{12}$
8. $\frac{9}{10}$
9. $\frac{5}{6}$
10. $\frac{3}{14}$
11. $1\frac{15}{16}$
12. $1\frac{31}{63}$
13. $5\frac{7}{10}$
14. $1\frac{1}{12}$
15. $\frac{9}{14}$
16. $2\frac{2}{5}$
17. 2
18. $3\frac{5}{24}$
19. $3\frac{1}{3}$
20. $14\frac{7}{10}$
21. $3\frac{18}{35}$
22. $\frac{7}{8}$
23. $1\frac{1}{15}$
24. 10
25. $\frac{2}{3}$
26. $1\frac{1}{4}$
27. $\frac{3}{5}$
28. $1\frac{7}{20}$
29. $4\frac{1}{2}$
30. $1\frac{3}{22}$

Chapter 1 Fractions—Posttest 2, pp. 27-28

1. $1\frac{1}{12}$
2. $4\frac{1}{10}$
3. $3\frac{2}{21}$
4. $5\frac{11}{40}$
5. $4\frac{19}{24}$
6. $11\frac{4}{5}$
7. $3\frac{1}{2}$
8. $\frac{1}{9}$
9. $1\frac{7}{8}$
10. $1\frac{5}{6}$
11. $2\frac{5}{16}$
12. $1\frac{1}{2}$
13. $3\frac{9}{10}$
14. $\frac{3}{5}$
15. $\frac{4}{21}$
16. $6\frac{1}{5}$
17. $1\frac{1}{3}$
18. $1\frac{17}{18}$
19. $\frac{1}{1000}$
20. 36
21. $3\frac{1}{2}$
22. $11\frac{1}{4}$
23. $\frac{27}{32}$
24. $\frac{21}{26}$
25. $6\frac{2}{9}$
26. $\frac{1}{49}$
27. $\frac{5}{8}$
28. $\frac{21}{32}$
29. $1\frac{11}{16}$
30. $1\frac{1}{8}$

Chapter 2 Decimals—Pretest, pp. 29-31

1. Four hundredths
2. One and six tenths
3. Sixteen and six thousand seven hundred thirty-four hundred thousandths
4. One and fifteen thousandths
5. Nine thousandths
6. 0.02
7. 0.004
8. 1.6
9. 2.082
10. 0.003
11. 25.376
12. 324.3
13. 1012.867
14. 150.6736
15. 84.565
16. 1.078
17. 1.008
18. 759.4
19. 1.7
20. 10.946
21. 0.0567
22. 6.6472
23. 1.9425
24. 29.5336
25. 186.543
26. 0.21
27. 17.95
28. 0.01
29. 627
30. 0.02
31. $\frac{1}{125}$
32. $\frac{1}{4}$
33. $\frac{161}{500}$
34. $\frac{1}{250}$
35. $\frac{17}{50}$
36. 0.6
37. 0.67
38. 0.01
39. 0.35
40. 0.625, 0.63

Chapter 2 Decimals—Work Sheet, pp. 41-46

1. Two tenths
2. Nine and sixty-eight hundredths
3. Three ten thousandths
4. One thousand nine hundred sixty-eight and three hundred forty-two thousandths
5. Two hundredths
6. 0.25
7. 0.45
8. 0.98
9. 0.68
10. 1.8
11. 7.44
12. 0.6
13. 0.0003
14. 1.0022
15. 0.08
16. 0.007
17. 3.006

Addition, pp. 41-42

1. 41.755
2. 372.675
3. 40.9787
4. 39.073
5. 894.842
6. 67.137
7. 26.62
8. 37.9
9. 55.117
10. 142.218

Subtraction, p. 42

1. 1257.87
2. 1.849
3. 0.71
4. 174.804
5. 7.418
6. 4.144
7. 0.461
8. 0.988
9. 62.022
10. 287.371

Multiplication, p. 43

1. 16.25
2. 609.6
3. 52.052
4. 56.1144
5. 41.92
6. 33.6
7. 103.983
8. 409.0318
9. 0.15113
10. 23.5971

Multiply by 10, p. 43

1. 0.9
2. 2.0
3. 1.8
4. 3.0
5. 6.25
6. 23.3

Multiply by 100, p. 43

1. 2.3
2. 150
3. 0.4
4. 12.5
5. 865
6. 7640

Multiply by 1000, p. 43

1. 200
2. 5
3. 187
4. 9650
5. 460
6. 489

Multiply by 0.1, p. 44

1. 3.0
2. 0.069
3. 0.17
4. 0.095
5. 0.0138
6. 0.567

Multiply by 0.01, p. 44

1. 0.0026
2. 0.908
3. 0.055
4. 0.112
5. 0.00875
6. 0.633

Multiply by 0.001, p. 44

1. 0.056
2. 0.01255
3. 0.1265
4. 0.0333
5. 0.009684
6. 0.241

Round to the nearest tenth, p. 44

1. 0.3
2. 0.9
3. 2.4
4. 0.7
5. 58.4
6. 8.1

Round to the nearest hundredth, p. 44

1. 2.56
2. 4.28
3. 0.28
4. 3.92
5. 6.53
6. 2.99

Round to the nearest thousandth, p. 44

1. 27.863
2. 5.925
3. 2.157
4. 0.849
5. 321.087
6. 455.768

Division, pp. 44-45

1. 1.17
2. 4140
3. 7.8
4. 400
5. 0.02
6. 0.13
7. 82.6
8. 4.53
9. 0.48
10. 2.52

Divide by 10, p. 45

1. 0.6
2. 0.02
3. 0.98
4. 0.005
5. 0.0375
6. 0.099

Divide by 100, p. 45

1. 0.007
2. 0.0811
3. 7
4. 0.0019
5. 0.12
6. 0.302

Divide by 1000, p. 45

1. 0.0018
2. 0.36
3. 0.00025
4. 0.0546
5. 0.0075
6. 7.14

Divide by 0.1, p. 45

1. 28
2. 1
3. 6.5
4. 9.87
5. 150
6. 82.5

Divide by 0.01, p. 45

1. 3600
2. 16
3. 48
4. 959
5. 80
6. 9.7

Divide by 0.001, p. 45

1. 6200
2. 839,000
3. 5000
4. 860
5. 13,800
6. 15.6

Decimal fractions to proper fractions, p. 46

1. $\frac{3}{50}$
2. $\frac{4}{5}$
3. $\frac{17}{25}$
4. $\frac{1}{400}$
5. $\frac{5}{8}$
6. $\frac{1}{4}$
7. $\frac{16}{25}$
8. $\frac{1}{200}$
9. $\frac{1}{100}$
10. $\frac{11}{250}$

Proper fractions to decimal fractions, p. 46

1. 0.125, 0.13
2. 0.67
3. 0.64
4. 0.6
5. 0.04
6. 0.33
7. 0.8
8. 0.875, 0.88
9. 0.01
10. 0.83

Chapter 2 Decimals—Posttest 1, pp. 47-48

1. Six hundred thirty-four and eighteen hundredths
2. Nine tenths
3. Sixty-four and two hundred thirty-one thousandths
4. 0.15
5. 0.6666
6. 54.66
7. 8.89
8. 6.352
9. 6.104
10. 2152.626
11. 0.339
12. 1.4532
13. 323.08
14. 43.6077
15. 0.211
16. 702.4472
17. 0.13904
18. 162
19. 44.278
20. 0.585
21. 16.8
22. 1481.67
23. 627
24. 1.41
25. 55.19
26. $\frac{9}{100}$
27. $\frac{1}{400}$
28. $\frac{3}{8}$
29. $\frac{2}{5}$
30. $\frac{3}{500}$
31. 0.71
32. 0.01
33. 0.004
34. 0.125, 0.13
35. 0.09

Chapter 2 Decimals—Posttest 2, pp. 49-50

1. Five hundred sixteen thousandths
2. Four and two ten thousandths
3. One hundred twenty-three and sixty-nine hundredths
4. 0.86
5. 1.222
6. 456.8191
7. 16.055
8. 33.209
9. 47.725
10. 339
11. 612.969
12. 0.587
13. 2.766
14. 2.513
15. 1.085
16. 167.04
17. 104,552
18. 1.01574
19. 83.2
20. 161.975
21. 1.11
22. 5
23. 15,500
24. 0.30
25. 2.47
26. $\frac{1}{200}$
27. $\frac{7}{20}$
28. $\frac{1}{8}$
29. $\frac{17}{20}$
30. $\frac{3}{5}$
31. 0.17
32. 0.003
33. 0.875, 0.88
34. 0.007
35. 0.008

Chapter 3 Percents—Pretest, pp. 51-53

Fractions to percents, p. 51

1. $1\frac{2}{3}\%$, 1.6666%
2. $71\frac{3}{7}\%$, 71.4285%
3. $12\frac{1}{2}\%$, 12.5%
4. 30%
5. $133\frac{1}{3}\%$, 133.3333%

Decimals to percents, p. 51

6. 0.6%
7. 35%
8. 42.7%
9. 382.1%
10. 70%

Percents to fractions, p. 52

11. $\frac{1}{200}$
12. $\frac{3}{4}$
13. $\frac{19}{200}$
14. $\frac{31}{125}$
15. $\frac{3}{800}$

Percents to decimals, p. 52

16. 0.0116
17. 0.075
18. 0.133
19. 0.0088
20. 0.63

What percent of, pp. 52-53

21. 375%
22. $16\frac{2}{3}\%$, 16.6666%
23. 65%
24. $\frac{1}{5}\%$, 0.2%
25. $33\frac{1}{3}\%$, 33.333%
26. $12\frac{32}{189}\%$, 12.1693%
27. $43\frac{7}{26}\%$, 43.2692%
28. 10%
29. $7\frac{1}{7}\%$, 7.1428%
30. $1\frac{209}{291}\%$, 1.7182%

What is, p. 53

31. 1.8
32. 0.15
33. 2.565
34. 0.68
35. 3.08
36. 4.278
37. 0.05999
38. 19.36
39. 11.856
40. 15

Chapter 3 Percents—Work Sheet, pp. 61-63

Fractions to percents, p. 61

1. 75%
2. $37\frac{1}{2}\%$
3. 80%
4. 32%
5. $\frac{3}{10}\%$
6. $3\frac{1}{2}\%$
7. $2\frac{1}{4}\%$
8. 15%
9. 6%
10. $68\frac{3}{4}\%$
11. $83\frac{1}{3}\%$
12. $\frac{3}{4}\%$

Decimals to percents, p. 61

1. 40.2%
2. 3.67%
3. 16.3%
4. 98%
5. 30%
6. 14.5%
7. 70%
8. 42%
9. 15.9%
10. 67.3%
11. 37.12%
12. 220%

Percents to fractions, p. 62

1. $\frac{7}{200}$
2. $\frac{3}{400}$
3. $\frac{1}{800}$
4. $\frac{1}{10}$
5. $\frac{1}{150}$
6. $\frac{101}{500}$
7. $\frac{3}{25}$
8. $\frac{1}{400}$
9. $\frac{19}{800}$
10. $\frac{1}{16}$
11. $\frac{21}{1000}$
12. $\frac{2}{3}$

Percents to decimals, p. 62

1. 0.375
2. 0.03
3. 0.0675
4. 0.0042
5. 0.0025
6. 0.025
7. 0.0023
8. 0.726
9. 0.16
10. 0.003125
11. 0.005
12. 0.0058

What percent of, p. 63

1. 55%
2. $7\frac{7}{8}\%$, 7.875%
3. 2%
4. 12%
5. 5%
6. 15%
7. 20%
8. 10%
9. 45%
10. 1%
11. $2\frac{2}{25}\%$, 2.08%
12. 20%

What is, p. 63

1. 119.5
2. 3.4
3. 14.28
4. 0.14
5. 999.9 or 1000
6. 0.13
7. 0.585
8. 0.12
9. 540.02
10. 0.17
11. 11.07
12. 10.752

Chapter 3 Percents—Posttest 1, pp. 65-66

Fractions to percents, p. 65

1. $87\frac{1}{2}\%$, 87.5%
2. 55%
3. $\frac{3}{10}\%$, 0.3%

Decimals to percents, p. 65

4. 25.6%
5. 0.4%
6. 90%

Percents to fractions, p. 65

7. 17/20
8. 3/1000
9. 7/200

Percents to decimals, p. 65

10. 0.863
11. 0.04625
12. 0.0036

What percent of, pp. 65-66

13. 10%
14. 5%
15. 1/3%, 0.33%
16. 12%
17. 42 6/7%, 42.8571%
18. 20%
19. 50%
20. 7 1/2%, 7.5%
21. 8%

What is, p. 66

22. 520
23. 36
24. 0.09
25. 170
26. 42.3
27. 292.5
28. 0.15
29. 2.408
30. 0.4576

Chapter 3 Percents—Posttest 2, pp. 67-68

Fractions to percents, p. 67

1. 12 1/2%, 12.5%
2. 40%
3. 16 2/3%, 16.6666%

Decimals to percents, p. 67

4. 6.5%
5. 0.5%
6. 20%

Percents to fractions, p. 67

7. 3/1000
8. 33/200
9. 1/400

Percents to decimals, p. 67

10. 0.0375
11. 0.07
12. 0.0555

What percent of, pp. 67-68

13. 22 2/9%, 22.2222%
14. 50%
15. 2 2/5%, 2.4%
16. 80%
17. 7 1/2%, 7.5%
18. 10%
19. 41 7/23%, 41.3043%
20. 12 1/2%, 12.5%
21. 126 62/63%, 126.9841%

What is, p. 68

22. 227.5
23. 0.29
24. 42.3
25. 9.68
26. 14.4
27. 19.575
28. 10.9215
29. 0.56
30. 97.232

Chapter 4 Ratios—Pretest, p. 69

1. 1/3, 0.3333, 33.33%
2. 143 : 200, 143/200, 71.5%
3. 2 : 5, 0.4, 40%
4. 1 : 8, 1/8, 0.125
5. 1/20, 0.05, 5%
6. 5 : 32, 0.15625, 15.625%
7. 143 : 500, 143/500, 28.6%
8. 5 : 7, 5/7, 0.714
9. 13 : 80, 13/80, 0.1625
10. 231 : 500, 231/500, 46.2%

Chapter 4 Ratios—Work Sheet, pp. 75-78

Fractions to ratios, p. 75

1. 3 : 4
2. 2 : 3
3. 1 : 2
4. 14 : 25
5. 2 : 5
6. 31 : 100
7. 5 : 8
8. 1 : 4
9. 16 : 27
10. 10 : 1
11. 7 : 30
12. 1 : 1

Decimals to ratios, pp. 75-76

1. 112 : 125
2. 24 : 25
3. 3 : 50
4. 3 : 5
5. 252 : 625
6. 37 : 50
7. 83 : 500
8. 13 : 50
9. 123 : 250
10. 19 : 20
11. 47 : 200
12. 43 : 250

Percents to ratios, p. 76

1. 1 : 10
2. 1 : 3
3. 3 : 800
4. 27 : 1000
5. 11 : 25
6. 157 : 1000
7. 31 : 400
8. 11 : 2500
9. 39 : 500
10. 1 : 100
11. 3 : 500
12. 6 : 175

Ratios to fractions, p. 77

1. $\frac{1}{16}$
2. $\frac{1}{200}$
3. $\frac{1}{50}$
4. $1\frac{1}{2}$
5. 1
6. $\frac{1}{3}$
7. $3\frac{1}{5}$
8. $\frac{1}{2}$
9. $\frac{8}{45}$
10. $1\frac{6}{11}$
11. $\frac{37}{67}$
12. $\frac{82}{127}$

Ratios to decimal numbers, pp. 77-78

1. 0.5
2. 0.25
3. 0.375
4. 0.3333
5. 6.25
6. 0.5
7. 1.5
8. 0.1
9. 0.4
10. 0.9
11. 0.027
12. 3.5

Ratios to percents, p. 78

1. 50%
2. $3\frac{1}{33}$%, 3.0303%
3. 10%
4. 20%
5. $37\frac{1}{27}$%, 37.037%
6. $\frac{1}{10}$%, 0.1%
7. 25%
8. $52\frac{1}{12}$%, 52.0833%
9. $\frac{1}{5}$%, 0.2%
10. $66\frac{2}{3}$%, 66.6666%
11. $55\frac{5}{9}$%, 55.5555%
12. $2133\frac{1}{3}$%, 2133.3333%

Chapter 4 Ratios—Posttest 1, p. 79

1. $\frac{7}{8}$, 0.875, 87.5%
2. 1 : 250, $\frac{1}{250}$, 0.4%
3. 13 : 20, 0.65, 65%
4. 9 : 400, $\frac{9}{400}$, 0.0225
5. 7 : 20, $\frac{7}{20}$, 35%
6. 6 : 25, 0.24, 24%
7. $\frac{27}{40}$, 0.675, 67.5%
8. 3 : 1000, $\frac{3}{1000}$, 0.003
9. 41 : 200, $\frac{41}{200}$, 20.5%
10. 4 : 11, 0.3636, 36.36%

Chapter 4 Ratios—Posttest 2, p. 81

1. $\frac{7}{10}$, 0.7, 70%
2. 5 : 16, 0.3125, 31.25%
3. 3 : 40, $\frac{3}{40}$, 7.5%
4. 3 : 50, $\frac{3}{50}$, 0.06
5. 3 : 800, $\frac{3}{800}$, 0.00375
6. 1 : 150, 0.0066, 0.66%
7. 7 : 1000, $\frac{7}{1000}$, 0.7%
8. $\frac{2}{7}$, 0.2857, 28.57%
9. 161 : 500, $\frac{161}{500}$, 32.2%
10. 91 : 500, $\frac{91}{500}$, 0.182

Chapter 5 Proportions—Pretest, pp. 83-84

1. 100
2. $7\frac{1}{2}$ or 7.5
3. $\frac{1}{600}$
4. 3.2
5. 128
6. 4
7. 400 or 399.9
8. $\frac{1}{2}$
9. $\frac{3}{7}$
10. 8
11. 80
12. $\frac{1}{6}$
13. 14
14. 48
15. $\frac{3}{10}$
16. 80
17. 10
18. 126
19. $\frac{1}{150}$
20. $16\frac{1}{4}$ or 16.25

Chapter 5 Proportions—Work Sheet, pp. 89-92

1. 84
2. 28.125
3. $1\frac{1}{5}$
4. $52\frac{1}{2}$
5. $1\frac{1}{2}$ or 1.5
6. $\frac{3}{4}$
7. 1
8. $4\frac{4}{5}$
9. $1\frac{1}{2}$
10. 2000
11. 1
12. 80
13. 600
14. 40
15. 0.032
16. 0.2
17. 960
18. 25
19. 20
20. $\frac{1}{2}$ or 0.5
21. 1.2
22. 1.17
23. 3
24. 15
25. 48
26. 0.9
27. 16
28. 6
29. $1\frac{1}{3}$
30. 3.6
31. 450
32. $\frac{657}{1100}$ or 0.597
33. $\frac{3}{5}$ or 0.6
34. $2\frac{7}{10}$
35. 171.43
36. 500
37. 10
38. $12\frac{1}{2}$ or 12.5
39. 240
40. $18\frac{3}{4}$
41. 6
42. 180
43. $12\frac{1}{2}$
44. 80
45. $\frac{1}{32}$, 0.03125
46. 1620

Chapter 5 Proportions—Posttest 1, pp. 93-94

1. 2
2. $\frac{35}{48}$
3. 6
4. 6.25
5. 32
6. $\frac{1}{2}$
7. $2\frac{1}{2}$ or 2.5
8. 2
9. $\frac{5}{9}$
10. 36
11. 4
12. 4
13. 8
14. 1500
15. 42
16. $\frac{4}{9}$
17. 4
18. 100
19. 1
20. 3.2

Chapter 5 Proportions—Posttest 2, pp. 95-96

1. 225
2. $1\frac{7}{25}$, 1.28
3. 120
4. 6.84
5. $13\frac{1}{3}$
6. 56
7. 1
8. 3.8
9. $\frac{3}{20}$
10. 40
11. 3.6
12. 105
13. $2\frac{7}{10}$
14. $\frac{35}{72}$
15. 10
16. 360
17. 15
18. 72
19. $1\frac{2}{25}$ or 1.08
20. 150

Mathematics Review Posttest, pp. 97-101

1. mixed
   whole
2. $\frac{7}{6}$
   $\frac{6}{3}$
   $\frac{9}{9}$
3. fraction
4. $\frac{1}{2}/4$
   $\frac{3}{7}/\frac{4}{2}$
   $21/\frac{2}{3}$
5. relationship
6. two
7. 4 : 12
8. 24 : 100
9. 3 : 100
10. 13 : 8
11. 22 : 1000 or 2.2 : 100
    (same value)
12. 124 : 100
13. denominator
14. 2 / ③
15. 4 ÷ ⑧
16. 10 : ⑤
17. ④)12
18. 14 / ⑧
19. 6 ÷ ㉔
20. ㊷)7
21. 7 : ⑩
22. numerator
23. 10
24. 10
25. $\frac{436}{1000}$
26. $\frac{51}{1000}$
27. $1\frac{42}{10,000}$
28. $\frac{9684}{10,000}$
29. $\frac{19}{10,000}$
30. $1\frac{2064}{100,000}$
31. $1\frac{28}{45}$
32. $7\frac{1}{12}$
33. $5\frac{5}{6}$
34. $5\frac{1}{2}$
35. 8.52
36. 46.29
37. 234.93
38. 459.56
39. $\frac{1}{6}$
40. $1\frac{13}{21}$
41. $\frac{41}{45}$
42. $5\frac{11}{18}$
43. 23.9
44. 0.1
45. 4.1
46. 1.0
47. $5\frac{5}{8}$
48. $\frac{2}{3}$
49. $8\frac{26}{27}$
50. $26\frac{3}{5}$
51. 1.93

52. 1.97
53. 4.48
54. 181.79
55. $1\frac{31}{32}$
56. $\frac{18}{35}$
57. $\frac{1}{225}$
58. $\frac{473}{576}$
59. 5.654
60. 0.001
61. 80,000
62. 17.349
63. 0.014, 0.048, 0.407, 0.45, 1.46, 2.401
64. 0.015, 0.15, 0.155, 1.0015, 1.015, 1.15
65. 0.090, 0.90, 0.99, 9.009, 9.09, 90.90
66. 0.24, 0.4, 0.44, 0.52, 0.6, 0.7
67. 0.021, 0.1091, 0.191, 0.2, 0.201, 0.21
68. 0.83
69. 0.56
70. 0.56
71. 0.01
72. $\frac{9}{40}$
73. $\frac{93}{200}$
74. $\frac{3}{50}$
75. $\frac{93}{250}$
76. 27.5%
77. 37.5%
78. $\frac{21}{50}$
79. 62 : 10,000
80. 12.5%
81. 25%
82. 15%
83. 0.24
84. 54.6
85. 149.5
86. 2 : 9
87. 3 : 8
88. 73 : 125
89. 2 : 3
90. 12 : 25
91. 270
92. 1.68
93. 13.04
94. 1.13
95. 150
96. 484
97. 198.33
98. $533\frac{1}{3}$ or 533.33
99. 27
100. 3.75

PART II UNITS AND MEASUREMENTS FOR THE CALCULATION OF DRUG DOSAGES

Chapter 6 Metric and Household Measurements—Pretest, pp. 105-106

1. 0.8 g
2. 3000 mcg
3. 0.255 g
4. 46,000 mcg
5. 3 mg
6. 680 mg
7. 0.326 L
8. 72.6 lb
9. 2100 mg
10. 3 kg
11. 100 mL
12. 116.6 lb
13. 5 cc
14. 800 g
15. 0.25 mg
16. 300 mL
17. 10,000 g
18. 630 mL
19. 0.733 kg
20. 1,250,000 mcg
21. 0.06 g
22. 250 mcg
23. 250 mL
24. 20.45 kg
25. 0.01 g
26. 1200 g
27. 300 mL
28. 710 mg
29. 0.48 L
30. $1\frac{43}{100}$ lb

Chapter 6 Metric and Household Measurements—Work Sheet, pp. 113-116

1. 0.00023 g
2. 5000 mcg
3. 2,500,000 mcg
4. 4 mg
5. 330 mg
6. 6000 g
7. 0.725 L
8. 0.002 g
9. 30 mm
10. 0.62 kg
11. 36 mL
12. 0.46 L
13. 660 mcg
14. 500,000 mcg
15. $1\frac{1}{2}$ feet
16. 0.35 g
17. 0.025 g
18. 1460 mL
19. 2500 g
20. 12,000 mcg
21. 3400 g
22. 0.00092 g
23. 2.5 cm
24. 0.3 mg
25. 160 mL
26. 10 mg
27. 0.5 mg
28. 0.36 g
29. 1700 mL
30. 450 mg
31. 0.24 L
32. 10 mL
33. 7.5 cm
34. 405 mL
35. 320 mL
36. 160 mL
37. 270 mL
38. $17\frac{3}{5}$ lb
39. 8.415 lb
40. 17.5 cm
41. 1.36 kg
42. $26\frac{2}{5}$ lb
43. $3\frac{2}{25}$ lb
44. 30 inches
45. 68.18 kg

Chapter 6 Metric and Household Measurements—Posttest 1, pp. 117-118

1. 0.005 g
2. 10,000 mcg
3. 810 mL
4. 0.035 g
5. 30 inches
6. 120,000 mcg
7. $35\frac{1}{5}$ lb
8. 0.28 L
9. 400 g
10. $3\frac{1}{2}$ feet
11. 12727.27 g
12. 10 cm
13. 0.5 g
14. 0.037 L
15. 20 cc
16. 216 mL
17. 2500 mg
18. 12 mL
19. 6.7 kg
20. 300 mL
21. 4000 mcg
22. $5\frac{18}{25}$ lb
23. 360 mL
24. 200 mL
25. 0.533 L
26. 1,500,000 mcg
27. 0.62 g
28. 2300 g
29. $1\frac{1}{4}$ feet
30. 3.18 kg

Chapter 6 Metric and Household Measurements—Posttest 2, pp. 119-120

1. 4 mg
2. 0.15 kg
3. 450 mL
4. $1\frac{19}{25}$ lb
5. $96\frac{4}{5}$ lb
6. 0.76 g
7. 550 mL
8. 3.5 cm
9. 80 mL
10. 965.909 g
11. 100 mL
12. 32,000 mcg
13. 0.618 L
14. 0.1 g
15. $2\frac{1}{3}$ feet
16. 0.714 L
17. 0.35 g
18. 0.25 g
19. 870 mg
20. 7000 mcg
21. 0.37 mg
22. 1400 mL
23. 780 mg
24. 0.225 mg
25. 4.5 kg
26. 200 mL
27. 40 inches
28. 40 mL
29. 2,600,000 mcg
30. 33.18 kg

Chapter 7 Apothecary and Household Measurements—Pretest, p. 121

1-2. $1\frac{1}{4}$ pt, $\frac{5}{8}$ qt
3-4. 80 fl oz, $2\frac{1}{2}$ qt
5-6. $1\frac{3}{4}$ gal, 14 pt
7. 24 fl oz
8. $1\frac{1}{2}$ pt
9. 12 fl oz
10. 15 fl oz

Chapter 7 Apothecary and Household Measurements—Work Sheet, pp. 127-128

Arabic to Roman numerals, p. 127

1. xxii
2. ix
3. iii
4. xxx
5. xiv
6. vi
7. xv
8. xii

Roman to Arabic numerals, p. 127

1. 29
2. 7
3. 20
4. 6
5. 16
6. 4
7. 25
8. 240

Equivalents within the apothecary system, p. 127

1. $\frac{5}{32}$ pt
2. $\frac{15}{16}$ pt
3. 64 fl oz, 2 qt
4. 40 fl oz
5. 4 qt, 1 gal
6. 8 fl oz
7. $\frac{3}{4}$ gal, 6 pt
8. 20 pt, $2\frac{1}{2}$ gal

Household measures to equivalents in the apothecary system, p. 128

9. 16 fl oz
10. 3 fl oz
11. 26 fl oz
12. 12 fl oz

Chapter 7 Apothecary and Household Measurements—Posttest 1, p. 129

1-2. $\frac{3}{4}$ qt, $1\frac{1}{2}$ pt
3-4. 3 pt, $1\frac{1}{2}$ qt
5-6. $1\frac{1}{4}$ gal, 10 pt
7-8. 7 qt, 224 fl oz
9. 12 fl oz
10. $4\frac{1}{2}$ fl oz

Chapter 7 Apothecary and Household Measurements—Posttest 2, p. 131

1-2. 3 pt, $1\frac{1}{2}$ qt
3-4. 72 fl oz, $2\frac{1}{4}$ qt
5-6. $1\frac{1}{2}$ gal, 192 fl oz
7-8. 10 qt, 20 pt
9. 18 fl oz
10. 4 fl oz

Chapter 8 Equivalents between Apothecary and Metric Measurements—Pretest, pp. 133-134

1. 50 kg
2. 0.5 L
3. $79\frac{1}{5}$ lb
4. 5250 mL
5. 3 fl oz
6. 1.75 L
7. 6 g
8. $18\frac{1}{25}$ lb
9. 3909.0909 g
10. 1125 mL
11. 210 mL
12. 0.6666 g
13. $5\frac{1}{2}$ qt
14. $3\frac{13}{25}$ lb
15. 240 mg
16. 12 fl oz
17. $1\frac{1}{5}$ pt
18. $12\frac{1}{10}$ lb
19. $\frac{2}{3}$ fl oz
20. $\frac{1}{5}$ gr
21. 0.2 mg
22. 38.6363 kg
23. $\frac{1}{150}$ gr
24. 5.57 kg
25. $4\frac{1}{5}$ qt
26. 45 mL
27. 12 mg
28. 69 gr
29. 37.1° C
30. 105.8° F
31. 36.4° C
32. 101.3° F
33. 37.7° C
34. 103.3° F
35. 39.2° C
36. 104.4° F

Chapter 8 Equivalents between Apothecary and Metric Measurements—Work Sheet, pp. 139-141

1. $3\frac{1}{3}$ gr
2. 10 kg
3. 10 g
4. 1750 mL
5. 7 fl oz
6. 22 lb
7. $3\frac{1}{2}$ pt
8. 15 mL
9. 270 mg
10. $9\frac{6}{25}$ lb
11. 7 gr
12. 3000 mL
13. $3\frac{1}{2}$ qt
14. 300 mg
15. 5 fl oz
16. $1\frac{1}{2}$ lb
17. 3090.909 g
18. 11.25 mL
19. 165 mg
20. 2.2727 kg
21. $5\frac{2}{5}$ pt
22. $5\frac{2}{3}$ gr
23. 2.5 L
24. $8\frac{3}{100}$ lb
25. 120 mL
26. 5454.5454 g
27. 34.0909 kg
28. 2125 mL
29. $1\frac{2}{3}$ gr
30. $3\frac{1}{2}$ qt
31. 90 mg
32. 55 lb
33. 37.6° C
34. 38.8° C
35. 40.1° C
36. 36.3° C
37. 104.7° F
38. 95.7° F
39. 98.2° F
40. 102.6° F
41. 91.4° F
42. 36.9° C
43. 106.2° F
44. 39.8° C
45. 105.1° F
46. 39° C
47. 99.3° F
48. 38° C

Chapter 8 Equivalents between Apothecary and Metric Measurements—Posttest 1, pp. 143-144

1. 180 mg
2. 5 g
3. 90 mL
4. 750 mL
5. 1/4 gr
6. 1½ qt
7. 3409.0909 g
8. 1 7/10 qt
9. 0.3333 g
10. 9.0909 kg
11. 10 mg
12. 2 pt
13. 1/200 gr
14. 45 gr
15. 2 fl oz
16. 5 47/50 lb
17. 150 mL
18. 70 2/5 lb
19. 1/12 gr
20. 5.33 g
21. 2.75 L
22. 18 fl oz
23. 35.2° C
24. 96.1° F
25. 39.6° C
26. 105.4° F
27. 40.1° C
28. 99° F
29. 37.4° C
30. 92.8° F

Chapter 8 Equivalents between Apothecary and Metric Measurements—Posttest 2, pp. 145-146

1. 27.2727 kg
2. 2½ qt
3. 625 mL
4. 15 mg
5. 1¼ qt
6. 1/3 gr
7. 9.09 kg
8. 375 mL
9. 2375 mL
10. 45 gr
11. 0.5 mg
12. 0.4666 g
13. 3.5 L
14. 3 pt
15. 2 16/25 lb
16. 1/75 gr
17. 92 2/5 lb
18. 3 mg
19. 1515.1515 g
20. 15 2/5 lb
21. 19½ gr
22. 1590.909 g
23. 35.7° C
24. 100.8° F
25. 98.2° F
26. 36.6° C
27. 104.7° F
28. 38.2° C
29. 106.5° F
30. 39.6° C

PART III CALCULATION OF DRUG DOSAGES

Chapter 9 Interpretation of the Physician's Orders—Posttest, p. 155

#	Date	Medication	Dose	Route	Interval	Times				
1	1/12	Cefuroxime	1g	IV	q 8 hours	08		16		24
2	1/12	Lasix	40 mg	p.o.	b.i.d.		09		21	
3	1/12	Slow-K	10 mEq	p.o.	b.i.d.		09		21	

Chapter 10 How to Read Drug Labels—Posttest 1, pp. 161-162

1. Glucophage
   metformin hydrochloride
   500 mg
   tablets
   500 tablets
2. Diabinese
   chlorpropamide
   250 mg
   tablets
   250 tablets
3. Robinul
   glycopyrrolate
   0.4 mg/2 mL or 0.2 mg/mL
   milliliters
   IM or IV
4. Cefobid
   cefoperazone sodium
   10 g
   milliliters
   intravenous

Chapter 10 How to Read Drug Labels—Posttest 2, pp. 163-164

1. Furadantin
   nitrofurantoin
   5 mg/mL
   suspension
   oral
   60 mL
2. Decadron
   dexamethasone
   1.5 mg
   tablets
3. Capoten
   captopril
   25 mg
   tablet
   100 tablets
4. Kefzol
   cefazolin sodium
   225 mg/mL
   milliliters after reconstitution
   injection

Chapter 11 Dimensional Analysis and the Calculation of Drug Dosages—Work Sheet, pp. 172-174

1. $x \text{ tablet} = \dfrac{1 \text{ tablet}}{5 \text{ mg}} \times 10 \text{ mg}$

$x = \dfrac{1 \times 10}{5}$

$x = 2$ tablets

2. $x \text{ mL} = \dfrac{5 \text{ mL}}{25 \text{ mg}} \times 60 \text{ mg}$

$x = \dfrac{5 \times 60}{25}$

$x = 12$ mL

3. $x \text{ tablet} = \dfrac{1 \text{ tablet}}{50 \text{ mg}} \times \dfrac{1000 \text{ mg}}{1 \text{ g}} \times 0.025 \text{ g}$

$x = \dfrac{1 \times 1000 \times 0.025}{50}$

$x = \dfrac{25}{50}$

$x = \frac{1}{2}$ tablet

4. $x \text{ tablet} = \dfrac{1 \text{ tablet}}{\frac{1}{4} \text{ gr}} \times \dfrac{1 \text{ gr}}{60 \text{ mg}} \times 30 \text{ mg}$

$x = \dfrac{1 \times 1 \times 30}{\frac{1}{4} \times 60}$

$x = \dfrac{30}{15}$

$x = 2$ tablets

5. $x \text{ capsule} = \dfrac{1 \text{ capsule}}{250 \text{ mg}} \times \dfrac{1000 \text{ mg}}{1 \text{ g}} \times 0.5 \text{ g}$

$x = \dfrac{1 \times 1000 \times 0.5}{250}$

$x = \dfrac{500}{250}$

$x = 2$ capsules

6. $x \text{ mL} = \dfrac{1 \text{ mL}}{4 \text{ mg}} \times 3 \text{ mg}$

$x = \dfrac{1 \times 3}{4}$

$x = \dfrac{3}{4}$ or 0.75 mL

7. $x \text{ mL} = \dfrac{1 \text{ mL}}{0.05 \text{ mg}} \times \dfrac{1 \text{ mg}}{1000 \text{ mcg}} \times 40 \text{ µg}$

$x = \dfrac{1 \times 1 \times 40}{0.05 \times 1000}$

$x = \dfrac{40}{50}$

$x = 0.8$ mL

8. $x \text{ mL} = \dfrac{1 \text{ mL}}{2 \text{ mg}} \times 1 \text{ mg}$

$x = \dfrac{1}{2}$

$x = 0.5$ mL

9. $x \text{ mL} = \dfrac{1 \text{ mL}}{5000 \text{ U}} \times 2500 \text{ U}$

$x = \dfrac{1 \times 2500}{5000}$

$x = \dfrac{2500}{5000}$ or 0.5 mL

10. $x \text{ tablet} = \dfrac{1 \text{ tablet}}{500 \text{ mg}} \times \dfrac{1000 \text{ mg}}{1 \text{ g}} \times 2 \text{ g}$

$x = \dfrac{1 \times 1000 \times 2}{500 \times 1}$

$x = \dfrac{2000}{500}$

$x = 4$ tablets

11. $x \text{ gtt/min} = \frac{20 \times 100 \times 1}{1 \times 1 \times 60}$

$x \text{ gtt/min} = \frac{2000}{60}$

$x = 33.3$ or 33 gtt/min

12. $x \text{ gtt/min} = \frac{10 \times 500 \times 1}{1 \times 2 \times 60}$

$x \text{ gtt/min} = \frac{5000}{120}$

$x = 41.6$ or 42 gtt/min

13. $x \text{ mL/h} = \frac{250 \times 1400}{25{,}000 \times 1}$

$x \text{ mL/h} = \frac{350{,}000}{25{,}000}$

$x = 14$ mL/h

14. $x \text{ mL/h} = \frac{100 \times 8}{50 \times 1}$

$x \text{ mL/h} = \frac{800}{50}$

$x = 16$ mL/h

Chapter 12 Oral Dosages—Work Sheet, pp. 187-216

Proportion / **Formula**

1. 1 mg : 1 cap : : 2 mg : x cap
   1 : 1 : : 2 : x
   $x = 2$ capsules

   $\frac{2 \text{ mg}}{1 \text{ mg}} \times 1 \text{ cap} = 2$ capsules

2. 20 mg : 5 mL : : 30 mg : x mL
   20 : 5 : : 30 : x
   $20x = 150$
   $x = 7.5$ mL

   $\frac{30 \text{ mg}}{20 \text{ mg}} \times 5 \text{ mL} =$

   $\frac{30}{\cancel{20}_{4}} \times \frac{\cancel{5}^{1}}{1} = \frac{30}{4}$

   $\frac{30}{4} = 7.5$ mL

3. 0.05 mg : 1 tab : : 0.2 mg : x tab
   0.05 : 1 : : 0.2 : x
   $0.05x = 0.2$
   $x = \frac{0.2}{0.05}$
   $x = 4$ tablets

   $\frac{0.2 \text{ mg}}{0.05 \text{ mg}} \times 1 \text{ tab} =$

   $\frac{0.2}{0.05} = 4$ tablets

   0.05 mg : 1 tab : : 0.15 mg : x tab
   0.05 : 1 : : 0.15 : x
   $0.05x = 0.15$
   $x = \frac{0.15}{0.05}$
   $x = 3$ tablets

   $\frac{0.15 \text{ mg}}{0.05 \text{ mg}} \times 1 \text{ tab} =$

   $\frac{0.15}{0.05} = 3$ tablets

4. 250 mg : 1 tab : : 500 mg : x tab
   250 : 1 : : 500 : x
   $250x = 500$
   $x = \frac{500}{250}$
   $x = 2$ tablets

   $\frac{500}{250} \times 1 \text{ tab} =$

   $\frac{\cancel{500}^{2}}{\cancel{250}_{1}} \times \frac{1}{1} =$

   $\frac{2}{1} \times \frac{1}{1} = 2$ tablets

Proportion	Formula
5. 5 mg:5 mL::2.5 mg:x mL 5:5::2.5:x $5x = 12.5$ $x = \frac{12.5}{5}$ $x = 2.5$ mL	$\frac{2.5 \text{ mg}}{5 \text{ mg}} \times 5 \text{ mL} =$ $\frac{2.5}{\cancel{5}_1} \times \frac{\cancel{5}^1}{1} = \frac{2.5}{1} = 2.5 \text{ mL}$

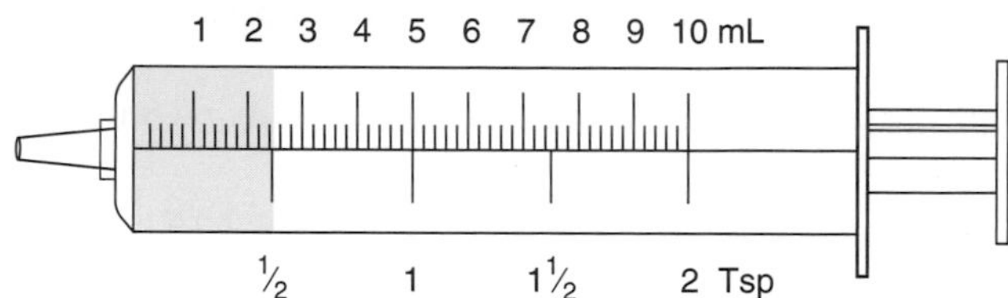

Proportion	Formula
6. 1 mg:1 tab::2 mg:x tab 1:1::2:x $x = 2$ tablets	$\frac{2 \text{ mg}}{1 \text{ mg}} \times 1 \text{ tab} =$ $\frac{2}{1} \times 1 = 2$ tablets
7. 10 mg:1 tab::20 mg:x tab 10:1::20:x $10x = 20$ $x = 2$ tablets	$\frac{20}{10} \times 1 \text{ tab} =$ $\frac{\cancel{20}^2}{\cancel{10}_1} \times 1 = 2$ tablets
8. 0.5 g:1 tab::1 g:x tab 0.5:1::1:x $0.5x = 1$ $x = 2$ tablets	$\frac{1 \text{ g}}{0.5 \text{ g}} \times 1 \text{ tab} =$ $\frac{1}{0.5} = 2$ tablets
9. 20 mg:5 mL::40 mg:x mL 20:5::40:x $20x = 200$ $x = \frac{200}{20}$ $x = 10$ mL	$\frac{40}{20} \times 5 \text{ mL} =$ $\frac{\cancel{40}^{10}}{\cancel{20}_{\cancel{4}_1}} \times \frac{\cancel{5}^1}{1} =$ $\frac{10}{1} = 10$ mL
10. 0.5 mg:1 tab::1 mg: x tab 0.5:1::1:x $0.5x = 1$ $x = 2$ tablets	$\frac{1 \text{ mg}}{0.5 \text{ mg}} \times 1 \text{ tab} =$ $\frac{1}{0.5} = 2$ tablets

Proportion	Formula
11. 60 mg : 1 gr : : x mg : 5 gr 60 : 1 : : x : 5 $x = 300$ mg	
300 mg : 1 tab : : 300 : x tab 300 : 1 : : 300 : x $300x = 300$ $x = \frac{300}{300}$ $x = 1$ tablet	$\frac{300 \text{ mg}}{300 \text{ mg}} \times 1 \text{ tab} =$ $\frac{300}{300} = 1$ tablet
12. 1000 mg : 1 gr : x mg : 0.6 g 1000 : 1 : : x : 0.6 $x = 600$ mg	
300 mg : 1 tab : : 600 mg : x tab 300 : 1 : : 600 : x $300x = 600$ $x = \frac{600}{300}$ $x = 2$ tablets	$\frac{600 \text{ mg}}{300 \text{ mg}} \times 1 \text{ tab} =$ $\frac{600}{300} \times 1 = 2$ tablets
600 mg : 1 dose : : x mg : 2 dose 600 : 1 : : x : 2 $x = 1200$ mg	
13. 1000 mg : 1 g : : x mg : 0.25 g 1000 : 1 : : x : 0.25 $x = 250$ mg	
500 mg : 1 tab : : 250 mg : x tab 500 : 1 : : 250 : x $500x = 250$ $x = \frac{250}{500}$ $x = \frac{1}{2}$ tablet	$\frac{250 \text{ mg}}{500 \text{ mg}} \times 1 \text{ tab} = \frac{1}{2}$ tablet
14. 50 mg : 1 tab : : 25 mg : x tab 50 : 1 : : 25 : x $50x = 25$ $x = \frac{25}{50}$ $x = \frac{1}{2}$ tablet	$\frac{25 \text{ mg}}{50 \text{ mg}} \times 1 \text{ tab} =$ $\frac{25}{50} = \frac{1}{2}$ tablet

Proportion	Formula
15. 60 mg : 1 gr : : x mg : 5 gr 60 : 1 : : x : 5 $x = 300$ mg	
300 mg : 1 tab : : 300 mg : x tab 300 : 1 : : 300 : x $300x = 300$ $x = \frac{300}{300}$ $x =$ 1 tablet	$\frac{300 \text{ mg}}{300 \text{ mg}} \times 1 \text{ tab} =$ $\frac{300}{300} = 1$ tablet
16. 0.5 g : 1 tab : : 4 g : x tab 0.5 : 1 : : 4 : x $0.5x = 4$ $x = \frac{4}{0.5}$ $x = 8$ tablets	$\frac{4 \text{ g}}{0.5 \text{ g}} \times 1 \text{ tab} =$ $\frac{4}{0.5} = 8$ tablets
0.5 g : 1 tab : : 2 g : x tab 0.5 : 1 : : 2 : x $0.5x = 2$ $x = \frac{2}{0.5}$ $x = 4$ tablets	$\frac{2 \text{ g}}{0.5 \text{ g}} \times 1 \text{ tab} =$ $\frac{2}{0.5} = 4$ tablets
17. 400 mg : 1 tab : : 800 mg : x tab 400 : 1 : : 800 : x $400x = 800$ $x = \frac{800}{400}$ $x = 2$ tablets	$\frac{800 \text{ mg}}{400 \text{ mg}} \times 1 \text{ tab} =$ $\frac{\overset{2}{\cancel{800}}}{\underset{1}{\cancel{400}}} \times \frac{1}{1} = 2$ tablets
18. 30 mL = 1 fl oz each dose 4 fl oz given each day	
19. 12.5 mg : 5 mL : : 30 mg : x mL 12.5 : 5 : : 30 : x $12.5x = 150$ $x = \frac{150}{12.5}$ $x = 12$ mL	$\frac{30 \text{ mg}}{12.5 \text{ mg}} \times \frac{5 \text{ mL}}{1} =$ $\frac{30}{12.5} \times \frac{5}{1} =$ $\frac{150}{12.5} = 12$ mL

Proportion / **Formula**

20. Proportion:

60 mg : 1 gr : : x mg : ¼ gr

$$x = \frac{\overset{15}{\cancel{60}}}{1} \times \frac{1}{\underset{1}{\cancel{4}}}$$

$x = 15$ mg

15 mg = ¼ gr = 1 tablet

15 mg : 1 tab : : 60 mg : x tab

15 : 1 : : 60 : x

$15x = 60$

$$x = \frac{60}{15}$$

$x = 4$ tablets

Formula:

$$\frac{60\text{ mg}}{15\text{ mg}} \times 1\text{ tab} =$$

$$\frac{60}{15} = 4\text{ tablets}$$

21. Proportion:

125 mg : 5 mL : : x mg : 5.5 mL

125 : 5 : : x : 5.5

$5x = 125 \times 5.5$

$5x = 687.5$

$$x = \frac{687.5}{5}$$

$x = 137.5$ mg

Formula:

$$\frac{x\text{ mg}}{125\text{ mg}} \times 5\text{ mL} = 5.5\text{ mL}$$

$$\frac{x}{\underset{25}{\cancel{125}}} \times \frac{\overset{1}{\cancel{5}}}{1} = 5.5$$

$$\frac{x}{25} = 5.5$$

$$\frac{\overset{1}{\cancel{25}}}{1} \times \frac{x}{\underset{1}{\cancel{25}}} = 5.5 \times 25$$

$x = 137.5$ mg

22. Proportion:

40 mg : 1 tab : : 80 mg : x tab

40 : 1 : : 80 : x

$40x = 80$

$$x = \frac{80}{40}$$

$x = 2$ tablets

Formula:

$$\frac{80\text{ mg}}{40\text{ mg}} \times 1\text{ tab} =$$

$$\frac{80}{40} = 2\text{ tablets}$$

23. Proportion:

0.4 mg : 1 tab : : x mg : 2 tab

0.4 : 1 : : x : 2

$x = 0.4 \times 2$

$x = 0.8$ mg

Formula:

$$\frac{x}{0.4} \times 1\text{ tab} = 2\text{ tablets}$$

$$\frac{x}{0.4} = 2$$

$x = 2 \times 0.4$

$x = 0.8$

Proportion	Formula

24. 0.5 mg : 5 mL : : 1.5 mg : x mL
0.5 : 5 : : 1.5 : x
$0.5x = 7.5$
$x = \frac{7.5}{0.5}$
$x = 15$ mL

30 mL : 1 fl oz : : 15 mL : x fl oz
30 : 1 : : 15 : x
$30x = 15$
$x = \frac{15}{30}$
$x = ½$ fl oz

$$\frac{1.5 \text{ mg}}{0.5 \text{ mg}} \times \frac{5 \text{ mL}}{1} =$$
$$\frac{1.5}{0.5} \times \frac{5}{1} = \frac{7.5}{0.5}$$
$$\frac{7.5}{0.5} = 15 \text{ mL}$$

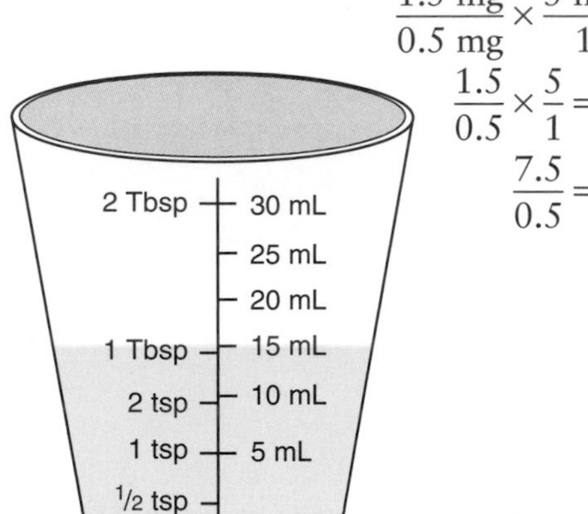

25. 10 mg : 5 mL : : 15 mg : x mL
10 : 5 : : 15 : x
$10x = 75$
$x = \frac{75}{10}$
$x = 7.5$ mL

$$\frac{15 \text{ mg}}{10 \text{ mg}} \times 5 \text{ mL} =$$
$$\frac{15}{\cancel{10}_{2}} \times \frac{\cancel{5}^{1}}{1} = \frac{15}{2}$$
$$\frac{15}{2} = 7.5 \text{ mL}$$

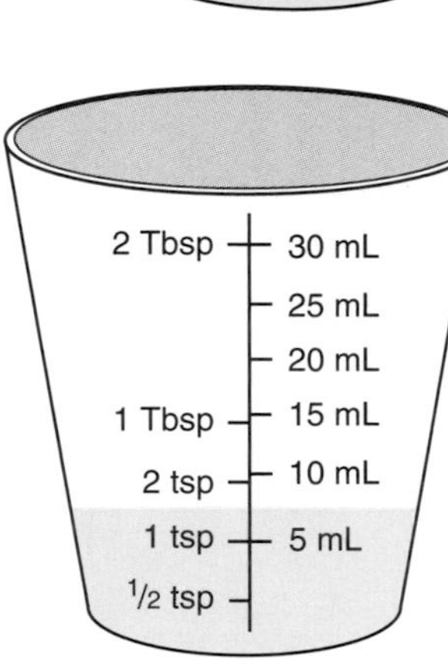

26. 50 mg : 1 tab : : 25 mg : x tab
50 : 1 : : 25 : x
$50x = 25$
$x = \frac{25}{50}$
$x = ½$ tablet

$$\frac{25 \text{ mg}}{50 \text{ mg}} \times 1 \text{ tab} =$$
$$\frac{25}{50} = ½ \text{ tablet}$$

27. 30 mL = 1 fl oz
Order is for 1 fl oz
Supplied in 12-oz bottle
1 fl oz : 1 dose : : 12 fl oz : x dose
1 : 1 : : 12 : x
$x = 12$ doses

28. 100 mg : 1 tab : : 200 mg : x tab
100 : 1 : : 200 : x
$100x = 200$
$x = \frac{200}{100}$
$x = 2$ tablets

$$\frac{200 \text{ mg}}{100 \text{ mg}} \times 1 \text{ tab} =$$
$$\frac{200}{100} = 2 \text{ tablets}$$

Proportion | **Formula**

29. 60 mg : 1 gr : : x mg : ½ gr
60 : 1 : : x : ½

$$x = \frac{\overset{30}{\cancel{60}}}{1} \times \frac{1}{\underset{1}{\cancel{2}}}$$

x = 30 mg = ½ gr

30 mg : 1 tab : : 15 mg : x tab
30 : 1 : : 15 : x
30x = 15

$$x = \frac{15}{30}$$

x = ½ tablet

Formula:

$$\frac{15 \text{ mg}}{30 \text{ mg}} \times 1 \text{ tab} =$$

$$\frac{15}{30} = ½ \text{ tablet}$$

30. 250 mg : 5 mL : : 125 mg : x mL
250 : 5 : : 125 : x
250x = 625

$$x = \frac{625}{250}$$

x = 2.5 mL

Formula:

$$\frac{125 \text{ mg}}{250 \text{ mg}} \times 5 \text{ mL} =$$

$$\frac{\overset{1}{\cancel{125}}}{\underset{2}{\cancel{250}}} \times \frac{5}{1} = \frac{5}{2}$$

$$\frac{5}{2} = 2.5 \text{ mL}$$

31. 50 mg : 1 tab : : 25 mg : x tab
50 : 1 : : 25 : x
50x = 25

$$x = \frac{25}{50}$$

x = ½ tablet

Formula:

$$\frac{25 \text{ mg}}{50 \text{ mg}} \times 1 \text{ tab} =$$

$$\frac{25}{50} = ½ \text{ tablet}$$

32. 1000 mg : 1 g : : x mg : 0.6 g
1000 : 1 : : x : 0.6
x = 0.6 × 1000
x = 600 mg

200 mg : 1 tab : : 600 mg : x tab
200 : 1 : : 600 : x
200x = 600

$$x = \frac{600}{200}$$

x = 3 tablets

Formula:

$$\frac{600 \text{ mg}}{200 \text{ mg}} \times 1 \text{ tab} =$$

$$\frac{600}{200} = 3 \text{ tablets}$$

3 tablets : 1 dose : : x tab : 6 doses
3 : 1 : : x : 6
x = 18 tablets

Proportion | **Formula**

33. 6.25 mg : 5 mL : : 12.5 mg : x mL
6.25 : 5 : : 12.5 : x
$6.25x = 62.5$
$x = \frac{62.5}{6.25}$
$x = 10$ mL

$\frac{12.5 \text{ mg}}{6.25 \text{ mg}} \times 5 \text{ mL} =$
$\frac{\overset{2}{\cancel{12.5}}}{\underset{1}{\cancel{6.25}}} \times \frac{5}{1} =$
$\frac{2 \times 5}{1} = 10 \text{ mL}$

34. 500 mg : 5 mL : : 750 mg : x mL
500 : 5 : : 750 : x
$500x = 3750$
$x = \frac{3750}{500}$
$x = 7.5$ mL

$\frac{750 \text{ mg}}{500 \text{ mg}} \times 5 \text{ mL} =$
$\frac{\overset{15}{\cancel{750}}}{\underset{2}{\cancel{500}\ \cancel{100}}} \times \frac{\overset{1}{\cancel{5}}}{1} =$
$\frac{15}{2} = 7.5 \text{ mL}$

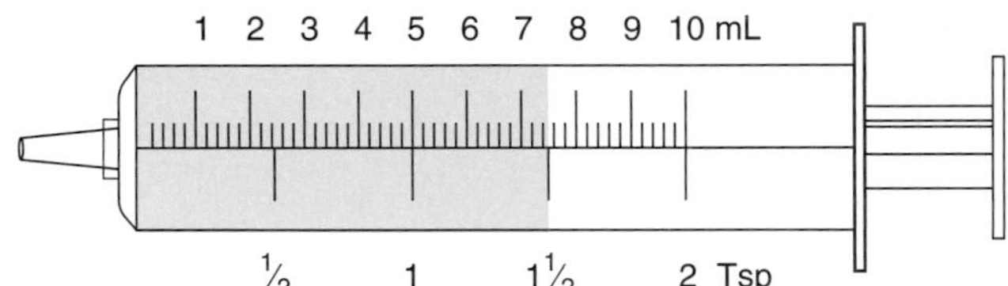

35. 20 mg : 5 mL : : 100 mg : x mL
20 : 5 : : 100 : x
$20x = 500$
$x = \frac{500}{20}$
$x = 25$ mL

$\frac{100 \text{ mg}}{20 \text{ mg}} \times \frac{5}{1} \text{ mL} =$
$\frac{100}{\underset{4}{\cancel{20}}} \times \frac{\overset{1}{\cancel{5}}}{1} =$
$\frac{100}{4} = 25 \text{ mL}$

36. 40 mEq : 15 mL : : 80 mEq : x mL
40 : 15 : : 80 : x
$40x = 1200$
$x = \frac{1200}{40}$
$x = 30$ mL

$\frac{80}{\underset{8}{\cancel{40}}} \times \frac{\overset{3}{\cancel{15}}}{1} =$
$\frac{240}{8} = 30 \text{ mL}$

37. 2.5 mg : 1 tab : : 7.5 mg : x tab
2.5 : 1 : : 7.5 : x
$2.5x = 7.5$
$x = \frac{7.5}{2.5}$
$x = 3$ tablets

$\frac{7.5 \text{ mg}}{2.5 \text{ mg}} \times 1 \text{ tab} =$
$\frac{7.5}{2.5} = 3 \text{ tablets}$

Proportion	Formula
38. 1000 mg:1 g::x mg:0.2 g 1000:1::x:0.2 $x = 200$ mg	
100 mg:1 tab::200 mg:x tab 100:1::200:x $100x = 200$ $x = \frac{200}{100}$ $x = 2$ tablets	$\frac{200 \text{ mg}}{100 \text{ mg}} \times 1 \text{ tab} =$ $\frac{200}{100} = 2$ tablets
39. 60 mg:1 gr::x mg:5 gr 60:1::x:5 $x = 300$ mg	
160 mg:5 mL::300 mg:x mL 160:5::300:x $160x = 1500$ $x = 9.375$ mL or 9.38 mL	$\frac{300 \text{ mg}}{160 \text{ mg}} \times 5 \text{ mL} =$ $\frac{300}{\cancel{160}_{32}} \times \frac{\cancel{5}^{1}}{1} = \frac{300}{32}$ $\frac{300}{32} = 9.375$ mL or 9.38 mL

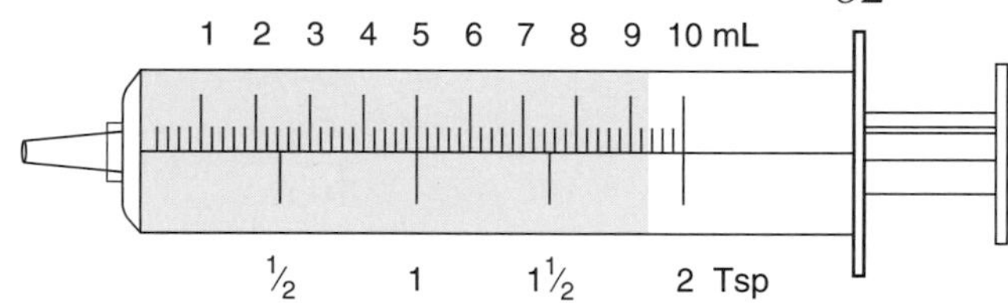

Proportion	Formula
40. 0.25 mg:1 tab::0.5 mg:x tab 0.25:1::0.5:x $0.25x = 0.5$ $x = \frac{0.5}{0.25}$ $x = 2$ tablets	$\frac{0.5 \text{ mg}}{0.25 \text{ mg}} \times 1 \text{ tab} =$ $\frac{0.5}{0.25} = 2$ tablets
41. 5 mg:1 tab::10 mg:x tab 5:1::10:x $5x = 10$ $x = \frac{10}{5}$ $x = 2$ tablets	$\frac{10 \text{ mg}}{5 \text{ mg}} \times 1 \text{ tab} =$ $\frac{10}{5} = 2$ tablets
42. 50 mg:1 tab::100 mg:x tab 50:1::100:x $50x = 100$ $x = \frac{100}{50}$ $x = 2$ tablets	$\frac{100 \text{ mg}}{50 \text{ mg}} \times 1 \text{ tab} =$ $\frac{100}{50} = 2$ tablets

Proportion	Formula
43. grss = ½ gr = 30 mg 30 mg : 1 tab : : 30 mg : x tab 30 : 1 : : 30 : x $30x = 30$ $x = \frac{30}{30}$ $x = 1$ tablet	$\frac{30 \text{ mg}}{30 \text{ mg}} \times 1 \text{ tab} =$ $\frac{30}{30} = 1$ tablet
44. 0.125 mg : 1 tab : : 0.25 : x tab 0.125 : 1 : : 0.25 : x $0.125x = 0.25$ $x = \frac{0.25}{0.125}$ $x = 2$ tablets	$\frac{0.25 \text{ mg}}{0.125 \text{ mg}} \times 1 \text{ tab} =$ $\frac{0.25}{0.125} = 2$ tablets
45. 250 mg : 1 cap : : 500 mg : x cap 250 : 1 : : 500 : x $250x = 500$ $x = \frac{500}{250}$ $x = 2$ capsules 2 cap : 1 dose : : x cap : 4 dose 2 : 1 : : x : 4 $x = 8$ capsules	$\frac{500 \text{ mg}}{250 \text{ mg}} \times 1 \text{ cap} =$ $\frac{500}{250} = 2$ capsules
46. 10 mg : 1 tab : : 5 mg : x tab 10 : 1 : : 5 : x $10x = 5$ $x = \frac{5}{10}$ $x = ½$ tablet	$\frac{5 \text{ mg}}{10 \text{ mg}} \times 1 \text{ tab} =$ $\frac{5}{10} = ½$ tablet
47. 60 mg : 1 gr : : x mg : 1½ gr 60 : 1 : : x : 1½ $x = \frac{\overset{30}{\cancel{60}}}{1} \times \frac{3}{\underset{1}{\cancel{2}}}$ $x = 90$ mg 30 mg : 1 tab : : 90 mg : x tab 30 : 1 : : 90 : x $30x = 90$ $x = 3$ tablets	$\frac{90 \text{ mg}}{30 \text{ mg}} \times 1 \text{ tab} =$ $\frac{90}{30} = 3$ tablets

Proportion	Formula
48. 40 mEq : 15 mL : : 2 mEq : x mL 40 : 15 : : 2 : x $40x = 30$ $x = \frac{30}{40}$ $x = 0.75$ mL	$\frac{2 \text{ mEq}}{40 \text{ mEq}} \times 15 \text{ mL} =$ $\frac{2}{40} \times \frac{15}{1}$ $\frac{2}{\cancel{40}_{8}} \times \frac{\cancel{15}^{3}}{1} = \frac{6}{8}$ $\frac{6}{8} = 0.75$ mL
49. 65 mg : 1 gr : : x mg : 10 gr 65 : 1 : : x : 10 $x = 650$ mg	
325 mg : 1 tab : : 650 mg : x tab 325 : 1 : : 650 : x $325x = 650$ $x = \frac{650}{325}$ $x = 2$ tablets	$\frac{650 \text{ mg}}{325 \text{ mg}} \times 1 \text{ tab} =$ $\frac{650}{325} = 2$ tablets
50. 15 mg : 1 mL : : 150 mg : x mL 15 : 1 : : 150 : x $15x = 150$ $x = \frac{150}{15}$ $x = 10$ mL	$\frac{150 \text{ mg}}{15 \text{ mg}} \times \frac{1}{1} \text{ mL} =$ $\frac{\cancel{150}^{10}}{\cancel{15}_{1}} \times \frac{1}{1} = 10$ mL
51. 250 mg : 1 cap : : 1000 mg : x cap 250 : 1 : : 1000 : x $250x = 1000$ $x = \frac{1000}{250}$ $x = 4$ capsules	$\frac{1000 \text{ mg}}{250 \text{ mg}} \times 1 \text{ cap} =$ $\frac{1000}{250} \times 1 =$ $\frac{1000}{250} = 4$ capsules
52. 60 mg : 1 gr : : x mg : 5 gr 60 : 1 : : x : 5 $x = 300$ mg 0.3 g = 300 mg	
324 mg : 1 tab : : 300 mg : x tab 324 : 1 : : 300 : x $324x = 300$ $x = \frac{300}{324} = 0.93$ tablet $x = 1$ tablet	$\frac{300 \text{ mg}}{324 \text{ mg}} \times 1 \text{ tab} =$ $\frac{300}{324} = 0.93$ tablet; give 1 tablet

Proportion	Formula
53. 10 mg : 1 cap : : 20 mg : x cap 10 : 1 : : 20 : x $10x = 20$ $x = \frac{20}{10}$ $x = 2$ capsules	$\frac{20\text{ mg}}{10\text{ mg}} \times 1\text{ cap} =$ $\frac{20}{10} = 2$ capsules
54. 10 mg : 5 mL : : 30 mg : x mL 10 : 5 : : 30 : x $10x = 150$ $x = \frac{150}{10}$ $x = 15$ mL	$\frac{30\text{ mg}}{10\text{ mg}} \times 5\text{ mL} =$ $\frac{\overset{15}{\cancel{30}}}{\underset{\underset{1}{\cancel{2}}}{\cancel{10}}} \times \frac{\overset{1}{\cancel{5}}}{1} =$ $\frac{15}{1} = 15$ mL
55. 1000 mg : 1 g : : x mg : 0.75 g 1000 : 1 : : x : 0.75 $x = 1000 \times 0.75$ $x = 750$ mg	
250 mg : 1 tab : : 750 mg : x tab 250 : 1 : : 750 : x $250x = 750$ $x = \frac{750}{250}$ $x = 3$ tablets	$\frac{750\text{ mg}}{250\text{ mg}} \times 1\text{ tab} =$ $\frac{750}{250} = 3$ tablets
56. 12.5 mg : 1 tab : : 25 mg : x tab 12.5 : 1 : : 25 : x $12.5x = 25$ $x = \frac{25}{12.5}$ $x = 2$ tablets	$\frac{25\text{ mg}}{12.5\text{ mg}} \times 1\text{ tab} =$ $\frac{25}{12.5} = 2$ tablets
57. 25 mg : 5 mL : : 15 mg : x mL 25 : 5 : : 15 : x $25x = 75$ $x = \frac{75}{25}$ $x = 3$ mL	$\frac{15\text{ mg}}{25\text{ mg}} \times 5\text{ mL} =$ $\frac{15}{\underset{5}{\cancel{25}}} \times \frac{\overset{1}{\cancel{5}}}{1} = \frac{15}{5}$ $\frac{15}{5} = 3$ mL

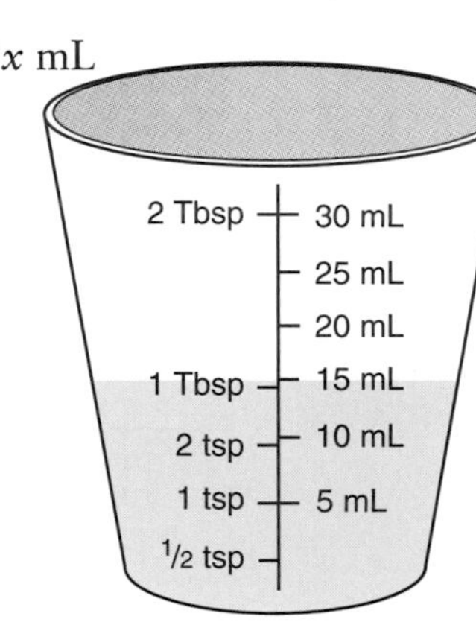

Proportion	Formula
58. 50 mg:1 tab::100 mg:x tab 50:1::100:x $50x = 100$ $x = \frac{100}{50}$ $x = 2$ tablets	$\frac{100\text{ mg}}{50\text{ mg}} \times 1\text{ tab} =$ $\frac{\overset{2}{\cancel{100}}}{\underset{1}{\cancel{50}}} \times \frac{1}{1} = \frac{2}{1}$ $\frac{2}{1} = 2$ tablets
59. 100 mg:1 cap::200 mg:x cap 100:1::200:x $100x = 200$ $x = \frac{200}{100}$ $x = 2$ capsules	$\frac{200}{100} \times 1\text{ cap} =$ $\frac{\overset{2}{\cancel{200}}}{\underset{1}{\cancel{100}}} \times \frac{1}{1} = 2$ capsules
60. 150 mg:5 mL::250 mg:x mL 150:5::250:x $150x = 1250$ $x = \frac{1250}{150}$ $x = 8.33$ mL	$\frac{250\text{ mg}}{150\text{ mg}} \times 5\text{ mL} =$ $\frac{250}{\underset{30}{\cancel{150}}} \times \frac{\overset{1}{\cancel{5}}}{1} = \frac{250}{30}$ $\frac{250}{30} = 8.33$ mL

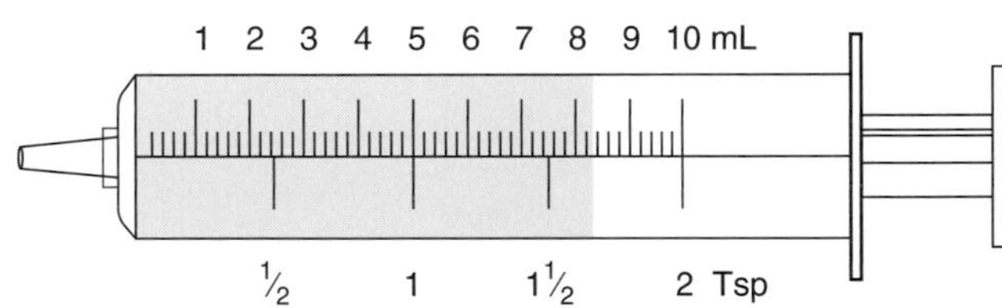

Proportion	Formula
61. 50 mg:5 mL::100 mg:x mL 50:5::100:x $50x = 500$ $x = \frac{500}{50}$ $x = 10$ mL	$\frac{100\text{ mg}}{50\text{ mg}} \times 5\text{ mL} =$ $\frac{100}{\underset{10}{\cancel{50}}} \times \frac{\overset{1}{\cancel{5}}}{1} =$ $\frac{100}{10} = 10$ mL
62. 50 mg:1 tab::25 mg:x tab 50:1::25:x $50x = 25$ $x = \frac{25}{50}$ $x = ½$ tablet	$\frac{25\text{ mg}}{50\text{ mg}} \times 1\text{ tab} =$ $\frac{25}{50} = ½$ tablet

Proportion / **Formula**

63. 80 mg:1 tab::240 mg:x tab
80:1::240:x
$80x = 240$
$x = \frac{240}{80}$
$x = 3$ tablets

$\frac{240 \text{ mg}}{80 \text{ mg}} \times 1 \text{ tab} =$
$\frac{240}{80} = 3$ tablets

64. 1000 mcg:1 mg::x mcg:0.05 mg
1000:1::x:0.05
$x = 50$ mcg

50 mcg:1 mL::90 mcg:x mL
50:1::90:x
$50x = 90$
$x = \frac{90}{50}$
$x = 1.8$ mL

$\frac{90 \text{ mcg}}{50 \text{ mcg}} \times 1 \text{ mL} =$
$\frac{90}{50} = 1.8$ mL

65. 12.5 mg:5 mL::x mg:10 mL
12.5:5::x:10
$5x = 125$
$x = \frac{125}{5}$
$x = 25$ mg

$\frac{x \text{ mg}}{12.5 \text{ mg}} \times \frac{5}{1} = 10 \text{ mL}$
$\frac{x}{12.5} \times \frac{5}{1} = 10$
$\frac{12.5}{1} \times \frac{x}{12.5} \times \frac{5}{1} = \frac{10}{1} \times 12.5$
$5x = 125$
$x = \frac{125}{5}$
$x = 25$ mg

66. 1000 mg:1 g::x mg:0.5 g
1000:1::x:0.5
$x = 500$ mg

500 mg:1 tab::500 mg:x tab
500:1::500:x
$500x = 500$
$x = \frac{500}{500}$
$x = 1$ tablet

$\frac{500 \text{ mg}}{500 \text{ mg}} \times 1 \text{ tab} =$
$\frac{500}{500} = 1$ tablet

67. 60 mg:1 gr::x mg:1.5 gr
60:1::x:1.5
$x = 60 \times 1.5$
$x = 90$ mg

30 mg:1 cap::90 mg:x cap
30:1::90:x
$30x = 90$
$x = \frac{90}{30}$
$x = 3$ capsules

$\frac{90 \text{ mg}}{30 \text{ mg}} \times 1 \text{ cap} =$
$\frac{90}{30} = 3$ capsules

Proportion	Formula
68. 40 mg : 1 tablet : : 40 : x tablet 40 : 1 : : 40 : x $40x = 40$ $x = \frac{40}{40}$ $x = 1$ tablet	The other strengths of the medication would require swallowing more pills.
69. 20 mEq : 15 mL : : 10 mEq : x mL 20 : 15 : : 10 : x $20x = 150$ $x = \frac{150}{20}$ $x = 7.5$ mL	$\frac{10 \text{ mEq}}{20 \text{ mEq}} \times \frac{15 \text{ mL}}{1} =$ $\frac{10}{\cancel{20}_{4}} \times \frac{\cancel{15}^{3}}{1} = \frac{30}{4}$ $\frac{30}{4} = 7.5$ mL

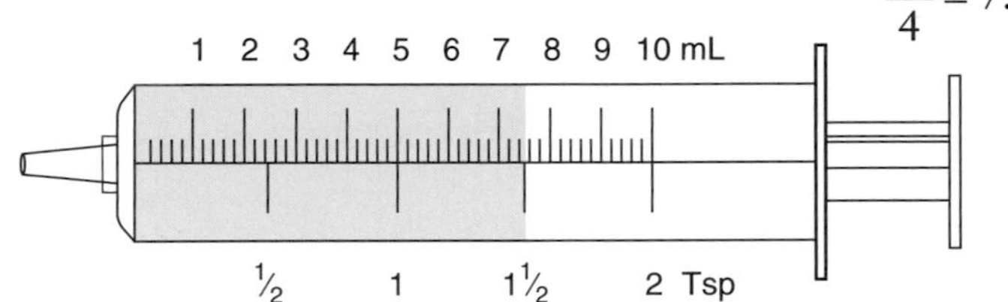

Proportion	Formula
70. 600 mg : 1 tab : : 300 mg : x tab 600 : 1 : : 300 : x $600x = 300$ $x = \frac{300}{600}$ $x = ½$ tablet	$\frac{300 \text{ mg}}{600 \text{ mg}} \times 1$ tab $=$ $\frac{300}{600} = ½$ tablet
71. 0.25 mg : 1 tab : : 0.5 mg : x tab 0.25 : 1 : : 0.5 : x $0.25x = 0.5$ $x = \frac{0.5}{0.25}$ $x = 2$ tablets	$\frac{0.5 \text{ mg}}{0.25 \text{ mg}} \times 1$ tab $=$ $\frac{0.5}{0.25} = 2$ tablets
72. 325 mg : 10.15 mL : : 650 mg : x mL 325 : 10.15 : : 650 : x $325x = 6597.5$ $x = \frac{6597.5}{325}$ $x = 20.3$ mL	$\frac{\cancel{650}^{2} \text{ mg}}{\cancel{325}_{1} \text{ mg}} \times 10.15$ mL $=$ $\frac{2}{1} \times \frac{10.15}{1} = \frac{20.30}{1} =$ 20.3 mL
73. 0.25 mg : 1 tab : : 0.5 mg : x tab 0.25 : 1 : : 0.5 : x $0.25x = 0.5$ $x = \frac{0.5}{0.25}$ $x = 2$ tablets	$\frac{0.5 \text{ mg}}{0.25 \text{ mg}} \times 1$ tab $=$ $\frac{0.5}{0.25} = 2$ tablets

Proportion	Formula
74. 30 mL:1 fl oz::x mL:½ fl oz 30:1::x:½ $x = \frac{30}{1} \times \frac{1}{2}$ x = 15 mL	
75. 50 mg:5 mL::30 mg:x mL 50:5::30:x $50x = 150$ $x = \frac{150}{50}$ x = 3 mL	$\frac{30\text{ mg}}{50\text{ mg}} \times 5\text{ mL} =$ $\frac{30}{\cancel{50}_{10}} \times \frac{\cancel{5}^{1}}{1} = \frac{30}{10}$ $\frac{30}{10} = 3\text{ mL}$

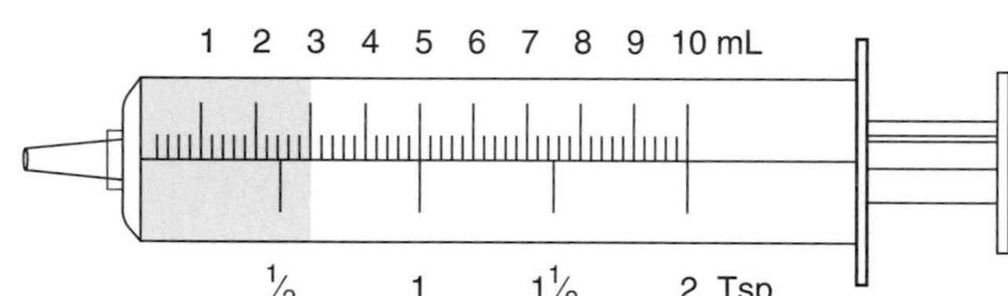

Proportion	Formula
76. 60 mg:1 gr::x mg:$\frac{1}{200}$ gr 60:1::x:$\frac{1}{200}$ $x = \frac{60}{1} \times \frac{1}{200}$ $x = \frac{60}{200}$ x = 0.3 mg	
0.15 mg:1 tab::0.3 mg:x tab 0.15:1::0.3:x $0.15x = 0.3$ $x = \frac{0.3}{0.15}$ x = 2 tablets of 0.15 mg	$\frac{0.3\text{ mg}}{0.15\text{ mg}} \times 1\text{ tab} =$ $\frac{0.3}{0.15}$ = 2 tablets of 0.15 mg
77. 5 mg:1 tab::7.5 mg:x tab 5:1::7.5:x $5x = 7.5$ $x = \frac{7.5}{5}$ x = 1.5 tablet	$\frac{7.5\text{ mg}}{5\text{ mg}} \times 1\text{ tab} =$ $\frac{7.5}{5}$ = 1.5 tablet

Proportion	Formula

78. 125 mg : 5 mL : : 250 mg : x mL

$125:5::250:x$

$125x = 1250$

$x = \frac{1250}{125}$

$x = 10$ mL

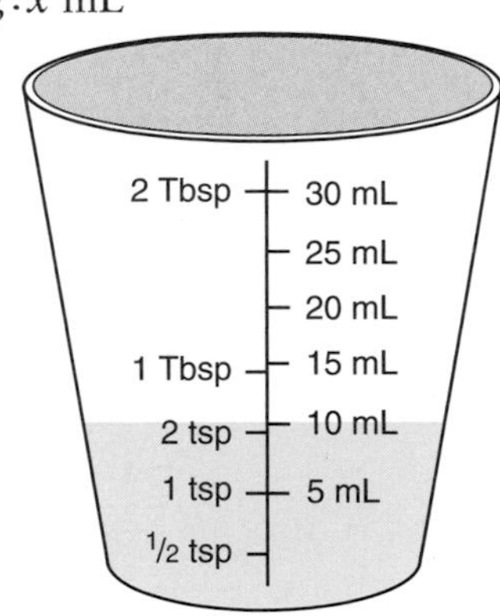

Formula

$\frac{250 \text{ mg}}{125 \text{ mg}} \times 5 \text{ mL} =$

$\frac{\overset{2}{\cancel{250}}}{\underset{1}{\cancel{125}}} \times \frac{5}{1} = \frac{10}{1}$

$\frac{10}{1} = 10$ mL

79. 50 mg : 1 cap : : 250 mg : x cap

$50:1::250:x$

$50x = 250$

$x = \frac{250}{50}$

$x = 5$ capsules

Formula

$\frac{250 \text{ mg}}{50 \text{ mg}} \times 1 \text{ cap} =$

$\frac{250}{50} = 5$ capsules

80. 15 mEq : 11.25 mL : : x mEq : 15 mL

$15:11.25::x:15$

$11.25x = 225$

$x = \frac{225}{11.25}$

$x = 20$ mEq

Formula

$\frac{x \text{ mEq}}{15 \text{ mEq}} \times 11.25 =$

$\frac{x}{15} \times \frac{11.25}{1} = 15$

$\frac{15}{1} \times \frac{x}{15} \times 11.25 = \frac{15}{1} \times \frac{15}{1}$

$11.25x = 225$

$x = \frac{225}{11.25}$

$x = 20$ mEq

81. 20 mg : 5 mL : : 55 mg : x mL

$20:5::55:x$

$20x = 275$

$x = \frac{275}{20}$

$x = 13.75$ mL

Formula

$\frac{55 \text{ mg}}{20 \text{ mg}} \times 5 \text{ mL} =$

$\frac{55}{\underset{4}{\cancel{20}}} \times \frac{\overset{1}{\cancel{5}}}{1} = \frac{55}{4}$

$\frac{55}{4} = 13.75$ mL

82. 125 mg : 1 tab : : 250 mg : x tab

$125:1::250:x$

$125x = 250$

$x = \frac{250}{125}$

$x = 2$ tablets

Formula

$\frac{250 \text{ mg}}{125 \text{ mg}} \times 1 \text{ tab} =$

$\frac{250}{125} = 2$ tablets

Proportion	Formula
83. 0.05 mg : 1 tab : : 0.05 mg : x tab 0.05 : 1 : : 0.05 : x $0.05x = 0.05$ $x = \frac{0.05}{0.05}$ $x = 1$ tablet	$\frac{0.05 \text{ mg}}{0.05 \text{ mg}} \times 1 \text{ tab} =$ $\frac{0.05}{0.05} = 1$ tablet
84. 1000 mg : 1 g : : x mg : 0.2g 1000 : 1 : : x : 0.2 $x = 200$ mg Give 1 tablet of 200 mg 200 mg : 1 dose : : x mg : 3 doses $x = 600$ mg will be given per day	$\frac{200 \text{ mg}}{200 \text{ mg}} \times 1 \text{ tab} =$ $\frac{200}{200} = 1$ tablet
85. 5 mg : 1 tab : : 15 mg : x tab 5 : 1 : : 15 : x $5x = 15$ $x = \frac{15}{5}$ $x = 3$ tablets	$\frac{15 \text{ mg}}{5 \text{ mg}} \times 1 \text{ tab} =$ $\frac{15}{5} = 3$ tablets
86. 300 mg : 1 dose : : x mg : 4 doses 300 : 1 : : x : 4 $x = 1200$ mg given per day	
87. 15 mg : 1 cap : : 30 mg : x cap 15 : 1 : : 30 : x $15x = 30$ $x = \frac{30}{15}$ $x = 2$ capsules	$\frac{30 \text{ mg}}{15 \text{ mg}} \times 1 \text{ cap} =$ $\frac{30}{15} = 2$ capsules
88. 25 mg : 1 tab : : 50 mg : x tab 25 : 1 : : 50 : x $25x = 50$ $x = \frac{50}{25}$ $x = 2$ tablets	$\frac{50 \text{ mg}}{25 \text{ mg}} \times 1 \text{ tab} =$ $\frac{50}{25} = 2$ tablets
89. 30 mg : 1 mL : : 40 mg : x mL 30 : 1 : : 40 : x $30x = 40$ $x = \frac{40}{30}$ $x = 1.33$ mL	$\frac{40 \text{ mg}}{30 \text{ mg}} \times 1 \text{ mL} =$ $\frac{40}{30} = 1.33$ mL

Proportion	Formula
90. 10 mg:1 mL:x mg:0.6 mL 10:1::x:0.6 $x = 10 \times 0.6$ $x = 6$ mg	$\frac{x \text{ mg}}{10 \text{ mg}} \times 1 = 0.6$ mL $\frac{x}{10} \times 1 = 0.6$ $\frac{10}{1} \times \frac{x}{10} \times 1 = 0.6 \times 10$ $x = 6$ mg
91. 75 mg:1 cap::150 mg:x cap 75:1::150:x $75x = 150$ $x = \frac{150}{75}$ $x = 2$ capsules	$\frac{150 \text{ mg}}{75 \text{ mg}} \times 1$ cap = $\frac{150}{75} = 2$ capsules
92. 0.1 mg:1 tab::0.05 mg:x tab 0.1:1::0.05:x $0.1x = 0.05$ $x = \frac{0.05}{0.1}$ $x = 0.5$ or ½ tablet	$\frac{0.05 \text{ mg}}{0.1 \text{ mg}} \times 1$ tab = $\frac{0.05}{0.1} = 0.5$ or ½ tablet
93. 2.5 mg:1 tab::10 mg:x tab 2.5:1::10:x $2.5x = 10$ $x = \frac{10}{2.5}$ $x = 4$ tablets	$\frac{10 \text{ mg}}{2.5 \text{ mg}} \times 1$ tab = $\frac{10}{2.5} = 4$ tablets
94. 1000 mg:1 g::x mg:0.25 g 1000:1::x:0.25 $x = 1000 \times 0.25$ $x = 250$ mg	
250 mg:1 tab::250 mg:x tab 250:1::250:x $250x = 250$ $x = 1$ tablet	$\frac{250 \text{ mg}}{250 \text{ mg}} \times 1$ tab = $\frac{250}{250} = 1$ tablet

Proportion	Formula
95. 60 mg : 1 gr : : x mg : ⅙ gr 60 : 1 : : x : ⅙ $x = \frac{\overset{10}{\cancel{60}}}{1} \times \frac{1}{\underset{1}{\cancel{6}}}$ $x = 10$ mg	
10 mg : 1 tab : : 25 mg : x tab 10 : 1 : : 25 : x $10x = 25$ $x = \frac{25}{10}$ $x = 2.5$ tablets	$\frac{25 \text{ mg}}{10 \text{ mg}} \times 1 \text{ tab} =$ $\frac{25}{10} = 2.5$ tablets
96. 10 mg : 1 tab : : 30 mg : x tab 10 : 1 : : 30 : x $10x = 30$ $x = \frac{30}{10}$ $x = 3$ tablets	$\frac{30 \text{ mg}}{10 \text{ mg}} \times 1 \text{ tab} =$ $\frac{\overset{3}{\cancel{30}}}{\underset{1}{\cancel{10}}} \times 1 = 3$ tablets
97. 5 mg : 1 tab : : 15 mg : x tab 5 : 1 : : 15 : x $5x = 15$ $x = \frac{15}{5}$ $x = 3$ tablets	$\frac{15 \text{ mg}}{5 \text{ mg}} \times 1 \text{ tab} =$ $\frac{15}{5} = 3$ tablets
98. 1000 mg : 1 g : : x mg : 0.015 g 1000 : 1 : : x : 0.015 $x = 1000 \times 0.015$ $x = 15$ mg	
15 mg : 1 cap : : 15 mg : x cap 15 : 1 : : 15 : x $15x = 15$ $x = \frac{15}{15}$ $x = 1$ capsule	$\frac{15 \text{ mg}}{15 \text{ mg}} \times 1 \text{ cap} =$ $\frac{15}{15} = 1$ capsule

Proportion

99. 20 mEq : 15 mL : : 40 mEq : x mL

20 : 15 : : 40 : x

$20x = 600$

$x = \dfrac{600}{20}$

$x = 30$ mL

Formula

$\dfrac{40\text{ mEq}}{20\text{ mEq}} \times \dfrac{15\text{ mL}}{1} =$

$\dfrac{40}{\underset{4}{\cancel{20}}} \times \dfrac{\overset{3}{\cancel{15}}}{1} = \dfrac{120}{4}$

$\dfrac{120}{4} = 30$ mL

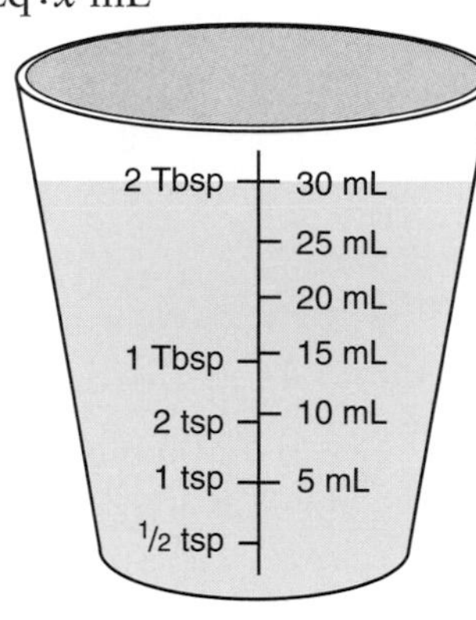

100. 40 mg : 1 tab : : 20 mg : x tab

40 : 1 : : 20 : x

$40x = 20$

$x = \dfrac{20}{40}$

$x = ½$ tablet

$\dfrac{20\text{ mg}}{40\text{ mg}} \times 1$ tab $=$

$\dfrac{20}{40} \times 1 = ½$ tablet

Chapter 12 Oral Dosages—Posttest 1, pp. 217-222

Proportion

1. 5 gr : 1 tab : : 15 gr : x tab

5 : 1 : : 15 : x

$5x = 15$

$x = \dfrac{15}{5}$

$x = 3$ tablets

Formula

$\dfrac{15\text{ gr}}{5\text{ gr}} \times 1$ tab $=$

$\dfrac{15}{5} = 3$ tablets

2. 1000 mg : 1 g : : x mg : 0.5 g

1000 : 1 : : x : 0.5

$x = 500$ mg

500 mg : 1 cap : : 500 mg : x cap

500 : 1 : : 500 : x

$500x = 500$

$x = \dfrac{500}{500}$

$x = 1$ capsule

$\dfrac{500\text{ mg}}{500\text{ mg}} \times 1$ cap $=$

$\dfrac{500}{500} = 1$ capsule

3. 500 mg : 1 cap : : 1000 mg : x cap

500 : 1 : : 1000 : x

$500x = 1000$

$x = \dfrac{1000}{500}$

$x = 2$ capsules

$\dfrac{1000\text{ mg}}{500\text{ mg}} \times 1$ cap $=$

$\dfrac{1000}{500} = 2$ capsules

Proportion	Formula

4. 30 mg : 1 tab : : 60 mg : x tab

30 : 1 : : 60 : x

$30x = 60$

$$x = \frac{\overset{2}{\cancel{60}}}{\underset{1}{\cancel{30}}}$$

$x = 2$ tablets

Formula:

$$\frac{60 \text{ mg}}{30 \text{ mg}} \times 1 \text{ tab} =$$

$$\frac{\overset{2}{\cancel{60}}}{\underset{1}{\cancel{30}}} \times \frac{1}{1} = 2 \text{ tablets}$$

5. 0.5 g = 500 mg

500 mg : 1 tab : : 500 : x tab

500 : 1 : : 500 : x

$500x = 500$

$$x = \frac{500}{500}$$

$x = 1$ tablet

Formula:

$$\frac{500 \text{ mg}}{500 \text{ mg}} \times 1 \text{ tab} =$$

$$\frac{500}{500} = 1 \text{ tablet}$$

6. 10 mg : 5 mL : : 25 mg : x mL

10 : 5 : : 25 : x

$10x = 125$

$$x = \frac{125}{10}$$

$x = 12.5$ mL

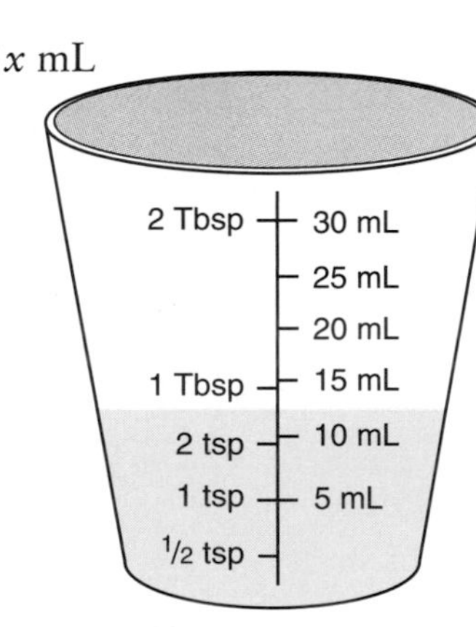

Formula:

$$\frac{25 \text{ mg}}{10 \text{ mg}} \times \frac{5}{1} \text{ mL} =$$

$$\frac{25}{\underset{2}{\cancel{10}}} \times \frac{\overset{1}{\cancel{5}}}{1} = \frac{25}{2}$$

$$\frac{25}{2} = 12.5 \text{ mL}$$

7. 120 mg : 1 tab : : 60 mg : x tab

120 : 1 : : 60 : x

$120x = 60$

$$x = \frac{60}{120}$$

$x = ½$ tablet

Formula:

$$\frac{60 \text{ mg}}{120 \text{ mg}} \times \frac{1}{1} \text{ tab} =$$

$$\frac{\overset{1}{\cancel{60}}}{\underset{2}{\cancel{120}}} \times \frac{1}{1} = ½ \text{ tablet}$$

8. 60 mg : 1 gr : : x mg : ½ gr

60 : 1 : : x : ½

$$x = \frac{60}{2}$$

$x = 30$ mg

30 mg : 1 tab : : 30 mg : x tab

30 : 1 : : 30 : x

$30x = 30$

$$x = \frac{30}{30}$$

$x = 1$ tablet

Formula:

$$\frac{30 \text{ mg}}{30 \text{ mg}} \times 1 \text{ tab} =$$

$$\frac{30}{30} = 1 \text{ tablet}$$

Proportion	Formula

9. 25 mg : 5 mL : : 50 mg : x mL
25 : 5 : : 50 : x
$25x = 250$
$x = \frac{250}{25}$
$x = 10$ mL

$\frac{50 \text{ mg}}{25 \text{ mg}} \times 5 =$

$\frac{\not{50}^{10}}{\not{25}_{\not{5}_1}} \times \frac{\not{5}^{1}}{1} =$

$\frac{10}{1} = 10$ mL

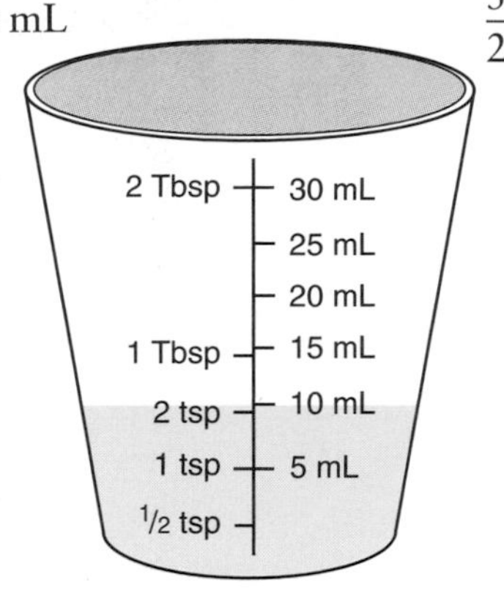

10. 1000 mg : 1 g : : x mg : 0.25 g
1000 : 1 : : x : 0.25
$x = 250$ mg
Each dose equals one 250 mg tablet. The patient will receive a total of 2 tablets each day

11. $\frac{1}{300}$ gr : 1 tab : : $\frac{1}{600}$ gr : x tab
$\frac{1}{300} : 1 : : \frac{1}{600} : x$
$\frac{1}{300}x = \frac{1}{600}$
$x = \frac{300}{600}$
$x = ½$ tablet

$\frac{\frac{1}{600} \text{ gr}}{\frac{1}{300} \text{ gr}} \times 1 \text{ tab} =$

$\frac{1}{600} \div \frac{1}{300} =$

$\frac{1}{600} \times \frac{300}{1} = \frac{300}{600}$

$\frac{300}{600} = ½$ tablet

12. 30 mEq : 22.5 mL : : 20 mEq : x mL
30 : 22.5 : : 20 : x
$30x = 450$
$x = \frac{450}{30}$
$x = 15$ mL

$\frac{20 \text{ mEq}}{30 \text{ mEq}} \times 22.5 =$

$\frac{\not{20}^{2}}{\not{30}_{3}} \times \frac{22.5}{1} = \frac{450}{30}$

$\frac{\not{450}^{15}}{\not{30}_{1}} = 15$ mL

13. 0.5 g : 1 tab : : 2 g : x tab
0.5 : 1 : : 2 : x
$0.5x = 2$
$x = 2 \div 0.5$
$x = 4$ tablets

$\frac{2 \text{ g}}{0.5 \text{ g}} \times 1 \text{ tab} =$

$\frac{2}{0.5} = 4$ tablets

14. 50 mg : 1 cap : : 100 mg : x cap
50 : 1 : : 100 : x
$50x = 100$
$x = \frac{100}{50}$
$x = 2$ capsules

$\frac{100 \text{ mg}}{50 \text{ mg}} \times 1 \text{ cap} =$

$\frac{100}{50} = 2$ capsules

Proportion	Formula

15. 10 mg : 1 mL :: 9 mg : x mL

10 : 1 :: 9 : x

$10x = 9$

$x = \frac{9}{10}$ or 0.9 mL

$\frac{9 \text{ mg}}{10 \text{ mg}} \times 1 \text{ mL} =$

$\frac{9}{10} = 0.9 \text{ mL}$

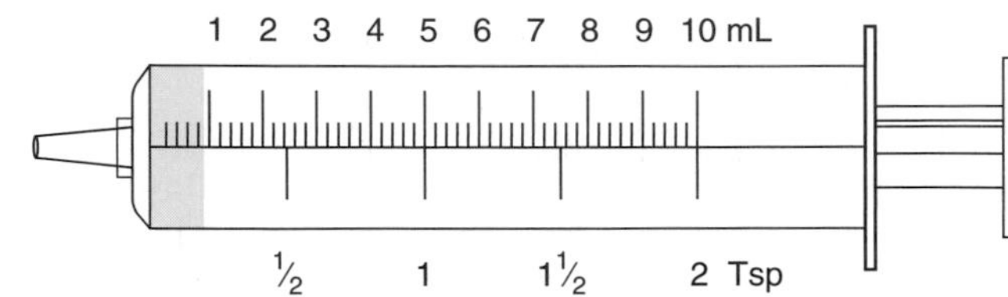

16. 125 mg : 5 mL :: 100 mg : x mL

125 : 5 :: 100 : x

$125x = 500$

$x = \frac{500}{125}$

$x = 4$ mL

$\frac{100 \text{ mg}}{125 \text{ mg}} \times 5 \text{ mL} =$

$\frac{100}{\cancel{125}_{25}} \times \frac{\cancel{5}^{1}}{1} = \frac{100}{25}$

$\frac{100}{25} = 4 \text{ mL}$

17. 10 mg : 1 tab :: 30 mg : x tab

10 : 1 :: 30 : x

$10x = 30$

$x = \frac{30}{10}$

$x = 3$ tablets

$\frac{30 \text{ mg}}{10 \text{ mg}} \times 1 \text{ tab} =$

$\frac{30}{10} = 3$ tablets

18. 40 mg : 1 tab :: 80 mg : x tab

40 : 1 :: 80 : x

$40x = 80$

$x = \frac{80}{40}$

$x = 2$ tablets

$\frac{80 \text{ mg}}{40 \text{ mg}} \times 1 \text{ tab} =$

$\frac{80}{40} = 2$ tablets

19. 10 mg : 1 tab :: 20 mg : x tab

10 : 1 :: 20 : x

$10x = 20$

$x = \frac{20}{10}$

$x = 2$ tablets

$\frac{20 \text{ mg}}{10 \text{ mg}} \times 1 \text{ tab} =$

$\frac{20}{10} = 2$ tablets

Proportion | **Formula**

20. 60 mg : 1 gr : : x mg : 1½ gr
60 : 1 : : x : 3/2

$$x = \frac{\overset{30}{\cancel{60}}}{1} \times \frac{3}{\underset{1}{\cancel{2}}}$$

x = 90 mg = 1½ gr

60 mg : 1 tab : : 90 mg : x tab
60 : 1 : : 90 : x
$60x = 90$

$$x = \frac{90}{60}$$

x = 1½ tablets per dose

1½ tab : 1 dose : : x tab : 3 doses

3/2 : 1 : : x : 3

$$x = \frac{3}{2} \times \frac{3}{1}$$

$$x = \frac{9}{2}$$

x = 4½ tablets per day

Formula:

$$\frac{90 \text{ mg}}{60 \text{ mg}} \times 1 \text{ tab} =$$

$$\frac{90}{60} = 1½ \text{ tablets per dose}$$

Chapter 12 Oral Dosages—Posttest 2, pp. 223-228

Proportion | **Formula**

1. 10 mg : 1 cap : : 20 mg : x
10 : 1 : : 20 : x
$10x = 20$

$$x = \frac{20}{10}$$

x = 2 capsules

Formula:

$$\frac{20 \text{ mg}}{10 \text{ mg}} \times 1 \text{ cap} =$$

$$\frac{20}{10} = 2 \text{ capsules}$$

2. 4 mg : 5 mL : : 8 mg : x mL
4 : 5 : : 8 : x
$4x = 40$

$$x = \frac{40}{4}$$

x = 10 mL

Formula:

$$\frac{8 \text{ mg}}{4 \text{ mg}} \times 5 \text{ mL} =$$

$$\frac{\overset{2}{\cancel{8}}}{\underset{1}{\cancel{4}}} \times \frac{5}{1} = \frac{10}{1} = 10 \text{ mL}$$

Proportion	Formula
3. 160 mg : 5 mL : : 30 mg : x mL 160 : 5 : : 30 : x $160x = 150$ $x = \frac{150}{160}$ $x = 0.9375$ mL	$\frac{30 \text{ mg}}{160 \text{ mg}} \times 5 \text{ mL} =$ $\frac{\overset{3}{\cancel{30}}}{\underset{16}{\cancel{160}}} \times \frac{5}{1} = \frac{15}{16}$ $\frac{15}{16} = 0.9375$ mL

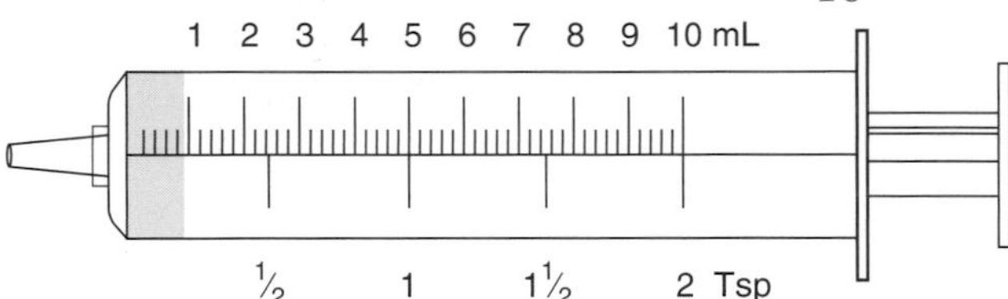

Proportion	Formula
4. 10 mg : 1 tab : : 15 mg : x tab 10 : 1 : : 15 : x $10x = 15$ $x = \frac{15}{10}$ $x = 1\frac{1}{2}$ tablets	$\frac{15 \text{ mg}}{10 \text{ mg}} \times 1$ tab $\frac{15}{10} \times \frac{1}{1} = \frac{15}{10}$ $\frac{15}{10} = 1\frac{1}{2}$ tablets
5. 20 mEq : 30 mL : : 5 mEq : x mL 20 : 30 : : 5 : x $20x = 150$ $x = \frac{150}{20}$ $x = 7.5$ mL	$\frac{5 \text{ mEq}}{20 \text{ mEq}} \times 30 \text{ mL} =$ $\frac{5}{\underset{2}{\cancel{20}}} \times \frac{\overset{3}{\cancel{30}}}{1} = \frac{15}{2}$ $\frac{15}{2} = 7.5$ mL

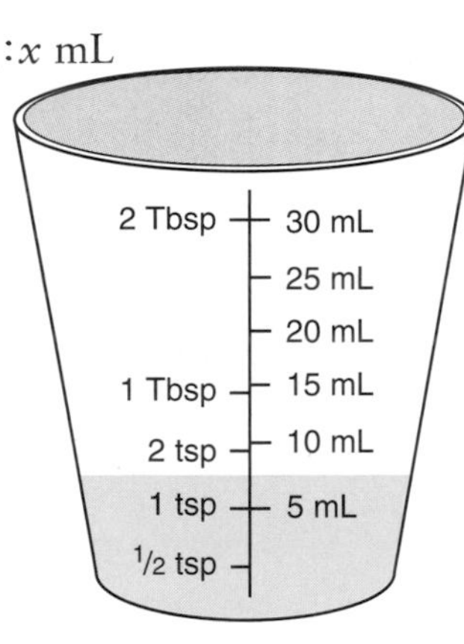

Proportion	Formula
6. 1000 mg : 1 g : : x mg : 0.25 g 1000 : 1 : : x : 0.25 $x = 250$ mg	
250 mg : 1 cap : : 250 mg : x cap 250 : 1 : : 250 : x $250x = 250$ $x = \frac{250}{250}$ $x = 1$ capsule	$\frac{250 \text{ mg}}{250 \text{ mg}} \times 1 \text{ cap} =$ $\frac{250}{250} = 1$ capsule

Proportion	Formula
7. 2.5 mg : 1 tab : : 7.5 mg : x tab 2.5 : 1 : : 7.5 : x $2.5x = 7.5$ $x = \frac{7.5}{2.5}$ $x = 3$ tablets	$\frac{7.5 \text{ mg}}{2.5 \text{ mg}} \times 1 \text{ tab} =$ $\frac{7.5}{2.5} = 3$ tablets
8. 0.05 mg : 1 mL : : 0.05 mg : x mL 0.05 : 1 : : 0.05 : x $0.05x = 0.05$ $x = \frac{0.05}{0.05}$ $x = 1$ mL	$\frac{0.05 \text{ mg}}{0.05 \text{ mg}} \times 1 \text{ mL} =$ $\frac{0.5}{0.5} = 1$ mL
9. 1000 mg : 1 g : : x mg : 0.1 g 1000 : 1 : : x : 0.1 $x = 1000 \times 0.1$ $x = 100$ mg	
50 mg : 1 capsule : : 100 mg : x cap 50 : 1 : : 100 : x $50x = 100$ $x = \frac{100}{50}$ $x = 2$ capsules	$\frac{100 \text{ mg}}{50 \text{ mg}} \times 1 \text{ cap} =$ $\frac{100}{50} = 2$ capsules
10. 60 mg : 1 gr : : x mg : 6 gr 60 : 1 : : x : 6 $x = 360$ mg	
325 mg : 1 tab : : 360 mg : x tab 325 : 1 : : 360 : x $325x = 360$ $x = \frac{360}{325}$ $x = 1.11$ tablet; give 1 tablet	$\frac{360 \text{ mg}}{325 \text{ mg}} \times 1 \text{ tab} =$ 1.11 tablet; give 1 tablet
11. 60 mg : 1 gr : : x mg : ¾ gr 60 : 1 : : x : ¾ $x = \frac{\overset{15}{\cancel{60}}}{1} \times \frac{3}{\underset{1}{\cancel{4}}}$ $x = 45$ mg = ¾ gr	
50 mg : 1 tab : : 45 mg : x tab 50 : 1 : : 45 : x $50x = 45$ $x = \frac{45}{50}$ $x = \frac{9}{10}$ tablet; give 1 tablet	$\frac{45 \text{ mg}}{50 \text{ mg}} \times 1 \text{ tab} =$ $\frac{45}{50} = \frac{9}{10}$ tablet; give 1 tablet

Proportion / **Formula**

12. $125 \text{ mg} : 5 \text{ mL} :: 250 \text{ mg} : x \text{ mL}$

$125 : 5 :: 250 : x$

$125x = 1250$

$x = \frac{1250}{125}$

$x = 10 \text{ mL}$

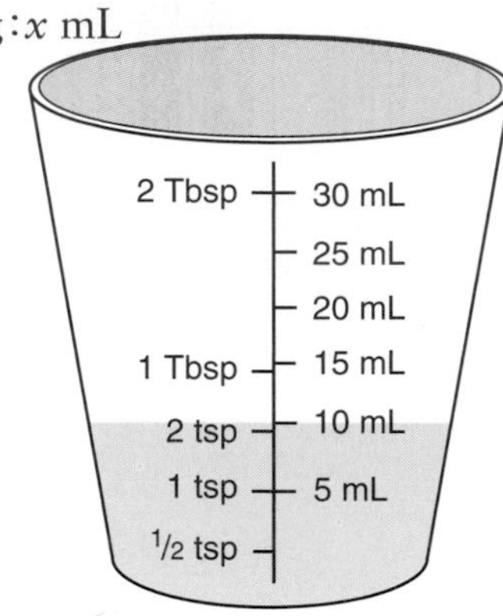

$\frac{250 \text{ mg}}{125 \text{ mg}} \times 5 \text{ mL} =$

$\frac{250}{\cancel{125}_{25}} \times \frac{\cancel{5}^{1}}{1} = \frac{250}{25}$

$\frac{250}{25} = 10 \text{ mL}$

13. $5 \text{ mg} : 1 \text{ tab} :: 20 \text{ mg} : x \text{ tab}$

$5 : 1 :: 20 : x$

$5x = 20$

$x = \frac{20}{5}$

$x = 4$ tablets of 5 mg/tab

$\frac{20 \text{ mg}}{5 \text{ mg}} \times 1 \text{ tab} =$

$\frac{20}{5} = 4$ tablets of 5 mg/tab

14. $0.125 \text{ mg} : 1 \text{ tab} :: 0.25 \text{ mg} : x \text{ tab}$

$0.125 : 1 :: 0.25 : x$

$0.125x = 0.25$

$x = \frac{0.25}{0.125}$

$x = 2$ tablets

$\frac{0.25 \text{ mg}}{0.125 \text{ mg}} \times 1 \text{ tab} =$

$\frac{0.25 \text{ mg}}{0.125} = 2$ tablets

15. $20 \text{ mg} : 5 \text{ mL} :: x \text{ mg} : 25 \text{ mL}$

$20 : 5 :: x : 25$

$5x = 500$

$x = \frac{500}{5}$

$x = 100 \text{ mg}$

$\frac{x \text{ mg}}{20 \text{ mg}} \times 5\text{mL} = 25\text{mL}$

$\frac{x}{\cancel{20}_{4}} \times \frac{\cancel{5}^{1}}{1} = 25$

$\frac{x}{4} = 25$

$\frac{\cancel{4}^{1}}{1} \times \frac{x}{\cancel{4}_{1}} = \frac{25}{1} \times \frac{4}{1}$

$x = 100 \text{ mg}$

16. $1000 \text{ mg} : 1 \text{ g} :: x \text{ mg} : 0.6 \text{ g}$

$1000 : 1 :: x : 0.6$

$x = 600 \text{ mg}$

$325 \text{ mg} : 1 \text{ tab} :: 600 \text{ mg} : x \text{ tab}$

$325 : 1 :: 600 : x$

$325x = 600$

$x = \frac{600}{325}$

$x = 1.85$ tablets; give 2 tablets

$\frac{600 \text{ mg}}{325 \text{ mg}} \times 1 \text{ tab} =$

$\frac{600}{325} = 1.85$ tablets; give 2 tablets

Proportion	Formula
17. 40 mg : 1 tab : : 80 mg : x tab 40 : 1 : : 80 : x $40x = 80$ $x = \frac{80}{40}$ $x = 2$ tablets	$\frac{80\text{ mg}}{40\text{ mg}} \times 1\text{ tab} =$ $\frac{\overset{2}{\cancel{80}}}{\underset{1}{\cancel{40}}} = 2$ tablets
18. 0.5 g : 1 tab : : 1.5 g : x tab 0.5 : 1 : : 1.5 : x $0.5x = 1.5$ $x = \frac{1.5}{0.5}$ $x = 3$ tablets	$\frac{1.5\text{ g}}{0.5\text{ g}} \times 1\text{ tab} =$ $\frac{1.5}{0.5} = 3$ tablets
19. 15 mg : 1 tab : : 30 mg : x tab 15 : 1 : : 30 : x $15x = 30$ $x = \frac{30}{15}$ $x = 2$ tablets	$\frac{30\text{ mg}}{15\text{ mg}} \times 1\text{ tab} =$ $\frac{30}{15} = 2$ tablets
20. 250 mg : 1 tab : : 750 mg : x tab 250 : 1 : : 750 : x $250x = 750$ $x = \frac{750}{250}$ $x = 3$ tablets	$\frac{750\text{ mg}}{250\text{ mg}} \times 1\text{ tab} =$ $\frac{750}{250} = 3$ tablets

Chapter 13 Parenteral Dosages—Work Sheet, pp. 243-272

Proportion	Formula
1. 10 mg : 1 mL : : 30 mg : x mL $10x = 30$ $x = \frac{30}{10} = 3$ mL	$\frac{30\text{ mg}}{10\text{ mg}} \times \frac{1\text{ mL}}{1} = \frac{30}{10} = 3$ mL

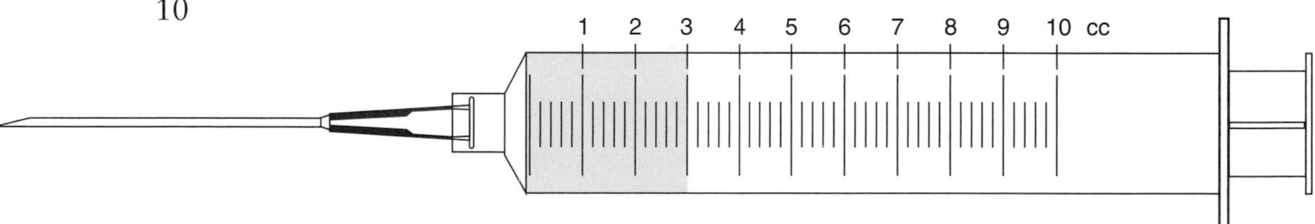

Proportion | **Formula**

2. 500 mcg : 2 mL : : 110 mcg : x mL

$500x = 220$

$x = \frac{220}{500}$

$x = 0.44$ mL

$$\frac{110 \text{ mcg}}{500 \text{ mcg}} \times \frac{2 \text{ mL}}{1} = \frac{220}{500} = 0.44 \text{ mL}$$

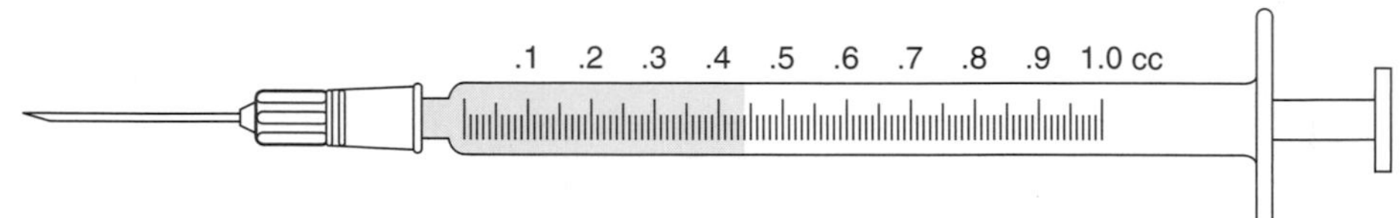

3. 60 mg : 1 gr : : x mg : $\frac{1}{200}$ gr

$x = \frac{60}{200}$

$x = 0.3$ mg

0.4 mg : 1 mL : : 0.3 mg : x mL

$0.4x = 0.3$

$x = \frac{0.3}{0.4}$

$x = 0.75$ mL

$$\frac{0.3}{0.4} \times \frac{1}{1} = 0.75 \text{ mL}$$

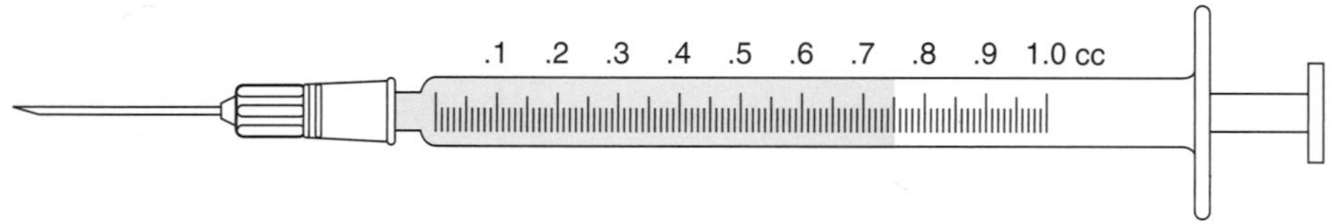

4. 5 mg : 1 mL : : 10 mg : x mL

$5x = 10$

$x = \frac{10}{5} = 2$ mL

$$\frac{10}{5} \times 1 = 2 \text{ mL}$$

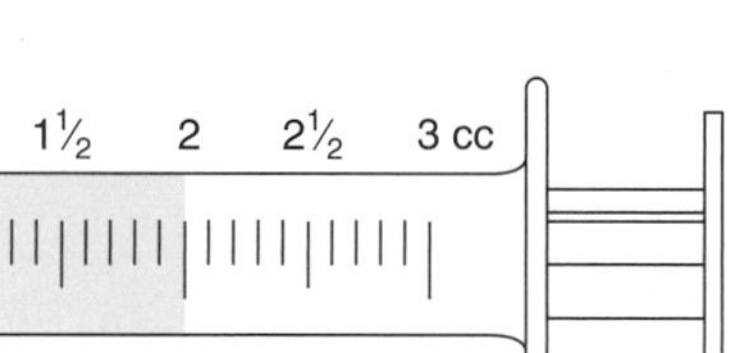

5. 75 mg : 1 mL : : 45 mg : x mL

$75x = 45$

$x = \frac{45}{75}$

$x = 0.6$ mL

$$\frac{45}{75} \times 1 = 0.6 \text{ mL}$$

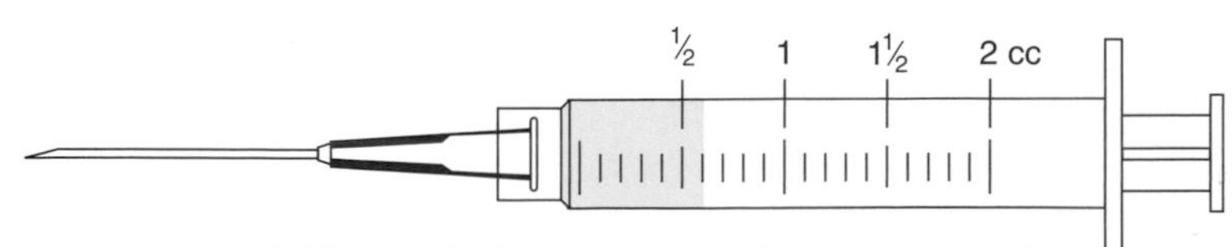

Proportion | **Formula**

6. 1 g : 2.5 mL : : 3 g : x mL
$x = 2.5 \times 3$
$x = 7.5$ mL

$\frac{3}{1} \times 2.5 = 7.5$ mL

7. 10 mg : 1 mL : : 5 mg : x mL
$10x = 5$
$x = \frac{5}{10} = 0.5$ mL

$\frac{5}{10} \times 1 = 0.5$ mL

8. 500 mg : 6 mL : : 1000 mg : x mL
$500x = 6000$
$x = \frac{6000}{500}$
$x = 12$ mL

$\frac{1000}{500} \times \frac{6}{1} = \frac{6000}{500} = 12$ mL

9. 40 mg : 4 mL : : 30 mg : x mL
$40x = 120$
$x = \frac{120}{40}$
$x = 3$ mL

$\frac{30}{\cancel{40}_{10}} \times \frac{\cancel{4}^{1}}{1} = \frac{30}{10} = 3$ mL

10. 30 mg : 1 mL : : 15 mg : x mL
$30x = 15$
$x = \frac{15}{30}$
$x = 0.5$ mL

$\frac{\cancel{15}^{1}\text{ mg}}{\cancel{30}_{2}\text{ mg}} \times \frac{1\text{ mL}}{1\text{ mL}} = ½$ or 0.5 mL

11. 44.6 mEq : 50 mL : : 25.8 : x mL
$44.6x = 1290$
$x = \frac{1290}{44.6}$
$x = 28.9$ mL or 29 mL

$\frac{25.8}{44.6} \times \frac{50}{1} =$
$0.58 \times 50 = 29$ mL

12. 25 mg : 1 mL : : 100 mg : x mL
$25x = 100$
$x = \frac{100}{25}$
$x = 4$ mL

$\frac{100}{25} \times 1 = 4$ mL

13. 100 mg : 20 mL : : 350 mg : x mL
$100x = 7000$
$x = \frac{7000}{100}$
$x = 70$ mL

$\frac{\cancel{350}^{70}\text{ mg}}{\cancel{100}_{\cancel{5}\ 1}\text{ mg}} \times \frac{\cancel{20}^{1}\text{ mL}}{1} =$

$\frac{70}{1} = 70$ mL

14. Proportion

15 gr = 1 g

2 g : 5 mL : : 1 g : x mL

2 : 5 : : 1 : x

$2x = 5$

$x = 2.5$ mL

Formula

$$\frac{1\text{ g}}{2\text{ g}} \times \frac{5}{1} = \frac{5}{2} = 2.5\text{ mL}$$

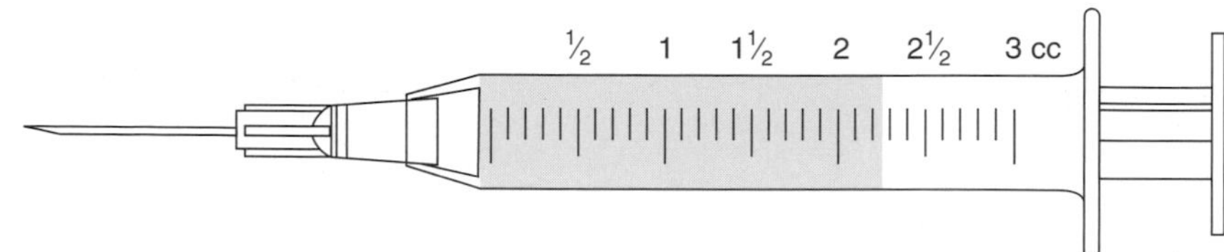

15. 250 mg : 2 mL : : 50 mg : x mL

$250x = 100$

$$x = \frac{100}{250}$$

$x = 0.4$ mL

$$\frac{50}{\cancel{250}_{125}} \times \frac{\cancel{2}^{1}}{1} = \frac{50}{125} = 0.4\text{ mL}$$

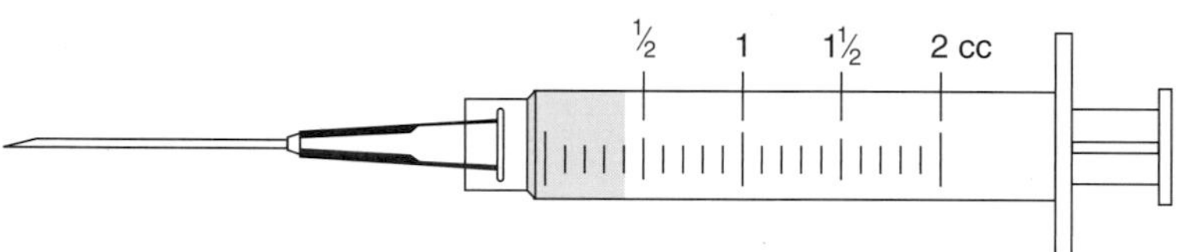

16. 120 mg : 1 mL : : 300 mg : x mL

$120x = 300$

$$x = \frac{300}{120}$$

$x = 2.5$ mL

$$\frac{300}{120} \times 1 = 2.5\text{ mL}$$

17. 300 mg : 2 mL : : 300 mg : x mL

$300x = 600$

$$x = \frac{600}{300}$$

$x = 2$ mL

$$\frac{300}{300} \times \frac{2}{1} = 2\text{ mL}$$

18. 5 mg : 1 mL : : 10 mg : x mL

$5x = 10$

$$x = \frac{10}{5}$$

$x = 2$ mL

$$\frac{10}{5} \times 1 = 2\text{ mL}$$

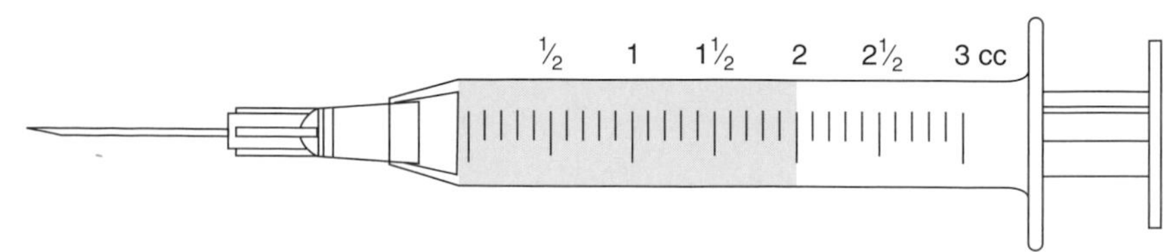

Proportion | **Formula**

19. $2 \text{ mg} : 1 \text{ mL} :: 0.5 \text{ mg} : x \text{ mL}$

$2x = 0.5$

$x = \dfrac{0.5}{2}$

$x = 0.25 \text{ mL}$

Formula: $\dfrac{0.5}{2} \times 1 = 0.25 \text{ mL}$

20. $4 \text{ mg} : 1 \text{ mL} :: 1 \text{ mg} : x \text{ mL}$

$4x = 1$

$x = 0.25 \text{ mL}$

Formula: $\dfrac{1}{4} \times 1 = 0.25 \text{ mL}$

21. $20 \text{ mg} : 1 \text{ mL} :: 10 \text{ mg} : x \text{ mL}$

$20x = 10$

$x = \dfrac{10}{20}$

$x = 0.5 \text{ mL}$

Formula: $\dfrac{10}{20} \times 1 = 0.5 \text{ mL}$

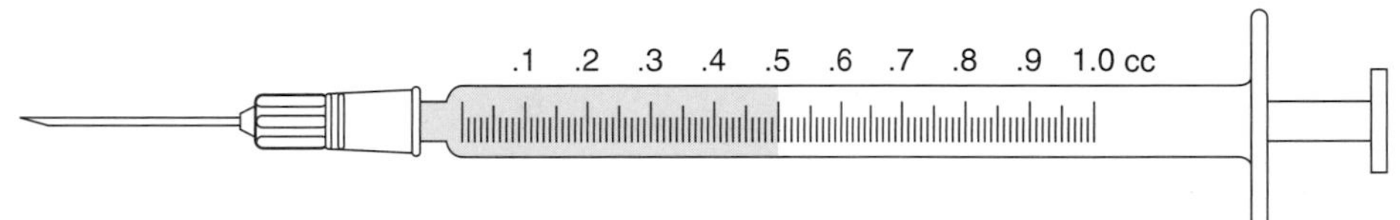

22. $2 \text{ mEq} : 1 \text{ mL} :: 30 \text{ mEq} : x \text{ mL}$

$2x = 30$

$x = \dfrac{30}{2}$

$x = 15 \text{ mL}$

Formula: $\dfrac{30}{2} \times \dfrac{1}{1} = \dfrac{30}{2} = 15 \text{ mL}$

23. $5 \text{ mg} : 1 \text{ mL} :: 10 \text{ mg} : x \text{ mL}$

$5x = 10$

$x = \dfrac{10}{5} = 2 \text{ mL}$

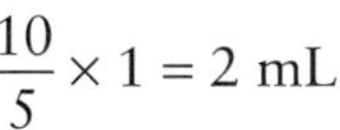

Formula: $\dfrac{10}{5} \times 1 = 2 \text{ mL}$

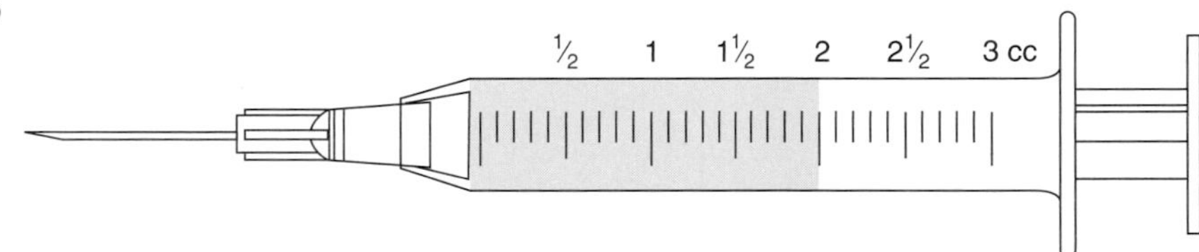

24. $\frac{1}{2} \text{ gr} : 1 \text{ mL} :: \frac{1}{4} \text{ gr} : x \text{ mL}$

$\frac{1}{2}x = \frac{1}{4}$

$x = \dfrac{1}{4} \times \dfrac{2}{1}$

$x = \dfrac{2}{4} = 0.5 \text{ mL}$

Formula: $\dfrac{\frac{1}{4}}{\frac{1}{2}} \times 1$

$\dfrac{1}{4} \div \dfrac{1}{2}$

$\dfrac{1}{4} \times \dfrac{2}{1} = \dfrac{2}{4} = 0.5 \text{ mL}$

Proportion	Formula
25. 10 mg : 1 mL : : 10 mg : x mL $10x = 10$ $x = 1$ mL	$\frac{10}{10} \times 1 = 1$ mL

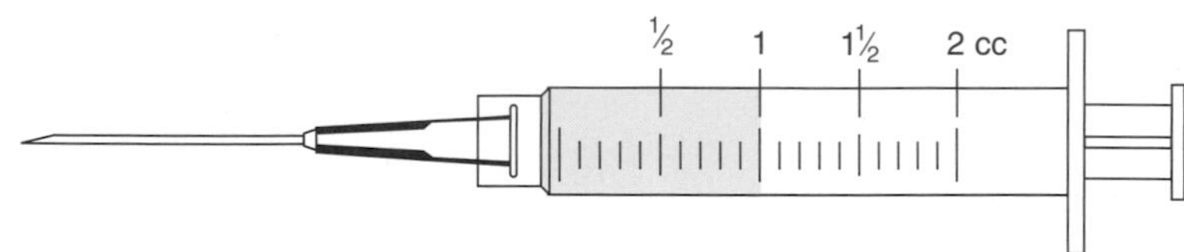

Proportion	Formula
26. 400 mg : 40 mL : : 300 mg : x mL $400x = 12{,}000$ $x = \frac{12{,}000}{400}$ $x = 30$ mL	$\frac{\overset{30}{\cancel{300}}}{\underset{\underset{1}{\cancel{10}}}{\cancel{400}}} \times \frac{\overset{1}{\cancel{40}}}{1} = 30$ mL
27. 15 mg : 1 mL : : 12 mg : x mL $15x = 12$ $x = \frac{12}{15}$ $x = 0.8$ mL	$\frac{\overset{4}{\cancel{12}}}{\underset{5}{\cancel{15}}} \times 1 = 0.8$ mL
28. 50 mg : 1 mL : : 100 mg : x mL $50x = 100$ $x = \frac{100}{50}$ $x = 2$ mL	$\frac{100}{50} \times 1 = 2$ mL
29. 500 mcg : 2 mL : : 100 mcg : x mL $500x = 200$ $x = \frac{200}{500}$ $x = 0.4$ mL	$\frac{100}{500} \times 2 = 0.4$ mL
30. 225 mg : 1 mL : : 500 mg : x mL $225x = 500$ $x = \frac{500}{225}$ $x = 2.22$ mL	$\frac{500}{225} \times 1 = 2.22$ mL

Proportion	Formula

31. 120 mg : 1 mL : : 300 mg : x mL

$$120x = 300$$
$$x = \frac{300}{120}$$
$$x = 2.5 \text{ mL}$$

Formula:
$$\frac{300}{120} \times 1 = 2.5 \text{ mL}$$

32. 250 mg : 2 mL : : 100 mg : x mL

$$250x = 200$$
$$x = \frac{200}{250}$$
$$x = 0.8 \text{ mL}$$

Formula:
$$\frac{100}{\cancel{250}_{125}} \times \frac{\cancel{2}^{1}}{1} = 0.8 \text{ mL}$$

33. 2.5 mEq : 1 mL : : 7.5 mEq : x mL

$$2.5x = 7.5$$
$$x = \frac{7.5}{2.5}$$
$$x = 3 \text{ mL}$$

Formula:
$$\frac{7.5}{2.5} \times \frac{1}{1} = 3 \text{ mL}$$

34. 50 mg : 1 mL : : x mg : 3 mL

$$x = 150 \text{ mg}$$

Formula:
$$\frac{x}{50} \times 1 = 3$$
$$x = 150 \text{ mg}$$

35. $\frac{1}{150}$ gr : 1 mL : : $\frac{1}{100}$ gr : x mL

$$\frac{1}{150}x = \frac{1}{100}$$
$$x = \frac{150}{100}$$
$$x = 1.5 \text{ mL}$$

Formula:
$$\frac{\frac{1}{100}}{\frac{1}{150}} \times \frac{1}{1} =$$
$$\frac{1}{100} \div \frac{1}{150}$$
$$\frac{1}{100} \times \frac{150}{1} = \frac{150}{100} = 1.5 \text{ mL}$$

36. 50 mg : 1 mL : : 50 mg : x mL

$$50x = 50$$
$$x = \frac{50}{50} = 1 \text{ mL}$$

Formula:
$$\frac{50}{50} \times 1 = 1 \text{ mL}$$

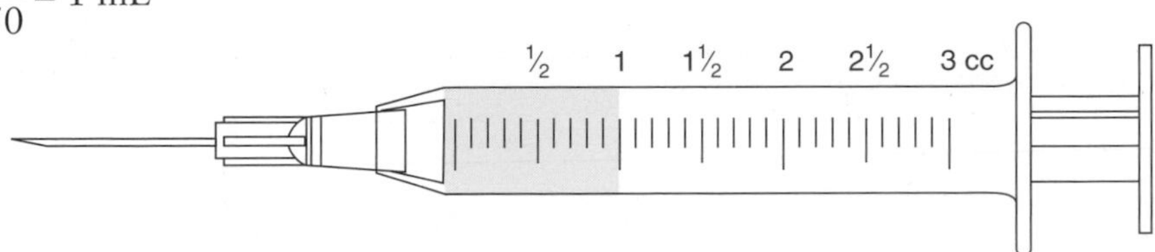

Proportion | **Formula**

37. 100 mg:2 mL::75 mg:x mL

$100x = 150$

$x = \frac{150}{100}$

$x = 1.5$ mL

$\frac{75}{100} \times 2 = \frac{150}{100} = 1.5$ mL

38. 25 mg:1 mL::75 mg:x mL

$25x = 75$

$x = \frac{75}{25}$

$x = 3$ mL

$\frac{75}{25} \times \frac{1}{1} = 3$ mL

39. 100 mg:2 mL::75 mg:x mL

$100x = 150$

$x = \frac{150}{100}$

$x = 1.5$ mL

$\frac{75}{100} \times \frac{2}{1} = \frac{150}{100} = 1.5$ mL

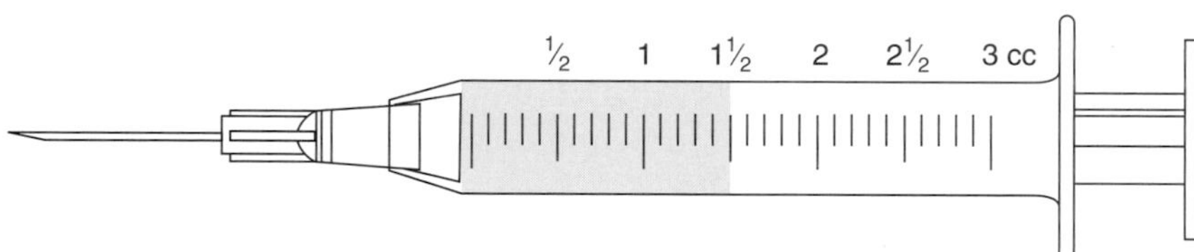

40. 5 mg:1 mL::10 mg:x mL

$5x = 10$

$x = \frac{10}{5}$

$x = 2$ mL

$\frac{10}{5} \times 1 = 2$ mL

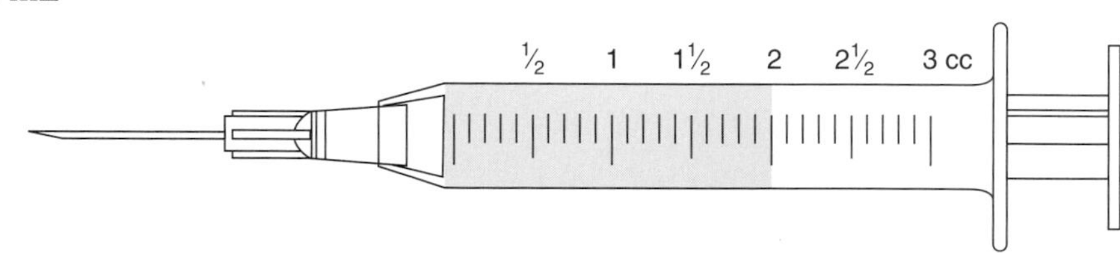

Proportion	Formula
41. 100 mg:2 mL::25 mg:x mL $100x = 50$ $x = \frac{50}{100}$ $x = 0.5$ mL	$\frac{25}{100} \times \frac{2}{1} = \frac{50}{100} = 0.5$ mL

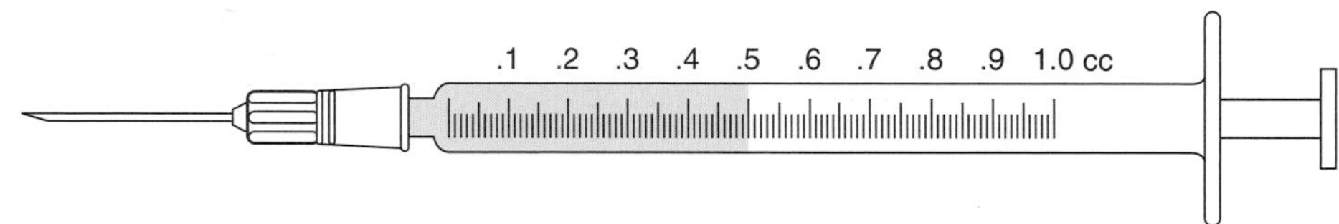

Proportion	Formula
42. 500 mg:2 mL::400 mg:x mL $500x = 800$ $x = \frac{800}{500}$ $x = 1.6$ mL	$\frac{400}{500} \times \frac{2}{1} = \frac{800}{500} = 1.6$ mL
43. 500 mg:1 mL::250 mg:x mL $500x = 250$ $x = \frac{250}{500}$ $x = 0.5$ mL	$\frac{250}{500} \times \frac{1}{1} = 0.5$ mL
44. 13.6 mEq:10 mL::5 mEq:x mL $13.6x = 50$ $x = \frac{50}{13.6}$ $x = 3.68$ mL	$\frac{5}{13.6} \times \frac{10}{1} = \frac{50}{13.6} = 3.68$ mL

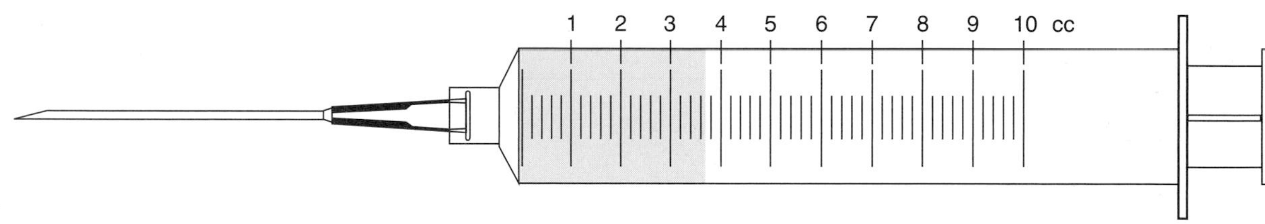

Proportion	Formula
45. 65 mg:1 mL::70 mg:x mL $65x = 70$ $x = \frac{70}{65}$ $x = 1.07$ or 1.1 mL	$\frac{70}{65} \times \frac{1}{1} = 1.07$ or 1.1 mL

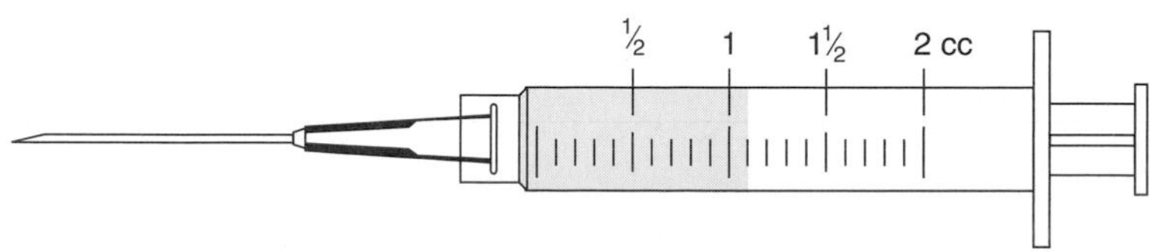

Proportion	Formula
46. 10 mg : 1 mL : : 200 mg : x mL $10x = 200$ $x = \frac{200}{10}$ $x = 20$ mL	$\frac{200}{10} \times \frac{1}{1} = 20$ mL
47. $\frac{1}{30}$ gr = 2 mg 4 mg : 1 mL : : 2 mg : x mL $4x = 2$ $x = \frac{2}{4} = 0.5$ mL	$\frac{2}{4} \times \frac{1}{1} = \frac{2}{4} = 0.5$ mL
48. 0.5 mg : 2 mL : : 0.2 mg : x mL $0.5x = 0.4$ $x = \frac{0.4}{0.5}$ $x = 0.8$ mL	$\frac{0.2}{0.5} \times \frac{2}{1} = \frac{0.4}{0.5} = 0.8$ mL

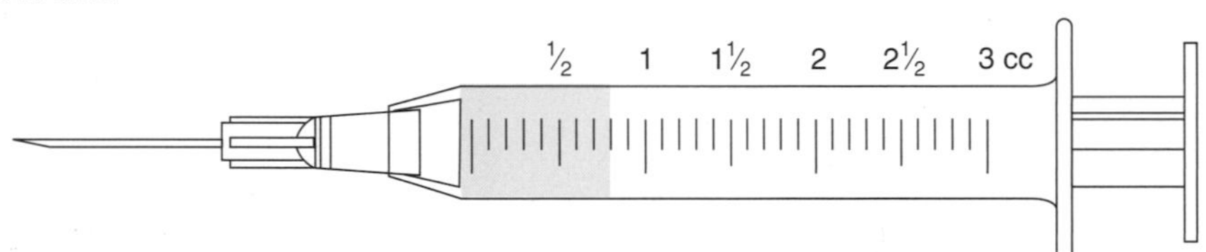

Proportion	Formula
49. 15 mg : 1 mL : : 10 mg : x mL $15x = 10$ $x = \frac{10}{15}$ $x = 0.66$ mL	$\frac{10}{15} \times 1 = 0.66$ mL
50. 5 mg : 1 mL : : 3 mg : x mL $5x = 3$ $x = \frac{3}{5}$ $x = 0.66$ mL	$\frac{3}{5} \times \frac{1}{1} = 0.66$ mL

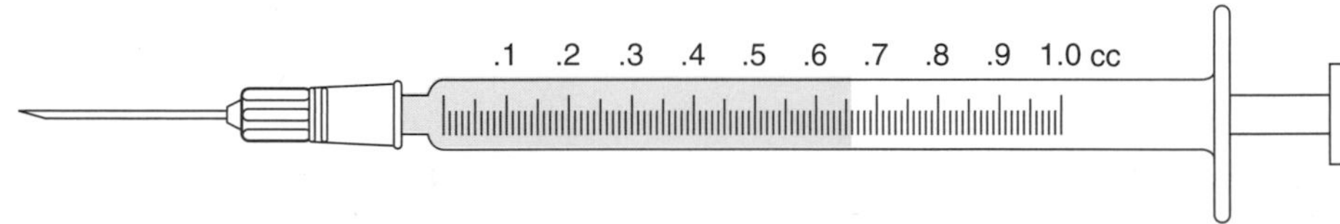

Proportion	Formula
51. 500 mg : 1.2 mL : : 600 mg : x mL $500x = 720$ $x = \frac{720}{500}$ $x = 1.44$ mL	$\frac{600}{500} \times 1.2 = 1.44$ mL

Proportion	Formula
52. 0.4 mg : 1 mL : : 0.9 mg : x mL $0.4x = 0.9$ $x = \frac{0.9}{0.4}$ $x = 2.25$ mL	$\frac{0.9}{0.4} \times \frac{1}{1} = 2.25$ mL
53. ½ gr : 1 mL : : ½ gr : x mL $\frac{1}{2}x = \frac{1}{2}$ $x = 1$ mL	$\frac{\frac{1}{2}}{\frac{1}{2}} \times 1 =$ $\frac{1}{2} \div \frac{1}{2} =$ $\frac{1}{2} \times \frac{2}{1} = 1$ mL
54. 65 mg : 1 mL : : 15 mg : x mL $65x = 15$ $x = \frac{15}{65}$ $x = 0.23$ mL	$\frac{15}{65} \times 1 = 0.23$ mL

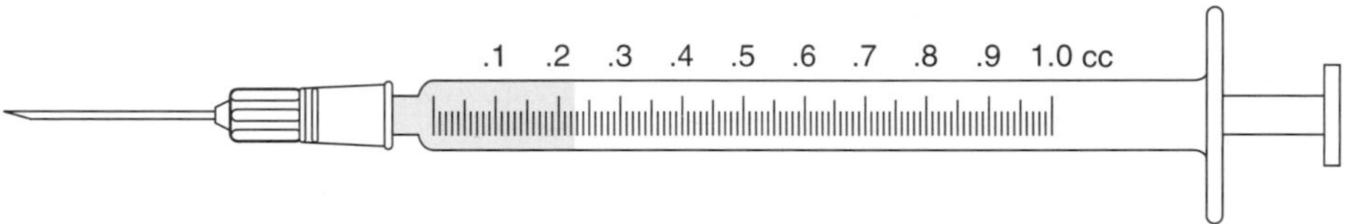

Proportion	Formula
55. 0.89 mEq : 1 mL : : 6 mEq : x mL $0.89x = 6$ $x = \frac{6}{0.89}$ $x = 6.74$ mL	$\frac{6}{0.89} \times 1 = 6.74$ mL

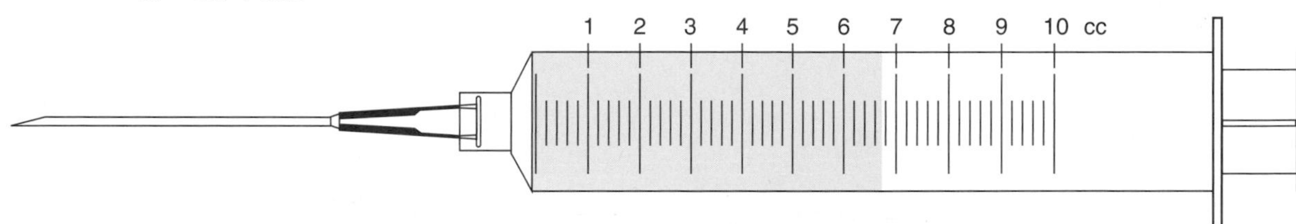

Proportion	Formula
56. 40 mg : 1 mL : : 20 mg : x mL $40x = 20$ $x = \frac{20}{40}$ $x = 0.5$ mL	$\frac{20}{40} \times 1 = 0.5$ mL
57. 25 mg : 1 mL : : x mg : 0.2 mL $x = 25 \times 0.2$ $x = 5$ mg	$\frac{x}{25} \times 1 = 0.2$ $\frac{x}{25} = 0.2$ $x = 0.2 \times 25$ $x = 5$ mg

Proportion	Formula
58. 100 mg : 1 mL : : 500 mg : x mL $100x = 500$ $x = \frac{500}{100}$ $x = 5$ mL	$\frac{500}{100} \times \frac{1}{1} = 5$ mL

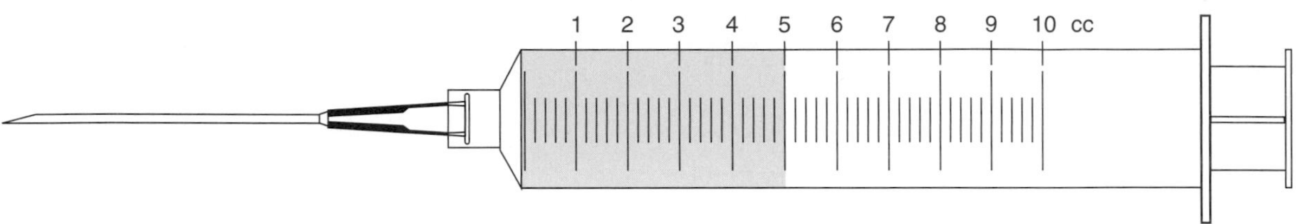

59. 100 mg : 1 mL : : 50 mg : x mL

$100x = 50$

$x = \frac{50}{100}$

$x = 0.5$ mL

$\frac{50}{100} \times \frac{1}{1} = 0.5$ mL

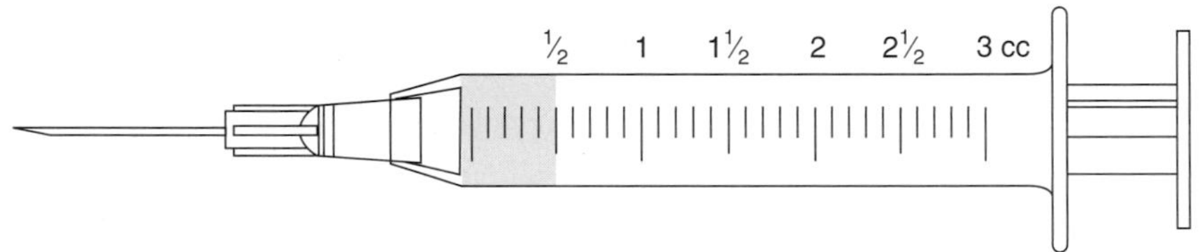

60. 2 mg : 1 mL : : 0.5 mg : x mL

$2x = 0.5$

$x = \frac{0.5}{2}$

$x = 0.25$ mL

$\frac{0.5}{2} \times 1 = 0.25$ mL

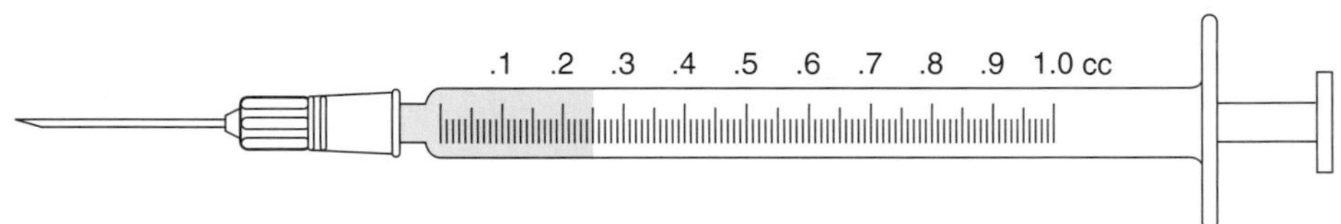

61. 0.25 g : 10 mL : : 0.2 g : x mL

$0.25x = 2$

$x = \frac{2}{0.25}$

$x = 8$ mL

$\frac{0.2}{0.25} \times \frac{10}{1} = \frac{2}{0.25} = 8$ mL

62. 30 mg : 1 mL : : 15 mg : x mL

$30x = 15$

$x = \frac{15}{30}$

$x = 0.5$ mL

$\frac{15}{30} \times \frac{1}{1} = 0.5$ mL

Proportion	Formula
63. 50 mg : 1 mL : : 100 mg : x mL $50x = 100$ $x = \frac{100}{50}$ $x = 2$ mL	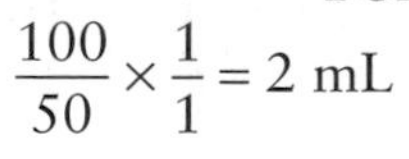 $\frac{100}{50} \times \frac{1}{1} = 2$ mL

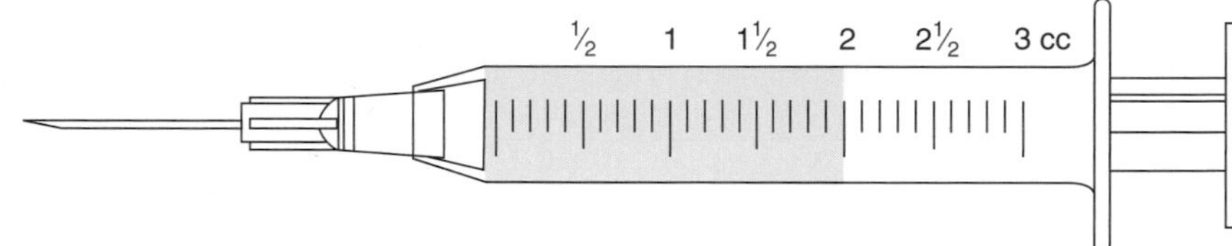

64. 0.5 mg : 2 mL : : 0.25 : x mL

$0.5x = 0.5$

$x = \frac{0.5}{0.5}$

$x = 1$ mL

$$\frac{0.25}{0.50} \times \frac{2}{1} = \frac{0.5}{0.5} = 1 \text{ mL}$$

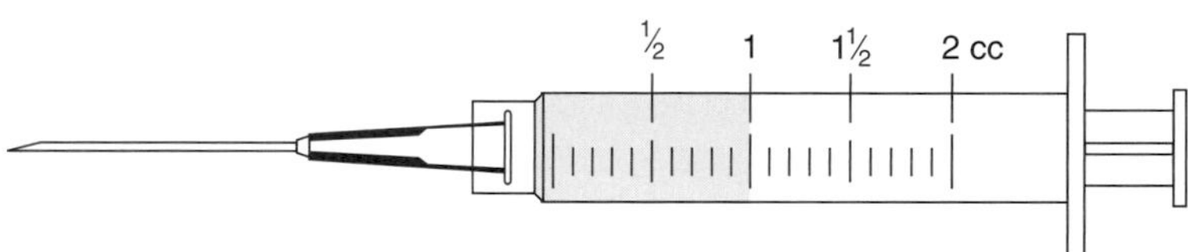

65. 25 mg : 0.5 mL : : 35 mg : x mL

$25x = 17.5$

$x = \frac{17.5}{25}$

$x = 0.7$ mL

$$\frac{\overset{7}{\cancel{35}}}{\underset{5}{\cancel{25}}} \times \frac{0.5}{1} = \frac{3.5}{5} = 0.7 \text{ mL}$$

66. 4.8 mEq : 10 mL : : 5 mEq : x mL

$4.8x = 50$

$x = \frac{50}{4.8}$

$x = 10.42$ mL

$$\frac{5}{4.8} \times \frac{10}{1} = \frac{50}{4.8} = 10.42 \text{ mL}$$

67. 150 mg : 1 mL : : 50 mg : x mL

$150x = 50$

$x = \frac{50}{150}$

$x = 0.33$ mL

$$\frac{50}{150} \times \frac{1}{1} = \frac{50}{150} = 0.33 \text{ mL}$$

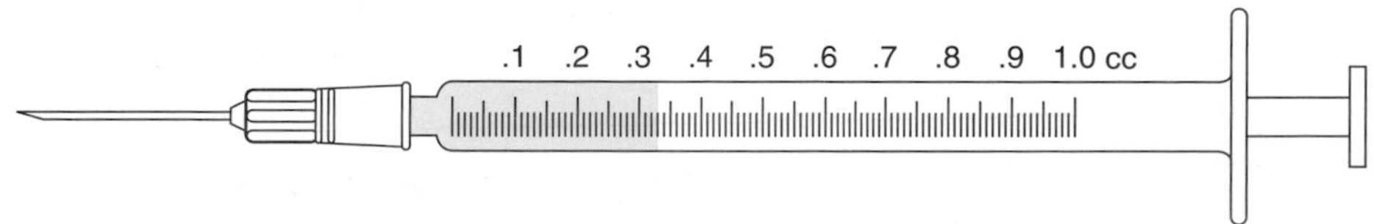

Proportion	Formula

68. 0.4 mg : 1 mL : : 0.2 mg : x mL

$0.4x = 0.2$

$x = \frac{0.2}{0.4}$

$x = 0.5$ mL

Formula: $\frac{0.2}{0.4} \times \frac{1}{1} = 0.5$ mL

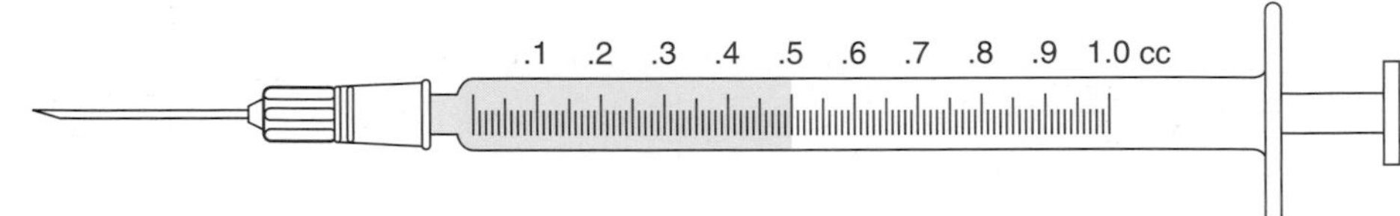

69. 40 mg : 1 mL : : 55 mg : x mL

$40x = 55$

$x = \frac{55}{40}$

$x = 1.38$ mL

Formula: $\frac{55}{40} \times \frac{1}{1} = 1.38$ mL

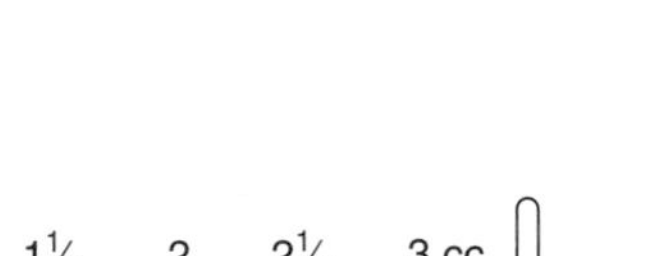

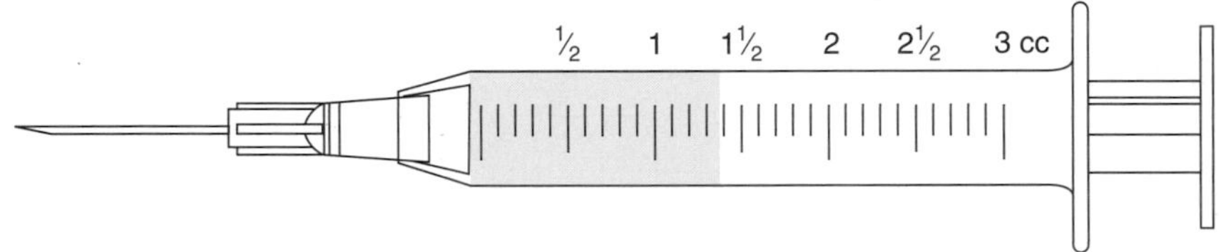

70. 65 mg : 1 mL : : 22 mg : x mL

$65x = 22$

$x = \frac{22}{65}$

$x = 0.34$ mL

Formula: $\frac{22}{65} \times \frac{1}{1} = 0.34$ mL

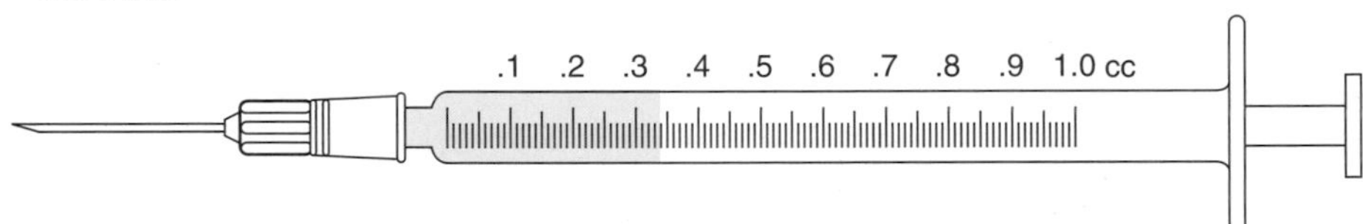

71. 15 mg : 1 mL : : 10 mg : x mL

$15x = 10$

$x = \frac{10}{15}$

$x = 0.66$ mL

Formula: $\frac{10}{15} \times \frac{1}{1} = 0.66$ mL

72. 1000 mcg : 1 mL : : 1000 mcg : x mL

$1000x = 1000$

$x = \frac{1000}{1000}$

$x = 1$ mL

Formula: $\frac{1000}{1000} \times \frac{1}{1} = 1$ mL

73. 325 mg : 1 mL : : 800 mg : x mL

$325x = 800$

$x = \frac{800}{325}$

$x = 2.46$ mL

Formula: $\frac{800}{325} \times \frac{1}{1} = 2.46$ mL

Proportion	Formula
74. 25 mg : 1 mL : : 12.5 mg : x mL $25x = 12.5$ $x = \frac{12.5}{25}$ $x = 0.5$ mL	$\frac{12.5}{25} \times \frac{1}{1} = 0.5$ mL

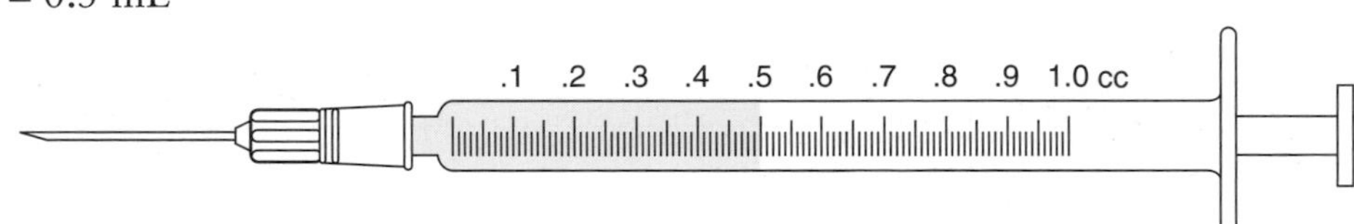

Proportion	Formula
75. 0.2 mg : 1 mL : : 0.28 mg : x mL $0.2x = 0.28$ $x = \frac{0.28}{0.2}$ $x = 1.4$ mL	$\frac{0.28}{0.2} \times \frac{1}{1} = 1.4$ mL
76. 25 mg : 1 mL : : 10 mg : x mL $25x = 10$ $x = \frac{10}{25}$ $x = 0.4$ mL	$\frac{\overset{2}{\cancel{10}}}{\underset{5}{\cancel{25}}} \times \frac{1}{1} = 0.4$ mL
77. 100 mEq : 40 mL : : 15 mEq : x mL $100x = 600$ $x = \frac{600}{100}$ $x = 6$ mL	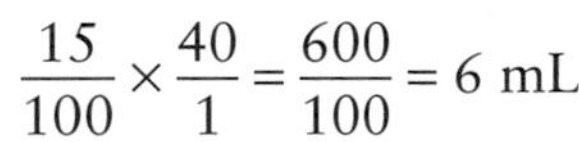 $\frac{15}{100} \times \frac{40}{1} = \frac{600}{100} = 6$ mL

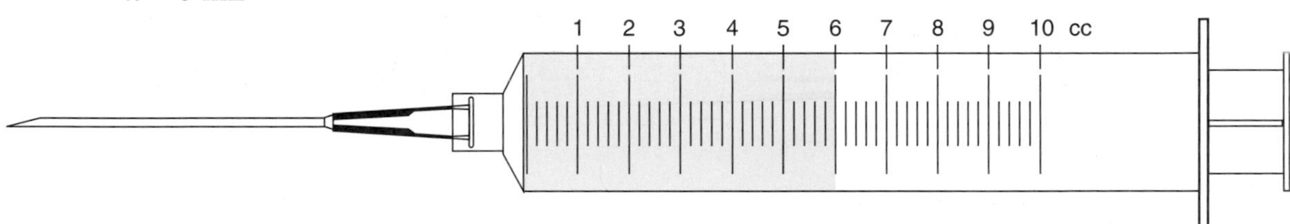

Proportion	Formula
78. 125 mg : 1 mL : : 250 mg : x mL $125x = 250$ $x = \frac{250}{125}$ $x = 2$ mL	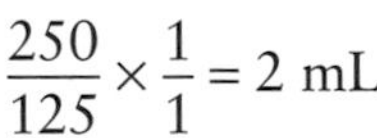 $\frac{250}{125} \times \frac{1}{1} = 2$ mL

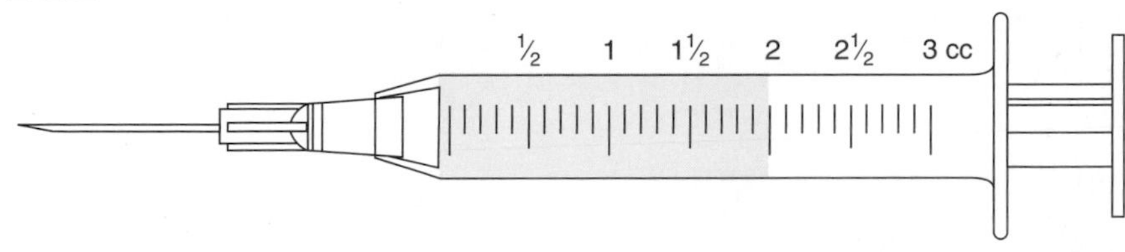

Proportion / Formula

79. 600 mg : 4 mL : : 300 mg : x mL

$600x = 1200$

$x = \frac{1200}{600}$

$x = 2$ mL

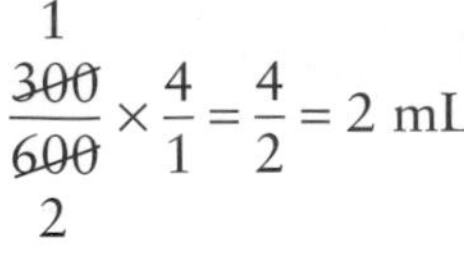

$\frac{\overset{1}{\cancel{300}}}{\underset{2}{\cancel{600}}} \times \frac{4}{1} = \frac{4}{2} = 2$ mL

80. 100 mg : 5 mL : : 75 mg : x mL

$100x = 375$

$x = \frac{375}{100}$

$x = 3.75$ mL

$\frac{75}{100} \times \frac{5}{1} = \frac{375}{100} = 3.75$ mL

81. 1 g : 2.6 mL : : 0.8 g : x mL

$x = 2.08$ mL

$\frac{0.8}{1} \times \frac{2.6}{1} = 2.08$ mL

82. 125 mg : 2 mL : : 100 mg : x mL

$125x = 200$

$x = \frac{200}{125}$

$x = 1.6$ mL

$\frac{\overset{4}{\cancel{100}}}{\underset{5}{\cancel{125}}} \times \frac{2}{1} = \frac{8}{5} = 1.6$ mL

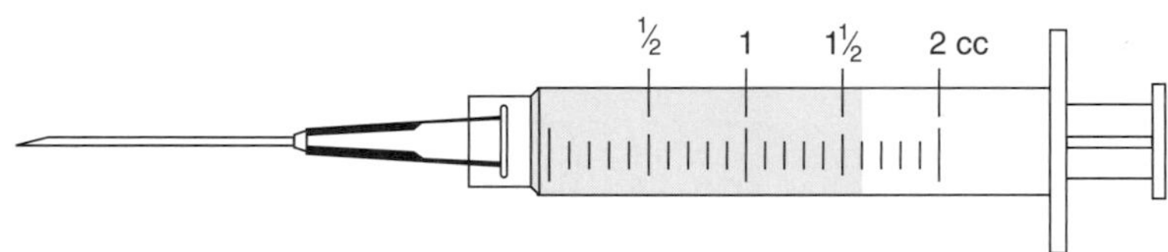

83. 50 mg : 1 mL : : 25 mg : x mL

$50x = 25$

$x = \frac{25}{50}$

$x = 0.5$ mL

$\frac{25}{50} \times \frac{1}{1} = 0.5$ mL

84. 0.4 mg : 1 mL : : 0.4 mg : x mL

$0.4x = 0.4$

$x = \frac{0.4}{0.4}$

$x = 1$ mL

$\frac{0.4}{0.4} \times \frac{1}{1} = 1$ mL

85. 25 mg : 1 mL : : x mg : 0.2 mL

$x = 5$ mg

$\frac{x}{25} \times \frac{1}{1} = 0.2$

$\frac{x}{25} = 0.2$

$x = 0.2 \times 25$

$x = 5$ mg

Proportion	Formula
86. 10 mg : 1 mL : : 1 mg : x mL $10x = 1$ $x = \frac{1}{10}$ or 0.1 mL	$\frac{1}{10} \times \frac{1}{1} = \frac{1}{10} = 0.1$ mL
87. 50 mg : 1 mL : : 50 mg : x mL $50x = 50$ $x = \frac{50}{50}$ $x = 1$ mL	$\frac{50}{50} \times \frac{1}{1} = \frac{50}{50} = 1$ mL

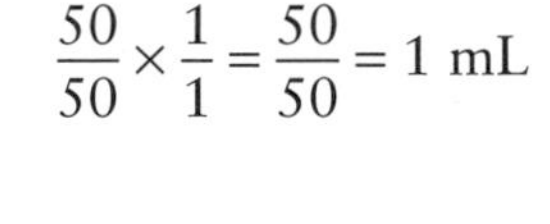

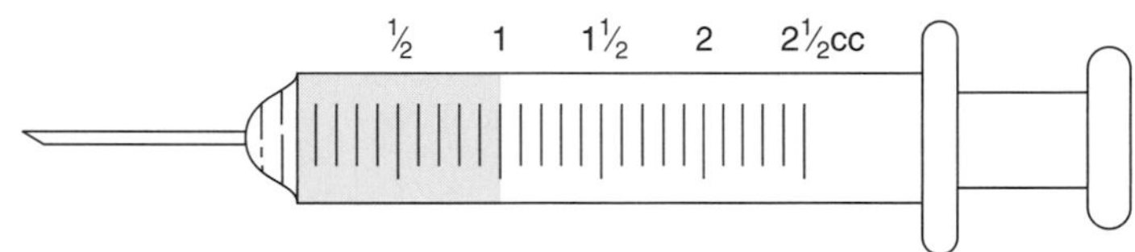

Proportion	Formula
88. 2 mEq : 1 mL : : 10 mEq : x mL $2x = 10$ $x = \frac{10}{2}$ $x = 5$ mL	$\frac{10}{2} \times \frac{1}{1} = \frac{10}{2} = 5$ mL
89. gr $\frac{1}{120} = 0.5$ mg 0.4 mg : 1 mL : : 0.5 mg : x mL $0.4x = 0.5$ $x = \frac{0.5}{0.4}$ $x = 1.25$ mL	$\frac{0.5}{0.4} \times \frac{1}{1} = 1.25$ mL

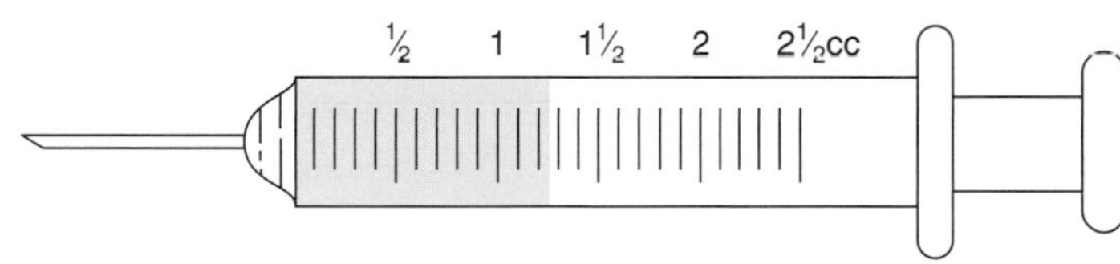

Proportion	Formula
90. 25 mg : 1 mL : : 15 mg : x mL $25x = 15$ $x = \frac{15}{25}$ $x = 0.6$ mL	$\frac{15}{25} \times \frac{1}{1} = 0.6$ mL
91. 250 mg : 5 mL : : 500 mg : x mL $250x = 2500$ $x = \frac{2500}{250}$ $x = 10$ mL	$\frac{500}{250} \times \frac{5}{1} = \frac{2500}{250} = 10$ mL

Proportion / **Formula**

92. 80 mg : 2 mL : : 90 mg : x mL

$80x = 180$

$x = 2.25$ mL

$$\frac{90}{\overset{}{\underset{40}{\cancel{80}}}} \times \frac{\overset{1}{\cancel{2}}}{1} = \frac{90}{40} = 2.25 \text{ mL}$$

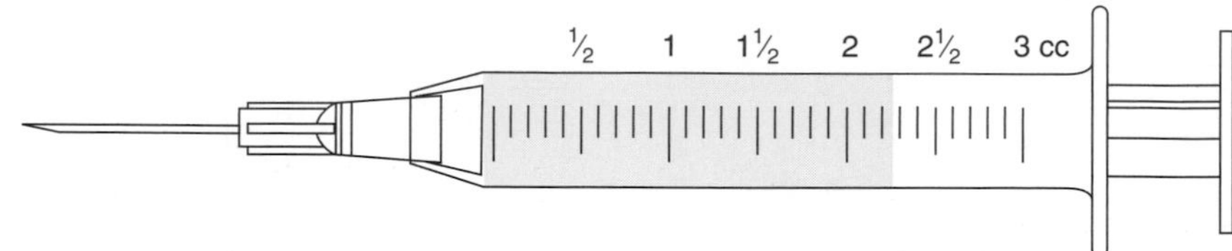

93. 5 mg : 1 mL : : 2 mg : x mL

$5x = 2$

$x = \frac{2}{5}$

$x = 0.4$ mL

$$\frac{2}{5} \times \frac{1}{1} = 0.4 \text{ mL}$$

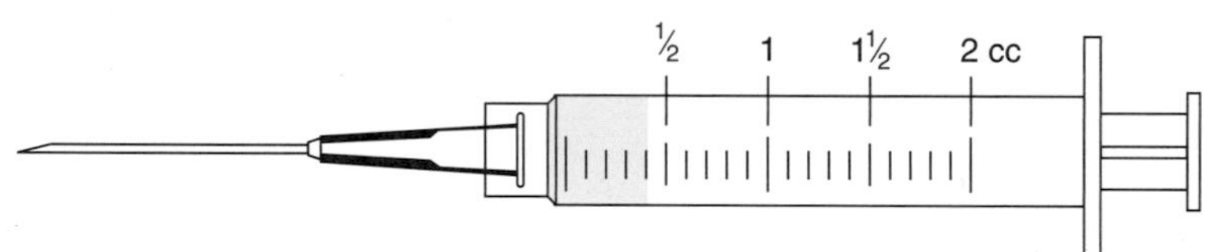

94. 100 mg : 1 mL : : 500 mg : x mL

$100x = 500$

$x = \frac{500}{100}$

$x = 5$ mL

$$\frac{500}{100} \times \frac{1}{1} = 5 \text{ mL}$$

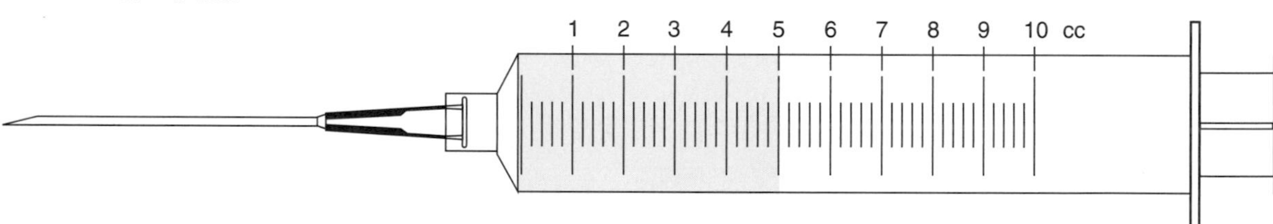

95. 400 mg : 1 mL : : 640 mg : x mL

$400x = 640$

$x = \frac{640}{400}$

$x = 1.6$ mL

$$\frac{640}{400} \times \frac{1}{1} = 1.6 \text{ mL}$$

96. 250 mg : 1 mL : : 500 mg : x mL

$250x = 500$

$x = \frac{500}{250}$

$x = 2$ mL

$$\frac{500}{250} \times \frac{1}{1} = 2 \text{ mL}$$

97. 1 mg : 5 mL : : 0.2 mg : x mL

$x = 1.0$ mL

$$\frac{0.2}{1} \times \frac{5}{1} = \frac{1.0}{1} = 1 \text{ mL}$$

Proportion

98. 25 mg:0.5 mL::100 mg:x mL

$$25x = 50$$
$$x = \frac{50}{25}$$
$$x = 2 \text{ mL}$$

Formula

$$\frac{100}{25} \times \frac{0.5}{1} = \frac{50}{25} = 2 \text{ mL}$$

99. 50 mg:1 mL::10 mg:x mL

$$50x = 10$$
$$x = \frac{10}{50}$$
$$x = 0.2 \text{ mL}$$

$$\frac{10}{50} \times \frac{1}{1} = 0.2 \text{ mL}$$

100. 10 mg:1 mL::4 mg:x mL

$$10x = 4$$
$$x = \frac{4}{10}$$
$$x = 0.4 \text{ mL}$$

$$\frac{4}{10} \times \frac{1}{1} = 0.4 \text{ mL}$$

Chapter 13 Parenteral Dosages—Posttest 1, pp. 273-278

Proportion

1. 50 mg:1 mL::25 mg:x mL

$$50x = 25$$
$$x = \frac{25}{50}$$
$$x = 0.5 \text{ mL}$$

Formula

$$\frac{25}{50} \times \frac{1}{1} = 0.5 \text{ mL}$$

2. 25 mg:1 mL::5.5 mg:x mL

$$25x = 5.5$$
$$x = \frac{5.5}{25}$$
$$x = 0.22 \text{ mL}$$

$$\frac{5.5}{25} \times \frac{1}{1} = \frac{5.5}{25} = 0.22 \text{ mL}$$

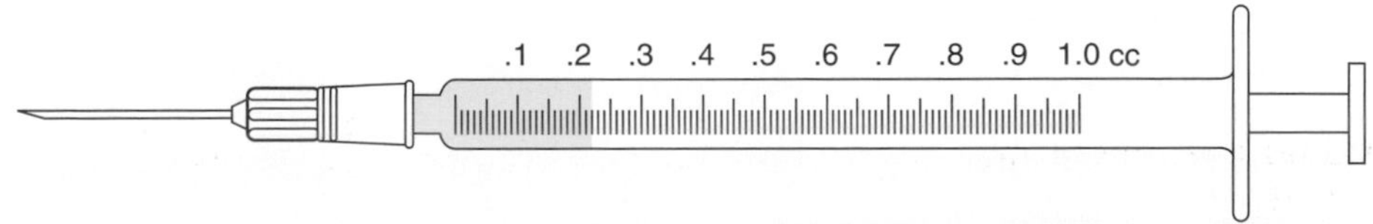

Proportion / **Formula**

3. 15 mg : 1 mL : : 30 mg : x mL

$15x = 30$

$x = \frac{30}{15}$

$x = 2$ mL

Formula: $\frac{30}{15} \times \frac{1}{1} = 2$ mL

4. 1000 mg : 10 mL : : 500 mg : x mL

$1000x = 5000$

$x = \frac{5000}{1000}$

$x = 5$ mL

Formula: $\frac{\overset{1}{\cancel{500}}}{\underset{2}{\cancel{1000}}} \times \frac{10}{1} = \frac{10}{2} = 5$ mL

5. 100 mg : 2 mL : : 50 mg : x mL

$100x = 100$

$x = \frac{100}{100}$

$x = 1$ mL

Formula: $\frac{50}{100} \times \frac{2}{1} = \frac{100}{100} = 1$ mL

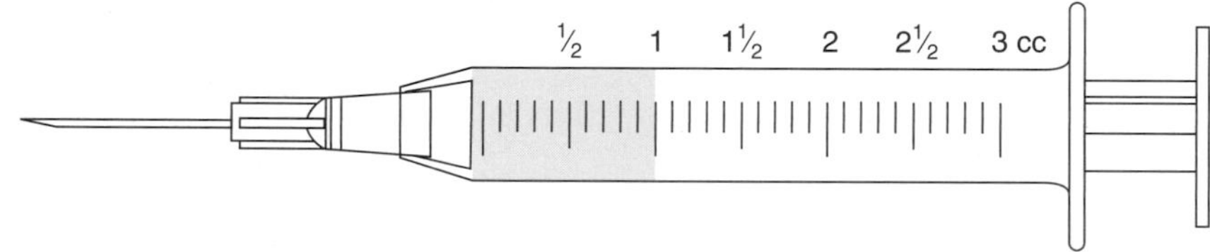

6. 2 mg : 1 mL : : 0.5 mg : x mL

$2x = 0.5$

$x = \frac{0.5}{2}$

$x = 0.25$ mL

Formula: $\frac{0.5}{2} \times \frac{1}{1} = 0.25$ mL

7. 120 mg : 1 mL : : 240 mg : x mL

$120x = 240$

$x = \frac{240}{120}$

$x = 2$ mL

Formula: $\frac{240}{120} \times \frac{1}{1} = 2$ mL

Proportion	Formula

8. $0.4\text{ mg}:1\text{ mL}::0.2\text{ mg}:x\text{ mL}$

$0.4x = 0.2$

$x = \frac{0.2}{0.4}$

$x = 0.5\text{ mL}$

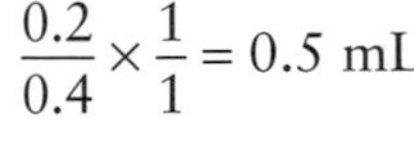

$\frac{0.2}{0.4} \times \frac{1}{1} = 0.5\text{ mL}$

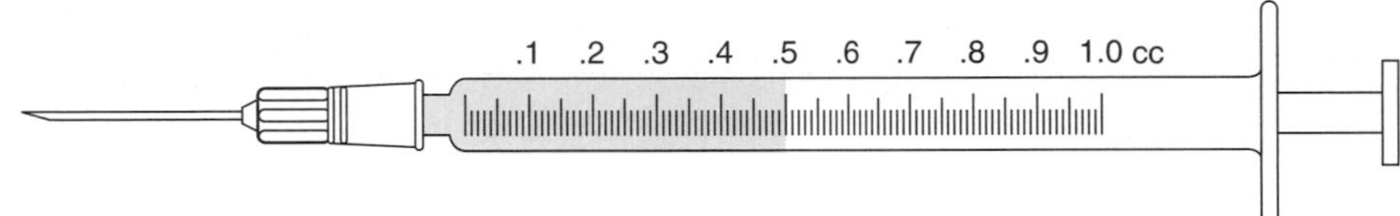

9. $25\text{ mg}:1\text{ mL}::100\text{ mg}:x\text{ mL}$

$25x = 100$

$x = \frac{100}{25}$

$x = 4\text{ mL}$

$\frac{100}{25} \times \frac{1}{1} = 4\text{ mL}$

10. $5\text{ mg}:1\text{ mL}::2\text{ mg}:x\text{ mL}$

$5x = 2$

$x = \frac{2}{5}$

$x = 0.4\text{ mL}$

$\frac{2}{5} \times \frac{1}{1} = 0.4\text{ mL}$

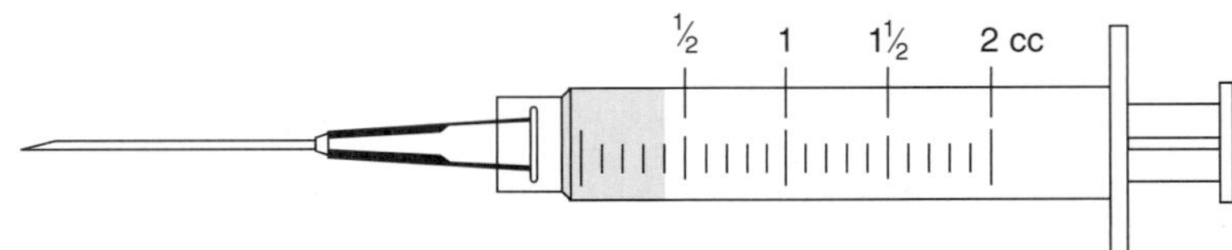

11. $0.5\text{ mg}:1\text{ mL}::0.7:x\text{ mL}$

$0.5x = 0.7$

$x = \frac{0.7}{0.5}$

$x = 1.4\text{ mL}$

$\frac{0.7}{0.5} \times \frac{1}{1} = 1.4\text{ mL}$

12. $50\text{ mg}:1\text{ mL}::25\text{ mg}:x\text{ mL}$

$50x = 25$

$x = \frac{25}{50}$

$x = 0.5\text{ mL}$

$\frac{25}{50} \times \frac{1}{1} = 0.5\text{ mL}$

13. $80\text{ mg}:1\text{ mL}:50\text{ mg}:4\text{ mL}$

$80x = 50$

$x = \frac{50}{80}$

$x = 0.625\text{ mL}$

$\frac{50}{80} \times \frac{1}{1} = 0.625\text{ mL}$

Proportion	Formula
14. 250 mg : 1 mL : : 500 mg : x mL $250x = 500$ $x = \frac{500}{250}$ $x = 2$ mL	$\frac{500}{250} \times \frac{1}{1} = \frac{500}{250} = 2$ mL
15. 1000 mg : 50 mL : : 300 mg : x mL $1000x = 15{,}000$ $x = \frac{15{,}000}{1000}$ $x = 15$ mL	$\frac{300}{\cancel{1000}_{20}} \times \frac{\cancel{50}^{1}}{1} = \frac{300}{20} = 15$ mL
16. 10 mg : 1 mL : : 6 mg : x mL $10x = 6$ $x = \frac{6}{10}$ $x = 0.6$ mL	$\frac{6}{10} \times \frac{1}{1} = 0.6$ mL
17. 10 mg : 1 mL : : 6 mg : x mL $10x = 6$ $x = \frac{6}{10}$ $x = 0.6$ mL	$\frac{6}{10} \times \frac{1}{1} = \frac{6}{10} = 0.6$ mL
18. 40 mg : 4 mL : : 10 mg : x mL $40x = 40$ $x = 1$ mL	$\frac{10}{\cancel{40}_{10}} \times \frac{\cancel{4}^{1}}{1} = \frac{10}{10} = 1$ mL

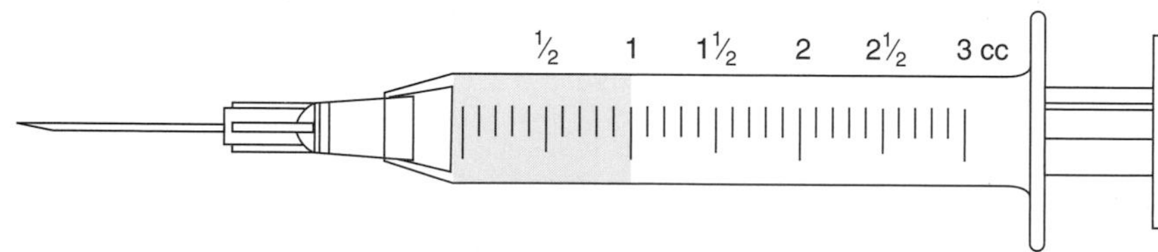

Proportion	Formula
19. 0.5 mg : 2 mL : : 0.3 mg : x mL $0.5x = 0.6$ $x = \frac{0.6}{0.5}$ $x = 1.2$ mL	$\frac{0.3}{0.5} \times \frac{2}{1} = \frac{0.6}{0.5} = 1.2$ mL

Proportion	Formula
20. 20 mEq : 1 mL : : 5 mEq : x mL $20x = 5$ $x = \frac{5}{20}$ $x = 0.25$ mL	$\frac{5}{20} \times \frac{1}{1} = 0.25$ mL

Chapter 13 Parenteral Dosages—Posttest 2, pp. 279-284

Proportion	Formula
1. 4 mg : 1 mL : : 2 mg : x mL $4x = 2$ $x = \frac{2}{4}$ $x = 0.5$ mL	$\frac{2}{4} \times \frac{1}{1} = 0.5$ mL
2. 4 mg : 1 mL : : 2 mg : x mL $4x = 2$ $x = \frac{2}{4}$ $x = 0.5$ mL	$\frac{2}{4} \times \frac{1}{1} = 0.5$ mL
3. 500 mg : 10 mL : : 400 mg : x mL $500x = 4000$ $x = \frac{4000}{500}$ $x = 8$ mL	$\frac{\overset{4}{\cancel{400}}}{\underset{5}{\cancel{500}}} \times \frac{10}{1} = \frac{40}{5} = 8$ mL

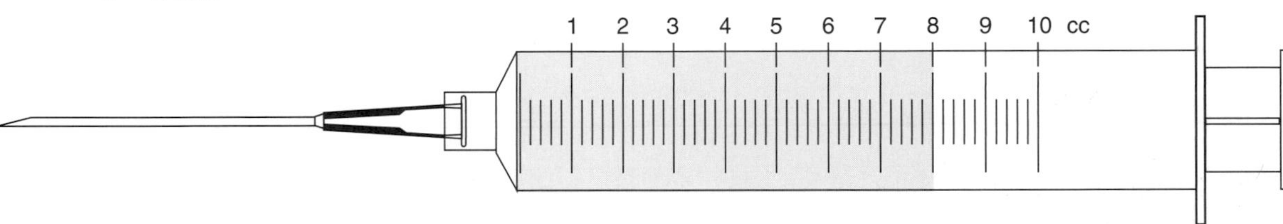

Proportion	Formula
4. 50 mg : 1 mL : : 75 mg : x mL $50x = 75$ $x = \frac{75}{50}$ $x = 1.5$ mL	$\frac{75}{50} \times \frac{1}{1} = 1.5$ mL
5. 30 mg : 1 mL : : 60 mg : x mL $30x = 60$ $x = \frac{60}{30}$ $x = 2$ mL	$\frac{60}{30} \times \frac{1}{1} = 2$ mL

Proportion | **Formula**

6. 25 mg:0.5 mL::15 mg:x mL

$25x = 7.5$

$x = \frac{7.5}{25}$

$x = 0.3$ mL

$\frac{15}{25} \times \frac{0.5}{1} = \frac{7.5}{25} = 0.3$ mL

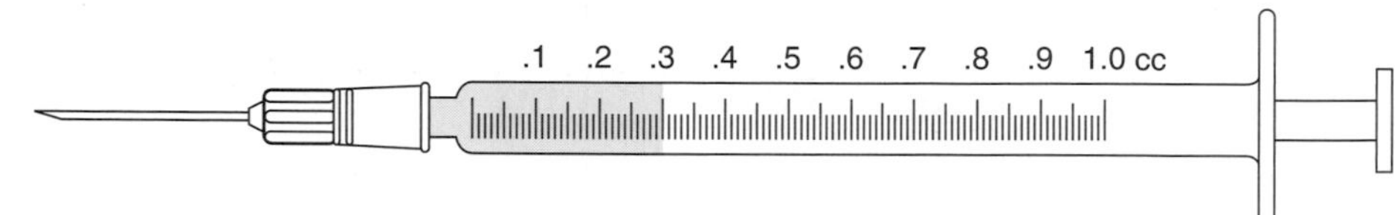

7. 0.4 mg:1 mL::0.3 mg:x mL

$0.4x = 0.3$

$x = \frac{0.3}{0.4}$

$x = 0.75$ mL

$\frac{0.3}{0.4} \times \frac{1}{1} = 0.75$ mL

8. 10 mg:1 mL::25 mg:x mL

$10x = 25$

$x = \frac{25}{10}$

$x = 2.5$ mL

$\frac{25}{10} \times \frac{1}{1} = 2.5$ mL

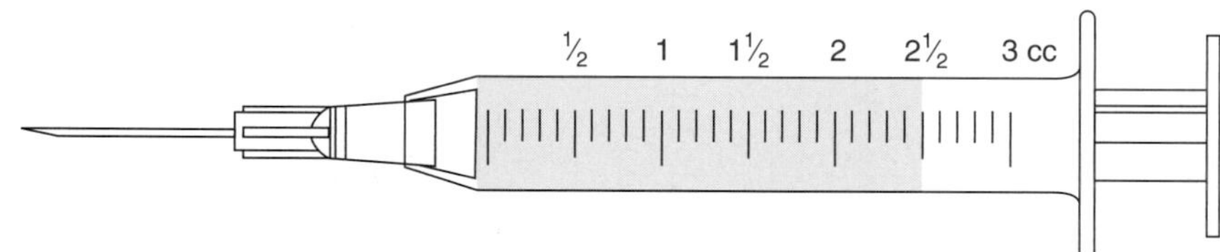

9. 40 mg:1 mL::55 mg:x mL

$40x = 55$

$x = \frac{50}{40}$

$x = 1.375$ mL

$\frac{\overset{11}{\cancel{55}}}{\underset{8}{\cancel{40}}} \times \frac{1}{1} = 1.375$ mL

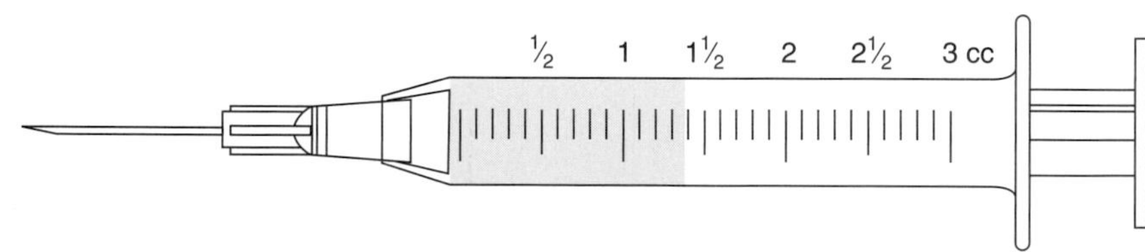

Proportion	Formula
10. 25 mg : 1 mL : : 30 mg : x mL $25x = 30$ $x = \frac{30}{25}$ $x = 1.2$ mL	$\frac{\overset{6}{\cancel{30}}}{\underset{5}{\cancel{25}}} \times \frac{1}{1} = 1.2$ mL

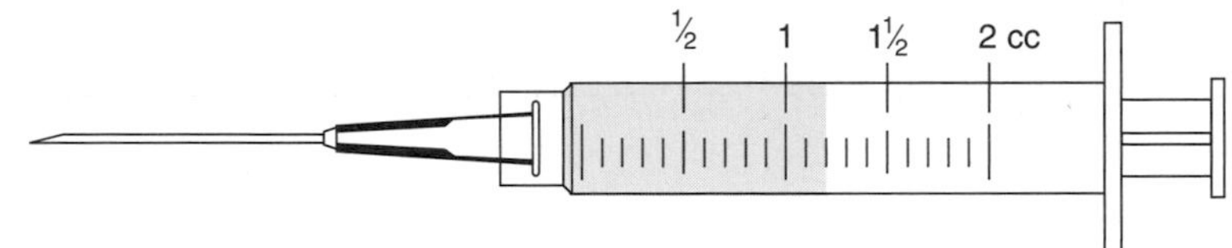

11. 100 mg : 1 mL : : 200 mg : x mL $100x = 200$ $x = \frac{200}{100}$ $x = 2$ mL	$\frac{200}{100} \times \frac{1}{1} = 2$ mL

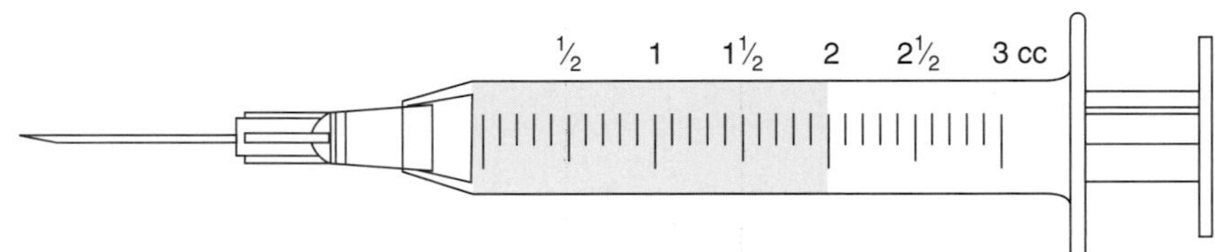

12. $\frac{1}{200}$ gr : 1 mL : : $\frac{1}{150}$ gr : x mL $\frac{1}{200}x = \frac{1}{150}$ $x = \frac{200}{150}$ $x = 1.33$ mL	$\frac{\frac{1}{150}}{\frac{1}{200}} \times \frac{15}{1} =$ $\frac{1}{150} \times \frac{200}{1} = \frac{200}{150}$ $\frac{200}{\underset{10}{\cancel{150}}} \times \frac{1}{1} = \frac{200}{150} = 1.33$ mL

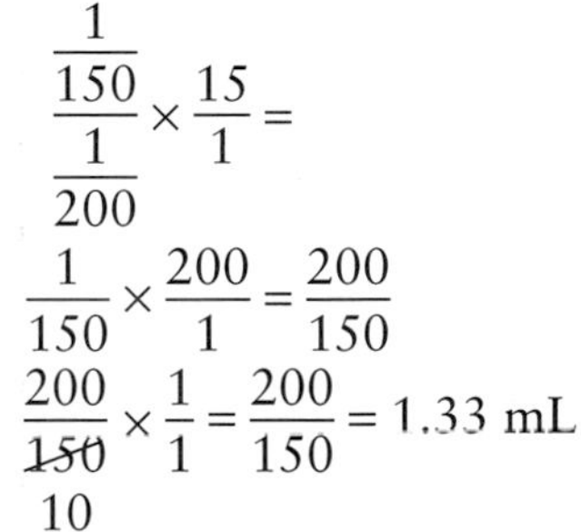

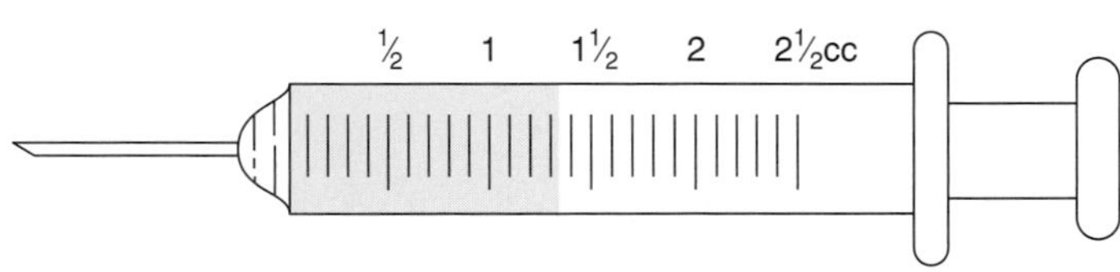

13. 1 g : 2.5 mL : : 2 g : x mL $x = 5$ mL	$\frac{2}{1} \times \frac{2.5}{1} = 5$ mL

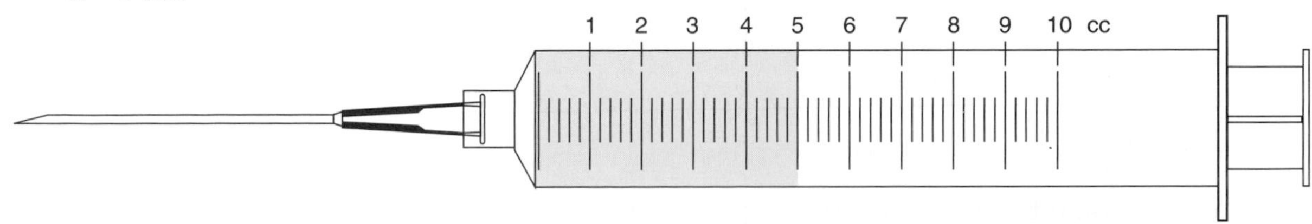

Proportion	Formula
14. 40 mg : 1 mL : : 26 mg : x mL $40x = 26$ $x = \frac{26}{40}$ $x = 0.65$ mL	$\frac{26}{40} \times \frac{1}{1} = 0.65$ mL
15. 60 mg : 0.6 mL : : 85 mg : x mL $60x = 51$ $x = \frac{51}{60}$ $x = 0.85$ mL	$\frac{85}{60} \times \frac{0.6}{1} = \frac{51}{60} = 0.85$ mL
16. 500 mcg : 2 mL : : 80 mcg : x mL $500x = 160$ $x = \frac{160}{500}$ $x = 0.32$ mL	$\frac{80}{500} \times \frac{2}{1} = \frac{160}{500} = 0.32$ mL
17. 8 mg : 1 mL : : 4 mg : x mL $8x = 4$ $x = \frac{4}{8}$ $x = 0.5$ mL	$\frac{4}{8} \times \frac{1}{1} = 0.5$ mL

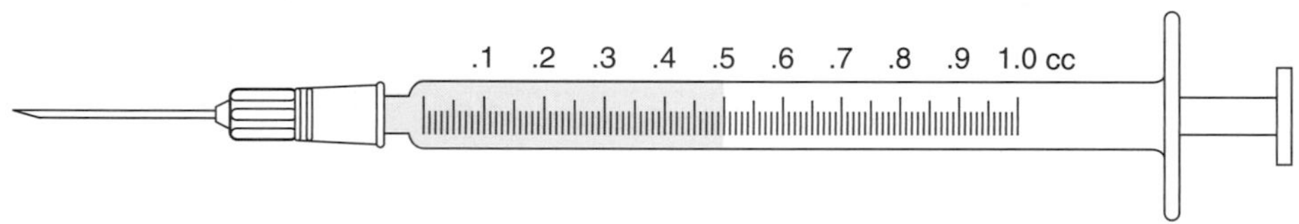

Proportion	Formula
18. 50 mg : 2 mL : : 100 mg : x mL $50x = 200$ $x = \frac{200}{50}$ $x = 4$ mL	$\frac{100}{50} \times \frac{2}{1} = \frac{200}{50} = 4$ mL

1 2 3 4 5 6 7 8 9 10 cc

Proportion	Formula
19. 120 mg : 1 mL : : 200 mg : x mL $120x = 200$ $x = \frac{200}{120}$ $x = 1.66$ mL	$\frac{200}{120} \times \frac{1}{1} = 1.66$ mL

Proportion	Formula

20. 13.6 mEq : 10 mL : : 10 mEq : x mL

$$13.64x = 100$$
$$x = \frac{100}{13.6}$$
$$x = 7.35 \text{ mL}$$

Formula:

$$\frac{10}{13.6} \times \frac{10}{1} = \frac{100}{13.6} = 7.35 \text{ mL}$$

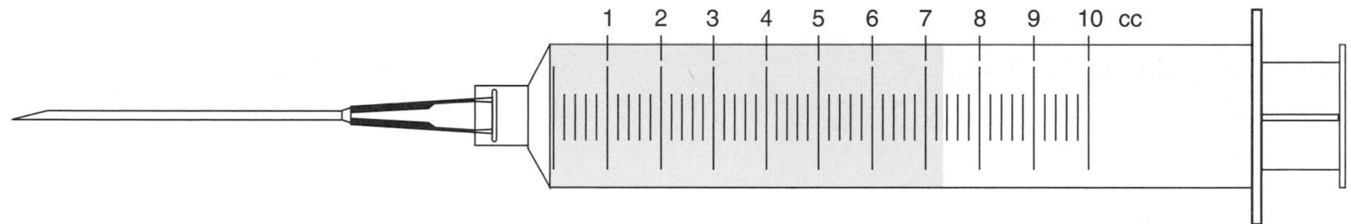

Chapter 14 Dosages Measured in Units—Work Sheet, pp. 293-299

Proportion	Formula

1. 400,000 U : 5 mL : : 200,000 U : x mL

$$400{,}000x = 1{,}000{,}000$$
$$x = \frac{1{,}000{,}000}{400{,}000}$$
$$x = 2.5 \text{ mL}$$

Formula:

$$\frac{200{,}000}{\cancel{400{,}000}_{\,80{,}000}} \times \frac{\cancel{5}^{\,1}}{1} =$$
$$\frac{200{,}000}{80{,}000} = 2.5 \text{ mL}$$

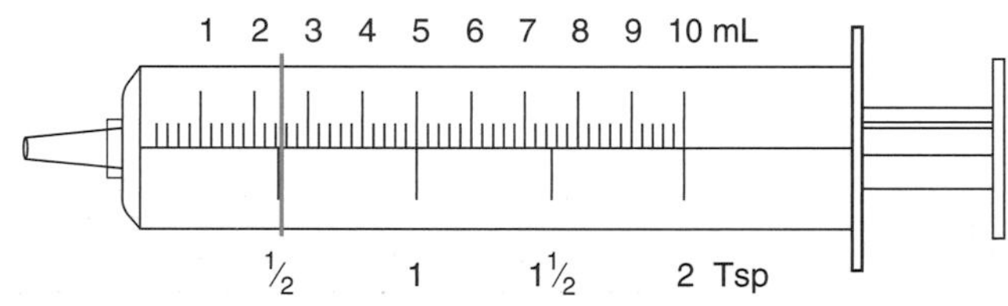

2. 5000 U : 1 mL : : 7500 U : x mL

$$5000x = 7500$$
$$x = \frac{7500}{5000}$$
$$x = 1.5 \text{ mL}$$

Formula:

$$\frac{7500}{5000} \times \frac{1}{1} = 1.5 \text{ mL}$$

3.

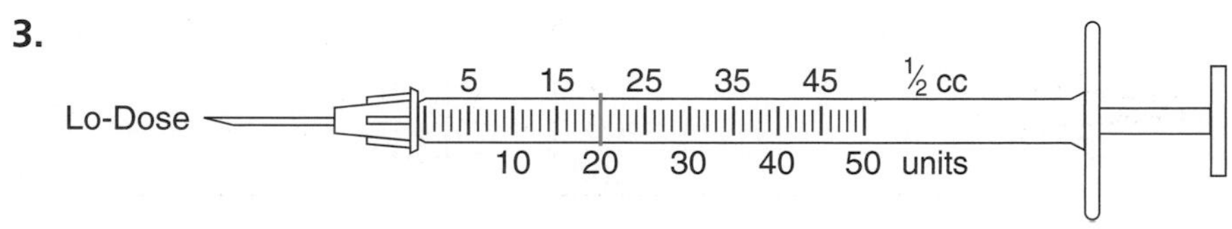

Proportion	Formula
4. Diluent 9.6 mL, 100,000 U/mL 100,000 U : 1 mL : : 500,000 U : x mL $100{,}000x = 500{,}000$ $x = \frac{500{,}000}{100{,}000}$ $x = 5$ mL	$\frac{500{,}000}{100{,}000} \times \frac{1}{1} = 5$ mL
Diluent 4.6 mL, 200,000 U/mL 200,000 U : 1 mL : : 500,000 U : x mL $200{,}000x = 500{,}000$ $x = \frac{500{,}000}{200{,}000}$ $x = 2.5$ mL	$\frac{500{,}000}{200{,}000} \times \frac{1}{1} = 2.5$ mL
Diluent 1.6 mL, 500,000 U/mL 500,000 U : 1 mL : : 500,000 U : x mL $500{,}000x = 500{,}000$ $x = \frac{500{,}000}{500{,}000}$ $x = 1$ mL	$\frac{500{,}000}{500{,}000} \times \frac{1}{1} = 1$ mL
5. 5000 U : 1 mL : : 2500 U : x mL $5000x = 2500$ $x = \frac{2500}{5000}$ $x = 0.5$ mL	$\frac{2500}{5000} \times \frac{1}{1} = 0.5$ mL

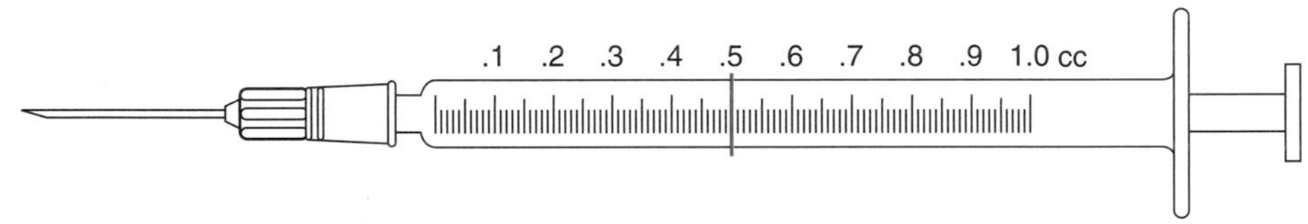

6.

Lo-Dose

5 15 25 35 45 ½ cc

10 20 30 40 50 units

Proportion	Formula
7. 10,000 U : 1 mL : : 5000 U : x mL $10{,}000x = 5000$ $x = \frac{5000}{10{,}000}$ $x = 0.5$ mL	$\frac{5000}{10{,}000} \times \frac{1}{1} = 0.5$ mL

Proportion | **Formula**

8. 200,000 U : 5 mL : : 400,000 U : x mL

$200{,}000x = 2{,}000{,}000$

$x = \dfrac{2{,}000{,}000}{200{,}000}$

$x = 10$ mL

$$\frac{400{,}000}{200{,}000} \times \frac{5}{1} = \frac{2{,}000{,}000}{200{,}000} = 10 \text{ mL}$$

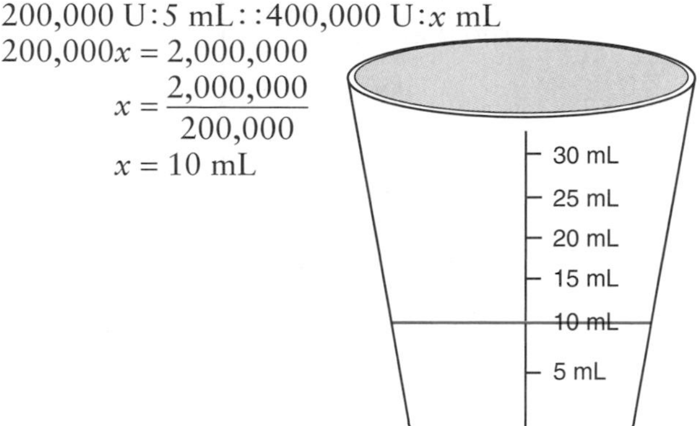

9.

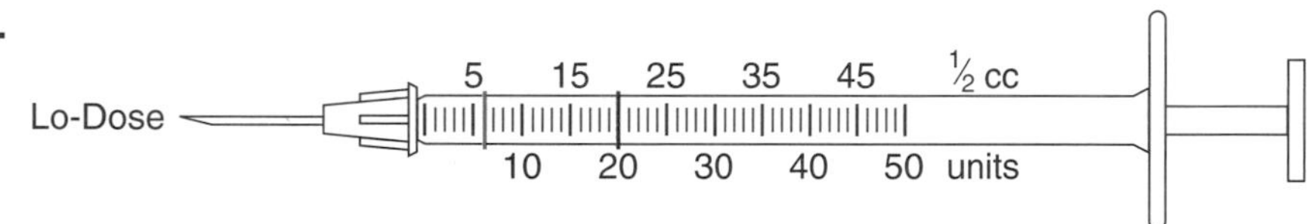

10. 400,000 U : 5 mL : : 300,000 U : x mL

$400{,}000x = 1{,}500{,}000$

$x = \dfrac{1{,}500{,}000}{400{,}000}$

$x = 3.75$ mL

$$\frac{300{,}000}{\cancel{400{,}000}_{\,80{,}000}} \times \frac{\cancel{5}^{\,1}}{1} =$$

$$\frac{300{,}000}{80{,}000} = 3.75 \text{ mL}$$

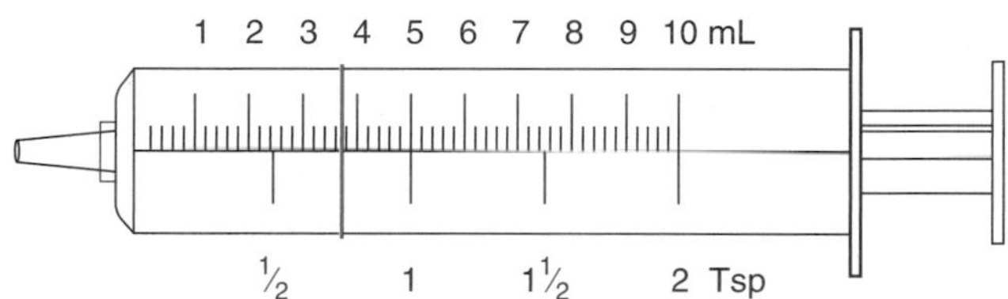

11. 10,000 U : 1 mL : : 6000 U : x mL

$10{,}000x = 6000$

$x = \dfrac{6000}{10{,}000}$

$x = 0.6$ mL

$$\frac{6000}{10{,}000} \times \frac{1}{1} = 0.6 \text{ mL}$$

12.

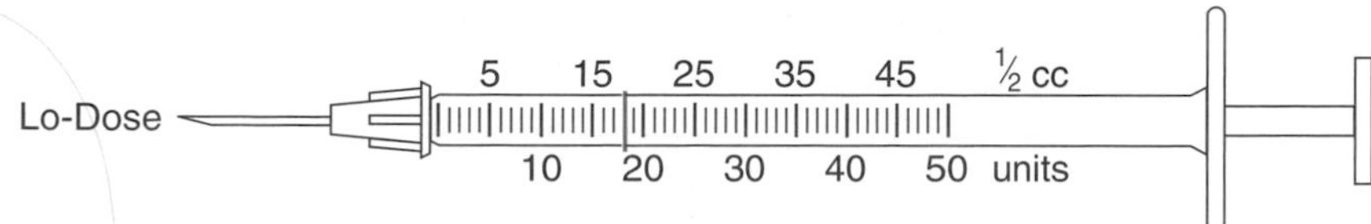

13.

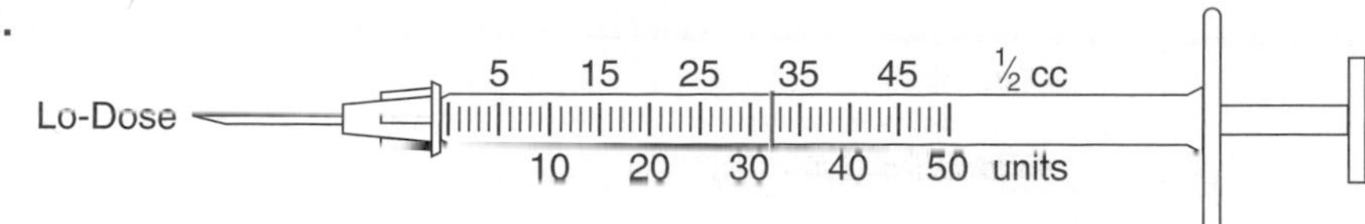

Proportion	Formula
14. Diluent 9.6 mL, 100,000 U/mL 100,000 U : 1 mL : : 600,000 U : x mL $100{,}000x = 600{,}000$ $x = \frac{600{,}000}{100{,}000}$ $x = 6$ mL	$\frac{600{,}000}{100{,}000} \times \frac{1}{1} = 6$ mL
Diluent 4.6 mL, 200,000 U/mL 200,000 U : 1 mL : : 600,000 U : x mL $200{,}000x = 600{,}000$ $x = \frac{600{,}000}{200{,}000}$ $x = 3$ mL	$\frac{600{,}000}{200{,}000} \times \frac{1}{1} = 3$ mL
Diluent 1.6 mL, 500,000 U/mL 500,000 U : 1 mL : : 600,000 : x mL $500{,}000x = 600{,}000$ $x = \frac{600{,}000}{500{,}000}$ $x = 1.2$ mL	$\frac{600{,}000}{500{,}000} \times \frac{1}{1} = 1.2$ mL
15. 5000 U : 1 mL : : 10,000 U : x mL $5000x = 10{,}000$ $x = \frac{10{,}000}{5000}$ $x = 2$ mL	$\frac{10{,}000}{5000} \times \frac{1}{1} = 2$ mL

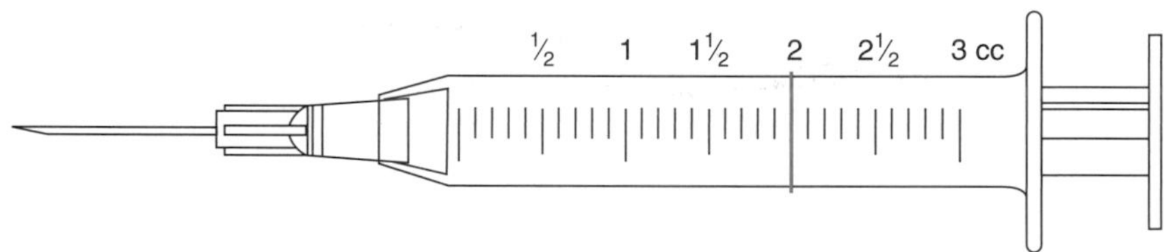

Proportion	Formula
16. 10,000 U : 1 mL : : 5000 U : x mL $10{,}000x = 5000$ $x = \frac{5000}{10{,}000}$ $x = 0.5$ mL	$\frac{5000}{10{,}000} \times \frac{1}{1} = 0.5$ mL

Proportion	Formula

17. 200,000 U : 5 mL : : 300,000 U : x mL

$200{,}000x = 1{,}500{,}000$

$x = \dfrac{1{,}500{,}000}{200{,}000}$

$x = 7.5$ mL

$\dfrac{300{,}000}{\cancel{200{,}000}_{40{,}000}} \times \dfrac{\cancel{5}^{1}}{1} =$

$\dfrac{300{,}000}{40{,}000} = 7.5$ mL

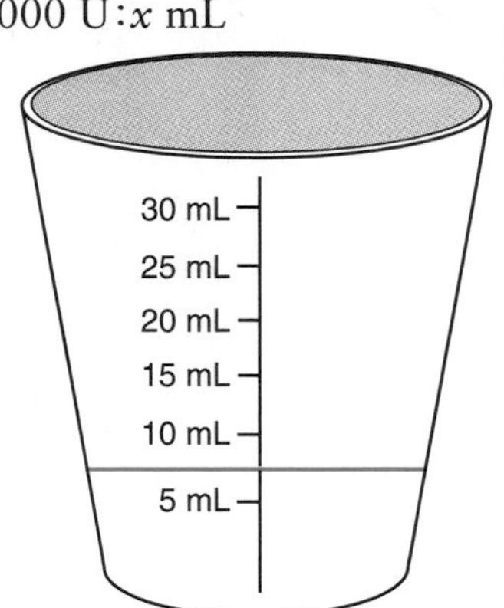

18.

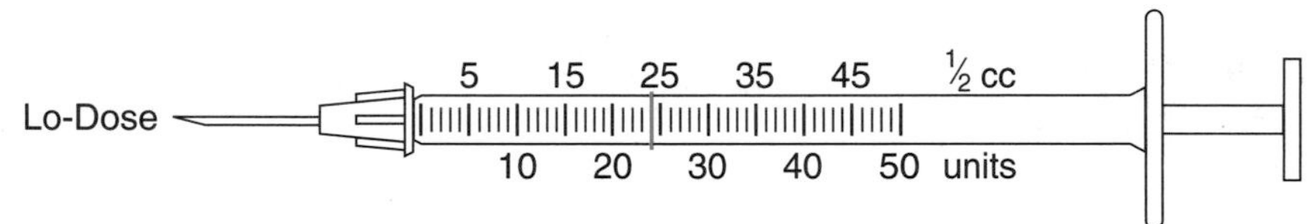

19. 10,000 U : 1 mL : : x U : 0.5 mL

$x = 5000$ U

$\dfrac{x}{10{,}000} \times \dfrac{1}{1} = 0.5$ mL

$\dfrac{x}{10{,}000} = 0.5$

$x = 0.5 \times 10{,}000$

$x = 5000$ U

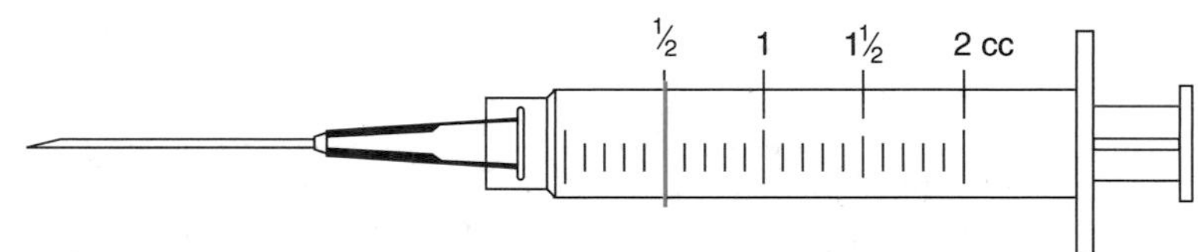

20. 250,000 U : 1 mL : : 200,000 U : x mL

$250{,}000x = 200{,}000$

$x = \dfrac{200{,}000}{250{,}000}$

$x = 0.8$ mL

$\dfrac{\cancel{200{,}000}^{4}}{\cancel{250{,}000}_{5}} \times \dfrac{1}{1} = 0.8$ mL

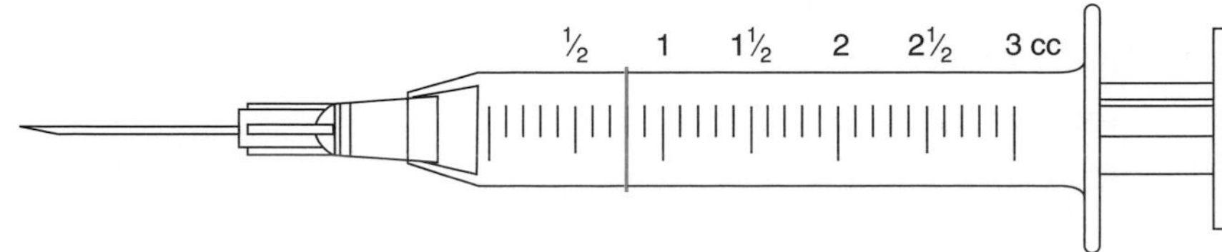

Chapter 14 Dosages Measured in Units—Posttest 1, pp. 301–305

Proportion / **Formula**

1. 400,000 U : 5 mL : : 500,000 U : x mL

$400{,}000x = 2{,}500{,}000$

$x = \frac{2{,}500{,}000}{400{,}000}$

$x = 6.25$ mL

Formula: $\frac{500{,}000}{400{,}000} \times \frac{5}{1} =$

$\frac{25}{4} = 6.25$ mL

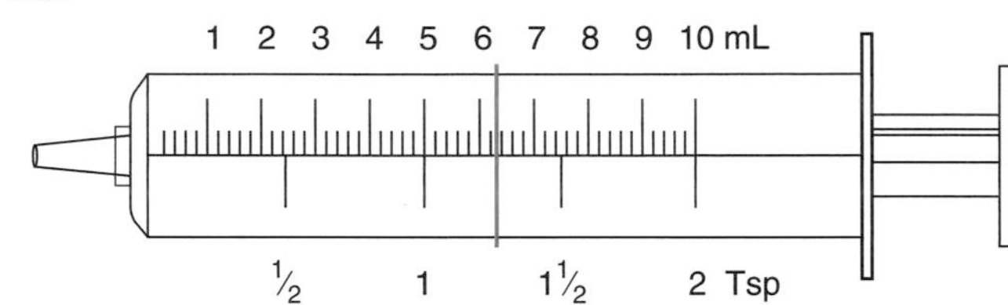

2.

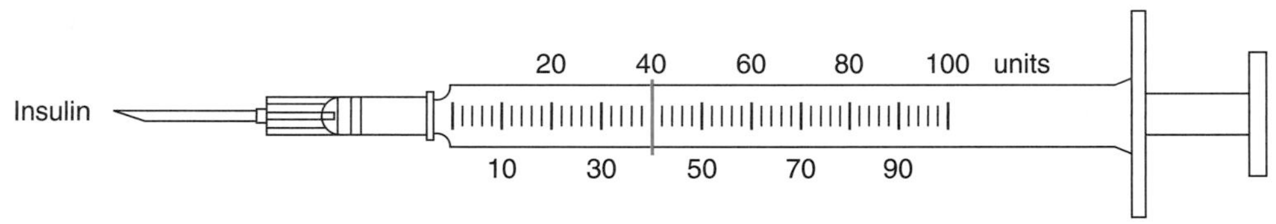

3. 5000 U : 1 mL : : 7500 U : x mL

$5000x = 7500$

$x = \frac{7500}{5000}$

$x = 1.5$ mL

Formula: $\frac{\overset{3}{7500}}{\underset{2}{5000}} \times \frac{1}{1} = 1.5$ mL

4.

5. 11.5 mL is best amount of diluent to add

1,000,000 U/mL

1,000,000 U : 1 mL : : 3,000,000 U : x mL

$1{,}000{,}000x = 3{,}000{,}000$

$x = \frac{3{,}000{,}000}{1{,}000{,}000}$

$x = 3$ mL

Formula: $\frac{3{,}000{,}000}{1{,}000{,}000} \times \frac{1}{1} = 3$ mL

6.

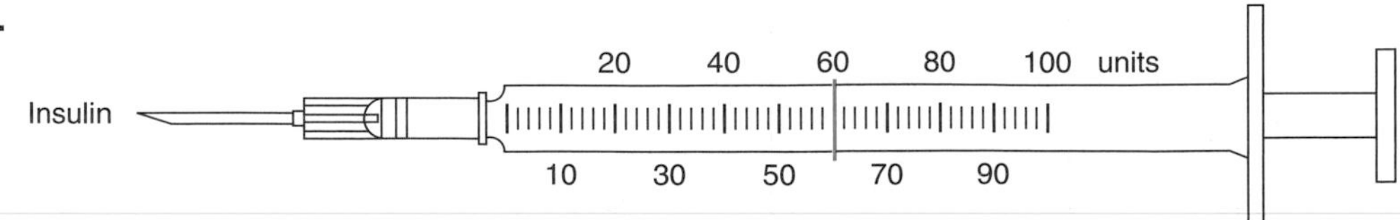

Proportion	Formula
7. 10,000 U:1 mL::20,000 U:x mL $10{,}000x = 20{,}000$ $x = \frac{20{,}000}{10{,}000}$ $x = 2$ mL	$\frac{20{,}000}{10{,}000} \times \frac{1}{1} = 2$ mL

8.

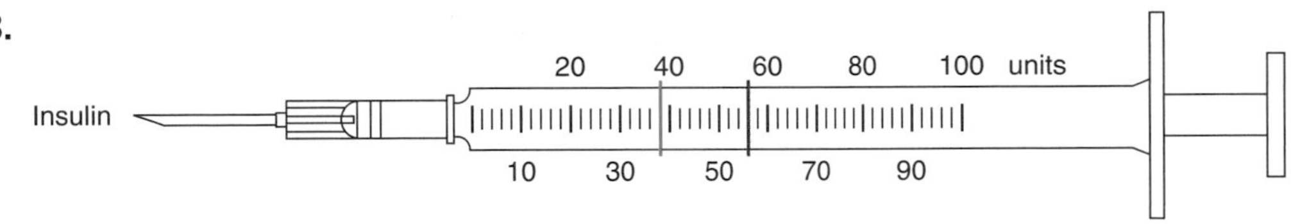

9. 200,000 U:5 mL::300,000 U:x mL

$200{,}000x = 1{,}500{,}000$

$x = \frac{1{,}500{,}000}{200{,}000}$

$x = 7.5$ mL

$\frac{\cancel{300{,}000}}{\cancel{200{,}000}} \times \frac{5}{1} =$

$\frac{15}{2} = 7.5$ mL

10. Diluent added = 11.5 mL

Concentration is 1,000,000 U/mL

1,000,000 mg:1 mL::1,200,000 mg:x

$1{,}000{,}000x = 1{,}200{,}000$

$x = \frac{1{,}200{,}000}{1{,}000{,}000}$

$x = 1.2$ mL

$\frac{1{,}200{,}000}{1{,}000{,}000} \times \frac{1}{1} = 1.2$ mL

11. 400,000 U:5 mL::200,000 U:x mL

$400{,}000x = 1{,}000{,}000$

$x = \frac{1{,}000{,}000}{400{,}000}$

$x = 2.5$ mL

$\frac{200{,}000}{400{,}000} \times \frac{5}{1} =$

$\frac{1{,}000{,}000}{400{,}000} = 2.5$ mL

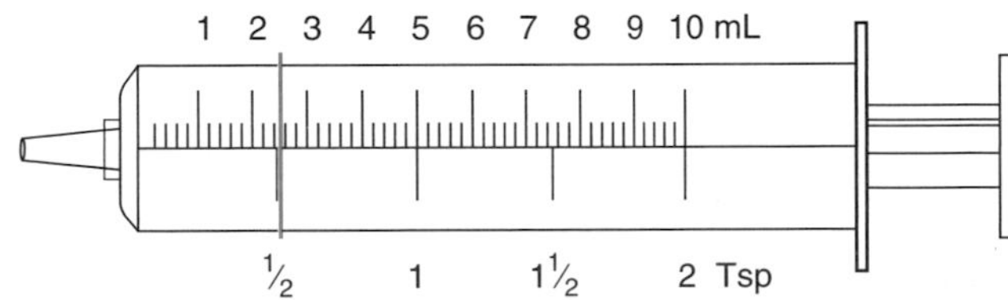

12. 5000 U:1 mL::7500 U:x mL

$5000x = 7500$

$x = \frac{7500}{5000}$

$x = 1.5$ mL

$\frac{7500}{5000} \times \frac{1}{1} = 1.5$ mL

13. 1,000,000 U:1 mL::500,000 U:x mL

$1{,}000{,}000x = 500{,}000$

$x = \frac{500{,}000}{1{,}000{,}000}$

$x = 0.5$ mL

$\frac{500{,}000}{1{,}000{,}000} \times \frac{1}{1} = 0.5$ mL

Proportion | **Formula**

14. Concentration is 100,000 U/mL
100,000 U : 1 mL : : 600,000 U : x mL
$100{,}000x = 600{,}000$
$x = \frac{600{,}000}{100{,}000}$
$x = 6$ mL

$$\frac{600{,}000}{100{,}000} \times \frac{1}{1} = 6 \text{ mL}$$

15. 10,000 U : 1 mL : : 5000 U : x mL
$10{,}000x = 5000$
$x = \frac{5000}{10{,}000}$
$x = 0.5$ mL

$$\frac{5000}{10{,}000} \times \frac{1}{1} = 0.5 \text{ mL}$$

Chapter 14 Dosages Measured in Units—Posttest 2, pp. 307-311

Proportion | **Formula**

1.

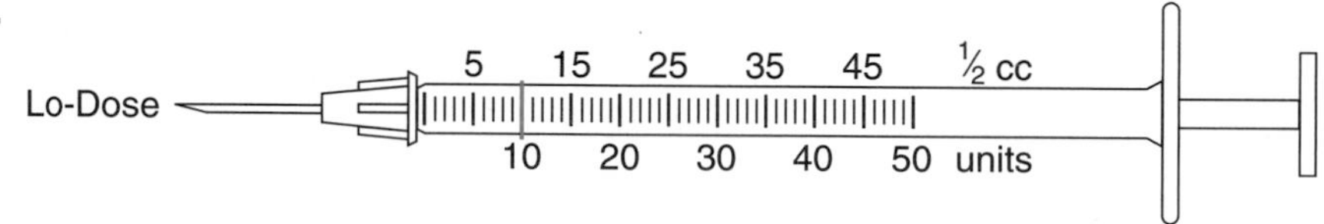

2. 10,000 U : 1 mL : : 1000 U : x mL
$10{,}000x = 1000$
$x = \frac{1000}{10{,}000}$
$x = 0.1$ mL

$$\frac{1000}{10{,}000} \times 1 \text{ mL} = 0.1 \text{ mL}$$

3. 200,000 U : 5 mL : : 500,000 : x mL
$200{,}000x = 2{,}500{,}000$
$x = \frac{2{,}500{,}000}{200{,}000}$
$x = 12.5$ mL

$$\frac{500{,}000}{\underset{40{,}000}{\cancel{200{,}000}}} \times \frac{\overset{1}{\cancel{5}}}{1} = 12.5 \text{ mL}$$

4.

Lo-Dose
5 15 25 35 45 ½ cc
10 20 30 40 50 units

5. 1000 U : 1 mL : : 1500 U : x mL
$1000x = 1500$
$x = \frac{1500}{1000}$
$x = 1.5$ mL

$$\frac{1500}{1000} \times \frac{1}{1} = 1.5 \text{ mL}$$

Proportion	Formula
6. 1,000,000 U:1 mL::1,200,000 U:x mL	$\frac{1,200,000}{1,000,000} \times \frac{1}{1} = 1.2$ mL

$$1,000,000x = 1,200,000$$
$$x = \frac{1,200,000}{1,000,000}$$
$$x = 1.2 \text{ mL}$$

7.

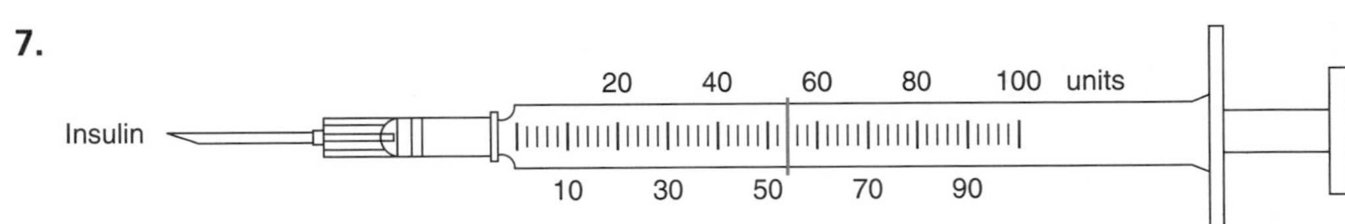

8.

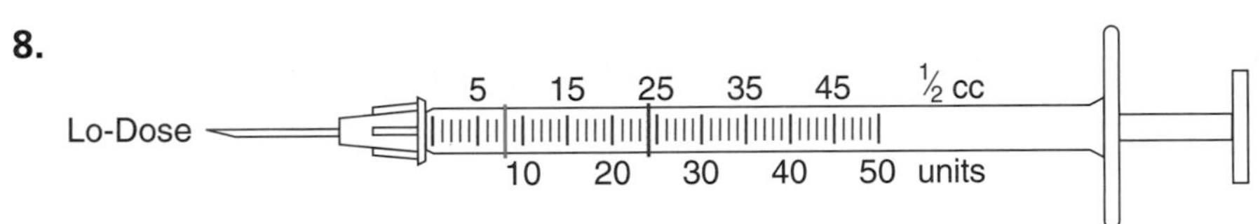

9. 400,000 U:5 mL::300,000 U:x mL

$$400,000x = 1,500,000$$
$$x = \frac{1,500,000}{400,000}$$
$$x = 3.75 \text{ mL}$$

$$\frac{300,000}{400,000} \times \frac{5}{1} =$$
$$\frac{1,500,000}{400,000} = 3.75 \text{ mL}$$

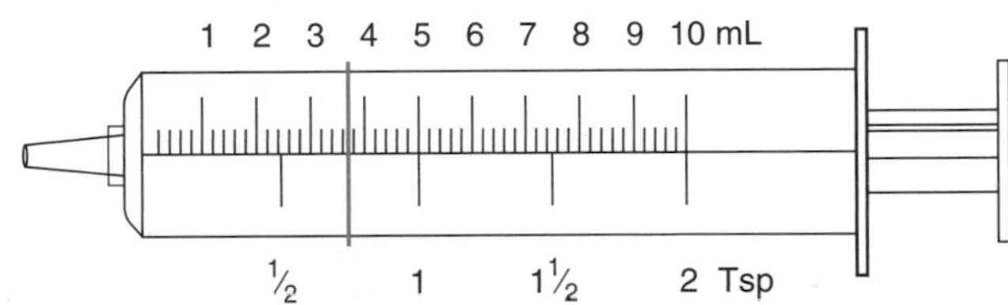

10. 5000 U:1 mL::6000 U:x mL

$$5000x = 6000$$
$$x = \frac{6000}{5000}$$
$$x = 1.2 \text{ mL}$$

$$\frac{6000}{5000} \times \frac{1}{1} = 1.2 \text{ mL}$$

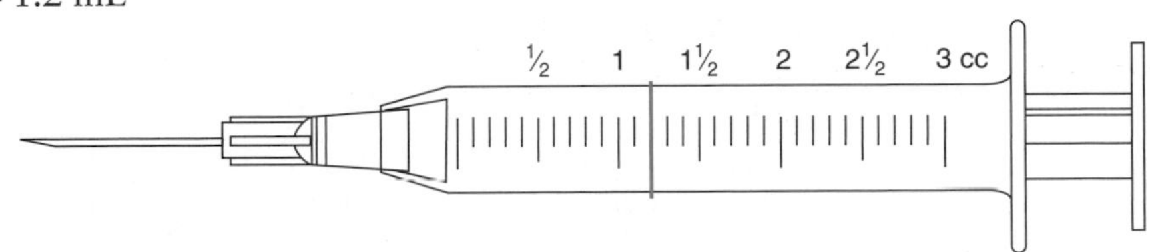

Proportion | **Formula**

11. 9.6 mL diluent, 100,000 U/mL

100,000 U:1 mL::600,000 U:x mL

$100{,}000x = 600{,}000$

$x = \dfrac{600{,}000}{100{,}000}$

$x = 6$ mL

Formula: $\dfrac{600{,}000}{100{,}000} \times \dfrac{1}{1} = 6$ mL

4.6 mL diluent, 200,000 U/mL

200,000 U:1 mL::600,000 U:x mL

$200{,}000x = 600{,}000$

$x = \dfrac{600{,}000}{200{,}000}$

$x = 3$ mL

Formula: $\dfrac{600{,}000}{200{,}000} \times \dfrac{1}{1} = 3$ mL

1.6 mL diluent, 500,000 U/mL

500,000 U:1 mL::600,000 U:x mL

$500{,}000x = 600{,}000$

$x = \dfrac{600{,}000}{500{,}000}$

$x = 1.2$ mL

Formula: $\dfrac{600{,}000}{500{,}000} \times \dfrac{1}{1} = 1.2$ mL

12. 5000 U:1 mL::10,000 U:x mL

$5000x = 10{,}000$

$x = \dfrac{10{,}000}{5000}$

$x = 2$ mL

Formula: $\dfrac{10{,}000}{5000} \times \dfrac{1}{1} = 2$ mL

13.

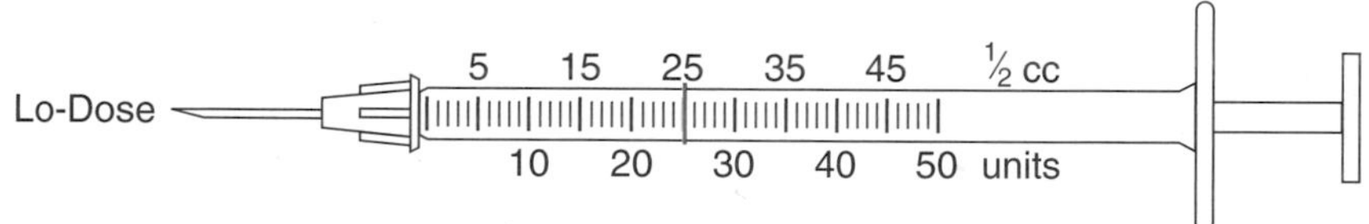

14. 5000 U:1 mL::7500 U:x mL

$5000x = 7500$

$x = \dfrac{7500}{5000}$

$x = 1.5$ mL

Formula: $\dfrac{7500}{5000} \times \dfrac{1}{1} = 1.5$ mL

½ 1 1½ 2 cc

15. 10,000 U:1 mL::20,000 U:x mL

$10{,}000x = 20{,}000$

$x = \dfrac{20{,}000}{10{,}000}$

$x = 2$ mL

Formula: $\dfrac{20{,}000}{10{,}000} \times \dfrac{1}{1} = 2$ mL

Chapter 15 Intravenous Flow Rates—Work Sheet pp. 327-331

1. $\frac{500}{24} = 20.8 \text{ or } 21 \text{ mL/h}$

2. $\frac{100}{1} = 100 \text{ mL/h}$

3. $\frac{100}{\underset{2}{\cancel{30}}} \times \overset{1}{\cancel{15}} = \frac{100}{2} = 50 \text{ gtt/min}$

4. $\frac{3000}{12} = 250 \text{ mL/h}$

5. $\frac{100}{\underset{3}{\cancel{30}}} \times \overset{1}{\cancel{10}} = \frac{100}{3} = 33.3 \text{ or } 33 \text{ gtt/min}$

6. $\frac{500}{6} = 83.3 \text{ or } 83 \text{ mL/h}$

7. $\frac{100}{\underset{6}{\cancel{60}}} \times \overset{1}{\cancel{10}} = \frac{100}{6} = 16.6 \text{ or } 17 \text{ gtt/min}$

Proportion	Formula
8. $60:250::20:x$ $60x = 5000$ $x = \frac{5000}{60}$ $x = 83.3 \text{ or } 83 \text{ mL/h}$	$\frac{\overset{2}{\cancel{20}}}{\underset{6}{\cancel{60}}} \times 250 \text{ mL} =$ $\frac{500}{6} = 83.3 \text{ or } 83 \text{ mL/h}$

9. $\frac{50}{\underset{1}{\cancel{30}}} \times \overset{2}{\cancel{60}} = \frac{100}{1} = 100 \text{ gtt/min}$

10. $\frac{1000}{10} = 100 \text{ mL/h}$

11. $\frac{50}{\underset{1}{\cancel{15}}} \times \overset{4}{\cancel{60}} = 200 \text{ gtt/min}$

Proportion	Formula
12. $400:200::200:x$ $400x = 40{,}000$ $x = \frac{40{,}000}{400}$ $x = 100 \text{ mL/h}$	$\frac{200}{\underset{2}{\cancel{400}}} \times \overset{1}{\cancel{200}} =$ $\frac{200}{2} = 100 \text{ mL/h}$

13. $\frac{1000}{\underset{6}{\cancel{60}}} \times \overset{1}{\cancel{10}} = \frac{1000}{6} = 16.6 \text{ or } 17 \text{ mL/h}$

14. $\frac{1000}{8} = 125 \text{ mL/h}$

Proportion | **Formula**

15. $\frac{25}{\cancelto{1}{15}} \times \cancelto{1}{15} = 25$ gtt/min

16. $20:100::0.5:x$

$20x = 50$

$x = \frac{50}{20}$

$x = 2.5$ mL/h

Formula:

$\frac{0.5}{\cancelto{1}{20}} \times \cancelto{5}{100} =$

$\frac{0.5}{1} \times 5 = 2.5$ mL/h

17. $\frac{25}{\cancelto{3}{15}} \times \cancelto{4}{20} = \frac{100}{3} = 33.3$ or 33 gtt/min

18. $2:100::1:x$

$2x = 100$

$x = \frac{100}{2}$

$x = 50$ mL/h

Formula:

$\frac{1}{\cancelto{1}{2}} \times \cancelto{50}{100} =$

$\frac{50}{1} = 50$ mL/h

19. $\frac{250}{\cancelto{12}{240}} \times \cancelto{1}{20} = \frac{250}{12} = 20.8$ or 21 gtt/min

20. $\frac{500}{\cancelto{24}{240}} \times \cancelto{1}{10} = \frac{500}{24} = 20.8$ or 21 gtt/min

21. $40:200::10:x$

$40x = 2000$

$x = \frac{2000}{40}$

$x = 50$ mL/h

Formula:

$\frac{10}{\cancelto{1}{40}} \times \cancelto{5}{200} =$

$\frac{10}{1} \times 5 = 50$ mL/h

22. $\frac{1350}{10} = 135$ mL/h

23. $2:50::1:x$

$2x = 50$

$x = \frac{50}{2}$

$x = 25$ mL/h

Formula:

$\frac{1}{\cancelto{1}{2}} \times \cancelto{25}{50} =$

$\frac{25}{1} = 25$ mL/h

Chapter 15 Intravenous Flow Rates—Posttest 1, pp. 333-335

Proportion | **Formula**

1. $\frac{500}{2} = 250$ mL/h

2. $\frac{500}{4} = 125$ mL/h

3. $\frac{120}{\underset{5}{\cancel{60}}} \times \overset{1}{\cancel{12}} = \frac{120}{5} = 24$ gtt/h

4. $\frac{1500}{8} = 187.5$ or 188 mL/h

5. $\frac{\overset{50}{\cancel{500}}}{\underset{24}{\cancel{240}}} \times 15 = \frac{750}{24} = 31.2$ or 31 gtt/min

6. $\frac{250}{\underset{15}{\cancel{180}}} \times \overset{1}{\cancel{12}} = \frac{250}{15} = 16.6$ or 17 gtt/min

7. $\frac{500}{\underset{24}{\cancel{360}}} \times \overset{1}{\cancel{15}} = \frac{500}{24} = 20.8$ or 21 gtt/min

8. Proportion:
   $4:250::2:x$
   $4x = 500$
   $x = \frac{500}{4}$
   $x = 125$ mL/h

   Formula:
   $\frac{\overset{1}{\cancel{2}}}{\underset{2}{\cancel{4}}} \times 250 =$
   $\frac{250}{2} = 125$ mL/h

9. $\frac{150}{\underset{1}{\cancel{60}}} \times \overset{1}{\cancel{60}} = \frac{150}{1} = 150$ gtt/min

10. $\frac{2500}{24} = 104.1$ or 104 mL/h

11. Proportion:
   $30:200::10:x$
   $30x = 2000$
   $x = \frac{2000}{30}$
   $x = 66.6$ or 67 mL/h

   Formula:
   $\frac{\overset{1}{\cancel{10}}}{\underset{3}{\cancel{30}}} \times 200 =$
   $\frac{200}{3} = 66.6$ or 67 mL/h

12. $\frac{25}{\underset{1}{\cancel{15}}} \times \overset{4}{\cancel{60}} = \frac{25}{1} \times 4 = 100$ gtt/min

Proportion	Formula
13. 100:200::15:x $100x = 3000$ $x = \frac{3000}{100}$ $x = 30$ mL/h	$\frac{15}{\cancel{100}_1} \times \overset{2}{\cancel{200}} =$ $\frac{15}{1} \times 2 = 30$ mL/h

14. $\frac{200}{4} = 50$ mL/h

15. $\frac{100}{\underset{1}{\cancel{60}}} \times \overset{1}{\cancel{60}} = 100$ gtt/min

Chapter 15 Intravenous Flow Rates—Posttest 2, pp. 337-339

Proportion	Formula
1. $\frac{200}{6} = 33.3$ or 33 mL/h	
2. $\frac{50}{\underset{3}{\cancel{30}}} \times \overset{1}{\cancel{10}} = \frac{50}{3} = 16.6$ or 17 gtt/min	
3. $\frac{200}{6} = 33.3$ or 33 mL/h	
4. $\frac{500}{\underset{18}{\cancel{180}}} \times \overset{1}{\cancel{10}} = \frac{500}{18} = 27.7$ or 28 gtt/min	
5. $\frac{500}{\underset{12}{\cancel{180}}} \times \overset{1}{\cancel{15}} = \frac{500}{12} = 41.6$ or 42 gtt/min	
6. $\frac{50}{0.5} = 100$ mL/h	
7. 100:100::8:x $100x = 800$ $x = \frac{800}{100}$ $x = 8$ mL/h	$\frac{8}{\underset{1}{\cancel{100}}} \times \overset{1}{\cancel{100}} =$ $\frac{8}{1} = 8$ mL/h
8. $\frac{50}{\underset{1}{\cancel{15}}} \times \overset{4}{\cancel{60}} = \frac{200}{1} = 200$ gtt/min	
9. $\frac{50}{\underset{1}{\cancel{15}}} \times \overset{1}{\cancel{15}} = \frac{50}{1} = 50$ gtt/min	
10. $\frac{1000}{6} = 166.6$ or 167 mL/h	

Proportion	Formula
11. $8:100::0.4:x$ $8x = 40$ $x = \frac{40}{8}$ $x = 5$ mL/h	$\frac{0.4}{\cancel{8}_{4}} \times \cancel{100}^{50} =$ $\frac{20}{4} = 5$ mL/h

12. $\frac{1200}{8} = 150$ mL/h

13. $\frac{25}{0.25} = 100$ mL/h

14. $\frac{1000}{\cancel{180}_{18}} \times \cancel{10}^{1} = \frac{1000}{18} = 55.5$ or 56 gtt/min

15. $\frac{1000}{12} = 83.3$ or 83 mL/h

Chapter 16 Critical Care IV Flow Rates—Work Sheet, pp. 347-351

Proportion	Formula
1. $25,000:250::1000:x$ $25,000x = 250,000$ $x = \frac{250,000}{25,000}$ $x = 10$ mL/h	$\frac{1000}{\cancel{25,000}_{100}} \times \cancel{250}^{1} =$ $\frac{1000}{100} = 10$ mL/h
2. $100:250::12:x$ $100x = 3000$ $x = \frac{3000}{100}$ $x = 30$ mL/h	$\frac{12}{\cancel{100}_{2}} \times \cancel{250}^{5} =$ $\frac{60}{2} = 30$ mL/h
3. $100:250::8:x$ $100x = 2000$ $x = \frac{2000}{100}$ $x = 20$ mL/h	$\frac{8}{\cancel{100}_{2}} \times \cancel{250}^{5} =$ $\frac{40}{2} = 20$ mL/h
4. $10,000:500::1000:x$ $10,000x = 500,000$ $x = \frac{500,000}{10,000}$ $x = 50$ mL/h	$\frac{1000}{\cancel{10,000}_{20}} \times \cancel{500}^{1} =$ $\frac{1000}{20} = 50$ mL/h

Proportion / **Formula**

5. $\frac{12 \times 75 \times 60}{4000} = \frac{54{,}000}{4000} = 13.5$ mL/h

6. $\frac{10 \times 60}{200} \times \frac{600}{200} = 3$ mL/h

7. $\frac{5 \times 80 \times 60}{8000} = \frac{24{,}000}{8000} = 3$ mL/h

8. Proportion:

$250{,}000:45::100{,}000:x$

$250{,}000x = 4{,}500{,}000$

$x = \frac{4{,}500{,}000}{250{,}000}$

$x = 18$ mL/h

Formula:

$\frac{\overset{10}{\cancel{100{,}000}}}{\underset{25}{\cancel{250{,}000}}} \times 45$

$\frac{450}{25} = 18$ mL/h

9. $\frac{0.5 \times 60}{1.8} = \frac{30}{1.8} = 16.6$ mL/h or 17 mL/h

10. $\frac{3 \times 70 \times 60}{200} = \frac{12{,}600}{200} = 63$ mL/h

11. $\frac{10 \times 100 \times 60}{4000} = \frac{60{,}000}{4000} = 15$ mL/h

12. $\frac{30 \times 75 \times 60}{15{,}000} = \frac{135{,}000}{15{,}000} = 9$ mL/h

13. $\frac{4 \times 60}{8} = \frac{240}{8} = 30$ mL/h

14. $\frac{10 \times 60}{8} = \frac{600}{8} = 75$ mL/h

15. $\frac{0.75 \times 60}{1.8} = \frac{45}{1.8} = 25$ mL/h

16. $\frac{15 \times 60}{16} = \frac{120}{16} = 15$ mL/h

17. $\frac{2 \times 60}{8} = \frac{120}{8} = 15$ mL/h

18. Proportion:

$25{,}000:500::7500:x$

$25{,}000x = 375{,}000$

$x = \frac{375{,}000}{25{,}000}$

$x = 15$ mL/h

Formula:

$\frac{750}{25{,}000} \times 500 =$

$\frac{750}{50} = 15$ mL/h

Proportion	Formula
19. $100:100::10:x$ $100x = 1000$ $x = \frac{1000}{100}$ $x = 10$ mL/h	$\frac{10}{100} \times 100 =$ $\frac{10}{1} = 10$ mL/h

20. $\frac{10 \times 90 \times 60}{8000} = \frac{54,000}{8000} = 6.75$ or 7 mL/h

Chapter 16 Critical Care IV Flow Rates—Posttest 1, pp. 353-355

Proportion	Formula
1. $500:500::9:x$ $500x = 4500$ $x = \frac{4500}{500}$ $x = 9$ mL/h	$\frac{9}{\cancel{500}_1} \times \overset{1}{\cancel{500}} =$ $\frac{9}{1} = 9$ mL/h
2. $50,000:50::800:x$ $50,000x = 400,000$ $x = \frac{400,000}{50,000}$ $x = 8$ mL/h	$\frac{800}{\cancel{50,000}_{100}} \times \overset{1}{\cancel{500}} =$ $\frac{800}{100} = 8$ mL/h

3. $\frac{5 \times 62 \times 60}{400} = \frac{18,600}{400} = 46.5$ mL/h

4. $\frac{5 \times 50 \times 60}{4000} = \frac{15,000}{4000} = 3.75 = 3.8$ mL/h

5. $\frac{20 \times 60}{200} = \frac{720}{200} = 3.6$ mL/h

6. $\frac{3 \times 60}{4} = \frac{180}{4} = 45$ mL/h

7. $\frac{5 \times 60}{4} = \frac{300}{4} = 75$ mL/h

8. $\frac{25 \times 50 \times 60}{10,000} = \frac{75,000}{10,000} = 7.5$ mL/h

Proportion | **Formula**

9. $25{,}000:250::1050:x$

$25{,}000x = 262{,}500$

$x = \dfrac{262{,}500}{25{,}000}$

$x = 10.5 \text{ mL/h}$

Formula: $\dfrac{1050}{\cancel{25{,}000}_{100}} \times \overset{1}{\cancel{250}} =$

$\dfrac{1050}{100} = 10.5 \text{ mL/h}$

10. $\dfrac{0.5 \times 60}{3.6} = \dfrac{30}{3.6} = 8.3 \text{ or } 8 \text{ mL/h}$

Chapter 16 Critical Care IV Flow Rates—Posttest 2, pp. 357-359

Proportion | **Formula**

1. $\dfrac{3 \times 85 \times 60}{4000} = \dfrac{15{,}300}{4000} = 3.82 \text{ or } 4 \text{ mL/h}$

2. $750{,}000:200::100{,}000:x$

$750{,}000x = 20{,}000{,}000$

$x = \dfrac{20{,}000{,}000}{750{,}000}$

$x = 26.66 \text{ or } 26.7 \text{ mL/h}$

Formula: $\dfrac{\overset{10}{\cancel{100{,}000}}}{\cancel{750{,}000}_{75}} \times 200 =$

$\dfrac{2000}{75} = 26.6 \text{ or } 27 \text{ mL/h}$

3. $\dfrac{50 \times 80 \times 60}{10{,}000} = \dfrac{240{,}000}{10{,}000} = 24 \text{ mL/h}$

4. $\dfrac{0.5 \times 60}{3.6} = \dfrac{30}{3.6} = 8.3 \text{ mL/h or } 8 \text{ mL/h}$

5. $\dfrac{10 \times 60}{8} = \dfrac{600}{8} = 75 \text{ mL/h}$

6. $\dfrac{4 \times 60}{4} = \dfrac{240}{4} = 60 \text{ mL/h}$

7. $\dfrac{7 \times 55 \times 60}{5000} = \dfrac{23{,}100}{5000} = 4.6 \text{ or } 5 \text{ mL/h}$

8. $\dfrac{2 \times 60}{2} = \dfrac{120}{2} = 60 \text{ mL/h}$

9. $20{,}000:200::1500:x$

$20{,}000x = 300{,}000$

$x = \dfrac{300{,}000}{20{,}000}$

$x = 15 \text{ mL/h}$

Formula: $\dfrac{1500}{\cancel{20{,}000}_{100}} \times \overset{1}{\cancel{200}} =$

$\dfrac{1500}{100} = 15 \text{ mL/h}$

Proportion	Formula
10. $50:100::8:x$ $50x = 800$ $x = \frac{800}{50}$ $x = 16$ mL/h	$\frac{\overset{}{8}}{\underset{1}{\cancel{50}}} \times \overset{2}{\cancel{100}} =$ $\frac{16}{1} = 16$ mL/h

Chapter 17 Pediatric Dosages—Work Sheet, pp. 371-377

1.a. 2.2 lb : 1 kg : : 50 lb : x kg
$2.2x = 50$
$x = \frac{50}{2.2}$
$x = 22.73$ kg

b. $25:1::x:22.73$
$x = 568.25$ or
$x = 568$ mg

$50:1::x:22.73$
$x = 1136.5$ or
$x = 1137$ mg
The safe range is 568-1137 mg in a 24-hour period.

250 mg : 1 dose : : x mg : 4 doses
$x = 1000$ mg in a 24-hour period

c. Yes, the order is safe.

d. 250 mg : 1 cap : : 250 mg : x cap
$250x = 250$
$x = \frac{250}{250}$
$x = 1$ capsule

2.a. 2.2 lb : 1 kg : 6.5 lb : x kg
$2.2x = 6.5$
$x = \frac{6.5}{2.2}$
$x = 2.95$ kg

b. 0.035 mg : 1 kg : : x mg : 2.95 kg
$x = 0.103$ mg

0.06 mg : 1 kg : : x mg : 2.95 kg
$x = 0.177$ mg
The safe range is 0.103-0.177 mg per day.

12.5 mg : 1 dose : : x mg : 1 dose
$x = 12.5$ mg/day

c. No, the order is not safe.

3.a. 2.2 lb : 1 kg : : 50 lb : x kg
$2.2x = 50$
$x = \frac{50}{2.2}$
$x = 22.73$ kg

b. 5 mg : 1 kg : : x mg : 22.73 kg
$x = 113.65$ mg/day

25 mg : 1 dose : : x mg : 4 doses
$x = 100$ mg

c. Yes, the order is safe.

d. 10 mg : 1 mL : : 25 mg : x mL
$10x = 25$
$x = \frac{25}{10}$
$x = 2.5$ mL/dose

4.a. 2.2 lb : 1 kg : : 44 lb : x kg
$2.2x = 44$
$x = \frac{44}{2.2}$
$x = 20$ kg

b. 0.55 mg : 1 kg : : x mg : 20 kg
$x = 11$ mg q6-8h/day
Total of 33-44 mg/day

10 mg : 1 dose : : x mg : 4 doses
$x = 40$ mg/day

c. Yes, the order is safe.

d. 25 mg : 1 mL : : 10 mg : x mL
$25x = 10$
$x = \frac{10}{25}$
$x = 0.4$ mL

5.a. 2.2 lb : 1 kg : : 78 lb : x kg
$2.2x = 78$
$x = \frac{78}{2.2}$
$x = 35.45$ kg

b. 2 mg : 1 kg : : x mg : 35.45 kg
$x = 70.9$ mg/day
60 mg <70.9 mg

c. Yes, the order is safe.

d. 40 mg : 1 tab : : 60 mg : x tab
$40x = 60$
$x = \frac{60}{40}$
$x = 1.5$ tablets

6.a. 2.2 lb : 1 kg : 30.31 lb : x kg
$2.2x = 30.31$
$x = 13.77$ kg

b. 2 mg : 1 kg : : x mg : 13.77 kg
$x = 27.54$ mg

10 mg/day <27.54 mg

c. Yes, the order is safe.

d. 5 mg : 1 mL : : 10 mg : x mL
$5x = 10$
$x = \frac{10}{5}$
$x = 2$ mL

7.a. 2.2 lb : 1 kg : : 28 lb : x kg
$2.2x = 28$
$x = \frac{28}{2.2}$
$x = 12.73$ kg

b. 12 mg : 1 kg : : x mg : 12.73 kg
$x = 152.76$ mg/day

16 mg : 1 dose : : x mg : 4 doses
$x = 64$ mg/day

c. Yes, the order is safe.

d. 11.25 mg : 1 mL : : 16 mg : x mL
$11.25x = 16$
$x = \frac{16}{11.25}$
$x = 1.42$ mL

8.a. 2.2 lb : 1 kg : : 66 lb : x kg
$2.2x = 66$
$x = \frac{66}{2.2}$
$x = 30$ kg

b. 5 mg : 1 kg : : x mg : 30 kg
$x = 150$ mg

7 mg : 1 kg : : x mg : 30 kg
$x = 210$ mg
The safe range is 150-210 mg per day.

75 mg : 1 dose : : x mg : 2 doses
$x = 150$ mg

c. Yes, the order is safe.

d. 50 mg : 1 tab : : 75 mg : x tab
$50x = 75$
$x = \frac{75}{50}$
$x = 1.5$ tablets

9.a. 2.2 lb : 1 kg : : 78 lb : x kg
$2.2x = 78$
$x = \frac{78}{2.2}$
$x = 35.45$ kg

b. 15 mg : 1 kg : : x mg : 35.45 kg
$x = 531.75$ mg

250 mg : 1 dose : : x mg : 2 doses
$x = 500$ mg/day

c. Yes, the order is safe.

d. 75 mg : 2 mL
: : 250 mg : x mL
$75x = 500$
$x = 6.67$ mL

$\frac{250 \text{ mg}}{75 \text{ mg}} \times \frac{2 \text{ mL}}{1} = x$
$x = \frac{500}{75} = 6.67$ mL

10.a. 2.2 lb : 1 kg : : 42 lb : x kg
$2.2x = 42$
$x = \frac{42}{2.2}$
$x = 19.09$ kg

b. 20 mg : 1 kg : : x mg : 19.09 kg
$x = 381.8$ mg/day

50 mg : 1 kg : : x mg : 19.09 kg
$x = 954.5$ mg/day
The safe range is 381.8-954.5 mg per day.

375 mg : 1 dose : : x mg : 3 doses
$x = 1125$ mg/day

c. No, the order is not safe.

11.a. 2.2 lb : 1 kg : : 63 lb : x kg
$2.2x = 63$
$x = \frac{63}{2.2}$
$x = 28.64$ kg

b. 2.5 mg : 1 dose : : x mg : 3 doses
$x = 7.5$ mg

5 mg : 1 dose : : x mg : 2 doses

2.2 lb : 1 kg : : 66 lb:x kg
$x = 10$ mg
The safe range is 7.5-10 mg per day.

c. Yes, the order is safe.

d. 5 mg : 5 mL : : 2.5 mg : x mL
$5x = 12.5$
$x = \frac{12.5}{5}$
$x = 2.5$ mL

$\frac{2.5 \not{mg}}{\not{5 mg}_1} \times \frac{\not{5}^1 \text{ mL}}{1} = 2.5 \text{ mL}$

12.a. 2.2 lb : 1 kg : : 58 lb : x kg
$2.2x = 58$
$x = \frac{58}{22}$
$x = 26.36$ kg

b. 10 mg : 1 kg : : x mg : 26.36 kg
$x = 263.6$ mg

20 mg : 1 kg : : x mg : 26.36 kg
$x = 527.2$ mg
The safe range is 263.6-527.2 mg per day.

150 mg : 1 dose : : x mg : 3 doses
$x = 450$ mg

c. Yes, the order is safe.

d. 100 mg : 5 mL : : 150 mg : x mL
$100x = 750$
$x = 7.5$ mL

$\frac{150 \not{mg}}{\not{100 mg}_{20}} \times \frac{\not{5}^1 \text{ mL}}{1} = \frac{150}{20}$
$= 7.5$ mL

13.a. 2.2 lb : 1 kg : : 36 lb : x kg
$2.2x = 36$
$x = \frac{36}{2.2}$
$x = 16.36$ kg

b. 0.03 mg : 1 kg : : x mg : 16.36 kg
$x = 0.49$ mg

0.08 : 1 kg : : x mg : 16.36 kg
$x = 1.31$ mg
The safe range is 0.49-1.31 mg q4-6 hours.

c. No, the order is not safe.

14.a. 2.2 lb : 1 kg : : 66 lb : x kg
$2.2x = 66$
$x = \frac{66}{2.2}$
$x = 30$ kg

b. 10 mg : 1 kg : : x mg : 30 kg
$x = 300$ mg

150 mg : 1 dose : : x mg : 2 doses
$x = 300$ mg
The safe range is 300 mg per day.

c. Yes, the order is safe.

d. 125 : 5 mL : : 150 mg : x mL
$125x = 750$
$x = \frac{750}{125}$
$x = 6$ mL

$\frac{150 \not{mg}}{\not{125 mg}_{25}} \times \frac{\not{5}^1 \text{ mL}}{1} = x$
$x = \frac{150}{25} = 6$ mL

15.a. 2.2 lb : 1 kg : : 81 lb : x kg
$2.2x = 81$
$x = \frac{81}{2.2}$
$x = 36.82$ kg

b. 25 mg : 1 kg : : x mg : 36.82 kg
$x = 920.5$ mg

50 mg : 1 kg : : x mg : 36.82 kg
$x = 1841$ mg
The safe range is 920.5-1841 mg per day.

350 mg : 1 dose : : x mg : 3 doses
$x = 1050$ mg

c. Yes, the order is safe.

d. 125 mg : 1 mL : : 350 mg : x mL
$125x = 350$
$x = \frac{350}{125}$
$x = 2.8$ mL

$\frac{350 \not{mg}}{125 \not{mg}} \times \frac{1 \text{ mL}}{1} = x$
$x = 2.8$ mL

16.a. 2.2 lb : 1 kg : : 16.5 lb : x kg
$2.2x = 16.5$
$x = \frac{16.5}{2.2}$
$x = 7.5$ kg

b. 10 mg : 1 kg : : x mg : 7.5 mg
$x = 75$ mg

20 mg : 1 kg : : x mg : 7.5 kg
$x = 150$ mg
The safe range is 75-150 mg per day.

100 mg : 1 dose : : x mg : 2 doses
$x = 200$ mg/day

c. No, the order is not safe.

17.a. 2.2 lb : 1 kg : : 13 lb : x kg
$2.2x = 13$
$x = \frac{13}{2.2}$
$x = 5.91$ kg

b. 6 mg : 1 kg : : x mg : 5.91 kg
$x = 35.46$ mg

7.5 mg : 1 kg : : x mg : 5.91 kg
$x = 44.33$ mg
The safe range is 35.46-44.33 mg per day.

16 mg : 1 dose : : x mg : 4 doses
$x = 64$ mg

c. No, the order is not safe.

18.a. 2.2 lb : 1 kg : : 19 lb : x kg
$2.2x = 19$
$x = \frac{19}{2.2}$
$x = 8.64$ kg

b. 0.05 mg : 1 kg : : x mg : 8.64 kg
$x = 0.432$ mg

2 mg : 1 kg : : x mg : 8.64 kg
$x = 17.28$ mg
The safe range is 0.432-17.28 mg per day.

8 mg : 1 dose : : x mg : 2 doses
$x = 16$ mg

c. Yes, the order is safe.

d. 5 mg : 5 mL
: : 16 mg : x mL
$5x = 80$
$x = \frac{80}{5}$
$x = 16$ mL

$$\frac{16 \text{ mg}}{\cancel{5}\,\cancel{\text{mg}}_{1}} \times \frac{\cancel{5}^{1} \text{ mL}}{1} = 16 \text{ mL}$$

19.a. 2.2 lb : 1 kg : : 22 lb : x kg
$2.2x = 22$
$x = \frac{22}{2.2}$
$x = 10$ kg

b. 30 mg : 1 kg : : x mg = 10 kg
$x = 300$ mg

50 mg : 1 kg : : x mg : 10 kg
$x = 500$ mg
The safe range is 300-500 mg per day.

75 mg : 1 dose : : x mg : 4 doses
$x = 300$ mg

c. Yes, the order is safe.

d. 125 mg : 5 mL
: : 75 mg : x mL
$125x = 375$
$x = \frac{375}{125}$
$x = 3$ mL

$$\frac{\cancel{75}^{3}\,\cancel{\text{mg}}}{\cancel{125}_{\cancel{25}_{1}}\,\cancel{\text{mg}}} \times \frac{\cancel{5}^{1} \text{ mL}}{1} = 3 \text{ mL}$$

20.a. 2.2 lb : 1 kg : : 32 lb : x kg
$2.2x = 32$
$x = \frac{32}{2.2}$
$x = 14.55$ kg

b. 100 mg : 1 kg : : x mg : 14.55 kg
$x = 14.55$ mg/day is safe

400 mg : 1 dose : : x mg : 3 doses
$x = 1200$ mg/day

c. Yes, the order is safe.

d. 330 mg : 1 mL
: : 400 mg : x mL
$330x = 400$
$x = \frac{400}{330}$
$x = 1.21$ mL

$$\frac{400 \cancel{\text{mg}}}{330 \cancel{\text{mg}}} \times \frac{1 \text{ mL}}{1} = 1.21 \text{ mL}$$

21. $\frac{250 \text{ mL}}{3 \text{ h}} = 83.3$ or 3 mL/h

22. Step 1: 10 mg : 1 mL : : 40 mg : x mL
$10x = 40$
$x = \frac{40}{10}$
$x = 4$ mL

Step 2: $40 \times \frac{1}{2} = 20 \text{ mL} \rightarrow 20 \text{ mL} - 4 \text{ mL} = 16 \text{ mL}$

Step 3: $\frac{20}{20} \times 60 = 60$ gtt/min

Chapter 17 Pediatric Dosages—Posttest 1, pp. 379-383

1.a. 2.2 lb : 1 kg : : 55 lb : x kg

$2.2x = 55$

$x = \frac{55}{2.2}$

$x = 25$ kg

b. 4 mg : 1 kg : : x mg : 25 kg

$x = 100$ mg

6 mg : 1 kg : : x mg : 25 kg

$x = 150$ mg

The safe range is 100-150 mg per day.

60 mg : 1 dose : : x mg : 2 doses

$x = 120$ mg/day

c. Yes, the order is safe.

d. 20 mg : 5 mL : : 60 mg : x mL

$20x = 300$

$x = \frac{300}{20}$

$x = 15$ mL

2.a. 2.2 lb : 1 kg : : 44 lb : x kg

$2.2x = 44$

$x = \frac{44}{2.2}$

$x = 20$ kg

b. 30 mg : 1 kg : : x mg : 20 kg

$x = 600$ mg

60 mg : 1 kg : : x mg : 20 kg

$x = 1200$ mg

The safe range is 600-1200 mg per day.

500 mg : 1 dose : : x mg : 4 dose

$x = 2000$ mg

c. No, the order is not safe.

3.a. 2.2 lb : 1 kg : : 6.75 lb : x kg

$2.2x = 6.75$

$x = \frac{6.75}{2.2}$

$x = 3.07$ kg

b. 50,000 U : 1 kg : : x U : 3.07 kg

$x = 153{,}500$ U/day

150,000 U <153,500

c. Yes, the order is safe.

d. 300,000 U : 1 mL : : 150,000 U : x mL

$300{,}000x = 150{,}000$

$x = \frac{150{,}000}{300{,}000}$

$x = 0.5$ mL

4.a. 2.2 lb : 1 kg : : 44 lb : x kg

$2.2x = 44$

$x = \frac{44}{2.2}$

$x = 20$ kg

b. 20 mg : 1 kg : : x mg : 20 kg

$x = 400$ mg

40 mg : 1 kg : : x mg : 20 kg

$x = 800$ mg

The safe range is 400-800 mg per day.

250 mg : 1 dose : : x mg : 3 doses

$x = 750$ mg

c. Yes, the order is safe.

d. 125 mg : 5 mL : : 250 mg : x mL

$125x = 1250$

$x = \frac{1250}{125}$

$x = 10$ mL

5.a. 2.2 lb : 1 kg : : 78 lb : x kg

$2.2x = 78$

$x = \frac{78}{2.2}$

$x = 35.45$ kg

b. 0.1 mg : 1 kg : : x mg : 35.45 kg

$x = 3.55$ mg

0.2 mg : 1 kg : : x mg : 35.45 kg

$x = 7.09$ mg

The safe range is 3.55-7.09 mg per day.

4 mg <7.09 mg

c. Yes, the order is safe.

d. 15 mg : 1 mL : : 4 mg : x mL

$15x = 4$

$x = \frac{4}{15}$

$x = 0.27$ mL

6.a. 2.2 lb : 1 kg : : 92 lb : x kg
$2.2x = 92$
$x = \frac{92}{2.2}$
$x = 41.82$ kg

b. 15 mg : 1 kg : : x mg : 41.82 kg
$x = 627.3$ mg per day is safe

300 mg : 1 dose : : x mg : 2 doses
$x = 600$ mg

c. Yes, the order is safe.

d. 125 mg : 5 mL : : 300 mg : x mL
$125x = 1500$
$x = 12$ mL

$$\frac{\overset{12}{\cancel{300\ \text{mg}}}}{\underset{\underset{1}{\cancel{25}}}{\cancel{125\ \text{mg}}}} \times \frac{\overset{1}{\cancel{5}}\ \text{mL}}{1} = 12\ \text{mL}$$

7.a. 2.2 lb : 1 kg : : 35 lb : x kg
$2.2x = 35$
$x = \frac{35}{2.2}$
$x = 15.91$ kg

b. 12 mg : 1 kg : : x mg : 15.91 kg
$x = 190.92$ mg

c. Yes, the order is safe.

d. 200 mg : 5 mL : : 180 mg : x mL
$200x = 900$
$x = \frac{900}{200}$
$x = 4.5$ mL

$$\frac{\overset{9}{\cancel{180\ \text{mg}}}}{\underset{\underset{2}{\cancel{40}}}{\cancel{200\ \text{mg}}}} \times \frac{\overset{1}{\cancel{5}}\ \text{mL}}{1} = 4.5\ \text{mL}$$

8.a. 2.2 lb : 1 kg : : 52 lb : x kg
$2.2x = 52$
$x = \frac{52}{2.2}$
$x = 23.64$ kg

b. 4 mg : 1 kg : : x mg : 23.64 kg
$x = 94.56$ mg
7 mg : 1 kg : : x mg : 23.64 kg
$x = 165.48$ mg
The safe range is 94.56-165.48 mg per day.
25 mg : 1 dose : : x mg : 4 doses
$x = 100$ mg

c. Yes, the order is safe.

d. 100 mg : 15 mL : : 25 mg : x mL
$100x = 375$
$x = \frac{375}{100}$
$x = 3.75$ mL

$$\frac{\overset{5}{\cancel{25\ \text{mg}}}}{\underset{\underset{4}{\cancel{20}}}{\cancel{100\ \text{mg}}}} \times \frac{\overset{3}{\cancel{15}}\ \text{mL}}{1} = \frac{15}{4} = 3.75\ \text{mL}$$

9.a. 2.2 lb : 1 kg : : 6.25 lb : x kg
$2.2x = 6.25$
$x = \frac{6.25}{2.2}$
$x = 2.84$ kg

b. 0.05 mg : 1 kg : : x mg : 2.84 kg
$x = 0.142$ mg

0.1 mg : 1 kg : : x mg : 2.84 kg
$x = 0.284$ mg
The safe range is 0.142-0.284 mg.

0.5 mg : 1 dose : : x mg : 4 doses
$x = 2$ mg

c. No, the order is not safe.

10.a. 2.2 lb : 1 kg : : 66 lb : x mg
$2.2x = 66$
$x = \frac{66}{2.2}$
$x = 30$ kg

b. 15 mg : 1 kg : : x mg : 30 kg
$x = 450$ mg per day is safe

525 mg : 1 dose : : x mg : 2 doses
$x = 1050$ mg

c. No, the order is not safe.

11. $\frac{100\ \text{mL}}{6\ \text{h}} = 16.6$ or 17 mL/h

12. Step 1: 250 mg : 1 mL : : 400 mg : x mL
$250x = 400$
$x = \frac{400}{250}$
$x = 1.6$ mL

Step 2: $400 \times \frac{1}{50} = 8\ \text{mL} \rightarrow 8\ \text{mL} - 1.6\ \text{mL} = 7.4\ \text{mL}$

Step 3: $\frac{8}{30} \times 60 = x$ gtt/min
$x = \frac{480}{30}$
$x = 16$ gtt/min

Chapter 17 Pediatric Dosages—Posttest 2, pp. 385-388

1.a. 2.2 lb : 1 kg : : 58 lb : x kg
$2.2x = 58$
$x = \frac{58}{2.2}$
$x = 26.36$ kg

b. 15 mg : 1 kg : : x mg : 26.36 kg
$x = 395$ mg

40 mg : 1 kg : x mg : 26.36 kg
$x = 1054$ mg
The safe range is 395-1054 mg per day.

225 mg : 1 dose : x mg : 4 doses
$x = 1000$ mg

c. Yes, the order is safe.

d. 150 mg : 1 mL : : 225 mg : x mL
$150x = 225$
$x = \frac{225}{150}$
$x = 1.5$ mL

2.a. 2.2 lb : 1 kg : : 70 lb : x kg
$2.2x = 70$
$x = \frac{70}{2.2}$
$x = 31.81$ kg

b. 5 mg : 1 kg : : x mg : 31.81 kg
$x = 159$ mg

7 mg : 1 kg : : x mg : 31.81 kg
$x = 222.67$ mg
The safe range is 159-222.67 mg per day.

50 mg : 1 dose : : x mg : 2 doses
$x = 100$ mg

c. No, 100 mg <159 mg is recommended.

3.a. 2.2 lb : 1 kg : : 58 lb : x kg
$2.2x = 58$
$x = \frac{58}{2.2}$
$x = 26.36$ kg

b. 20 mg : 1 kg : : x mg : 26.36 kg
$x = 527$ mg

40 mg : 1 kg : : x mg : 26.36 kg
$x = 1054$
The safe range is 527-1054 mg per day.
250 mg : 1 dose : x mg : 3 doses
$x = 750$ mg/day

c. Yes, the order is safe.

d. 125 mg : 5 mL : : 250 mg : x mL
$125x = 1250$
$x = \frac{1250}{125}$
$x = 10$ mL

4.a. 2.2 lb : 1 kg : : 99 lb : x kg
$2.2x = 99$
$x = \frac{99}{2.2}$
$x = 45$ kg

b. 25 mg : 1 kg : : x mg : 45 kg
$x = 1125$ mg

50 mg : 1 kg : : x mg : 45 kg
$x = 2250$ mg
The safe range is 1125-2250 mg per day.

500 mg : 1 dose : : x mg : 4 doses
$x = 2000$

c. Yes, the order is safe.

d. 250 mg : 1 cap : : 500 mg : x cap
$250x = 500$
$x = \frac{500}{250}$
$x = 2$ capsules

5.a. 2.2 lb : 1 kg : : 66 lb : x kg
$2.2x = 66$
$x = \frac{66}{2.2}$
$x = 30$ kg

b. 50 mg : 1 kg : : x mg : 30 kg
$x = 1500$ mg

100 mg : 1 kg : : x mg : 30 kg
$x = 3000$ mg
The safe range is 1500-3000 mg per day.

500 mg : 1 dose : : x mg : 4 doses
$x = 2000$ mg

c. Yes, the order is safe.

d. 125 mg : 1 mL : : 500 mg : x mL
$125x = 500$
$x = \frac{500}{125}$
$x = 4$ mL

6.a. 2.2 lb : 1 kg : : 39 lb : x kg
$2.2x = 39$
$x = \frac{39}{2.2}$
$x = 17.73$ kg

b. 15 mg : 1 kg : : x mg : 17.73 kg
$x = 265.95$ mg

30 mg : 1 kg : : x mg : 17.73 kg
$x = 531.9$ mg
The safe range is 265.95-531.9 mg per day.

250 mg : 1 dose : : x mg : 2 doses
$x = 500$ mg

c. Yes, the order is safe.

d. 200 mg : 5 mL : : 250 mg : x mL
$200x = 1250$
$x = \frac{1250}{200}$
$x = 6.25$ mL

$$\frac{\overset{25}{\cancel{250\text{ mg}}}}{\underset{4}{\cancel{200\text{ mg}}}} \times \frac{\overset{1}{\cancel{5}}\text{ mL}}{1} = \frac{25}{4} = 6.25\text{ mL}$$

7.a. 2.2 lb : 1 kg : : 42 lb : x kg
$2.2x = 42$
$x = \frac{42}{2.2}$
$x = 10.09$ kg

b. 20 mg : 1 kg : : x mg : 19.09 kg
$x = 381.8$ mg

50 mg : 1 kg : : x mg : 19.09 kg
$x = 954.5$ mg
The safe range is 381.8-954.8 mg per day.

400 mg : 1 dose : : x mg : 3 doses
$x = 1200$ mg

c. No, the order is not safe.

8.a. 2.2 lb : 1 kg : : 70 lb : x kg
$2.2x = 70$
$x = \frac{70}{2.2}$
$x = 31.82$ kg

b. 40 mg : 1 kg : : x mg : 31.82 kg
$x = 1272.8$ mg per day is safe

300 mg : 1 dose : : x mg : 4 doses
$x = 1200$ mg

c. Yes, the order is safe.

d. 250 mg : 5 mL : : 300 mg : x mL
$250x = 1500$
$x = \frac{1500}{250}$
$x = 6$ mL

$$\frac{\overset{6}{\cancel{300\text{ mg}}}}{\underset{1}{\cancel{250\text{ mg}}}} \times \frac{\overset{1}{\cancel{5}}\text{ mL}}{1} = 6\text{ mL}$$

9.a. 2.2 lb : 1 kg : : 53 lb : x kg
$2.2x = 53$
$x = \frac{53}{2.2}$
$x = 24.09$ kg

b. 0.1 mg : 1 kg : : x mg : 24.09 kg
$x = 2.41$ mg

0.2 mg : 1 kg : : x mg : 24.09 kg
$x = 4.82$ mg
The safe range is 2.41-4.82 mg per day.

0.9 mg 1 dose : : x mg : 6 doses
$x = 5.4$ mg

c. No, the order is not safe.

10.a. 2.2 lb : 1 kg : : 10.25 lb : x kg
$2.2x = 10.25$
$x = \frac{10.25}{2.2}$
$x = 4.66$ kg

b. 4 mg : 1 kg : : x mg : 4.66 kg
$x = 18.64$ mg per day is safe

9 mg : 1 dose : : x mg : 2 doses
$x = 18$ mg

c. Yes, the order is safe.

d. 10 mg : 1 mL : : 9 mg : x mL
$10x = 9$
$x = \frac{9}{10} = 0.9$ mL

$$\frac{9\ \cancel{\text{mg}}}{10\ \cancel{\text{mg}}} \times \frac{1\text{ mL}}{1} = 0.9\text{ mL}$$

11. $\frac{200}{6} = 33.3$ or 33 mL/h

12. Step 1: 50 mg : 1 mL : : 500 mg : x mL
$50x = 500$
$x = \frac{500}{50}$
$x = 10$ mL

Step 2: $500 \times \frac{1}{5} = 100 \rightarrow 100 - 10 = 90$

Step 3: $\frac{100}{60} \times 60 = x$ gtt/min

$\frac{6000}{60} = 100$ gtt/min

Comprehensive Posttest, pp. 407-421

Case 1, pp. 407-410

1. 2 tablets
2. Digoxin 0.25 mg
   EC ASA gr v
   Cimetidine 300 mg
   Slow-K 10 mEq
3. 400 mL of $D_5\frac{1}{2}$ NS per shift
4.

Date	Medication	Dose	Route	Interval						
2/3	Percocet	2	p.o.	q.4 h.	prn pain					
2/3	Tylenol	grX	p.o.	q.4 h.	prn pain or Temp >38°					
2/3	MOM	30 cc	p.o.	q.day	prn constipation					
2/3	Mylanta	30 cc	p.o.	q.4 h.	prn indigestion					
2/3	Restoril	15 mg	p.o.	q.h.s.	prn insomnia					

5.

Date	Medication	Dose	Route	Interval						
2/3	Digoxin	0.25 mg	p.o.	q.day	09					
2/3	E.C. ASA	gr V	p.o.	q.day	09					
2/3	Cimetidine	300 mg	p.o.	t.i.d.	09	13	17			
2/3	Lasix	20 mg	I.V.	q.8 h.	08		16		24	
2/3	Slow-K	10 mEq	p.o.	b.i.d.	09		17			

6. Restoril 15 mg po
7. 100 gtt/min
8. Milk of Magnesia 30 cc
9. Lasix 20 mg

Case 2, pp. 411-413

1. Synthroid 0.15 mg
   Tagamet 300 mg
2. 1 mL
3. 600 mL/shift
   1800 mL/day
4. ½ tablet
5. Demerol
   Tylenol
6. 0.5 mL
7. 2 tablets

8.

1	Synthroid			
	0.15 mg (dose)	p.o. (route)	q.day (interval)	
2	Tagamet			
	300 mg (dose)	p.o. (route)	q.day (interval)	

Case 3, pp. 414-415

1. Med $FESO_4$
amt 0.3 g

2. 300 cc

3. 0.5 mL

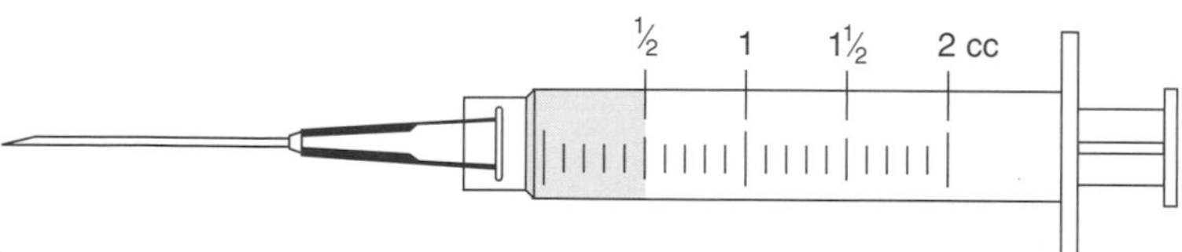

4. ½ tablet

5.

10	Ibuprofen			
	600 mg (dose)	p.o. (route)	q.6 h. (interval)	prn pain
11	Seconal			
	100 mg (dose)	IM (route)	q.h.s. (interval)	prn
12	Tucks			
	one (dose)	Peri (route)	(interval)	prn @ bedside
13	Senokot			
	one (dose)	p.o. (route)	qd prn (interval)	
14	Tylenol			
	650 mg (dose)	p.o. (route)	q.4 h. (interval)	prn pain

Case 4, pp. 416-418

1.

1	Allopurinol		
	50 mg (dose)	p.o. (route)	t.i.d. (interval)
2	Theophylline		
	16 mg (dose)	p.o. (route)	q.6 h. (interval)
3	Prednisone		
	2 mg/kg (dose)	p.o. (route)	q.day (interval)
4	Vincristine		
	5.0 mg/m² (dose)	I.V. (route)	x 1 now (interval)
5	MVI		
	1 (dose)	p.o. (route)	q.day (interval)

2.

7	Compazine			
	0.07 mg/kg (dose)	IM (route)	q.day (interval)	PRN Nausea
8	Tylenol			
	120 mg (dose)	p.o. (route)	t.i.d. (interval)	PRN pain

3. 1.42 mL
4. 0.5 mL
5. 12.73 kg
   2.5 mL
6. 50 gtt/min
7. 0.90 mL

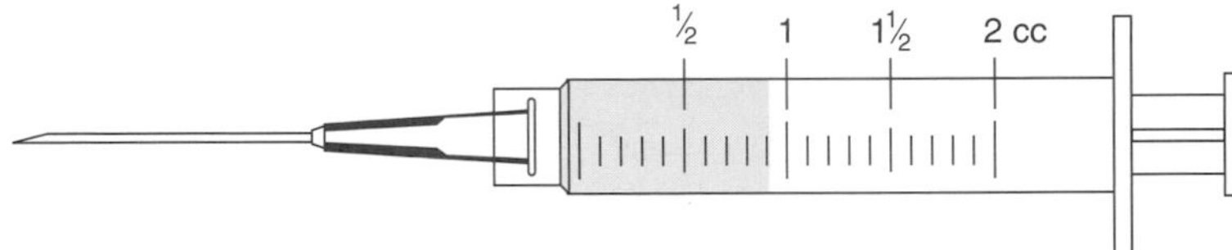

8. 200 cc
9. 0.66 mL

Case 5, pp. 419-421

1.

#	Medication	Dose	Route	Interval	Times			
1	Heparin	5000 U	SC	b.i.d.	09		21	
2	Cefuroxime	1 g	IVPB	q.8 h.	08	16		24

2.

#	Medication	Dose	Route	Interval	Notes
3	Torecan	10 mg	IM	q.4 h.	prn nausea
4	Mylanta	30 cc	p.o.		prn indigestion
5	Dulcolax Supp.	1	pr	q.shift	prn
6	Restoril	15 mg	p.o.	q.h.s.	prn insomnia
7	Tylenol #3	2	p.o.	q.4 h.	prn pain
8	Tylenol #3	1	p.o.	q.4 h.	prn pain
9	PCA-Demerol	10 mg	IV	q.10 min	250 mg/4 h. lockout

3. 0.5 mL

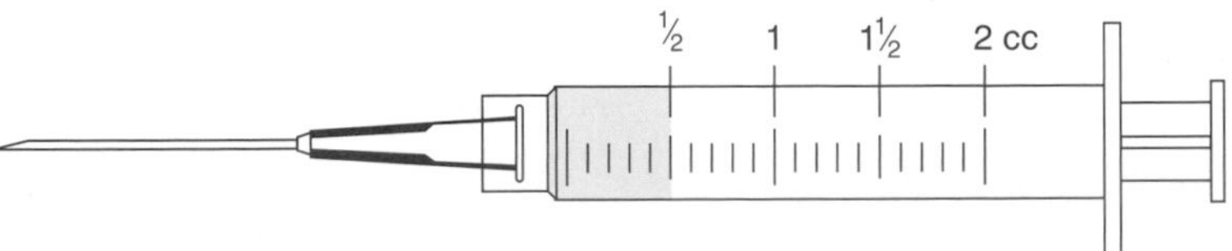

4. 1 mL/10 min
5. 1.0 mL
6. 400 cc/shift
   1200 cc/day
7. 200 mL/h
   3.33 mL/min
   200 gtt/min

Index

Page numbers followed by *f* or *t* refer to figures or tables, respectively.